AF530528

Veterinary and Livestock Sector : A Blueprint for Capacity Building

Veterinary and Livestock Sector : A Blueprint for Capacity Building

Editor
SUDHI RANJAN GARG
PhD, FIAVPHS
Professor & Ex-Head of Department
Department of Veterinary Public Health & Epidemiology.
College of Veterinary Sciences,
Lala Lajpat Rai University of Veterinary and Animal Sciences, Hisar

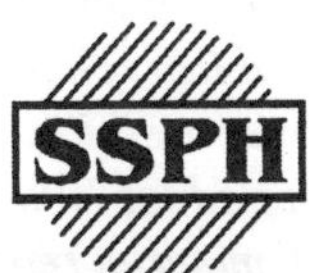

SATISH SERIAL PUBLISHING HOUSE
403, Express Tower, Commercial Complex, Azadpur, Delhi-110033 (India)
Phone : 011-27672852, Fax : 91-11-27672046
E-mail : info@satishserial.com, hkjain1975@yahoo.com
Website : www.satishserial.com

Published by :

SATISH SERIAL PUBLISHING HOUSE

403, Express Tower, Commercial Complex, Azadpur, Delhi-110033 (INDIA)
Phone : 011-27672852 Fax : 91-11-27672046
E-mail : info@satishserial.com, hkjain1975@yahoo.com

ISBN 978-93-81226-09-4

Typeset by : Harminder Singh Kharb *for* Laxmi Art Creation
Printed at: Salasar Imaging Systems, Delhi-110035

To my dear father Shri Narender Pal Garg

Preface

Livestock sector is vital for food security of a country and of the world in the widest sense. It also makes a major contribution to poverty alleviation, socioeconomic development and self-employment. Veterinary Services constitute its inseparable component to ensure livestock health, food safety and public health. The changing scenario of global food market, transborder animal infections, zoonotic diseases, public health threats, biological disasters have all put much greater responsibilities upon the Veterinary Services at national and international level. Besides sufficient and quality food production, veterinarians are engaged in the task of identifying and controlling risks that have adverse impact on animals, animal products and human health. It demands a wide range of organisational, legislative and technical competence in Veterinary Services that may not be restricted to the public sector alone but encompass the private sector too. A recent study by the World Organisation for Animal Health (OIE) reveals that though all the 108 countries responding to a survey have an institutional framework of Veterinary Services but it does not necessarily mean that it is operationally effective. Financial and human resource crunch is widespread. The budget allocation to Veterinary Services is grossly insufficient in developing countries despite high contribution of livestock sector to the country's Gross Domestic Product (GDP). In more than 60% of the countries, public investment in the Veterinary Services is less than USD 2 per capita per year. The study presented at the 79th General Session of the OIE World Assembly of National Delegates in Paris (France) in May 2011 shows that more than half of the countries have less than 35 public sector veterinarians and less than 100 private sector veterinarians per million inhabitants. Very few veterinarians have an animal health mandate, reflecting an overall weakness of surveillance systems in developing countries. The shortage of veterinary professionals poses a major constraint to the world food security and public health safety.

In India, a network of 27562 veterinary polyclinics, hospitals and dispensaries, and 25195 veterinary aid centers (including stockmen centers and mobile dispensaries) is functioning in the States and Union Territories, according to the Annual Report (2010-11) of the Department of Animal Husbandry, Dairying and Fisheries. About 250 disease diagnostic laboratories provide support for quick and reliable diagnosis of livestock diseases. There are 29 veterinary vaccine production units in the public and private sector producing the required quantity of vaccines for control of major livestock and poultry diseases through prophylactic vaccination. The picture may look quite impressive but actually, it is not as bright considering the nation's huge livestock and poultry population. The country ranks first in the world in respect of buffaloes, second in cattle and goats, third in sheep, fifth in ducks and chickens and tenth in camel population.

Inadequacy of veterinary resources has a direct adverse impact on the economy, animal health, animal welfare, and public health. It is imperative to undertake capacity building of Veterinary Services, veterinary professionals and the livestock sector at a fast pace to catch up with the growing global demands. It is time for the gap analysis and evolving strategic action plans for improvement.

This book is a humble attempt just in that direction. Leading academicians, researchers, and professionals, who are authorities in their respective fields, have provided the blueprints for strategies and action plans for capacity building in the areas that are very close to their hearts. They have enriched the chapters with their longstanding professional experience, own research findings and the latest data to develop the book into an unmatched resource. Simple language and lucid illustrations make the book quite comprehensible and a reading pleasure.

I express my deep sense of gratitude to the contributing authors who despite their time constraints extended all help to complete this task. The assistance provided by my colleague, Dr. Vijay J. Jadhav, during preparation of the manuscript is gratefully acknowledged.

The encouraging attitude and support of my wife, Dr. (Mrs.) Meenakshi Garg, through the years I worked on the book is praiseworthy.

Sudhi Ranjan Garg

List of Contributors

A. A. Kumar, Former Principal Scientist, Indian Veterinary Research Institute, Izatnagar-243122

A. K. Singh, Senior Scientist, National Dairy Research Institute, Karnal-132001

A. K. Srivastava, Director, National Dairy Research Institute, Karnal-132001

A. S. Khanna, Professor, Department of Animal Genetics & Breeding, College of Veterinary Sciences, Lala Lajpat Rai University of Veterinary and Animal Sciences, Hisar-125004

A. Sahoo, Principal Scientist and Head, Animal Nutrition Division, Central Sheep & Wool Research Institute, Avikanagar-304501

Abdul Samad, Dean & Director of Instructions, Maharashtra Animal and Fishery Sciences University, Nagpur-440006

Anshu Sharma, Senior Bacteriologist, College Central Laboratory, College of Veterinary Sciences, Lala Lajpat Rai University of Veterinary and Animal Sciences, Hisar-125004

Arun K. Sangwan, Professor, Department of Veterinary Parasitology, College of Veterinary Sciences, Lala Lajpat Rai University of Veterinary and Animal Sciences, Hisar-125004

B. R. Singh, Principal Scientist, Centre for Animal Disease Research and Diagnosis, Indian Veterinary Research Institute, Izatnagar-243122

B. Sunil, Associate Professor, Department of Veterinary Public Health, College of Veterinary and Animal Sciences, Mannuthy, Thrissur-680651

D. K. Singh, Principal Scientist, Division of Veterinary Public Health, Indian Veterinary Research Institute, Izatnagar-243122

D. Swarup, Director, Central Institute for Research on Goats, Makhdoom, Farah, Mathura-281122

D. V. Deshpande, General Manager, National Bank for Agriculture and Rural Development, Mumbai-400051

Deepika Lather, Assistant Professor, Department of Veterinary Pathology, College of Veterinary Sciences, Lala Lajpat Rai University of Veterinary and Animal Sciences, Hisar-125004

F. R. Sheriff, Former Professor & Head, Department of Poultry Science, Madras Veterinary College, Chennai-600007

Gaya Prasad, Assistant Director General (Animal Health), Indian Council of Agricultural Research, New Delhi-110001

J. John Kirubaharan, Professor, Department of Veterinary Microbiology, Tamil Nadu Veterinary and Animal Sciences University, Chennai-600007

J. Sahoo, Professor-cum-Head, Department of Livestock Products Technology, Guru Angad Dev Veterinary and Animal Sciences University, Ludhiana-141004

Jitender Mohindroo, Associate Professor, Department of Veterinary Surgery and Radiology, College of Veterinary Science, Guru Angad Dev Veterinary & Animal Sciences University, Ludhiana-141004

K. Vrinda Menon, Assistant Professor, Department of Veterinary Public Health, College of Veterinary and Animal Sciences, Mannuthy, Thrissur-680651

L. Gunaseelan, Professor and Head, Department of Veterinary Public Health & Epidemiology, Madras Veterinary College, Tamil Nadu Veterinary & Animal Sciences University, Chennai-600007

M. C. Sharma, Director & Vice Chancellor, Indian Veterinary Research Institute, Izatnagar-243122

M. L. Sangwan, Professor and Head, Department of Animal Biotechnology, College of Veterinary Sciences, Lala Lajpat Rai University of Veterinary and Animal Sciences, Hisar-125004

Minakshi, Professor, Department of Animal Biotechnology, College of Veterinary Sciences, Lala Lajpat Rai University of Veterinary & Animal Sciences, Hisar-125004

N. K. Kakker, Senior Scientist, Department of Veterinary Microbiology, College of Veterinary Sciences, Lala Lajpat Rai University of Veterinary & Animal Sciences, Hisar-125004

N. Kondaiah, Director, National Research Centre on Meat, Chengicherla, Hyderabad-500092

N. Punniamurthy, Professor and Head, Ethnoveterinary Herbal Training and Research Unit, Veterinary University Training and Research Centre, Tamil Nadu Veterinary and Animal Sciences University, Thanjavur-613006

Narinder Singh Saini, Professor-cum-Head, Department of Veterinary Surgery and Radiology, College of Veterinary Science, Guru Angad Dev Veterinary & Animal Sciences University, Ludhiana-141004

P. Dhanapalan, Professor and Head, Bioinformatics Centre & ARIS Cell, Madras Veterinary College, Tamil Nadu Veterinary and Animal Sciences University, Chennai-600007

P. K. Rout, Principal Scientist, Central Institute for Research on Goats, Makhdoom, Farah, Mathura-281122

P. Selvaraj, Associate Professor, Department of Veterinary Clinical Medicine, Ethics and Jurisprudence, Madras Veterinary College, Tamil Nadu Veterinary and Animal Sciences University, Chennai-600007

Prashant Murdeshwar, Infovet India, Thane-400605

R. C. Patra, Professor and Head, Department of Clinical Medicine, Ethics and Jurisprudence, College of Veterinary Science and Animal Husbandry, Orissa University of Agriculture and Technology, Bhubaneswar-751003

R. K. Chandolia, Professor, Department of Veterinary Gynaecology and Obstetrics, College of Veterinary Sciences, Lala Lajpat Rai University of Veterinary and Animal Sciences, Hisar-125004

R. P. Gupta, Professor and Head, Department of Veterinary Pathology, College of Veterinary Sciences, Lala Lajpat Rai University of Veterinary and Animal Sciences, Hisar-125004

R. P. Singh, Senior Scientist, Division of Biological Products, Indian Veterinary Research Institute, Izatnagar-243122

R. Prabakaran, Vice Chancellor, Tamil Nadu Veterinary and Animal Sciences University, Chennai-600007

R. Sharma, Senior Virologist, Department of Veterinary Microbiology, College of Veterinary Sciences, Lala Lajpat Rai University of Veterinary & Animal Sciences, Hisar-125004

Rajesh Chhabra, Assistant Scientist, College Central Laboratory, College of Veterinary Sciences, Lala Lajpat Rai University of Veterinary and Animal Sciences, Hisar-125004

Renu Gupta, Assistant Professor, Department of Veterinary Public Health and Epidemiology, College of Veterinary Sciences, Lala Lajpat Rai University of Veterinary and Animal Sciences, Hisar-125004

S. B. Shivachandra, Senior Scientist & Incharge, Clinical Bacteriology Laboratory, Indian Veterinary Research Institute, Mukteshwar-263138

S. R. Garg, Professor, Department of Veterinary Public Health and Epidemiology, College of Veterinary Sciences, Lala Lajpat Rai University of Veterinary and Animal Sciences, Hisar-125004

Sandeep Kumar, Assistant Scientist, Department of Veterinary Physiology and Biochemistry, College of Veterinary Sciences, Lala Lajpat Rai University of Veterinary and Animal Sciences, Hisar-125004

Shiv Prasad, Principal Scientist, National Dairy Research Institute, Karnal-132001

Smita Sirohi, Principal Scientist, National Dairy Research Institute, Karnal-132001

V. J. Jadhav, Assistant Professor, Department of Veterinary Public Health and Epidemiology, College of Veterinary Sciences, Lala Lajpat Rai University of Veterinary and Animal Sciences, Hisar-125004

Ved Prakash, Scientist, Central Sheep and Wool Research Institute, Avikanagar-304501

Vidya Singh, Scientist, National Research Centre on Mithun, Jharnapani-797106

Vikas Nehra, Assistant Professor, Department of Veterinary Pathology, College of Veterinary Sciences, Lala Lajpat Rai University of Veterinary and Animal Sciences, Hisar-125004

Zohaib Hameed, Department of Electrical and Computer Engineering, University of Alberta, Edmonton, Canada

□□□

Contents

Chapter 1

Diverse Roles of Contemporary Veterinarians

SUDHI RANJAN GARG
Department of Veterinary Public Health and Epidemiology, College of Veterinary Sciences, Lala Lajpat Rai University of Veterinary and Animal Sciences, Hisar-125004

Contents

1. Introduction

Indus Valley civilization is among the foremost contributors in the history of development of veterinary science and animal husbandry. Historically, Shalihotra (2350 BC), the first known veterinarian of the world, and known as 'Father of Veterinary Medicine' in India was an expert in horse husbandry and medicine and composed a text Haya Ayurveda. Sage Palakapya (1800 BC) was an expert dealing with elephants and composed a text Gaja Ayurveda. During Mahabharata period (1000 BC), Nakula and Sahadeva, the two Pandava brothers, were experts of horse and cattle husbandry, respectively. Lord Krishna was an expert caretaker and conservator of cow husbandry. Ancient holy Vedas, Puranas, Brahmanas, and other Indian epics are flooded with information on animal care, health management, and disease cure. Even the surgical treatment of animal diseases was quite developed during the Vedic period (Somvanshi 2006). The techniques of surgical operations along with instruments have been dealt in detail in Shalihotra's and Palakapya's works. The first known veterinary hospitals of the world are known to be erected by the great Emperor Ashoka (around 300 BC) in India.

In the modern era, the world's first Veterinary School was founded in 1761 in Lyon (France), shortly followed by the Alfort Veterinary School near Paris in 1764 on Claude Bourgelat's initiative. It led to the formal creation of the veterinary profession. Thus, the year 2011 marked the 250th world anniversary of veterinary training. Bourgelat also suggested that studying animal biology and pathology would help to improve our understanding of human biology and pathology, thus evolving the concept of comparative biopathology, without which modern medicine would never have emerged.

Conventionally, with the mention of a veterinarian, there emerges in mind the picture of a person who is engaged in veterinary practice and is responsible for healthcare of farm and pet animals. However, with the major demographic, political, environmental, technological, economic and epidemiological influences, the relevance of veterinary sciences has changed vastly and the true dimensions of the roles and contributions of veterinarians are much broader today than contemplated conventionally. The veterinary sciences today serve not only the traditional responsibility of animal healthcare but also take on the drastically expanding other global issues, many of which influence the human health. The total efforts of the veterinarians and veterinary services are contributing to the physical and mental well-being of human beings, whether by reducing malnutrition through improvement in the quantity and quality of animal products, controlling infection and disease, preserving the environment, improvement in animal production and reproduction, healthcare of the companion animals, or promoting humane values in the society (WHO 1975).

On completion of graduation, a veterinarian takes oath (Fig.1) to use his scientific knowledge and skills for the benefit of society by functioning in several different but largely interrelated contexts. With the changing global needs, the American Veterinary Medical Association has amended the Veterinarian's Oath recently in the year 2010 to highlight the priority of the profession in animal welfare (Box 1). Though the concept of animal welfare is not new, the amendment reinforces the veterinarians' responsibilities for animal welfare.

The working domain of the veterinarians thus includes not only animal health and welfare but also the public health and welfare activities. The veterinarians' obligations to the society include (1) Animal healthcare, (2) Animal welfare, (3) Animal resource conservation, (4) Public health promotion, and (5) Advancement of medical knowledge. The contemporary veterinarians fulfil their obligations by performing a diverse range of functions as discussed below.

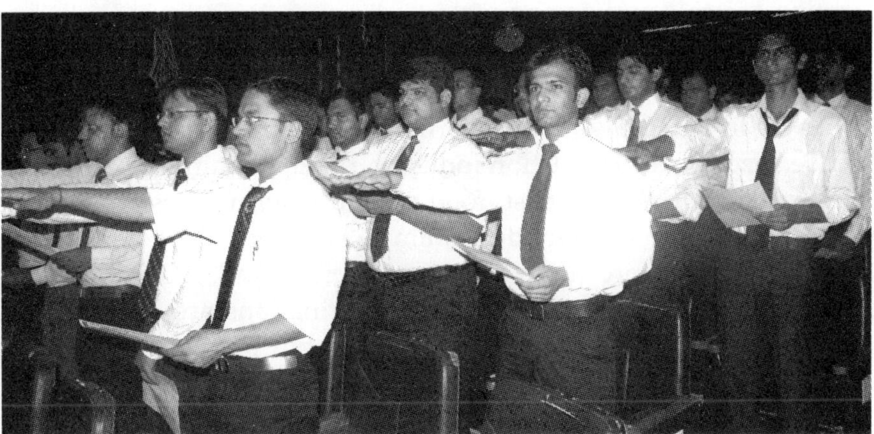

Fig. 1 : Veterinary graduates taking professional oath (Photo courtesy: Mr. Rakesh Bagga)

Box 1 : Veterinarian's Oath

Being admitted to the profession of veterinary medicine, I solemnly swear to use my scientific knowledge and skills for the benefit of society through the protection of animal health and welfare, the prevention and relief of animal suffering, the conservation of animal resources, the promotion of public health, and the advancement of medical knowledge.

I will practice my profession conscientiously, with dignity, and in keeping with the principles of veterinary medical ethics.

I accept as a lifelong obligation the continual improvement of my professional knowledge and competence.

2. Animal Healthcare

The most obvious role of the veterinarians is purely in the veterinary medicine context. It relates to the protection of animals from diseases, diagnosis of ailments, and treatment of sick animals. Consistent with the modern day's approach to veterinary practice, the contemporary veterinarians provide multifaceted, proficient and highly specialized services in animal healthcare.

2.1 Clinical treatment of sick animals

Treatment of sick and injured animals is historically the primary and original role of the veterinarians. By virtue of their professional training, the services rendered by the veterinarians in this area are unique and nobody else can substitute them. The main focus of the veterinarians engaged in treatment of sick animals, whether in government hospitals or in private practice, is on individual animals. The clientele of the general clinical veterinarians is very vast that includes domestic animals, farm animals, draught animals, pets, performing animals and zoo animals.

2.2 Livestock and poultry farm management and healthcare

With the livestock and poultry farming developing into a more organized and modernized food production industry, there is dramatic shift in the role of veterinarians too. In the past, food animal veterinarians were concerned only about the health of individual animals but today the veterinarians play valuable role in the productivity, sustainability and profitability of farm enterprises. In developed countries, the veterinarians are taking the role of consultants in not only a single or small farm but providing consultancy to several farms as herd health managers rather than as clinicians alone. Their emphasis is more on the prevention of diseases rather than cure of individual animals. Due to the current strict regulations regarding food safety, veterinarians have to consider all aspects of animal husbandry concerning consumer safety. Consistent with the demand of higher productivity, the role of the veterinarians in fertility management on dairy farms has also evolved from addressing individual clinical conditions alone to systematic herd fertility investigation and herd fertility management (Mee 2007). Apart from the services in animal disease treatment, reproduction, and preventive medicine, there is growing demand of veterinarians for advice on areas like data management, nutrition and the design of facilities on farms, particularly those that influence the health and welfare of livestock. The rural veterinary practices abroad are evolving into multi-disciplinary teams, which offer specialist knowledge and complete farm consultancy services to improve the future viability of farms.

2.3 Healthcare of pet and companion animals

The veterinary clinicians in rural areas while deal mainly with the treatment of domestic animals or livestock herds, their urban counterparts have more emphasis on the animals kept by the people for companionship, sport and leisure. A vast majority of the veterinarians who work in private practice in cities or big towns predominately or exclusively treat small animals which include companion animals as well as exotics. Veterinarians focusing on companion animals diagnose health problems, vaccinate against disease, medicate animals, treat and dress injuries, perform surgery, and advise the pet owners about various subjects like nutrition, behaviour and breeding.

2.4 Mobile veterinary services

Mobile veterinary units provide modern veterinary care at the doorstep of the clients on call for their comfort and convenience. These services quite commonly cater to the needs of the pet animal owners in urban areas. In developed countries, even mobile veterinary surgery units having a state of the art operating facilities are available. The mobile units also provide veterinary services to large animals in rural and remote areas, livestock farms and in emergencies. Similar services are also available for wildlife. The Wildlife Trust of India is running a Mobile Veterinary Service project to provide *in-situ* emergency relief to the displaced or distressed wild animals. These units comprise of a transport vehicle, a trained wildlife veterinarian, an animal attendant, equipment and supplies for medical attention to wild animals in need.

2.5 Veterinary diagnostic laboratory services

The veterinary diagnostic laboratories provide for diagnosing the cause of the diseases based on the diagnostic material submitted by the veterinary clinicians, practitioners and animal owners. These laboratories also extend similar support to other specialists engaged in animal disease control, wildlife management, and public health programmes. The diagnostic laboratories in veterinary institutions in addition also provide collaborative support in research and assist in training of veterinary graduate and postgraduate students.

2.6 Veterinary epidemiology

Veterinary epidemiology is an integral component of animal disease prevention and control strategies. It involves study of the distribution of diseases and determinants of the states or events related with animal health, welfare and production in specified populations and the application of this study to control the health problems. Veterinarians working in veterinary hospitals, diagnostic laboratories, research institutions and even slaughterhouses help in determining the origin, cause, mode of transmission, predisposing factors and pattern of diseases, ultimately facilitating the mitigation of the problem.

2.7 Veterinary surveillance

Emerging animal and zoonotic diseases and increasing international trade have resulted in an increased demand for veterinary surveillance systems. Veterinary surveillance is valuable in identifying the risks, setting priorities, and in allocating resources effectively and efficiently for protection of health of livestock and consumers (Stark *et al.* 2006). With the establishment of the World Trade Organization (WTO) and agreement on the application of sanitary and phytosanitary measures, the responsibility of veterinary services worldwide has become very crucial. The veterinarians fulfil a crucial role in protecting their country's animal health status, providing sound surveillance information on the occurrence of diseases within their territories, and conducting scientifically valid risk analyses to facilitate international trade according to the international standards and guidelines of the World Organization for Animal Health (OIE), Codex Alimentarius Commission (CAC), and other agencies (Zepeda *et al.* 2005).

2.8 Zoonotic disease identification and surveillance

A large number of human diseases have their origin in animals. Therefore, besides the prevention and control of the diseases affecting livestock, the veterinarians are also responsible for surveillance, detection, prevention and control of zoonotic diseases transmissible from animals to human beings, either directly or through animal products. The role of the veterinarians is not thus restricted to farms alone but has extended much beyond (Fig. 2).

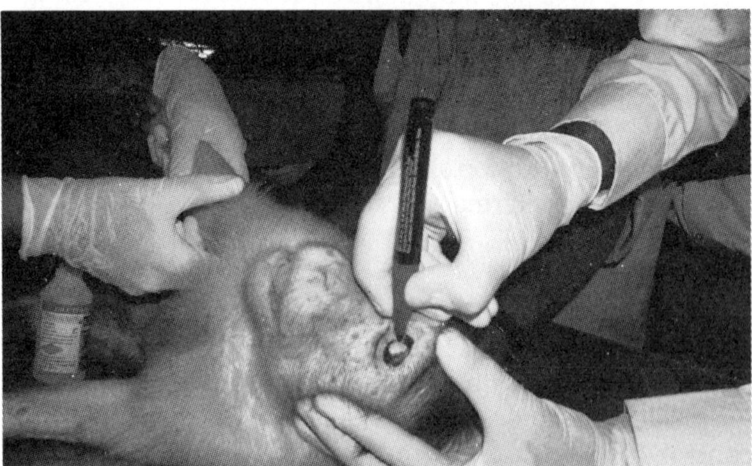

Fig. 2 : Tuberculosis testing in monkey (Photo courtesy: Dr. Chandrakant Galdhar, Veterinary Nuclear Medicine, Bombay Veterinary College)

2.9 Animal quarantine services

The role of veterinary professionals engaged in animal quarantine services is to prevent introduction of exotic diseases and disease agents into a country or a geographical area, to regulate the transborder movement of animals and animal products and by-products, and to establish and strengthen the disease surveillance system. Animal quarantine stations are provided at various entry points such as the seaports, airports and the border check posts to prevent the entry of dangerous pests and diseases by ensuring that the imported animals and animal products comply with the statutory requirements and are free from exotic diseases and disease agents that could affect the livestock industry and endanger public health in the country. Apart from animals, the animal products that may require sanitary import permits include meat and meat products; tissue or organs of animals; egg and egg powder; milk and milk products; animal embryos, ova or semen; and pet food products of animal origin.

2.10 Animal feed safety

Animal feed is a critical component of the food chain that has a direct impact on animal health and welfare and also on food safety and public health. The role of animal feed as a source of infections among animals was well known earlier too, however, the role of feed as a vector for zoonotic agents e.g. bovine spongiform encephalopathy (BSE), *Salmonella*, enterohaemorrhagic *E. coli* and other microorganisms has added a public health risk dimension to it. Among many other biological, chemical and physical hazards in feed, the residues of veterinary drugs may be a potential risk factor for food safety. Residues of veterinary drugs can be present in feed when it contains ingredients of animal origin (terrestrial and aquatic). The veterinarians, thus, have the direct role in mitigating this hazard by adopting good practices in the use of veterinary drugs.

Feed and feed ingredients are now widely traded internationally. Veterinary Services have also the responsibility of providing veterinary certificates for international trade in animal product-based feeds.

2.11 Detection of biohazard exposure

Biohazards include microorganisms or toxins derived from living organisms that have adverse effect on the health and life of living beings. They could be used against the livestock or poultry industries for causing economic devastation. State veterinary surveillance systems have great role in identifying such incidents quickly. Veterinarians and diagnostic laboratories contribute by reporting such events to the state functionaries for the protection of animal health in their respective states.

2.12 Veterinary disaster response

Well-planned and organised disaster plans for animals are essential to face any disaster event. These plans help in the protection, evacuation or rescue of the animals from hazardous situations and their sheltering, care and rehabilitation. Veterinarians and veterinary services are essential components of the disaster response teams.

2.13 Biomedical research and development of biological material

Veterinarians working in pharmaceutical and biomedical research organizations develop, test, and supervise the production of drugs, chemicals, and biological products, such as antibiotics and vaccines. Veterinarians also provide daily medical care to the animals involved in research and ensure that the animals are properly and humanely cared for. They use their expertise to improve surgical techniques for humans and animals. Research veterinarians work to find cures for diseases and sometimes test potential new drugs on the animals to determine if the drugs are effective and safe (AVMA 2007).

2.14 Army Veterinary Services

The Veterinary Corps is an integral part of the Armed Forces of a country and provides veterinary service to the Army, Air Force, Navy and Marines. Veterinarians here have three primary areas of focus: animal medicine, veterinary public health, and research and development. They provide care to military working dogs, ceremonial horses, working animals of different security organizations, and pets owned by service members. Besides providing clinical veterinary services, veterinarians also work for food safety and defence by supervising food defence programmes and performing sanitary audits of food production facilities. Veterinary Corps is also an essential component of the military medical research and development team.

The Remount and Veterinary Corps (RVC) in India accomplishes the task of procuring, rearing, breeding, training and issue of horses, mules and Army dogs along with prevention, control and treatment of infectious and contagious diseases. The veterinary public health component of their services involves inspection of food of animal origin and prevention of zoonotic diseases. Apart from this, the RVC also takes up the training of RVC Officers and other army personnel.

3. Animal Welfare

The veterinarians have responsibilities not only to protect, preserve and maintain animal health but also to prevent animal suffering and provide relief in distress. The animal welfare is not restricted to farm operations alone but also involves pet animals, draught animals, zoo animals, wildlife, performing animals and those kept for recreational purposes. It involves prevention of cruelty to all categories of animals. The veterinarians ensure that there is no cruelty to animals and they are handled humanely and compassionately during housing, transportation, working, training and even at the slaughterhouses. The veterinarians also undertake animal infrastructure assessment, animal population management and animal shelter operations.

3.1 Farm animal care

As the ultimate aim of the livestock farming activities is to provide food security and safety, the veterinarians have to ensure that human welfare does not get undue dominance over animals and that the intensification of animal production systems aiming to achieve lower production costs do not go against the animal welfare. The veterinarians have to face the challenge to look after not only their clients' interests but also have to fulfil their commitment to animal welfare and to ensure that their welfare is not compromised beyond an acceptable level (Edwards 2004).

3.2 Food animal welfare at abattoirs

The veterinarian is responsible to see that the animals meant for slaughter are handled humanely and slaughtered without inflicting unnecessary pain and suffering. They ensure that the animals are transported to abattoirs under appropriate conditions; they are given adequate rest, feed and water; and they do not suffer from injuries or painful conditions. Through ante-mortem inspection of the animals, the veterinarian also takes decision regarding emergency slaughter of any animal suffering from painful condition to relieve it from unnecessary prolonged distress. He also ensures efficient stunning of animals for painless slaughter operation.

3.3 Experimental animal care and management

Laboratory experimental animals are used frequently in research directed at enhancing human and animal health and protection of the environment. A variety of academic and research institutions, organizations, laboratories, hospitals and industries undertake animal experimentations. Many of these have facilities of breeding and raising their own experimental animals in animal houses. It is not only ethical but also mandatory that research animals must be used in a responsible manner. Experimental animals require adequate veterinary care and this responsibility in such institutions is given to veterinary professionals. Their primary roles include managing animal resources, providing adequate veterinary care, consulting with researchers on animal models, assisting in regulatory compliance, teaching and training. They are also responsible for diagnosing, treating and controlling diseases and injuries among research animals; performing surgery on sick and injured animals; prescribing and administering drugs, medicines and vaccines as appropriate; consulting with researchers and staff regarding the type and number of research animals needed; and providing instruction and assistance in the special care and treatment of animals.

Veterinary professionals may also carry out independent research and serve as consultants and collaborators to research investigators in a variety of disciplines. They also help and provide support to the institutions in planning and conducting research projects and in animal-health related issues.

3.4 Animal ethics committees

Veterinarians are generally a part of the Animal Ethics Committees in the institutions engaged in animal experimentations. Their role is to promote animal welfare and regulatory compliance. The duties include review of proposals to use animals for scientific purposes. They ensure that the use of animals in research is rational, humane, and without unnecessary pain or suffering or injury to animals during holding, experimentation and post-experimentation period. The Animal Ethics Committees also monitor the use of laboratory animals and the provision of proper housing, environment, feeding and veterinary care to them.

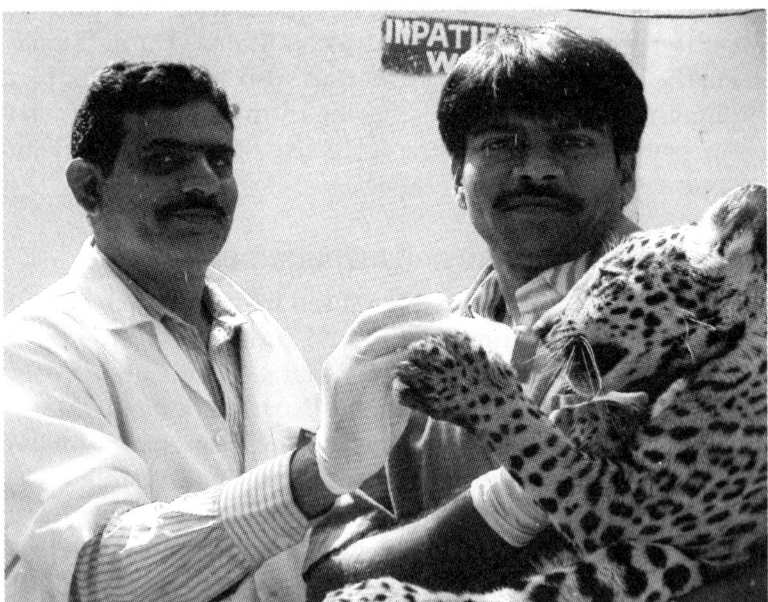

Fig. 3 : Zoo animal care (Photo courtesy: Dr. Pasham Srinivas, Nehru Zoological Park, Hyderabad)

3.5 Zoo animal care and management

Many veterinarians work in zoos and are responsible for the healthcare and welfare of wildlife animals (Fig. 3). They also assist in research projects by collecting baseline medical data on wild animals in captivity. They are also involved in investigating diseases, rehabilitating wild animals and conservation of wildlife. They participate in research to develop tools and methods for providing humane and compassionate treatment to animals during wildlife management activities. Zoo veterinarians also educate and train other fellow veterinarians, wildlife veterinarians and researchers.

3.6 Stray, abandoned and lost animal management

The control of stray animals, particularly dogs, is an important animal welfare issue. Such animals frequently suffer from hunger and illness. A check on the unrestricted growth of stray animal populations becomes essential due to the health risk posed by them. The veterinarians have a major role in devising and executing plans to control breeding of stray animals in a humane painless way instead of the people resorting to poisoning, electrocuting or shooting dogs inhumanely to eliminate them. For the abandoned or lost animals, veterinarians run animal shelters and strive to rehome such animals.

3.7 Public education, guidance and monitoring

The animal welfare cannot be accomplished without involvement of the total society, particularly the animal-keepers. A number of factors relating to the animal owners, such as the person's family, the specific human-animal interaction, socio-economical background and emotional mood, influence the attitude of the people towards animals. Similarly, the features of the animals such as breed, gender, age, socialization and training also have bearing on the animal-human interaction (Odendaal 1998). Thus, besides animals, the veterinarians have to fully realize the human aspect of veterinary practice as well, including people's concern about animal welfare and well-being. The veterinarians and the veterinary services, thus, have the responsibility to educate the society on the essentials of animal welfare, suggest methods for improving animal welfare as well as to assist in the compliance of legislative provisions. Veterinarians educate their clients about responsible pet ownership too.

4. Animal Resource Conservation

4.1 Farm animal genetic resource conservation

Conservation of animal genetic resources refers to all human activities including strategies, plans, policies and actions undertaken to ensure that the diversity of animal genetic resources is maintained to contribute to food and agricultural production and productivity, or to maintain other values of these resources (ecological, cultural) now and in the future. Sustainable management of farm animal genetic resources is of vital importance to food, nutrition and environment security. Their conservation and judicious use is critical for the survival as well as improved livelihood of resource constrained farmers. The veterinarians make a great contribution in conserving the animal breeds so that they do not face a threat of extinction.

4.2 Wildlife conservation

The global environmental changes have caused a huge loss of biodiversity leading to rise in the number of threatened or endangered species. Diseases also affect the wildlife conservation. The conservation of wildlife demands the intervention of wildlife veterinarians. By studying the ecological role of the host-parasite relationships and the host population dynamics, they help in taking corrective measures for biodiversity conservation (Lanfranchi *et al.* 2003).

Conservation medicine focuses on protection/reintroduction of endangered or threatened species and ecosystems. The role of veterinarian is not to provide medical care alone for the zoo's animal collection but also to participate in programmes that add to the knowledge base regarding the species, diseases, and management (Miller 2010). Zoo and wildlife veterinarians are in a vital position for developing programmes to address conservation medicine both *ex situ* and *in situ*. Veterinarians may also be involved in reintroduction programmes through assisting with safe capture and health assessments, medical care and health management of captive animals, development of disease-related protocols, and providing input on education materials and programmes.

5. Public Health Promotion

Many people perceive veterinary medicine solely as the science of preventing, diagnosing, and treating diseases and injuries of animals, failing to recognize the importance and responsibility of veterinary medicine as a human health activity. In fact, man's physical and mental well-being has been the ultimate concern and beneficiary of the veterinarian's total efforts. A strong relationship between veterinary medicine and public health is now well recognized and documented. As part of their Oath, veterinarians swear to use their scientific training to promote public health. Veterinary sciences exert direct influence on man's health by providing safe and nutritious food. Secondly, veterinary professionals safeguard the public health against zoonotic diseases, environmental hazards and biomedical hazards.

Veterinary public health constitutes an important component of public health activities devoted to the application of professional veterinary skills, knowledge, and resources to the protection and improvement of human health

(WHO 1975). Veterinary Public health unit within a department or Ministry of Health encourages the flow of information between veterinary sciences and human health disciplines strengthening intersectoral coordination in public health activities and larger interest of the society. A more recent WHO consultation in 1999 has defined veterinary public health as the sum of all contributions to the physical, mental, and social well-being of humans through an understanding and application of veterinary science. There is a recognized and fast growing role of veterinarians in protecting human health in the public and private sectors and at local, state, and national levels in several ways (Pappaioanou *et al.* 2003).

5.1 Food security

Animal production contributes to food security by providing a source of energy, dietary protein of high nutritional quality and micronutrients and by contributing directly and indirectly to the Gross Domestic Product (GDP) of a country. However, animal diseases or the contamination of animal products with microorganisms or xenobiotic substances have complex repercussions on food industry. The Veterinary Services, therefore, have the responsibility to identify and minimize the health risks in order to limit their impact on the livestock production sectors and on humans. In so doing, the Veterinary Services contribute to food security, economic development and human health protection (Bonnet *et al.* 2011). Advancement in livestock breeding, nutrition, animal healthcare, and biological products have contributed to substantial rise in animal productivity. Reduction in disease and animal mortality due to veterinary efforts has helped to reduce the cost of production.

5.2 Food protection

Food protection is one of the highest priority areas of veterinary public health activities. It embraces all the measures necessary for ensuring safety, wholesomeness, and soundness of food at all stages from its production to its final consumption. The Veterinary Services have an essential role to play in the minimization of food contamination and prevention and control of foodborne health risks due to microbial infections and intoxications, hazardous additives, pesticide residues, antimicrobial substances, hormonal substances, drug residues and heavy metals etc. Healthy animal production is the first and foremost step in this direction. The veterinarians are also responsible for implementation of sanitary and phytosanitary measures and good farming practices for animal production and food safety during production at farm. The veterinarians are directly associated not only with food production at farms but also with hygienic slaughter and processing of food animals. Veterinary Services contribute significantly in the control of meat-borne hazards through ante-mortem and post-mortem inspection of food animals.

Apart from this, veterinarians also carry out the inspection of animal products and food establishments.

5.3 Zoonotic disease prevention and control

Prevention and control of zoonotic diseases is an essential component of public health and it constitutes a major area of veterinary public health activities too. It is quite evident that it is impossible to achieve success in public health programmes against zoonotic diseases without the support of veterinary services. About 75% of the new diseases that have affected humans over the past 10 years have been caused by pathogens originating from an animal or from products of animal origin. Many of these diseases have the potential to spread through various means over long distances and to become global problems (WHO 2011). Such a scenario clearly points to the increasing importance of the Veterinary Services. Diagnosis, surveillance, epidemiology, prevention, control and elimination of zoonoses constitute the core domain of veterinary public health activities.

5.4 Epidemiological studies

Veterinary epidemiology is an integral component of animal health and veterinary public health. Epidemiology deals with populations rather than individuals. Medical and veterinary epidemiology, both use the same concepts. The veterinarians' role is not restricted to the epidemiological studies of animal diseases or zoonotic diseases only. Their versatility and broad public health background prepares them to function in many different public health arenas. Whether the public health issues relate to veterinary medicine, food safety, medical devices, or biologicals, Veterinary Epidemiologists play fascinating and important roles in national and international organizations.

5.5 Environmental health

The health of man largely depends upon his environment which includes all the external factors surrounding him. Many factors including unsafe water, unsafe food, polluted soil, unhygienic disposal of human and animal excreta, pollution from waste, poor housing and prevalence of insects, rodents and stray animals may affect human health adversely. The veterinarians contribute to environmental health of the people in many ways. They directly contribute to protection of drinking water and environment through safe disposal of animal farm waste, abattoir waste, livestock industry waste and dead animal carcasses; hygienic practices in safe food production; and control of insect vectors, rodents and stray animals. They may particularly help in regular monitoring of the drinking water quality, reporting about unsafe water, and educating people about the risk of waterborne diseases and the methods of their prevention and control.

5.6 Biohazard exposure and bioterrorism identification

Because most biological weapons developed for use against humans involve zoonotic agents, animals can serve as sentinels for disease. Veterinarians and veterinary diagnostic laboratories provide an important first line of detection for such agents, exposures and occurrence of some exotic diseases (Fitzpatrick and Bender 2000). They report any incidence of disease with human health implications to public health department for further investigation and actions for mitigation.

5.7 Occupational safety

The veterinary practitioners and those who handle animals or their products have the inherent risk of exposure to zoonotic agents. Veterinarians have to remain vigilant not only about their own safety, but they have a responsibility to provide a safe workplace and safety guidelines to the workers too who are associated with handling of animals, contaminated material and animal products. By warning about the risk potential of an animal or material and by suggesting safety guidelines, veterinarians directly protect the workers in veterinary hospitals, laboratories, animal houses, animal farms, abattoirs, animal industries and those handling stray animals and dead animal carcasses (Weese *et al.* 2002). The veterinarians also reduce the chances of occupational diseases through early recognition and appropriate management of infected (or potentially infected) animals, adequate training of support personnel, proper animal handling and housing, and, most importantly, personal hygiene.

5.8 Mental health promotion through companion animal healthcare

The human-companion animal relationship and bond continues to evolve. Pets often play a key role in the family structure, and the importance of the human-animal bond is well recognized to have positive effects on human well-being, health, stress, healing, and the immune system (Glaser and Kiecolt-Glaser 2005, McNicholas *et al.* 2005, Das and O'Keefe 2008). By providing veterinary healthcare to companion animals, the veterinary services indirectly benefit the pet-owners' mental and emotional well-being. Not only this, the healthcare provided to the guide or other working dogs for disabled persons ensures their physical well-being too.

5.9 Public health emergency and disaster response

During public health emergencies, the veterinarians by virtue of their knowledge of biology and medicine are able to provide leadership as well as emergency medical first aid to the people. This is very critical sometimes, particularly in the rural or remote areas. It has been shown that protection of animals through veterinary disaster response also enhances the ability of disaster response teams in evacuating the people and ensuring better public health and safety (Knight 2009).

5.10 Prevention of injury

The veterinarians being knowledgeable about the dangers of the biting, venomous or other hazardous animals provide guidance for protection from animal bite injuries, particularly dog bites.

5.11 Health education

The veterinarians are competent to provide general health education and guidance to their clients and other people regarding general health issues like obesity, diabetes, nutrition etc. Veterinarians also guide them about the risks associated with zoonoses, food safety, sanitation and personal hygiene.

5.12 Other functions

The other public health functions that veterinarians perform include pest and vector control, extension activities, disaster planning and management, health laboratory services and liaison role in development programmes. Due to their biomedical training, veterinarians are qualified for general public health roles concerned with administration, planning and coordination of public health programmes.

6. Advancement of Medical Knowledge

Veterinarians have a long and diverse training in biomedical sciences. Therefore, they are often associated in biomedical research and development where physicians and other public health professionals also work (Fig. 4).

6.1 Biomedical research

Veterinarians in academic institutions, research organizations and industry are often involved in a broad array of research including basic science research, biomedical research with applications to public health and medical product development without restricting them to animal health oriented research (Rosol *et al.* 2009). With their background and training, veterinarians have unique skill sets that enable them to serve as important members of interdisciplinary research teams dealing with different aspects of public health e.g. general epidemiology, health laboratory services, production and control of biological products, drug evaluation and control, general environmental health, radiological health, environmental physiology, reproductive physiology and fertility control etc. (WHO 1975).

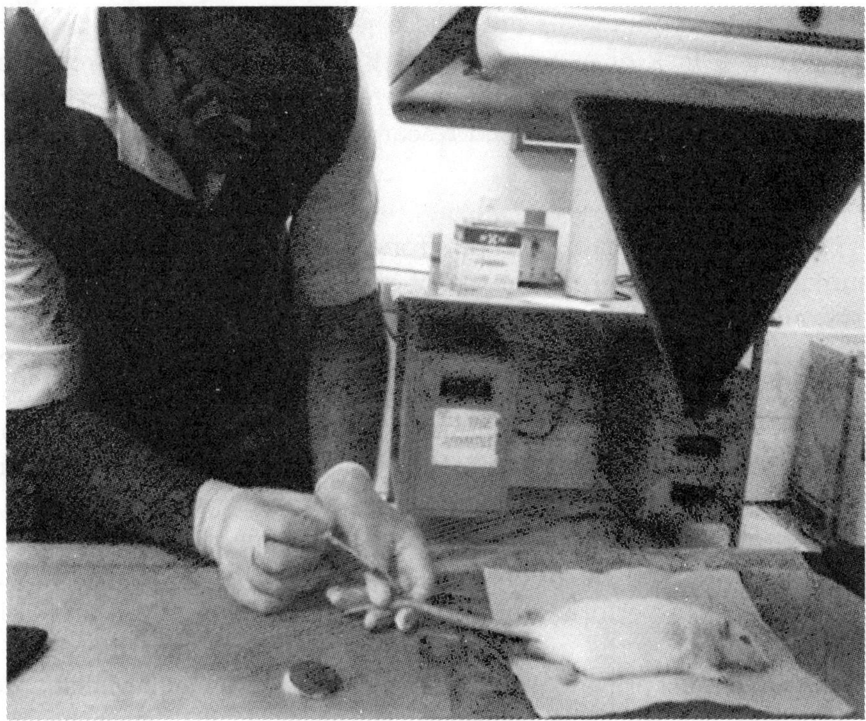

Fig. 4 : Biomedical research (Photo courtesy: Dr. Chandrakant Galdhar, Veterinary Nuclear Medicine, Bombay Veterinary College)

6.2 Comparative medicine

Comparative medicine involves the study of human disease by comparison with the diseases of animals, depending largely on work with naturally occurring diseases of animals that are models for human diseases. Comparative studies on the epidemiology of non-infectious diseases of animals may also be valuable in public health as the environmental or other factors may be common to man and lower animals (WHO 1975). Animal models of human disease are often an integral part of translational research. The laboratory mouse has become the preferred animal model for many diseases due to the availability of reagents and ease of manipulation of its genome. Mouse pathologists and laboratory animal veterinarians dramatically improve the ability of research teams to use mouse models of human disease to translate bench research to human medicine (Rosol *et al.* 2009). Laboratory animal veterinarians help select the best animal models for particular research projects, carry out research themselves, and play crucial roles in the support of biomedical research. Veterinary and medical pathologists (specializing in laboratory animal pathology) are central to the diagnosis of spontaneous diseases, understanding the mechanisms of disease induced by experimental procedures, and analyzing the phenotype of spontaneous or induced genetic modifications in animals. When there is a lack of expert pathology support on a research project, important information may be misinterpreted or go undiscovered, which reduces the impact of animal-based research (Ince *et al.* 2008).

7. Conclusion

With the growing realization of strong linkages between animal health and human health; frequent outbreaks of emerging and re-emerging zoonotic diseases; and growing demand for wholesome, nutritious and safe animal products, the veterinary profession is entrusted with much greater responsibilities. In addition to the traditional roles of taking care of animal health and welfare, veterinary professionals are today playing major role in production of food of animal origin for human consumption and in public health activities. Taking cognizance of the increasing responsibilities, the veterinary professionals and the veterinary services need to be proactive and willing to be involved in diverse roles in the public benefit. Veterinary community needs to perform ethically, independently and with professional competence to ensure the quality and integrity of all their missions. The Veterinary Oath must prevail over the harsh realities of the materialistic world. ".... I will practice my profession conscientiously, with dignity, and in keeping with the principles of veterinary medical ethics. I accept as a lifelong obligation the continual improvement of my professional knowledge and competence."

References

1. AVMA (2007). Veterinarians in biomedical research. American Veterinary Medical Association. http://www.avma.org/educators/teacher_guide/biomedical_bgnd.pdf. Accessed 6 June 2011.

2. Bonnet P, Lancelot R, Seegers H, Martinez D (2011). Contribution of veterinary activities to global food security for food derived from terrestrial and aquatic animals. 79th General Session, World Assembly, World Organisation for Animal Health (OIE), 22-27 May 2011, Paris. http://www.oie.int/fileadmin/Home/eng/Media_Center/docs/pdf/A_79SG_Food_Security.pdf. Accessed 6 June 2011.

3. Das S, O'Keefe JH (2008). Behavioral cardiology: recognizing and addressing the profound impact of psychosocial stress on cardiovascular health. Curr Hypertens Rep 10:374-381.

4. Edwards JD (2004). The role of the veterinarian in animal welfare - A global perspective. In: Proceedings- Global conference on animal welfare: an OIE initiative, 23-25 February 2004, Paris. Office for Official Publication of the European Communities, Luxembourg. p. 24-32.

5. Fitzpatrick AM, Bender JB (2000). Survey of chief livestock officials regarding bioterrorism preparedness in the United States. J Am Vet Med Assoc 217(9): 1315-1317.

6. Glaser R, Kiecolt-Glaser JK (2005). Stress-induced immune dysfunction: implications for health. Nat Rev Immunol 5:243-251.

7. Ince TA, Ward JM, Valli VE, Sgroi D, Nikitin AY, Loda M, Griffey SM, Crum CP, Crawford JM, Bronson RT, Cardiff RD (2008). Do-it-yourself (DIY) pathology. Nat Biotechnol 26:978-979.

8. Knight AP (2009). Elements for a disaster plan for animals. In: Wingfield WE, Palmer SB (eds) Veterinary disaster response. Wiley-Blackwell, Iowa, USA. p. 407-412.

9. Lanfranchi P, Ferroglio E, Poglayen G, Guberti V (2003). Wildlife veterinarian, conservation and public health. Vet Res Commun 27 Suppl 1:567-574.

10. McNicholas J, Gilbey A, Rennie A, Ahmedzai S, Dono JA, Ormerod E (2005). Pet ownership and human health: a brief review of evidence and issues. BMJ 331:1252-1254.

11. Mee JF (2007). The role of the veterinarian in bovine fertility management on modern dairy farms. Theriogenology 68 Suppl 1:S257-S265.

12. Miller MA (2010). The role of veterinarians in conservation medicine. 82nd Western Veterinary Conference V729. http://wvc.omnibooksonline.com/data/papers/2010_V729.pdf. Accessed 10 June 2011.

13. Odendaal JSJ (1998). The practicing veterinarian and animal welfare as a human endeavour. Applied Animal Behaviour Sci 59:85-91.

14. Pappaioanou M, Garbe PL, Glynn MK, Thacker SB (2003). Veterinarians and Public Health: The Epidemic Intelligence Service of the Centers for Disease Control and Prevention, 1951–2002. J Vet Med Educ 30(4):383-391.

15. Rosol TJ, Moore RM, Saville WJA, Oglesbee MJ, Rush LJ, Mathes LE, Lairmore MD (2009). The need for veterinarians in biomedical research. J Vet Med Educ 36(1):70-75. Author Manuscript at http://www.ncbi.nlm.nih.gov/pmc/articles/PMC2852242/pdf/nihms-183526.pdf.

16. Somvanshi R (2006). Veterinary medicine and animal keeping in ancient India. Asian Agri-History 10 (2):133-146.

17. Stark KDC, Regula G, Hernandez J, Knopf L, Fuchs K, Morris RS, Davies P (2006). Concepts for risk-based surveillance in the field of veterinary medicine and veterinary public health: Review of current approaches. BMC Health Services Research 6:20. http://www.biomedcentral.com/1472-6963/6/20. Accessed 6 June 2011.

18. Weese JS, Peregrine AS, Armstrong J (2002). Occupational health and safety in small animal veterinary practice: Part I - Nonparasitic zoonotic diseases. Can Vet J 43(8):631-636.

19. WHO (1975). The veterinary contribution to public health practice. Report of a Joint FAO/WHO Expert Committee on Veterinary Public Health. World Health Organization, Geneva.

20. WHO (2011). Zoonoses and veterinary public health. http://www.who.int/zoonoses/vph/en/. Accessed 10 June 2011.

21. Zepeda C, Salman M, Thiermann A, Kellar J, Rojas H, Willeberg P (2005). The role of veterinary epidemiology and veterinary services in complying with the World Trade Organization SPS agreement. Prev Vet Med 67(2-3):125-140.

❑❑❑

Chapter 2

Food Security and Sustainable Development through Livestock Products

J. SAHOO[1] AND S. R. GARG[2]

[1]Department of Livestock Products Technology, Guru Angad Dev Veterinary and Animal Sciences University, Ludhiana-141004 [2]Department of Veterinary Public Health and Epidemiology, College of Veterinary Sciences, Hisar-125004

Contents

1. Introduction

Food security refers to the availability of food and one's access to it. According to the Food and Agriculture Organization of the United Nations (FAO), food security exists when all people, at all times, have physical, social and economic access to sufficient, safe and nutritious food to meet their dietary needs and food preferences for an active and healthy life.

Food security is an urgent challenge for national and global governance. Based on the latest available data, the total number of undernourished people in the world is estimated to have reached 1023 million in 2009 and is estimated to have declined by 9.6 per cent to 925 million in 2010 owing to the recovery of global economy. Despite this decline, the number remains unacceptably high. Developing countries account for 98 per cent of the world's undernourished people and have a prevalence of undernourishment of 16 per cent (FAO 2010). The FAO Hunger Map reveals widespread prevalence of undernourishment in developing countries (FAO 2010). In India, it is rated as moderately high (15-24%) while in many African, Asian and South American countries it is even higher (25-34% or even more).

2. Food Security through Livestock Products

Livestock play particularly important role in farming systems in developing countries and contribute significantly to the total food production. Livestock provide over half the total value of agricultural output worldwide and one third in developing countries. In developed countries, about 60 per cent of dietary protein comes from animal products compared to only 22 per cent in developing countries where diets are composed of only a small number of staple foods. Animal products, therefore, assume great importance in developing countries in preventing malnutrition as they constitute rich source of essential amino acids that are available only in limited quantities in the protein of staple vegetable foods. In developed countries animal proteins provide more than 30% of all calories in the diet, whilst in developing countries, this proportion is less than 10% (Sansoucy 1995, Ehui *et al.* 1998).

3. Role of Livestock Products in Sustainable Development

Twelve per cent of the world's population depends solely on livestock for its livelihood. Livestock farming besides providing nutritive food to the farmers constitutes a source of regular income, draught power, fertilizer and soil conditioner, household energy and a means of disposing of otherwise unwanted crop residues. Besides all these, the livestock sector is also a great generator of employment for the people. Thus, besides providing food security, livestock make a significant contribution to the economy of the farmers and the nation (Sansoucy *et al.* 1995).

3.1 Employment generation

According to the FAO estimates, global annual meat production is expected to expand from the current 228 million tons to 463 million tons by 2050 with the cattle population estimated to grow from 1.5 billion to 2.6 billion and that of goats and sheep from 1.7 billion to 2.7 billion (UN News Centre 2010). The growing demand for animal food products, thus, offers great opportunities for livestock sector to contribute to economic growth and poverty reduction. This is particularly relevant in Indian perspective as the country has 66% of economically active population engaged in agriculture. Livestock has a great complementary and supplementary role under mixed farming systems prevalent in the country. This has fostered rapid expansion of livestock output such as milk, meat and eggs.

Despite the growth of livestock sector, per capita consumption of meat is only 17.7 kg/year, compared to 81.6 kg/year in developed countries. The strong demand for animal food products naturally offers significant opportunities for livestock to contribute to employment generation and poverty reduction.

3.2 Foreign exchange earnings

Rapid growth and transformation of the livestock sector can offer substantial economic benefits. The higher volume of production allows developing countries to reduce imports and even to become exporters. This helps in freeing foreign exchange resources for other development priorities. The developing countries have potential to increase their participation in international trade. They need to take into consideration the requirements of international market regarding food quality and safety to realize the potential gains from international trade.

4. Indian Perspective

4.1 Livestock population

India has been bestowed with abundant livestock resources in terms of number of animals as shown in Table 1. The livestock population review (1997-2009) indicates that the population of buffaloes, small ruminants, pigs and poultry has increased in the country, though the cattle population has shown some decline during the last decade. While possessing 53.6% of world's buffaloes, 12.4% cattle, 6.1% sheep, 14.5% goats, 1.46% pigs and 3.3% chicken, India ranks first in the world in cattle, goat and buffalo population. Interestingly, buffalo population has shown an increasing trend despite the slaughter rate of 9.7%. The poultry industry has come up from the backyard farming to most organized industry.

Table 1 : Trend in livestock population in India

Species	Year 1997 (million)	Year 2009 (million)	Trend
Cattle	198.9	172.4	decline
Buffalo	89.9	106.6	rise
Sheep	57.5	65.7	rise
Goat	122.7	126	rise
Pig	13.3	13.8	rise
Chickens	315.4	613	rise

Source : FAOSTAT database. www.faostat.fao.org

4.2 Meat production

Meat animals in India comprise sheep, goats, poultry (chicken and duck), pigs, buffaloes, cattle and rabbits. India ranks seventh in meat production in the world. The major portion of meat production in the country is from large ruminants, including buffalo and cattle meat. Most of the buffalo meat has export demand while beef is consumed in the domestic market. Indian poultry has shown phenomenal growth. The country ranks fifth in the world in poultry meat production. The tremendous growth in livestock products that has taken place during the period 1980-2007 in the country is reflected in Table 2 and 3. The data show that despite doubling of meat production in India between 1980 and 2007, the country's overall meat production levels remain low in the global context (FAO 2009a).

Table 2 : Production of livestock products in India and the world (year 1980 and 2007)

Region	Meat (million ton)		Milk (million ton)		Eggs (million ton)	
	1980	2007	1980	2007	1980	2007
India	2.6	6.3	31.6	102.9	0.6	2.7
World	136.7	285.7	465.5	671.3	27.4	67.8
India's part in world production (%)	1.9	2.2	6.8	15.3	2.2	4.0

Source : FAO (2009a,b)

Table 3 : Production of main categories of meat in India and the world (year 1980 and 2007)

Region	Pig meat (million ton)		Poultry meat (million ton)		Cattle meat (million ton)		Sheep & goat meat (million ton)	
	1980	2007	1980	2007	1980	2007	1980	2007
India	0.4	0.5	0.2	2.3	1.0	1.3	0.6	0.8
World	63.6	115.5	35.9	86.8	50.9	61.9	8.6	14.0
India's part in world production	0.6%	0.4%	0.6%	2.6%	2.0%	2.1%	7.0%	5.7%

Source: FAO (2009a,b)

4.3 Milk production

Dairy industry is of crucial importance to India. The country is the world's largest milk producer, accounting for more than 15% of world's total milk production. The milk production in the country has tripled between 1980 and 2007 (Table 2).

Dairy products are a major source of cheap and nutritious food to millions of people in India and the only acceptable source of animal protein for large vegetarian segment of the population, particularly among the landless, small and marginal farmers and women. The huge volume of milk produced in the country is consumed almost entirely within the country. Consequently, despite the largest milk production, India is a very minor player in the world market. India was primarily an import dependent country till early seventies. In the 1990s, the country started exporting surplus dairy commodities.

4.4 Livestock product consumption

The average animal protein intake in developing countries is only 15 g (10 g from meat and 5 g from milk) per person per day compared to almost 60 g in developed countries (Heinz 1995). The consumption of animal products is relatively much lower at 10.8 g per person per day in India. The scenario of per capita consumption of meat, milk and eggs in India and the world is given in Table 4 which shows wide margin between the world and India's averages.

Table 4 : Per capita consumption of livestock products in India and the world (years 1980 and 2005)

Region	Meat (kg/capita/year)		Milk (kg/capita/year)		Eggs (kg/capita/year)	
	1980	2005	1980	2005	1980	2005
India	3.7	5.1	38.5	65.2	0.7	1.8
World	30.0	41.2	75.7	82.1	5.5	9.0

Source: FAO (2009a,b)

4.5 Livestock product requirement

A person's daily protein intake should be about 1 g per kg bodyweight for adequate nutrition and 30 to 50 per cent of it should ideally be animal protein to provide optimal levels of amino acids. The Expert Committee of the Indian Council of Medical Research (ICMR) has recommended 60 g of protein per day with net protein utilization (NPU) of 65. It would not be possible to achieve it without substituting vegetable protein in the diet with adequate amount of animal protein. Thus a minimum requirement of animal protein would be targeted at 20 g per person per day compared to the present availability of 10 g and the world average of 25 g. It can be provided in vegetarians through milk and in non-vegetarians through milk, meat, fish and eggs. The requirements of different animal products for an estimated population of 1226 million (858 million non-vegetarians and 368 million vegetarians) in the year 2020 would be: milk 165.81 million tons, total meat 10.65 million tons, fish 10.65 million tons and eggs 103 billion. Demand for meat and dairy products is also expected to grow in tune with the population growth, rising incomes and increasing urbanization.

4.6 Livestock product export from India

The value of total exports of animal products during 2009-10 was Rs. 7200.72 crore (Table 5). The rise in meat export due to increasing international demand has resulted in establishment of more number of integrated meat processing plants with modern abattoirs as well as meat processing plants without abattoir facilities. India has also become one of the largest producers of milk and value-added milk products in the world though its share in the international trade is quite negligible (Table 5 & 6).

Table 5 : Three year export statement of APEDA for animal products

Product	2007-08		2008-09		2009-10	
	Quantity (ton)	Value (Rs. in lacs)	Quantity (ton)	Value (Rs. in lacs)	Quantity (ton)	Value (Rs. in lacs)
Buffalo meat	483478.29	354978.47	462749.62	483970.99	495019.71	548060.08
Sheep/goat meat	8908.72	13409.96	37790.64	49336.94	52868.01	74720.07
Poultry products	1355246.31	44108.55	1057016.47	42205.8	1016783.1	37211.85
Dairy products	69415.44	86656.36	70146.77	98086.06	34379.97	40268.39
Animal casings	619.68	684.14	1823.72	884.32	2020.56	3152.74
Processed meat	1245.47	1296.13	857.63	1014.4	716.19	958.51
Swine meat	1710.89	2463.69	817.82	917.23	1117.96	1034.9
Natural honey	12231.19	9329.64	15587.53	14896.37	13310.77	14665.42
Total	1932855.99	512926.94	1646790.2	691312.11	1616216.27	720071.96

Source: APEDA Agri Exchange (2011), DGCIS Annual Data

Table 6 : Three year export statement of APEDA for different dairy products

Dairy product	2007-2008		2008-2009		2009-2010	
	Quantity (ton)	Value (Rs. in lacs)	Quantity (ton)	Value (Rs. in lacs)	Quantity (ton)	Value (Rs. in lacs)
Skimmed milk in powder, granules and other sold forms (Fat <1.5%)	32050.05	45070.53	24360.5	37655.18	12173.5	13705.15
Other ghee	3701.55	5526.68	4213.82	6854.42	3084.23	7218.86
Other milk powder (Fat < 1.5%)	5454.52	7369.97	5618.74	8014.52	6227.41	6967.62
Butter	4491.82	5760.11	8174.51	11646.85	1275.52	1998.99
Fresh (unripened/uncured) cheese, including whey cheese, & curd	546.59	652.78	820.42	1024.01	1163.33	1558.03

Milk and cream of a fat content, by weight, exceeding 1%	7088.6	1564.47	8138.42	2156.0	5176.45	1509.4
Processed cheese, not grated/powdered	977.89	1922.84	1269.37	2342.34	1052.59	1474.09
Whole milk (Fat >1.5%)	1723.77	2368.73	6121.67	9696.79	679.1	1071.06
Other	277.58	340.2	729.22	1604.33	495.25	919.23
Other cheese	302.49	493.05	741.08	1410.07	450.89	787.29
Other	436.66	691.29	161.12	334.88	391.98	658.61
Other milk for babies	102.22	138.71	204.06	304.3	172.88	475.9
Milk food for babies (Fat < 1.5%)	1010.57	1750.39	601.25	1209.49	334.05	432.5
Whey, dry, blocks and powdered	3785.11	3411.14	1727.71	1490.12	574.56	396.48
Other butter oil	872.86	1297.03	4644.01	7796.7	214.18	359.45
Other	233.25	329.96	383.09	461.25	100.07	154.11
Other	3265.9	4290.85	180.38	193.15	95.72	86.51
Milk and cream of a fat content, by weight, not exceeding 1%	203.3	202.89	114.07	103.76	293.69	83.2
Other condensed Milk (Fat >1.5%)	10.47	5.93	61.03	39.53	56.49	82.25
Not containing added sugar or other sweetening matter (>1.5%)	603.89	1037.02	1294.02	2248.42	53.54	77.26
Other whey	04.51	75.38	62.06	31.65	113.95	69.52
Other whole milk	2.15	2.95	68.53	155.8	39.27	66.94
Milk and cream of a fat content, by weight, exceeding 6%	112.84	115.51	101.66	63.45	93.71	43.45
Other butter milk	9.15	14.67	18.4	13.41	38.79	15.92
Other condensed milk	5.47	5.23	17.21	16.35	11.79	15.8
Grated/powdered cheese, of all kinds	13.04	19.2	0.52	1.92	5.85	15.19
Condensed milk (Fat >1.5%)	8.55	11.11	4.42	11.1	4.97	13.46
Dairy spreads	2.06	1.5	14.96	22.94	5.38	10.33
Whey, concentrated, evaporated or condensed, liquid or semi-solid	508.99	640.26	135.65	99.64	0.57	0.89
Yogurt	0.11	0.23	13.25	953.38	0.2	0.75
Blue-veined cheese	4	8.9	7.15	13.46	0.05	0.14
Other	1505.47	1536.85	144.48	116.83	0	0

Source: APEDA Agri Exchange (2011), DGCIS Annual Data

5. Conclusion

The availability of animal products to common people is far less than the requirement and rising demand in India. The country's share in the global export is also quite negligible. Greater food security and economic development can be attained by increasing the production of livestock products. It is also essential to satisfy the escalating concern about food quality and safety among domestic as well as global consumers. Serious efforts are required to adhere to the global standards in order to improve access of our products to the international markets. Institutional policies must establish transparent mechanisms for defining, monitoring and enforcing standards and regulations that also take into account the differing needs of each market. New policy initiatives are needed to address the rapidly growing and changing impact of livestock production on economic development, social equity, the environment and public health (FAO 2005). Effective policies can maximize the benefits and minimize the costs associated with increased livestock production. It includes strengthening of economy, increased employment avenues, reduced prices, improved balance of trade, sustainable improvement in the livelihood of farmers, and poverty reduction. It will also help in controlling environmental degradation, better dietary diversity, greater food safety and improved animal health besides lowering the risk of foodborne illnesses among consumers and less vulnerability of livestock to disease epidemics.

References

1. APEDA Agri Exchange (2011). India exports statistics. Indian Agri Tradejunction, The Agricultural and Processed Food Products Export Development Authority, http://apeda.gov.in/agriexchange/indexp/exportstatement.aspx. Accessed 23 January 2011.

2. Ehui S, Li-Pun H, Mares V, Shapiro B (1998). The role of livestock in food security and environmental protection. Outlook on Agriculture 27:81-87.

3. FAO (2005). FAO Livestock policy briefs. No 1: Responding to the 'Livestock Revolution' - the case for livestock public policies. Livestock Information, Sector Analysis and Policy Branch, Animal Production and Health Division, FAO, Rome, Italy.

4. FAO (2009a). The state of food and agriculture. Livestock in the balance. Food and Agriculture Organization of the United Nations, Rome, Italy.

5. FAO (2009b). FAOSTAT statistical database. Rome, Italy. www.faostat.fao.org

6. FAO (2010). The state of food insecurity in the world- Addressing food insecurity in protracted crises. Food and Agriculture Organization of the United Nations, Rome, Italy.

7. Heinz G (1995). Preservation and processing technologies to improve availability and safety of meat and meat products in developing countries. World Animal Review 84/85 http://www.fao.org/docrep/V8180T/V8180T00.htm

8. Sansoucy R (1995). Livestock - a driving force for food security and sustainable development. World Animal Review 84/85 (4-5):5-17.

9. Sansoucy R, Jabbar MA, Ehui S, Fitzhugh H (1995). Keynote paper: The contribution of livestock to food security and sustainable development. In: Livestock development strategies for low income countries. FAO/ILRI, Rome/Nairobi. FAO Corporate Document Repository http://www.fao.org/wairdocs/ilri/x5462e/x5462e04.htm

10. UN News Centre (2010). More investment needed to ensure more sustainable livestock sector – UN report 18 February 2010. http://www.un.org/apps/news/story.asp?NewsID=33809&Cr=&Cr1=

❑❑❑

Chapter 3

Dairy Research and Development : Challenges Ahead

A. K. SRIVASTAVA, SHIV PRASAD, A. K. SINGH AND SMITA SIROHI
National Dairy Research Institute, Karnal-132001

Contents

1. Introduction

Dairying is one of the most important means of providing livelihood and nutritional security to the rural masses. The livestock activities, among which dairy farming predominates, employ about 18.5 million workers in the country. Milk production of the country has registered impressive growth during the post-independence era, increasing from 19.4 million ton in 1951 to more than 109 million ton at present (GOI 2010). The decadal rate of growth in milk production in India (3.6%) is substantially higher than the world average of 1.5 per cent. The share of livestock sector in agriculture GDP has increased mainly due to the enhanced rate of milk production which accounts for 67 per cent of the value of output from livestock sector. The increased production of milk has improved the per capita milk availability to 261 g per day; which is slightly higher than the recommended per capita nutritional requirement of 250 g by ICMR. However, there are considerable regional variations in per capita availability of milk (Table 1). In some states like Haryana, Punjab and Gujarat, the per capita availability far exceeds the recommended level, while in several other states, especially in the eastern part of the country, the same falls way behind the recommended level.

Dairy farmers, scientists, cooperative agencies and development departments have all played a crucial role in ushering in the 'White Revolution' in the country. In the times to come, the demand for food from animal origin is slated to rise at a very rapid pace. Milk is most preferred item, claiming 70 per cent of the expenditure on livestock based foods. The domestic demand for milk is expected to increase to 180 million ton by 2021-22 (Dalal 2010). In addition, trade liberalization coupled with rising income in several developing countries has opened up new vistas of international trade for the nation's dairy sector. In order to tap the economic benefits of growing domestic and global demand of milk and milk products, the Indian dairy sector has to gear itself by increasing the milk production at the rate close to 7 per cent as against 3.5-4.0 per cent at present, enhancing the production of value added dairy products and by providing complete quality assurance. Achieving higher growth in milk production is also crucial to attain and sustain the growth rate of 4 per cent in agriculture as envisaged in the National Agriculture Policy. The dairy scientists have a great role to play in meeting these targets and ensuing challenges in dairy production, processing and management.

Table 1 : Regional variations in milk availability

Region/State	Per capita availability (g/day)
Northern Region	
Punjab	957
Haryana	645
Himachal Pradesh	365
Jammu & Kashmir	362
Uttaranchal	352
Uttar Pradesh	279
Western Region	
Gujarat	403
Rajasthan	399
Maharashtra	188
Goa	99
Central Region	
Madhya Pradesh	271
Chhattisgarh	106
Southern Region	
Andhra Pradesh	317
Tamil Nadu	234
Karnataka	215
Kerala	197
Eastern Region	
Bihar	172
Jharkhand	132
West Bengal	131
Orissa	115
North-eastern Region	
Sikkim	226
Manipur	90
Meghalaya	83
Tripura	75
Assam	70
Nagaland	66
Arunachal Pradesh	55
Mizoram	48

Source: National Dairy Development Board (www.nddb.org) and Department of Animal Husbandry, Dairying & Fisheries, Ministry of Agriculture, Government of India

2. Dairy Production

The major challenges in milk production system are low productivity levels of dairy animals in India. Despite holding the number one position in milk production in the world for over a decade, the milk productivity in the country remains one of the lowest as compared to many leading countries of the world (Table 2). With about 17% of the world dairy animal stock, India accounts for 15% of the world milk production, while USA is producing 12.5% of the total world milk from merely 6% of the world cattle population (FAOSTAT). In India, the average milk productivity of crossbred cows, indigenous cows and buffaloes is only 6.5, 2.1 and 4.4 kg/day, respectively (GOI 2009) indicating the vast scope for improving the milk yield of dairy animals.

Table 2 : Productivity of cows in selected countries

Country	Lactation yield (Kg)
Israel	9833.3
United States of America	9219.1
Denmark	8288.2
Canada	7961.7
Netherlands	7449.7
United Kingdom	7187.3
Germany	6923.4
Australia	5132.6
New Zealand	3817.2
Ukraine	3675.2
Greece	3647.4
China	3108.7
Thailand	2973.4
Indonesia	1685.8
Brazil	1223.5
Pakistan	1199.5
India	1108.9

Source: FAOSTAT

The research efforts aimed at enhancing milk productivity require close synergies between various scientific aspects viz. animal breeding, genetics, biotechnology, nutrition, health care and management.

2.1 Animal genetics

As the genetic merit of our dairy stock is in general poor, the genetic tools to improve selection in commercial livestock populations for important production traits would have to be developed. The interactions among genetics and environment need to be worked out to understand and formulate the effective selection criteria for bulls and cows of different breeds. Concerted research efforts need to be directed towards identifying genetic markers for selecting superior males at an early age.

There is tremendous scope for identifying the unique genes specific to indigenous dairy animal genetic resources using the molecular techniques. It is expected that by the use of such technologies more number of superior animals per unit time can be obtained by reduction in generation interval which could further increase the pace of genetic advances by providing opportunities for increasing the selection intensity.

2.2 Cloning

Buffalo has been the strength of Indian dairy farming sector that needs to be capitalized on. The focus in buffalo breeding should be on constant improvement of area specific breeds using selective breeding. Cloning of buffalo calves, pioneered by the National Dairy Research Institute with birth of world's first buffalo female and male calves, can give an edge to the breed improvement programme for raising high producing breeds of buffaloes (Fig. 1 and 2). The technology has the potential to multiply elite breed of buffaloes and cattle without loss of parental traits. It may also prove to be a very fast way of creating new breeds.

Other advantage of cloning will be to save many vulnerable species of dairy animals. The population of well-known indigenous breeds Sahiwal, Red Sindhi, Tharparker, Gir etc. is dwindling very fast. In the times to come, the scientists face the challenge of responding to the requirement of improving of India's animal stock and germplasm conservation through cloning of animals.

2.3 Animal nutrition

Livestock productivity cannot be enhanced only by increasing the genetic potential of bovines. It is equally necessary to improve animal nutrition so that livestock can produce milk commensurate to their genetic potential. The dry fodder, green fodder and concentrate production in the country is 394, 462 and 35 million ton, repectively. Judging by the present requirements and availability of fodders, the deficit in terms of dry fodder, green fodder and concentrates is 11.20%, 27.66% and 34.45% which may persist and even aggravate unless adequate measures are undertaken to augment their resources (GOI 2007). Crop residues, such as rice and wheat straw and sorghum stover, represent the largest component of animal feed but tend to be low in nutritive value and cannot on their own support high levels of production.

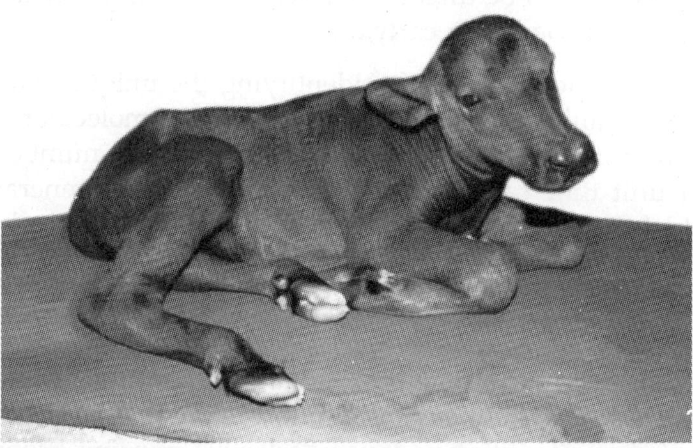

Fig. 1 : Cloned female buffalo calf: Garima (Photo courtesy : NDRI Photography Unit)

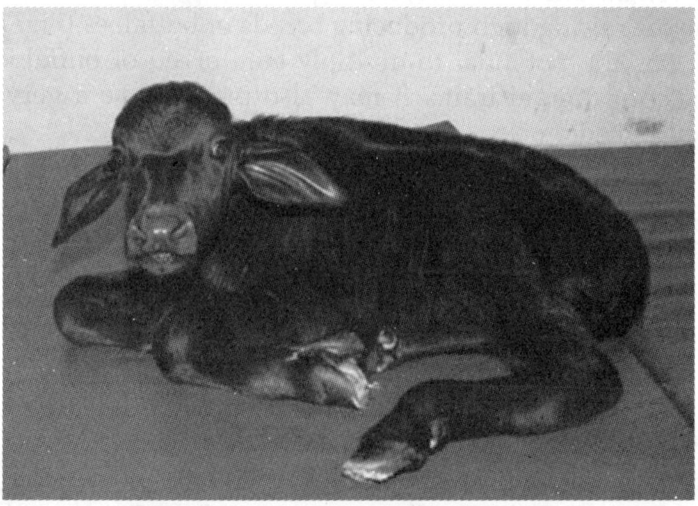

Fig. 2 : Cloned female buffalo calf: Shrestha (Photo courtesy : NDRI Photography Unit)

In order to meet the nutritional requirements of animals, the challenge before the researchers is to increase the bioavailability of the feeds and fodders using chemical, biological and biotechnological approaches. Also, it is necessary to improve the productivity of the land for meeting out the feed and fodder requirements from the limited area available for this purpose. Continuous mining of nutrients from the soil and application of fertilizers in a large scale coupled with lowering groundwater level and reduction in the irrigation capacity has posed constraints in increasing the crop production to feed the rising human population. Against the prevalence of deficiency of one or two nutrients, especially nitrogen in 1960s, today the soil is deficient in more than 15 nutrients, thus, on one hand, limiting the productivity, and on the other, posing nutrient deficiency in the livestock and human consuming the food produced from the deficient soils. The deficiency of nutrients, especially micronutrients, in the feed and fodder along with deficiency in total dry matter availability poses a complex problem for livestock production. A great challenge exists before the researchers and development agencies to address this issue, which is the base line for effective livestock production.

Research and developmental initiatives are required to enrich crop residues. There are a number of biotechnologies which use microorganisms to 'bioprocess' feeds and fodder with a view to improving nutritional quality, including digestibility. Important feed ingredients for dairy cattle can be nutritionally enhanced through genetic manipulation. Specifically, marker-based technologies can be used to understand the genetic diversity in forages and in other crops; the technology also has potential use in field crops in ways that ensure that food yields and qualities are preserved or enhanced while at the same time improving the feed attributes.

Rumen biotechnology has the potential to improve the nutritive value of ruminant feedstuffs that are fibrous, low in nitrogen and of limited nutritional value for other animal species. Methods for improving digestion in ruminants include the use of probiotics, supplementation with chelated minerals, and the transfer of rumen microorganisms from other species. Biotechnology can alter the amount and availability of carbohydrate and protein in plants as well as the rate and extent of fermentation and metabolism of these nutrients in the rumen. The potential applications of biotechnology to rumen microorganisms are many and research is needed in the following areas: isolation and taxonomic identification of strains for inoculation and DNA recombination; isolation and characterization of candidate enzymes; level of production, localization and efficiency of secretion of the recombinant enzyme; stability of the introduced gene; fitness, survival and functional contribution of introduced new strains.

2.4 Livestock health

The health and reproductive disorders, frequent susceptibility to diseases and high embryonic mortality are other potent challenges facing the animal scientists. Stem cell research is one of the latest and most promising areas having immense potential for addressing the health problems facing human as well as livestock species. These cells have the unique capacity of dividing and replenishing the damaged tissues so long as the animal is alive. Each new stem cell after division has the potential to either remain a true stem cell or get converted into a specialized cell. This unique property of these cells to get modified into different functional adult cell types has made them very special and they serve as a potential source of replacement cells to treat numerous diseases. Diseases exhibiting degeneration of tissues are the potential candidates for stem cell based therapies.

Embryonic mortality accounts for a considerable proportion of reproductive disorders. Several autocrine factors, like embryo secretary proteins, and paracrine factors, like prostaglandin, play crucial role in embryonic survival. The role of heat shock proteins (HSP), interferons (IFN-t), and embryo secretary proteins (early pregnancy factor, pregnancy specific protein-B, pregnancy associated glycoprotein, trophoblastic proteins etc.) on embryonic survival has been studied to some extent in normal animals (Thatcher *et al.* 1989, Athanasas *et al.* 1991, Semambo *et al.* 1992, Breukelman *et al.* 2005, Hansen 2007) but it needs to be studied in detail.

Antibiotics are known to reduce the immunity of the animal, especially the mucosal immunity in uterus. Considering the disadvantages of the antibiotics (withdrawal period for milk and meat; antibiotic resistance; cost; organic animal husbandry etc.), alternatives (immunomodulators) have to be evolved. The basic idea is to enhance the animal's immunity, so that it will automatically resist the infection. Several such alternative therapies like *E. coli* lipopolysaccharide, colostral whey, interleukins, neem oil etc. have to be evaluated in case of uterine infection.

3. Dairy Processing

The level of milk processing and value addition is quite low in India. About 35% of the milk produced is retained at producer's level and remaining 65% is traded (CII 2009). The share of organized sector in milk handling is only 16-17%. The majority of milk is traded in unorganized sector and around 50-52% of it is used for the manufacture of traditional dairy products. The changing life styles and dietary pattern indicate that the future demand will be towards the low fat-based products, milk based beverages, fermented milks, convenience mixes, cheese and indigenous dairy products. Food safety which is another major concern across the world has led to Sanitary and

Phytosanitary (SPS) agreements under the ambit of World Trade Organization. It is therefore, necessary that research priorities in the country should concentrate on manufacture of quality milk and milk products and greater value addition for imparting competitive edge to the Indian dairy industry. Only through research initiatives it would be possible to develop novel dairy products, indigenous processing equipments, appropriate packaging systems and rapid and reliable quality control methods.

3.1 Newer functional dairy foods with nutraceuticals

Milk delivers all essential nutrients required for growth and development, and can serve as excellent carrier for certain micronutrients like, calcium, iron, zinc, vitamin A, vitamin D and vitamin B groups. Liquid milk which is the major form of consumption can serve as an ideal medium for fortification or enrichment of such micronutrients. The technology of fortification or enrichment should yield a product that can provide micronutrients in bioavailable forms at cost effective manner. Probiotic dairy products are endowed with wide array of beneficial microbes and bioactive metabolites that assist in maintaining the healthy digestive tract and immune system. Recent research investigations also suggest that probioitic dairy products exhibit various putative pharmacological functions (Iyer *et al.* 2010). However, selection of suitable probiotic microorganisms for specific bioactivity and then its incorporation and delivery in dairy foods is a challenging task. Moreover, success of such novel products depends largely on perceived health benefits by consumers. Hence, validation of claimed therapeutic effects through *in vivo* studies is inevitable to generate confidence of the industry and consumers. In the present era of functional foods, dairy based novel ingredients such as bioactive peptides, lactose derivatives, whey proteins and milk minerals can be an attractive option for food formulators in designing of specialty foods meant for specific target groups. Whey proteins isolated from whey are known to improve body's immune and digestive system. Several research reports have suggested that whey proteins have immunostimulatory and anti-carcinogenic properties (Severin and Wenshui 2009). In addition, many other milk fractions offer tremendous scope for value addition and if scientifically exploited, they can bring enormous commercial returns to the Indian pharmaceutical and dairy industry.

3.2 Convenience dairy foods

Adding convenience to the existing dairy delicacies is another important research challenge for product development. It requires application of existing and emerging processing technologies coupled with innovative packaging of dairy products (Fig. 3). Aseptic processing, ohmic heating, osmotic dehydration, high pressure processing besides the existing conventional processing technologies viz. sterilization, concentration and drying could be attempted effectively for product development with longer shelf life and convenience. Application of these alternative technologies in processing of milk and milk products is in infancy and it requires thorough scientific investigations before becoming a reality at commercial scale.

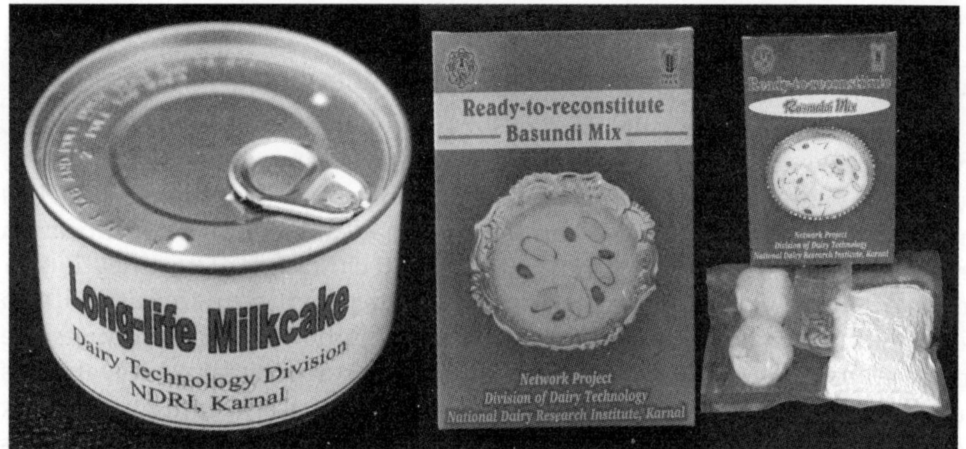

Fig. 3 : Ready-to-eat dairy products (Photo courtesy : NDRI Photography Unit)

3.3 Traditional dairy products

India has a rich tradition of making indigenous dairy products, particularly a large variety of *Channa* and *Khoa* based sweets. Although, several of these products are commercialized by the traditional sweet manufacturers (*halwaies*) and creameries, yet their market is predominantly localised due to short shelf life of products, improper packaging, non-conformity with the consumer safety standards etc. The availability of a few branded indigenous products (buttermilk, sweets) from Amul, Haldiram and others, is extremely limited to selected urban centres. The commercial potential of the vast knowledgebase of recipes of sweets and other milk based products has not been adequately exploited. Many traditional delicacies have not yet been scientifically revalidated and characterized for their commercialization. Also their manufacturing by conventional methods has inherent disadvantages like inefficient use of energy, poor hygiene and sanitation, variable product quality etc. To overcome these inherited problems and to ensure uniform quality of the products, mechanization is urgently required. Some of such machines are already in commercial use in certain dairies (Fig. 4). Mechanized processes have been developed for *khoa* and *khoa*-based products, *chhanna* and *paneer* and such efforts need to be done for other products as well.

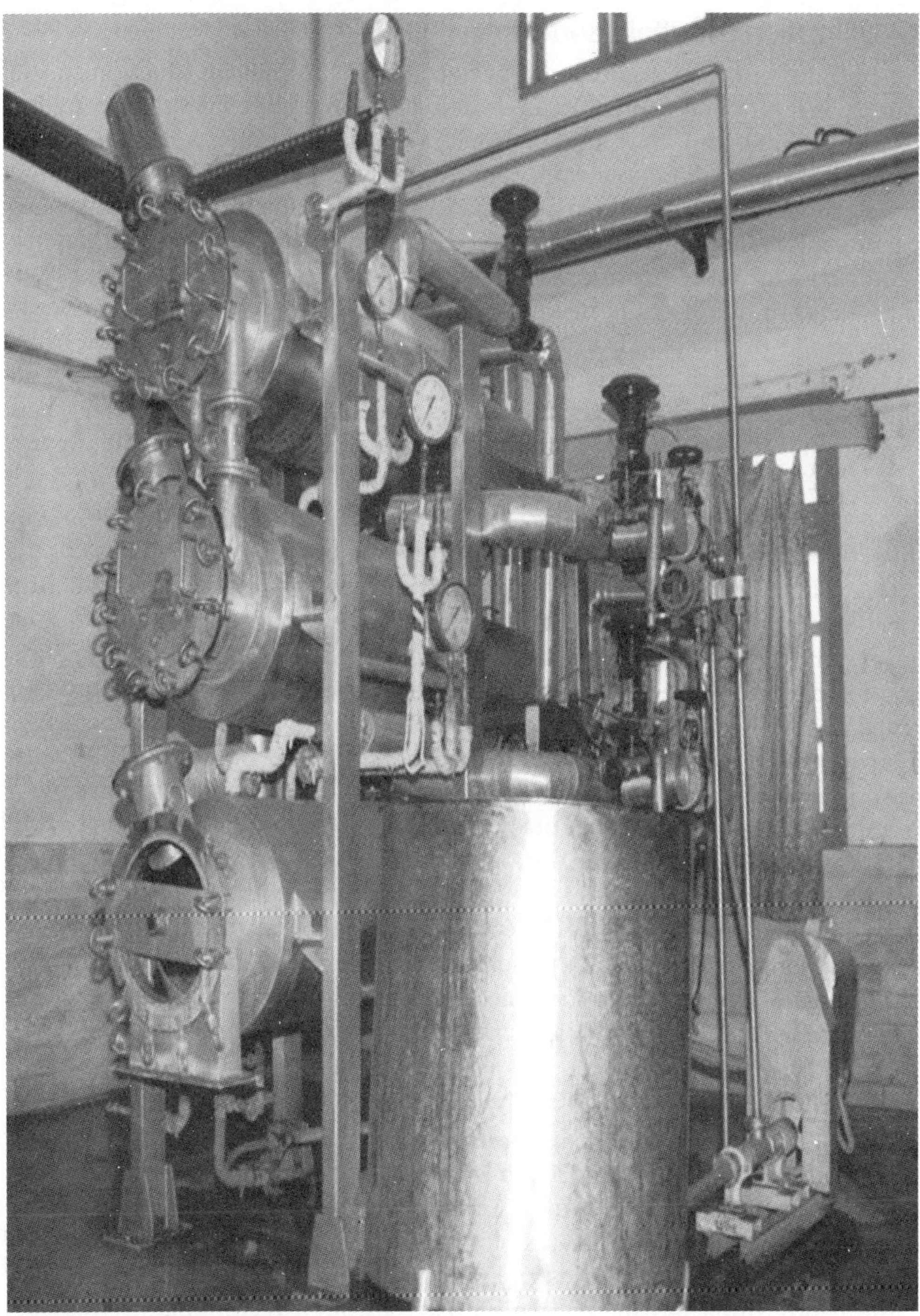

Fig. 4 : Three-stage scraped heat exchanger for continuous manufacturing of *khoa*
(Photo courtesy : NDRI Photography Unit)

3.4 Utilization of buffalo and camel milk

Buffalo milk that accounts for about 55% of the milk production in the country is high in fat content and has many bio-protective factors. It contains 92% higher calcium, 38% higher iron, 117% higher phosphorus and 50% lower cholesterol than cow milk (Pandya and Haenlein 2009). The unique compositional profile of buffalo milk and its superior whitening property makes it more suitable for the production of UHT cream, mozzarella cheese, dairy whiteners and edible casein as compared to cow milk. The comparative advantages of buffalo milk need to be further exploited for developing new value added products. Also, the medicinal values of camel milk have to be exploited at commercial level. It has been reported that camel milk has several pharmacological endogenous substances which act against many diseases and increase the cellular and humoral body defence mechanisms (El Agami *et al.* 1992).

3.5 Packaging and processing technique

Application of novel packaging techniques for improving shelf life, functionality and safety is required as an integral part of research for product development. Development of packaging materials with better functionality, non-toxicity and biodegradability should be prioritized on the basis of product range, marketing and consumer needs. In the area of membrane processing, microfiltration (MF), ultrafiltration (UF), reverse osmosis (RO), and nanofiltration (NF) have emerged as environment-friendly and energy saving technologies for the manufacture of excellent quality dairy products. MF besides being effective in separation of native casein and whey protein and peptides improves the microbiological quality of raw milk that can be utilized for UHT processing. UF technology is mainly employed for protein fractionation, and for the manufacture of cheeses and lactose powder. RO has been effectively applied for concentration of milk for bulk transportation whereas NF is an energy efficient process for demineralization of whey.

3.6 Application of biotechnology

Biotechnology offers great opportunities for value addition through modification of starters, improved enzymes for dairy processing and cost effective bioprocesses for nutraceutical production. It has potential for developing tests for rapid detection of pathogens and food contaminants like antibiotics, heavy metals, industrial pollutants and pesticides. Biotechnology significantly impacted the cheese industry through recombinant chymosin and novel cheese starters that led to enhanced organoleptic quality with substantial reduction in ripening time.

4. Dairy Management

In the changing global scenario, some of the vital issues and challenges that require research attention of subject matter specialists in dairy management include the management of quality of milk and its products, providing economic benefits to the millions of small milk producers, use of information and communication for effective dissemination of dairy technologies, and responding to the market challenges through appropriate policies.

4.1 Quality management

Rising liberalization of agro-industrial markets and the worldwide integration of food supply chains require new approaches and systems for assuring food safety. Food processors and retailers are sourcing their ingredients worldwide and it can be hard to track the region let alone the producer of the ingredient. For these reasons and others, global retailers, distributors, food manufacturers and food service companies are now concerned more about the safety of their food supply chain than ever before. Hence, appropriate risk management strategies need to be put in place to balance the producers' and consumers' concerns about quality of dairy products. In the Indian context, the adulteration of milk poses a serious threat to provisioning of safe dairy products to the consumers. The most commonly encountered adulterants in milk and milk products are salt, sugar, urea, neutralizer, maltodextrin, nitrates, pond water, hydrogen peroxide, formalin, vegetable oils, animal body fat, detergents, soya milk etc. These adulterants are injurious to health and detrimental to dairy business. This malpractice needs to be checked efficiently for which some rapid methods are required. In this context, researchers must put all their efforts to develop rapid diagnostic methods that can check the quality of milk.

4.2 Structural change in value chain

The unprecedented increase in the demand for milk and milk products will present opportunities for poor people, who rear, process or market livestock and livestock products to improve their livelihoods. However, if the soaring demand coupled with increasingly stringent requirements of product quality intensifies the industrialization of livestock sector, the small producers will find it increasingly difficult to compete with the industrial sub-sector and thus, risk losing a significant means of livelihood. Therefore, there is need to enhance the participation of small holder livestock producers in market led growth so that benefits of the market integration in globalised set up can percolate to them. In this context, there is a need to explore alternative institutional arrangements for efficient integration of smallholder producer in the value chain.

4.3 Preparedness for international negotiations

The reductions in distortions in the livestock products trade by developed countries, particularly in case of dairy products, are far from sufficient to provide a level playing field to the developing countries like India in the international markets. The tariff rates in developed countries are much higher as compared to India for almost all the livestock products. The continuance of high tariffs, domestic support and export subsidies by developed nations on the livestock products restricts the product access to their markets and makes very few Indian products internationally competitive. This calls for India to take up the critical issue of negotiating for more liberal trade environment. Currently, the WTO trade talks are at a standstill but, India along with other developing countries must continue to work on the agenda of seeking 'freer trade' for their products in future rounds of the trade talks.

Similarly, sometimes SPS measures are used to shield domestic producers from economic competition. An SPS measure which is not actually required for health reasons can be a very effective protectionist device, and because of its technical complexity, a particularly deceptive and difficult barrier to challenge. In several instances, SPS measures do not appear to be compatible with Codex Standards. For example, the requirement for aflatoxin content in groundnut is set at 15 parts per billion (ppb) by CAC. However, EC has a stricter standard of 4 ppb. Thus, even if Indian standards of 30 ppb are harmonized with CAC standards, EC standards prevent any import of groundnut from countries like India.

Drawing from over a decade of experiences in the implementation of SPS measures, the member countries, particularly the developing nation, should be more prepared to meet the international standards and continuously update their knowledge base. At the same time, they ought to renegotiate for introducing greater transparency in the application of the SPS rules and regulations. In this endeavour, the research support to the policymakers is imperative to understand the welfare impact of alternative policy measures.

4.4 Developing innovative approaches to disseminate technologies

The research efforts of the dairy scientists engaged in the development of production and processing technologies need to be firmly complemented and supplemented by the innovative extension approaches for transferring of the technologies to its end-users. For instance, for health care and breeding technologies, lack of a working institutional arrangement to facilitate their delivery can be a major impediment in the dairy development. The nature of these technologies requires the engagement of a large number of stakeholders, usually necessitating complex partnership arrangements for biosafety and intellectual property management. Consortia or networks of strategic international collaborators (including public research institutions and the private sector) and national partners are almost invariably essential for success. It may provide a platform of shared state-of-the-art research facilities and capacity for application of biosciences in dairy production. This shall also help in a transformation from "technology users" to "technology innovators".

4.5 Understanding and responding to market signals

Globalization of Indian economy warrants that the current Indian market scenario needs to be understood in right perspective to prepare itself to respond to emerging market trends. Furthermore, there is need to provide direction for restructuring the government policies to enhance competitiveness of the milk production and processing sectors through vertical integration in production, processing, value addition, and marketing of dairy products in domestic as well as global markets. The researchers have to work for formulation of macro, meso and micro level policies and programmes to control cost of milk production and processing, facilitate flow of milk to the organised sector, strengthen the legitimate interests of various stakeholders in dairy sector at national and international level.

5. Conclusion

Dairy sector in India faces a number of challenges that need to be appropriately tackled by the dairy scientists so as to capitalize on one of the fastest growing commodity market for milk and milk products. This is also in line of the National Policy on Agriculture which advocates avoiding mono-cropping and taking up animal husbandry as ancillary economic activity. India is a unique country where we have to go for the modern and latest technologies along with the traditional system for the long time to come. Therefore, the research and experimentation efforts to develop the technologies for all levels of livestock sector - production, procurement, processing, manufacturing, should be designed in a way so that the latest technologies are used and the efficiency of the traditional system is also improved.

References

1. Athanasas-Platsis S, Morton H, Dunglison GF, Kaye PL (1991). Antibodies to early pregnancy factor retard embryonic development in mice *in vivo.* J Reprod Fertil 92:443-451.

2. Breukelman SP, Perényi Zs, de Ruigh L, van Wagtendonk-de Leeuw AM, Jonker FH, Vernooij JCM, Beckers JF, van der Weijden GC, Vos, PLAM, Dieleman SJ, Taverne

MAM (2005). Plasma concentrations of bovine pregnancy-associated glycoprotein (bPAG) do not differ during the first 119 days between ongoing pregnancies derived by transfer of in vivo and in vitro produced embryos. Theriogenology 63:1378-1389.

3. CII (2009). Indian Dairying: Challenges and Opportunities. Background Paper. Conference on Indian Dairy Industry, Confederation of Indian Industries, Karnal, 22 October 2009.
4. Dalal SK (2010). National Dairy Plan: Potential Opportunities for entrepreneurs. In: Sirohi Smita and Chauhan AK (Eds.) Dairy entrerenureship development for economic and social change, Winter School Compendium of Lectures, National Dairy Research Institute, Karnal.
5. El-Agamy EI, Ruppanner R, Ismail A (1992). Antibacterial and antiviral activity of camel milk protective proteins. J Dairy Res 59(2): 169-175.
6. FAOSTAT. FAO Statistics Division, Food and Agricultural Organisation, www.fao.org.
7. GOI (2007). Report of the Working Group on Animal Husbandry and Dairying for the Eleventh Five Year Plan (2007-2012). Planning Commission, Government of India.
8. GOI (2009). Basic Animal Husbandry Statistic 2008. Department of Animal Husbandry, Dairying & Fisheries, Ministry of Agriculture, Government of India, New Delhi.
9. GOI (2010). Annual Report 2009-10. Department of Animal Husbandry, Dairying & Fisheries, Ministry of Agriculture, Government of India, New Delhi.
10. Hansen PJ (2007). To be or not to be - Determinants of embryonic survival following heat shock. Theriogenology 68S:S40-S48.
11. Iyer R, Tomar SK, Kapila S, Mani J, Singh R (2010). Probiotic properties of folate producing *Streptococcus thermophilus* strains. Food Research International 43: 103-110.
12. Pandya AJ, Haenlein GFW (2009). Bioactive components in buffalo milk. In: Park YW (ed) Bioactive component in milk and dairy products, Wiley-Blackwell Publishing, Iowa (USA), p. 105-158.
13. Semambo DKN, Eckersall PD, Sasser RG, Ayliffe TR (1992). Pregnancy-specific protein B and progesterone in monitoring viability of the embryo in early pregnancy in the cow after experimental infection with *Actinomyces pyogens*. Theriogenology 37:741-748.
14. Severin S, Wenshui X (2005). Milk Biologically Active Components as nutraceuticals: Review. Critical Rev Food Sci Nutr 45:645-656.
15. Thatcher WW, Macmillan KL, Hansen PJ, Drost M (1989). Concepts for regulation of corpus luteum function by the conceptus and ovarian follicles to improve fertility. Theriogenology 31:149-164.

□□□

Chapter 4

Sheep and Goat Research : Accomplishments and Future Strategies

P. K. ROUT[1], D. SWARUP[1] AND M. C. SHARMA[2]
[1] Central Institute for Research on Goats, Makhdoom, Farah, Mathura-281122
[2] Indian Veterinary Research Institute, Izatnagar-243122

Contents

1. Introduction

Livestock or 'farm animals' play multifaceted role in sustenance and sustainability of human society. Farm animals, mainly consisting of large ruminants like cattle and buffaloes and small ruminants such as sheep and goats, have contributed immensely to the socio-economic and cultural development of human society at least since the time of 'Neolithic Agricultural Revolution' around 10 millennia ago. Besides providing food, fur and fibre to human society, these animals have played crucial role in evolution of crop cultigens and expansion of agriculture system by providing crucial draught power for agricultural works and contributing to maintaining soil fertility. Being the sole source of milk and meat, the farm animals are categorized as 'food producing animals' in western countries. It is estimated that 30% of total protein requirement for human-being is derived from the livestock production system. Further boost in demand of livestock products is expected globally due to sustained economic growth and increase in per capita income.

The nature of livestock production in Indian subcontinent varies with environment and culture and the importance of livestock production goes beyond its food production function. In India, livestock sector contributes significantly to the national GDP. Besides milk and meat, farm animals are an important source of farm draught power, fibre and fur, organic manure, dung as fuel and other by-products such as leather, bone and horn. It is reported that income from livestock production accounts for 15-40 per cent of the total farm household's income in different states, which is expected to increase further with the growing demand of livestock products in the country due to expanding economy and higher population growth. In the year 2020, the demand would reach 147.26 million ton milk, 12.72 million ton mutton and goat meat, 1.15 million ton beef and buffalo meat, 0.81 million ton chicken and 2.58 million ton eggs (Dastagiri 2004). The current situation, therefore, presents a unique opportunity to reduce poverty through livestock production and marketing. However, in the changing socio-economic and agro-climatic conditions, the livestock sector has to expand to meet out the demand of the growing population by adapting to the changes in environment. Being a handy source of income and by virtue of their better adaptability to difficult agro-geo-climatic conditions, small ruminants can be a better choice to meet these challenges. Further, the changing consumption pattern and the increasing needs of livestock products also necessitate the use of new scientific technologies to achieve the goal of increased animal production efficiency.

2. Small Ruminant Sector-Growth and Production Trend

Small ruminants are spread all over the world adapting well to varied geographical regions Their importance for the development of mankind has been recognized since the dawn of civilization dating to Neolithic Period (Hole 1996). It is believed that goat was the first domesticated livestock species to produce edible products for human beings (Foote 2004). Since then, sheep and goat have served mankind by providing nutritional security as well as fibre and skin. Often in many catastrophic situations, these small ruminants have proved to be life saviour for farmers. Goats are particularly very useful and hardy animals and can be productive in the environmental conditions that do not support sheep and cattle rearing (Mason 1984). Currently, there are 830 million goats and 1086 million sheep in the world. The growth of the world mammalian population since 1980 reflected that during the last two decades of the century, goats have witnessed the largest increase in animal number. The distribution of sheep and goat varies between economically developed and developing countries. Sheep is almost equally distributed throughout the world. However, the population of goat is more in the low income countries (LRI) than in the high income countries (HRI) (Morand-Fehr *et al.* 2004). The total milk produced by goat in the world is about 11.91 million ton, whereas sheep produce about 7.11 million ton. However, the meat production trend is reverse as the total meat production from sheep is higher (7119 million ton) than the goat (3695 million ton) (FAO 2007).

During the early part of the 20th century, cattle or sheep farming was more popular than goat farming. Subsequently, cattle and sheep farming gained momentum, while goat farming was not popular and goat stocks fell due to industrialization of agriculture. However, during the second part of the century, the trend reversed and the number of goats around the world increased substantially. The trend of sheep and goat population and production in countries, categorized as low income (LRI) countries, intermediate income (IRI) countries and high income (HRI) countries indicated that 79.6% of goats were available in LRI, 19% in IRI and 1% in HRI countries. The per capita annual income was >$10,000 in HRI countries, between $10,000 and $1000 in IRI countries, and <$1000 in LRI countries (Morand-Fehr *et al.* 2004). The trend of sheep distribution showed that about 40% of sheep were in LRI, 34% in IRI and 27% in HRI countries. Surprisingly, HRI countries with only about 1% of goat population produced about 10% of world's goat milk while the LRI countries with 79.6% goat population contributed only 67% of world's goat milk. On the other hand, LRI countries produced 82% of goat meat and only 2% was produced by HRI countries. Approximately 47% of sheep milk was produced by IRI countries. The three categories of countries had equal share (33% each) of total sheep meat production in the world. Goat farming was primarily popular in LRI whereas sheep farming was evenly distributed over HRI, IRI and LRI countries (Fig. 1).

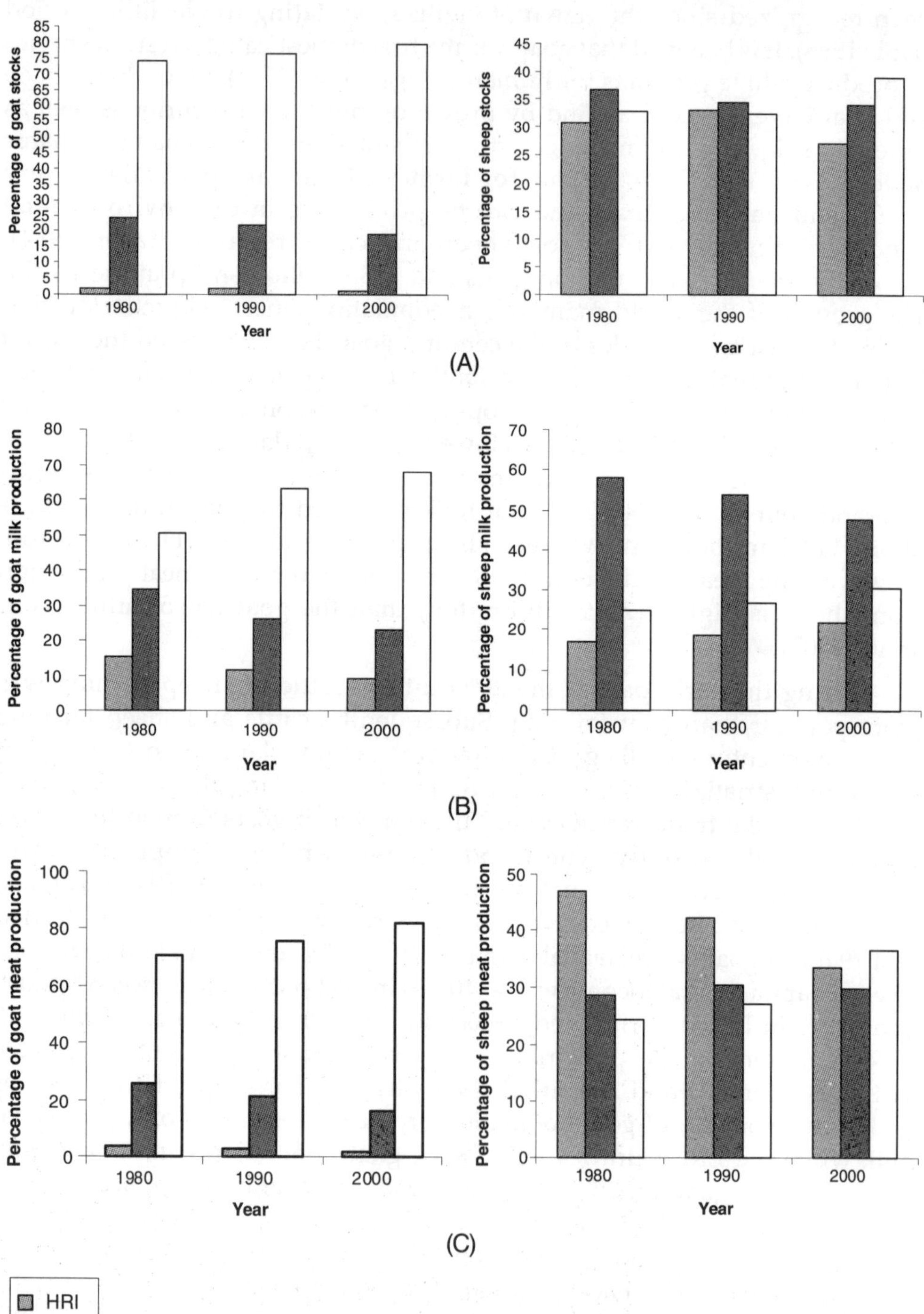

Fig. 1 : Changes in small ruminant stocks (A), milk production (B) and meat production (C) between 1980 and 2000 in countries with different levels of income

In India, goat population increased about 9.12% between the years 1990 and 2000, however, the population growth was slow (1.55% between the years 2000 and 2007) during the last decade. The corresponding increase in the world goat population was about 26.25% during 1990-2000 and 11.45% during 2000-2007 (FAO 2007). The sheep population in India was more than goat population with a growth of about 22.06% during 1990-2000 and 8.11% during 2000-2007. The world's sheep number, contrary to the Indian trend, declined by 12.38% during 1990-2000. However, the last decade (2000-2007) has shown a steady growth rate of 2.56% in sheep population (FAO 2007). In India, the goat population showed an annual growth rate of 1.33 million per annum between 1951 (47.1 million) and 2007 (125.45 million). Similarly, the increase in sheep population was 0.449 million per annum from 1951 (39 million) to 2007 (64.269 million). Goat showed about 166% growth over the base population whereas sheep recorded only 64% growth from the base population (Fig. 2) (FAO 2007 and DAHD 2008). The trend in sheep and goat population over the five year census period indicated negative growth rate in sheep during 1966-1972 and 1982-1987. Goats also showed the lowest growth rate (0.93 million per annum) during the period (Fig. 3). The pattern of growth rate in both the species indicated better resistance of goats to environmental effects and its adaptability to maintain the growth rate in the face of environmental vagaries.

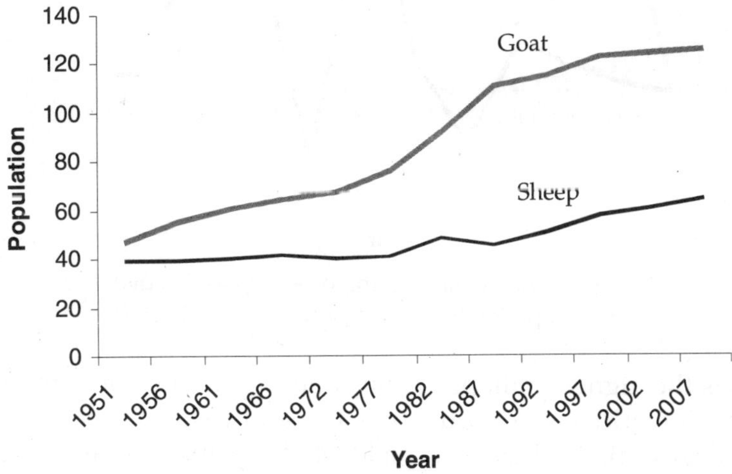

Fig. 2 : Trends in sheep and goat population (in million) in India during 1951-2007

In 2003, India was fifth in the world in respect to meat production with a total production of about 6.3 million ton. The contribution of cattle, buffalo, small ruminants (sheep and goats), pigs and poultry during this period was 31.1%, 30.5%, 14.9%, 10.0% and 13.4%, respectively (DAHD 2004). The number of sheep and goat slaughtered during 2003 was 47 million and 19.2 million, which was about 37.9% and 47.9% of the total population, respectively. Meat production by small ruminant sector over the last 20 years indicated that the rate of goat meat production doubled during 1997-2007 (18.6%) as compared to 9.3% during 1987-1997 (FAO 2007). However, the world goat meat production recorded an increase of about 43.45% during 1997-2007. The sheep meat production in India increased by about 5.38% during 1997-2007 as compared to 46.07% growth during 1987-1997 indicating a considerable decline in the last decade. On the contrary, the world sheep meat production has increased by about 15.7% from 1997 to 2007. In 2003, the share of goat and sheep meat to total meat production in India was 10% and 4.9%, respectively. During the last decade (1997-2007), buffalo (4.68%), pig (5.7%) and poultry (9.56%) meat production also showed an increasing trend in India, but the highest growth (15.7%) was noted in respect to goat meat (FAO 2007), indicating positive shift in goat production profile.

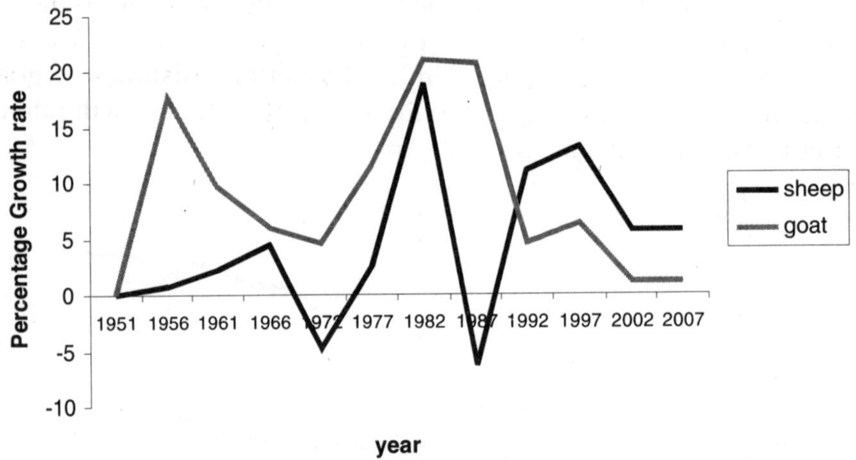

Fig. 3 : Trends in sheep and goat population over the 5 year period from base population 1951-2007

India is the highest milk producing country in the world and contributes nearly 13% of world's milk production. Generally sheep is not raised for milk production in India and as such yield of sheep milk is very less, although there was about 11.09% increase in world sheep milk production during 1997-2007. Interestingly, goat milk production in India has showed growth rate of about 31.53% during 1997-2007, whereas the world goat milk production increased to about 24.76% during this period. The average live weight did not show any significant increase over the years in both sheep and goat in India. The present goat skin production was about 129.96 thousand ton and that of sheep was 57.96 thousand tons. The goat and sheep skin production has increased about 3.14% and 17.19%, respectively during 1997-2007 (FAO 2008, DAHD 2008).

3. Genetic Research

The foundation of animal breeding research was started from the work of Mendel (1865). Principles of population genetics developed by Wright (1921) in guinea pigs were extended further for application to the breeding of farm animals. Lush (1937) developed "Animal Breeding Plans" and his work was later extended to sheep by Hazel (1943). The researchers used the concepts and methods of Lush to develop breeding objectives and effective genetic improvement programme. They estimated heritability and repeatability and developed selection index to carry out genetic improvement programme. Body growth, milk yield, fibre yield, feed conversion efficiency, meat quality traits have been developed by genetic methodology. The genetic research and breeding policies are also aimed at conservation of genetic resources.

3.1 Conservation of small ruminant genetic resource in India

The planned conservation programme of small ruminant in India is largely neglected. The sheep and goat breeds are adapted at high altitude and harsh environment, but no attention has been paid to the valuable traits like fecundity, disease resistance, grazing habit, cheese quality, meat quality and skin characteristics. The sheep and goat breeds should be conserved for those special characteristics in their home tract for future use (Baumung *et al.* 2004). The livestock sector is facing problems due to shortage of grazing land, availability of feed and fodder and loss of habitat. In India, goat breeds like Jamunapari, Surti, Jakhrana and Beetal are decreasing in number in their native tract. Jamunapari population has declined seriously and it is less than 8,500 (Rout *et al.* 2004) in its habitat due to different reasons. Beetal is drawing attention for conservation as the number is declining because of changing agricultural patterns in Punjab. Barbari is facing dilution in breed characteristics due to crossbreeding with Sirohi and Jamunapari breeds in its home tract. Due to decrease in natural browse and geographical restriction Surti and Jakhrana are decreasing in number. More weightage on improvement of some breeds and extensive use of the breeds such as Beetal, Barbari and Jamunapari could eliminate the other distinctive breeds by crossbreeding (Fig. 4 to 7).

Sheep breeds are also facing extinction in their native tract due to similar reasons as goats. Nilgiri and Kilakarsal are decreasing in number due to crossing with other breeds. Jaisalmeri, Pugal, Magra and Chokla are decreasing in number due to extensive use of Marwari breed for up-gradation in their native tract. Sheep breeds in Jammu & Kashmir are decreasing in number due to indiscriminate crossbreeding with exotic fine wool breeds. The other breeds such as Muzaffarnagari, Rampur Bushair, Bonpala, Gurej, Karnah, and Poonchi are decreasing in number due to various reasons in their home tract. Therefore, it is necessary to formulate an action plan for conservation and use of small ruminant genetic resources in our country.

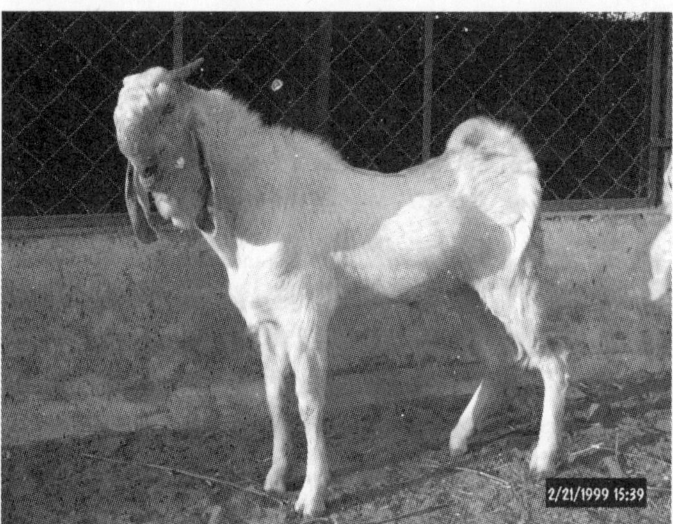

Fig. 4 : Elite Jamunapari buck for breed improvement programme

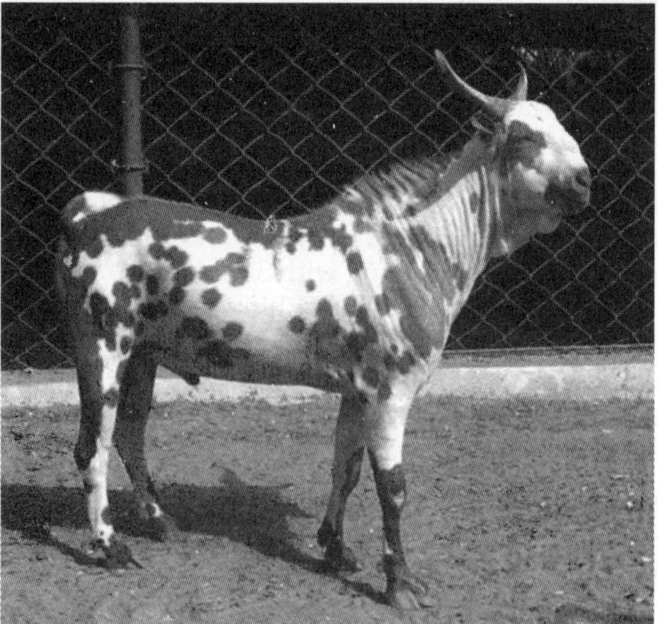

Fig. 5 : Barbari bucks for breed improvement programme

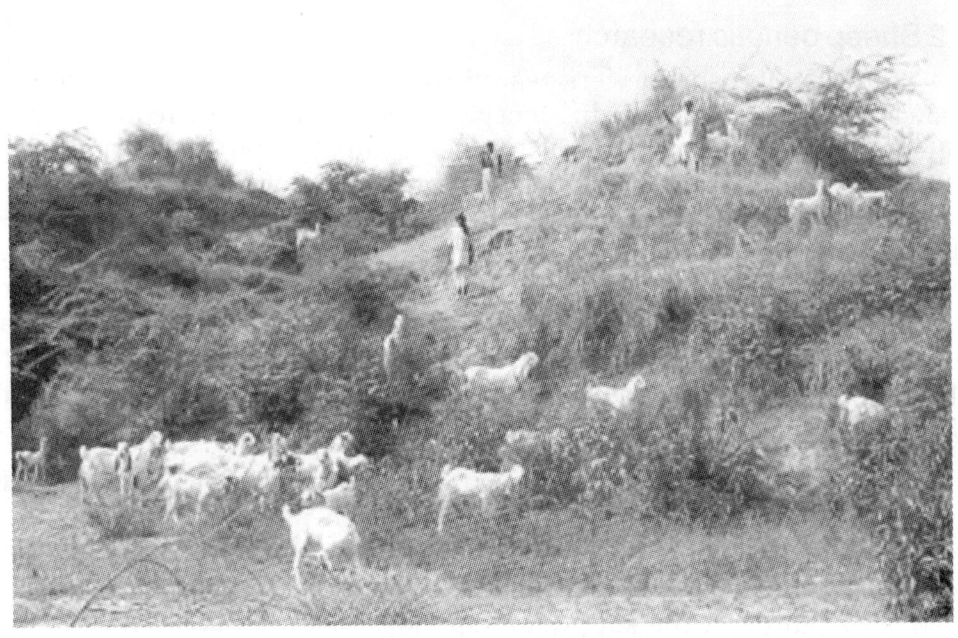

Fig. 6 : Grazing Jamunapari flock

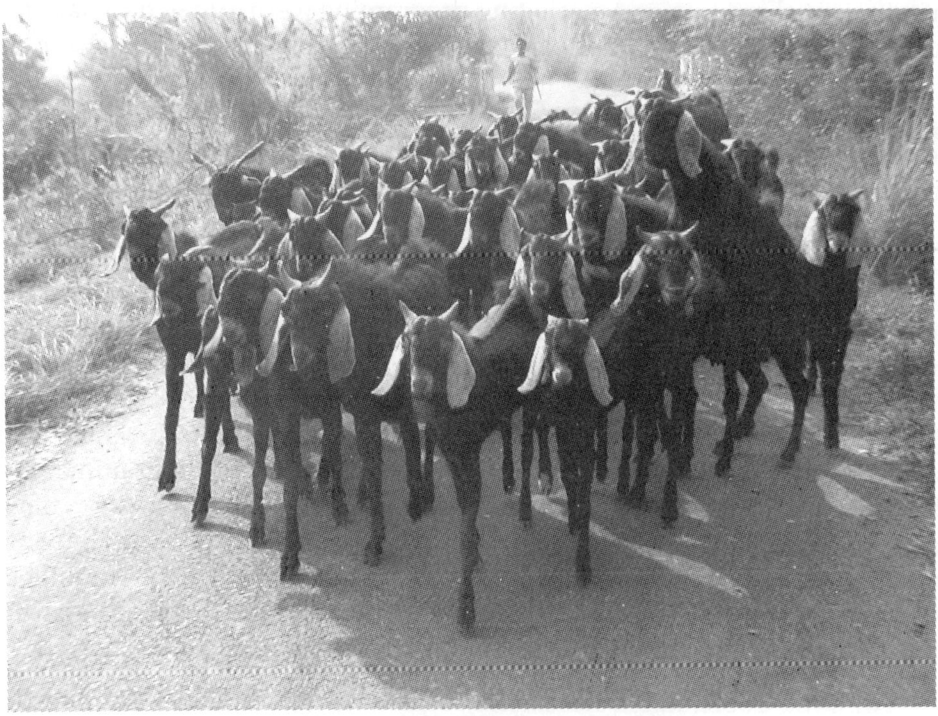

Fig. 7 : A flock of Jakhrana goats

3.2 Sheep genetic research

Traditionally, sheep were reared by farmers with their indigenous knowledge and maintaining different genotypes to fulfill their requirement in different agro-climatic zones. East India Company started crossbreeding during 19th century to improve the wool production of sheep. Cape Merino, exotic fine wool breed, was crossed with local breeds and 4000-5000 crossbred sheep were produced around Pune for superior quality wool production (NCA 1976). Nilgiri, a fine wool breed of sheep was evolved in the Nilgiri Hills of Tamil Nadu. Crossbreeding of indigenous sheep with Romeny Marsh was undertaken both in plains and hilly areas. Hisardale, a fine wool breed with about 75% exotic inheritance, was evolved by crossing of Bikaneri ewes with Merino rams at Government Livestock Farm at Hisar (HAU 1983).

During the first Five Year Plan, regional centres were set up in the hilly areas of Uttar Pradesh, Rajasthan and Deccan plateau where planned crossbreeding trials were undertaken. During the second Five Year Plan, wool extension centres were started in some states to carry out improvement in the field flocks through the supply of superior breeding rams. Wool testing laboratory was set up at each farm to assess the improvement in wool quality. Sheep and wool extension centres were established and a large scale sheep shearing, wool grading and marketing programme were initiated in Rajasthan during the third Plan. There were 84 sheep breeding farms, 602 sheep and wool extension centres and 52 supplementary sheep breeding centres in the country during the fourth Five Year Plan. The Ad-hoc Sheep Breeding Policy Committee suggested importing 20,000 exotic sheep of fine wool breeds to meet the shortage of stud rams in 1970. Indo-Australian sheep breeding farm was set up at Hissar with a foundation stock consisting of 3,000 ewes and 300 rams of Corriedale breed for production and distribution of Corriedale stud rams to different states to improve wool and mutton production. Corriedale did not perform well with respect to reproduction and survival and was replaced with exotic breed Rambouillet. Subsequently, Central sheep Breeding Farms were established in Jammu and Kashmir, Uttar Pradesh, Madhya Pradesh, Bihar, Andhra Pradesh and Karnataka to produce exotic purebred or crossbred rams. Intensive sheep development programmes were also initiated which included genetic upgrading using superior males, providing health care, improving pastures and machine shearing. Improved crossbred Hisardale was evolved by crossing Bikaneri ewes with Merino rams at Hisar. Kashmir Merino was evolved by crossing Gaddi, Bhakarwal, Rampurbushair, Poochhi, Kamah and Gurez with Merino.

All India Coordinated Research Programme (AICRP) on sheep breeding was launched by the ICAR in 1971. Sheep breeding work under AICRP for fine wool was started. The breeds involved were exotic fine-wool breeds, Soviet

Merino and Rambouillet and indigenous breeds, Gaddi, Nali, Chokla, Patanwadi, Nilgiri and Bonpala. The new stains of sheep were named as Avivastra, Nali-synthetic, Chokla-synthetic, Nilgiri-synthetic, Patanwadi-synthetic and Gaddi-synthetic. The details of sheep strains are described in Table 1. Crossbreeding was carried out to improve mutton production with exotic mutton breeds, Dorest and Suffolk. The indigenous breeds were Malpura, Sonadi, Muzzaffarnagari, Nellore, Mandya, Deccani and Madras Red. Avimaas (Mutton Synthetic) lambs attained 25 kg bodyweight at 130 days. Rambouillet was superior to other exotic breeds in crossbreeding experiments. The survival of half-breds was similar to that of indigenous breeds, but crosses containing higher exotic inheritance showed higher mortality. Improvement in fleece quality has been reflected by a decrease in the percentage of medullated fibres and average fibre diameter. Breeds like Bikaneri, Magra

Table 1 : Sheep strains developed in crossbreeding experiment

Genotypes with utility	Parent Breeds		Level of exotic inheritance (%)
	Indigenous	Exotic	
Bharar Merino for fine wool	Chokla, Nali, Malpura, Jaisalmeri	Rambouillet, Russian Merino	75
CSWRI Avikanagar for fine wool	Chokla, Nali	Rambouillet, Russian Merino	50
Nilgiri Synthetic, for apparel wool	Nilgiri	Rambouillet, Soviet Merino	62.5/75
Patanwadi Synthetic for carpet wool	Patanwadi	Rambouillet, Soviet Merino	50
Avikaln for carpet wool	Malpura	Rambouillet,	50
Avimaas for mutton	Malpura, Sonadi	Dorset, Sufolk	50
Indian Karakul for Pelt	Marwari, Malpura, Sonadi	Karakul	75
Kashmir Merino for fine wool	Gaddi, Bhakarwal, Poonchi	Delaine Merino Rambouillet, Soviet Merino	50-75
Hissardale for apparel wool	Bikaneri	Australian Merino	75

and Nali were used as improver breeds in Andhra Pradesh, Karnataka, Tamil Nadu and Uttar Preadesh for improving wool production and quality. This programme was not successful in the southern states as the rams did not survive long and did not adapt to the hot humid climate (Acharya 1982, Jain *et al.* 1998).

At the Central Sheep and Wool Research Institute, Avikanagar (CSWRI), the breeds involved were Rambouillet and three different indigenous breeds Chokla (a superior carpet wool breed), Jaisalmeri (a medium carpet wool breed) and Malpura (an extremely coarse and hairy wool breed). Research has also been undertaken at CSWRI for breeding sheep for pelt and Karakul. Garole, a prolific sheep breed, has been introduced at CSWRI to increase multiple births. The results indicated that twining per cent in Garole x Malpura (G x M) half-breds ewes was 52.24%. It was observed that the bodyweights at different ages of G x M half-breds were on lower side compared to contemporary Malpura lambs. The survivability of G x M sheep was almost equivalent to native Malpura sheep. Presently, the programme has been initiated for survey, evaluation and improvement of indigenous sheep breeds under native environment and different breeds of sheep are being improved through selection for wool and mutton production.

3.3 Goat genetic research

Goat improvement research was initiated by conducting pilot experiments in Haryana, Punjab, Uttar Pradesh and Tamil Nadu. Crossbreeding with exotic breeds like Alpine, Anglo-Nubian and Toggenburg was carried out with Beetal and Jamunapari (NCA 1976). For increasing goat productivity across the agro-climatic zone, a systematic effort was made by the Indian Council of Agriculture Research under the banner of All India Coordinated Research Project (AICRP) on Goat Improvement in 1971. The main objective was to improve the performance of goat for milk, meat and fibre (Pashmina) production in different parts of the country. Both crossbreeding and selective breeding approaches have been undertaken to improve the productive performance of goats.

3.3.1 Crossbreeding programme

Crossbreeding has been started in the country with exotic breeds to increase milk, meat and mohair production. Exotic breeds like Alpine, Saanen have been used for milk production and Angora for Mohair production. Alpine and Toggenberg exotic breeds have been crossed with Sirohi for improving milk and reproduction performance of the local breeds (Groot *et al.* 1992)

3.3.1.1 Milk production

Crossbreeding of Beetal and Malabari with exotic breeds Alpine and Saanen was carried out to increase milk production. Milk production and lactation length improved greatly in both the half-breds. The half-bred were better than 3/4th in both the crosses. Saanen breed showed better performance with both the indigenous breeds than Alpine. Saanen and Malabari cross produced average milk yield of 127.3 kg per lactation with an improvement of 128% over the native Malabari. The Saanen x Beetal crosses with 75% of exotic inheritance were the best, showing 103.4% improvement over purebred Beetal (AICRP 1985). The crosses of Alpine with Beetal and Malabari showed an improvement of 64% and 50% in lactation yields, respectively. However, the improvement in lactation length was relatively small (8 to 29%) in these crosses (Acharya 1992). The crosses of Beetal and Malabari with Alpine and Saanen have marginal differences with respect to age at first kidding, kidding interval and service period. Alpine x Beetal crossbreeds had higher age at first kidding, kidding efficiency and multiple births than Saanen x Beetal crossbreds. Similarly, the Saanen and Beetal crossbreeds also had less kid mortality than Alpine and Beetal crosses (AICRP 1985). However the age at first kidding, kidding efficiency, multiple births and survivability decreased in both the crossbreds as compared to purebreds. Therefore, the gain in production traits in the crossbreds was masked by the deterioration in the reproductive traits and survivability rate (AICRP 1985, Arora 1992).

Crossbreeding for improvement of milk production in Sirohi goat with Alpine and Toggenburg was carried out by Indo-Swiss Goat Production (ISGP; Groot *et al.* 1992). The lactation yield of 180 days was 130.1 kg for Sirohi, whereas, it was 160.3 kg for Alpine x Sirohi cross and 160.9 kg for Toggenburg x Sirohi cross. The differences in milk yield were significant between crossbred and purebreds, however, the observed increase in milk yield was less than expected. Subsequently, it was also observed that selective breeding in purebred was more effective and profitable than crossbreeding (Final Technical report PL-480 Project 1990).

3.3.1.2 Meat production

Jamunapari and Beetal as the improver breeds were used to cross with Black Bengal, Assam local, Sirohi and Sangamneri to improve the meat production. Crossbreeds of Black Bengal with Jamunapari and Beetal were much superior to Black Bengal, however, Beetal x Black Bengal cross performed better than Jamunapari x Black Bengal cross. There was improvement of 51.6% in pre-slaughter bodyweight, 8.7% in hot carcass weight and 17.4% in dressing percentage over purebred Black Bengal. The results of crossing between Beetal x Sirohi and Beetal x Assam local were quite encouraging. Beetal x Sirohi crosses attained about 32 kg of bodyweight at 6 months age under intensive feeding and 26.1 kg in semi-intensive system of management. However, the magnitude of improvement while crossing with Jamunapari was not so encouraging. The crossbreds of Beetal x Black Bengal exhibited 50.3% superiority at 3 months age over local Black Bengal. Beetal x Assam local crosses attainted about 11.5 kg bodyweight at 12 months age which showed an improvement of 31.5% over Assam local at 12 months age (AICRP 1985).

The combining ability of four important indigenous breeds was analysed in PL-480 project at RBS College, Agra involving Jamunapari, Black Bengal, Barbari and Beetal. Indigenous breeds, like Beetal and Jamunapari, were used as improver breeds for increasing both milk and meat production in different parts of the country. Jamunapari x Black Bengal crossbred performed better with respect to meat production while Beetal x Barbari crossbred performed better with respect to milk production. In another experiment at Hissar, the crosses of Beetal were superior to those of Jamunapari indicating Beetal to be better improver breed for enhancing production performance in this region.

3.3.1.3 Mohair production

Indian goat breeds do not produce mohair, however, crossbreeding was carried out in Sangamneri and Gaddi with an exotic goat breed, Angora. The crossbreds with 87.5 exotic inheritance were found to be the best amongst the crosses for mohair production under Indian condition. These crossbreeds produced about half of the mohair produced by purebred Angora contemporaries but with shorter staple length. The mohair yield of $7/8^{th}$ Angora crossbreed was 0.85 ± 0.05 kg in comparison to 1.45 kg yield of the purebred Angora. However, the crosses had higher mortality and the mohair production appeared to be uneconomical (AICRP 1985).

3.3.2 Selective breeding approach

As the indigenous breeds display great variation in relation to adaptability, productivity, feed utilization and disease resistance parameters, it was thought to conserve the uniqueness of the indigenous breeds and traditional characteristics for which they are valued. Selective breeding approach was, therefore, undertaken to improve the performance of indigenous breed in their home tract (CIRG 2007).

3.3.2.1 Milk production

Selective breeding has been practised at CIRG, Makhdoom for increasing the milk production in Jamunapari and Barbari goats since 1985. The average milk yield of Jamunapari goats at 90 days and 140 days was 111.30 ± 1.94 and 157.96 ± 2.66 litre, respectively. The 140 days milk yield has increased from 90.65 litres in 1985 to 148.60 litre indicating 63.38% increase over the years. Similarly in Barbari goats, the milk yield in 90 days and 140 days were 78.82 ± 1.95 and 122.37 ± 4.76 litre, respectively. The milk yield at 90 days has increased from 42.52 litres in base population to 78.82 litre indicating about 85.37% increase over the years in Barbari goats. The genetic parameters for 90 days milk yield, 140 days milk yield, lactational yield and lactation length have been estimated in both the breed.

3.3.2.2 Body growth

Selection for growth is continuing in Barbari and Jamunapari goats at CIRG, Makhdoom since 1985. The average bodyweights of Jamunapari kids at birth and at 3, 6, 9 and 12 months age were 2.96 ± 0.03, 10.52 ± 0.22, 17.24 ± 0.30, 23.34 ± 0.37 and 29.60 ± 0.44 kg, respectively. Feedlot kids attained 33.75 ± 1.01 kg and 41.85 ± 0.81 kg at 9 and 12 months of age, respectively. There was increase in bodyweight at 12 months age from 20.32 kg to 29.60 kg indicating the growth rate of 45.67% in bodyweight at 12 months of age over the years. The average bodyweights of Barbari goats at birth and at 3, 6, 9 and 12 months were 1.85 ± 0.02, 7.88 ± 0.10, 12.41 ± 0.19, 20.59 ± 0.36 and 24.44 ± 0.46 kg, respectively. There was an increase in 12 months bodyweight from 18.52 kg to 24.44 kg indicating increase of 31.96% over the years.

Genetic parameters for bodyweights at different ages have been estimated in both the breed. Breeding values of the bucks were estimated for bodyweight at 9 months age using BLUP method. Genetic, phenotypic and environmental trends for bodyweight have been estimated for both Jamunapari and Barbari goats. The differences between the bodyweights under two systems of feeding are clear indication that both Jamunapari and Barbari goats have lot of genetic potential to be exploited as evidenced from the difference between intensive and semi-intensive system.

3.3.2.3 Fibre production

Indian Pashmina is the finest and lightest natural fibre in the world produced by the Changthangi and Chegu breeds of goat. A sizable population of these breeds was maintained at Indian Veterinary Research Institute (IVRI), Mukteswar. The Pashmina yield varies from 78 g in first clip to 227 g in the third clip. Chegu and Changthangi goats showed an annual Pashmina production of 132 gm and 214 gm, respectively with average fibre diameter of 12.4 μ. Selection based on greasy fibre weight and fibre diameter combined into an index is likely to provide maximum genetic progress in improving Pashmina production (AICRP 1985).

3.4 Molecular genetics

Molecular genetics promises to have a great impact on small ruminant production in future. DNA from the individual organism is unique. The application of molecular tools has been recognized in the field of parentage identification and traceability of animal, genetic disorder screening, genetic disease monitoring, and sex determination. Marker assisted selection and gene introgression have been applied in the livestock selection programme. The practical applications of transgenesis in livestock production have been identified in the areas like enhancing prolificacy and reproductive performance, increased feed utilization and growth rate, improved carcass composition, improved milk production and composition, and increased resistance to disease. The most successful application of molecular genetics in sheep was cloning of Dolly, the first animal to be cloned from an adult somatic cell by using the process of nuclear transfer (Campbell *et al.* 1996). International Sheep Genomics consortium (comprising of partnership with USA, UK, Australia, New Zealand, France and Kenya) in November 2006 released virtual map of the sheep genome by using information from the cow, dog and human genome. Application of genomic information in livestock was the subject of a recent review by Sellner *et al.* (2007). The major achievements from the molecular genetics work are the DNA test for spider lamb syndrome carriers (Cockett *et al.* 1999, Cockett and Beever 2001), Booroola gene (FecB), the major gene for prolificacy identified in sheep (Wilson *et al.* 2001, McNatty *et al.* 2007) and woodlands ($FecX2^{w}$ mutation; Feary *et al.* 2007).

Animal pharming, the process of using transgenic animals to produce human drugs, is becoming more common and goat as an animal has become the most suitable choice. Currently transgenic goats are producing in their milk human protein C and antithrombin-III (AT-III) for the treatment of thrombosis, glutamic acid decarboxylase for the treatment of diabetes and human immunodeficiency virus. The spliced spider genes have been inserted into mammary gland of goats to manufacture silk in milk.

Goat map is very sparse and contains 731 loci with 271 genes and 423 microstaellites (Schibler *et al.* 1998). The last published goat map contains 622 mapped markers with the coverage of whole genome. The less available marker in goat map has become difficult to develop homology between sheep and cattle map (Maddox 2008). The application of gene-assisted selection has been applied to the αs1-casein (CSN1S1) gene in goats. The polymorphism for the αs1-casein in goat has strong effect on protein content, total protein output and other qualitative traits. The quantitative effects of αs1-casein variants on protein content have shown significant difference between the extreme genotypes AA and FF. The Indian goats exhibited αS1-CN (CSN1S1) A allele in higher frequency in all the breeds indicating the higher casein yield in their milk (Rout *et al.* 2010). It has been established that the allelic distributions of the CSN1S1 (αs_1-casein) in the Indian goats were quite different from the European goat breeds. Indian goat breeds are carrying better allelic combination to produce higher protein content in milk. Therefore, the variability at CSN1S1 locus can be utilized for conservation as well as genetic improvement of Indian goat breeds for increasing both quality and quantity of milk production (Kumar *et al.* 2007, Rout *et al.* 2010).

A more complex origin for domestic goats has been proposed by analyzing mitochondrial (mt DNA) HVRI (hyper variable) region in Indian goat breeds from different agro climatic region (Joshi *et al.* 2004). The study showed that there were additional lineages in Indian goats indicating that considerable additional diversity exists within Indian domestic goats. A novel divergent lineage was established in Indian goats. The usefulness of microsatellites for genetic diversity and breed differentiation study in Indian goats was carried out. The phylogenetic tree and the plot for principal component analysis grouped the Indian goats according to their geographic origin and the distances between populations were significantly different from each other (Joshi *et al.* 2004, Rout *et al.* 2008). Microsatellite markers for small ruminant genetic diversity has been studied as it is equally important for conservation decision, breed survival and adaptation to changing environment. Now the molecular genetic technology has showed the application of dense marker maps based on SNP for genetic improvement of various complex traits.

3.5 Genetic resistance to diseases in small ruminants

3.5.1 International scenario

The first indication of genetic variation for disease resistance often comes from the observation that some breeds or populations have the ability to tolerate endemic diseases or to survive an epidemic disease. The source of genetic variation in important diseases in farm animals will give an idea about the nature of variation and inheritance of the trait in the population. The application of breeding for resistance to diseases should consider all the factors in relation to impact on production, control strategy and zoonotic potential.

The susceptibility of sheep to ovine lentivirus infection such as Maedi/visna has long been known to be subject to distinct genetic variation. Scrapie is associated with major gene in sheep. British goats were more susceptible to capripox challenge than north Yemen Black goat. The susceptibility of British sheep breed to bluetongue virus infection revealed that Soya sheep were most susceptible and died before showing any clinical symptoms, whereas Dorset Horn and Merino developed several clinical signs before death. The indigenous sheep and cattle breeds of Kenya were relatively resistant to rift valley fever as compared to exotic animals imported for breed improvement programme.

Bacterial diseases that have been analysed for disease resistance include anthrax, brucellosis, caseous lymphadenitis, enterotoxaemia, pasterulosis, salmonellosis and dermatophilosis in sheep and mycoplasmosis in goat. Genetic variation to many bacterial diseases has been described in studies between small ruminant breeds and within breeds and flocks. Genetic resistance to foot rot in sheep has been well recognised and the heritability of resistance to foot rot has been reported in specifically designed experiment in Merino sheep. Breed differences in the susceptibility to Johne's disease in goat have been reported in different countries.

Genetic variation to parasites has been found both within and between host populations and for a number of important parasite species including nematode worms, coccidia, flies and ticks. Variation in resistance to gastrointestinal nematodes between breeds and within breeds have been reported and reviewed by Kassai and Streter (1992) and by Gray *et al.* (1995). In goats, the resistance to *H. Contortus* has been reported by different researchers (Baker 1998, Chauhan *et al.* 2003). In the case of small ruminants in the tropics this is well illustrated by the resistance and/or tolerance of a number of sheep breeds to gastrointestinal nematode infections including the Red Maasai in East Africa, the Djallonke in West Africa, the St. Croix and Barbados Blackbelly in the Caribbean, the Javanese Thin Tail in Indonesia & the Garole in India. The heritability estimates for resistance to gastrointestinal nematodes (assessed by faecal egg counts) estimated from the relatively susceptible Romney and Merino breeds in New Zealand and Australia. The potential impact of quantitative trait loci (QTL) associated with resistance to helminthes (*Trichostrongylus colubriformis*) infection has been carried out in Merino sheep, Thin tail sheep of Indonesia and Black face sheep of Scotland (Crawford *et al.* 2006, Davies *et al.* 2006, Bishop and Morris 2007).

3.5.2 National scenario

In small ruminants, some reports of breed differences to disease susceptibility from herds maintained by research institute and universities have been reported, however most of the studies are not aimed to assess genetic variation in the breeds. Comparative disease susceptibility to sheep pox, bluetongue, ovine adenovirus, FMD and haemonchosis has been reported. Malpura and Chokla breeds were less susceptible to sheep pox in comparison to Sonadi and Nali. Malpura, Marwari, Sonadi and Nali breeds were less susceptible to bluetongue in comparison to exotic breeds. Nellore, Mutton synthetic breeds of sheep were highly susceptible to FMD, whereas Malpura and Mandya were less susceptible to FMD. Similarly in goats, breed differences in resistance to goat pox, FMD, Johne's disease, colibacilosis have been reported. Results of analysis of data in natural infection revealed that Sirohi was less susceptible to goat pox in comparison to Kutchi and Marwari. Barbari was less susceptible to FMD than Jamunapari and Jakhrana. Jamunapari goats are less susceptible to Johne's disease than Barbari goats. Jamunapari kids were less susceptible to colibacilosis than Barbari kids. Barbari goats were more susceptible to pneumonia than Jamunapari goats under similar system of management.

Genetic resistance to gastrointestinal nematodes (*H. contortus*) in goats has been carried out at CIRG. Indicator traits for resistance to gastrointestinal nematodes have been established in Indian goats. The study showed the variability in resistance pattern in response to natural *H. contortus* infection in selected flocks of Barbari and Jamunapari goats and established genetic correlation with indicator traits and growth parameter. Age related immunity to nematodes (*H. contortus*) does not exist in Indian goats as observed in sheep. Genetic modelling including FEC, PCV and bodyweight at 9 months of age was proposed for getting optimum productivity as well as reduced pasture contamination, thereby fulfilling all the indicators of sustainable livestock production. Increase in parasite infection (particularly *H. contortus*) occurs during pregnant and lactating stages of goat and susceptibility to infection during pregnant and lactating stages varies with respect to breed. Therefore, the management decisions should be taken to get better kid weights and milk yield while the goats are under parasite challenge. Moreover, highly susceptible breeds should not be introduced in humid zones for breed improvement purpose.

Breeding for disease resistance experiment has been mainly conducted in temperate regions. The breeding objective for small ruminants in tropical production systems will be different from those in temperate production systems. The genetic variation among indigenous sheep or goat breeds in the tropics is likely to be larger than that found among the breeds in temperate regions. It is necessary to utilize the breed variation most efficiently to improve the performance of our stock and to check mortality as well as subclinical infection. We have not yet evaluated our genetic resources for genetically based resistance in different agro-climatic zones and production system.

4. Research in Reproduction, Health, Nutrition and Management Aspects

4.1 Reproduction

Reproduction is the major factor affecting profitability in commercial livestock production. It has been tried to optimize the reproductive efficiency by increasing ovulation rate, reducing embryo loss and reducing kid mortality. Artificial insemination (AI) has enormous impact worldwide in dairy cattle but less adopted by farmers in sheep and goat in both developed and developing countries. Vaginal and cervical insemination of ewes has been successful with fresh and diluted semen but not producing reliable result with frozen semen. Subsequently, researchers developed a laparoscopic method of inseminating ewes that generally has much greater rate of success. However, this technique is not routinely used by sheep breeders in the USA and other countries.

In India, a freezing method for *ex-situ* conservation of ram semen has been standardized at CSWRI, Avikanagar. A test for evaluating the fertilizing ability of frozen-thawed semen from individual rams has been developed. A success rate of 36 per cent in the pregnancy with cervical insemination of frozen-thawed semen in sheep has been achieved. A laparoscopic protocol for embryo collection has been perfected. Embryo can be preserved for 565 days in liquid nitrogen.

In goat, a modified freezing protocol has been developed at CIRG, Makhdoom for *ex-situ* conservation of buck semen and the post-thaw motility has been increased significantly. Good quality embryo (16 cell to morula) collections were successfully done through non-surgical (intra-cervical) technique. The conception rate in recipient goats varied from 25 to 40%. Caprine embryos could be successfully frozen by vitrified technique. Cryopreservation of oocyte and embryos showed better survivability than the vitrified oocytes and embryos. The 8-16 cell stage embryo (*in vitro* produced) on transfer at the tip of the uterine horn resulted in pregnancy and birth of kid (Sharma *et al.* 2006, Kharche *et al.* 2008).

Pregnancy detection in sheep by using ultrasound was first reported by Lindahl (1966). This technique has considerable impact by identifying ewes carrying single or multiple lambs for differential nutritional management to individuals by the farmer. Pregnancy diagnosis by ultrasound method has been standardized in goats at CIRG, Makhdoom. Prenatal loss such as loss of embryo within first 18 days of pregnancy affects the flock productivity. The reasons are different and the period is particularly sensitive to poor nutrition, overfeeding, toxins, high temperature and other stresses. Moreover the viability of fertlised egg is known to be breed dependent (Meyer 1985). Most perinatal losses occur within 15 days after parturition. The factors contributing to the losses include malformation, injuries, weak condition, infection, heat and cold exposure.

Breeding soundness of the male (buck/ram) for optimal performance is an important aspect of reproductive success. There are different aspects of thorough breeding soundness examination such as physical examination, and genitalia examination, semen evaluation. Rams/bucks should be tested for brucellosis and other diseases. Mating behaviour can be tested and observed in the field and organized farm. Low performance males should be identified and removed. Reasons for variation in male performance have been identified as genetic, social, and management related problems.

4.2 Health

Successful livestock production depends on maintaining animal health. There are several diseases affecting health and productivity of sheep and goat, however, some important diseases in India include PPR, HS, enterotoxaemia, coccidiosis, *E. coli* infection, Johne's disease and gastrointestinal nematode infection. Sheep flock health management calendar has been developed by CSWRI, Avikanagar and also adopted by farmers for better productivity. A low cost package of health practices has been developed which includes vaccination against PPR, ET, sheep pox, strategic drenching and one dipping for external parasites. A software programme FORGIN which simulates the lifecycle of *Haemonchus contortus* in sheep and on pasture for different agro-climatic conditions has been developed. FORGIN forecasts precisely the magnitude of parasitism 60 days in advance to execute deworming in the flocks. Biological control of worm in sheep by incorporating Chlamydospores fungus in poor quality roughage based complete feed block has been developed.

Similarly, goat health calendar has been developed by CIRG, Makhdoom for prevention of diseases and is being adopted by farmers in field condition. Health practices include vaccination against PPR, ET, HS, FMD, strategic drenching for pre and post-monsoon period and dipping for external parasites. PCR based diagnosis of JD, brucellosis and mycoplasmosis has been developed from clinical material, serum and milk. Several isolates of *Mycobacterium paratuberculosis* subsp. *avium* (MAP) have been characterized in organized and farmers' herd. A comb based dot-ELISA kit test has been developed for diagnosis of brucellosis and Johne's disease in goats. A latest agglutination test for quick and spot diagnosis has been applied to isolate *Mycoplasma capri*. Genetic resistance to different drugs to control internal parasites has been analysed in semi arid tropic. Herbal formulations have been developed and tested for controlling diseases in best possible manner.

4.3 Nutrition research

In order to implement genetic improvement, it is necessary for small ruminant farmers to improve the provision and nutritional contents of the daily feeding ration. Traditionally sheep and goats in India are grazing animals maintaining themselves on what they can find in the field. It is necessary to adopt controlled feeding for greater nutritional efficiency and to enhance individual animal productivity. The advantage of nutritional supplementation has been demonstrated in developing and developed countries (Haenlein and

Devendra 1983, Haenlein 1992, 2001) to improve the small ruminant productivity. The energy and protein requirement of sheep was attempted through feeding trials and extrapolation of cattle data during the period 1908 to 1933. Fraps and Cory published detailed articles on diet selection for sheep and analysed the nutritional values of forages and feeds (Fraps and Cory 1940). The maintenance energy requirement of sheep was published by NRC in 1957 (NRC 1957). Subsequently many experiments were carried out to determine more accurately the protein, energy, mineral and vitamin requirements of sheep in different stages of production. The energy and protein requirements of goats have been described (NRC 2007). The role of mineral and vitamins in sheep and goat nutrition have been less studied in India.

In India, nutrient requirements of sheep during different physiological stages and for mutton and wool production have been worked out. Complete feed and feeding system for maintenance and growth of animal using low grade roughage and agro-industrial by-products have been formulated. Under the prevailing field grazing conditions, a finishing bodyweight of 25 to 28 kg has been achieved in 6 months of age by feeding concentrate supplement at CSWRI, Avikanagar. In native Malpura lambs finishing weight of 33 kg at 6 months age under the challenged feeding conditions has been achieved. The finishing bodyweight of 30 kg at 6 months of marketing age has been achieved in weaned Malpura lambs under intensive feeding. Complete feed block technology with different combination of roughage and concentrate mixture has been developed for scarcity feeding. Nutritive value of blocks was found 33 per cent higher than the conventional feeds. Supplementary feeding schedule for field flock has been developed to optimize production in different physiological stages by CSWRI, Avikanagar. Area specific mineral mixture for semiarid region of Rajasthan has been prepared (CSWRI 2007).

In goats, economic feeding ration for goats has been developed based on tree leaves. Tree leaves based complete feeds in pelleted form have been developed by CIRG, Makhdoom. Milk replacers were developed and tested successfully in pre-weaning Barbari kids. Area specific mineral mixture has been developed for the ruminants. Complete feed pellets with 60% Cajanus straw and 40% concentrate mash were developed and found to be effective in lactating does. Three models of silvi-pasture system were evaluated for maximum biomass production, the sown pasture system consisting of *Cenchrus ciliaris, Cenchrus setigerus, Stylosenthes hamata* and *S. scabra* and tree component consisting of *Dalbergia sisoo, Acacia nilotica, Leucaena leucocephala* and *Azadirachta indica* was found best. *Acacia nilotica* (desi babool) survived well under irrigation with saline water grasses like Napier and Anjan and fodders like barley and oats were found most tolerant under saline water irrigation (CIRG 2007).

4.4 Management

Several management strategies have been developed and adopted by the farmers and industry to enhance the productivity and to decrease the kid mortality caused due to environmental variation and diseases. Practices for keeping pregnant ewes and does indoors, weaning at early age, providing artificial respiration to kids and applying tincture iodine during naval cord separation, feeding colostrum, rearing with different type ration are better practices for increasing profitability to owners. Grazing management is not generally practised in small flocks, however, providing better nutrition during pregnancy and lactating animals for better kid growth is a usual practice in field condition also.

In India, housing requirements in terms of floor space for different age groups and different physiological stages have been determined. Similarly ventilation space in different seasons has been determined for providing a comfortable environment to individuals. A set of 11 feeding and watering devices were developed which are quite suitable for sheep and goat farms. The benefit of predominantly black/dark coat color in desert goats in energy economy has been worked out. The breed variation to sustain water deprivation and its effect on feed utilization has been worked out. It has been discovered that physiologically Sirohi bucks are best suited to combat the thermal stress in semi-arid climate.

5. Research in Products, Product Technology and Marketing

5.1 Meat research

Different studies have evaluated the carcass characteristics, palatability and chemical composition of the meat of different breeds in different production system. Similarly, the effects of sex, age, slaughter weight, diet, feed additives, stress and post slaughter treatment on meat production and quality have been analysed. Generally, intensive system of management has resulted in higher bodyweight and carcass weight compared with the sheep and goats raised on pasture (Ryan *et al.* 2007).

The dressing yield of 50-55% in finisher lambs and 40-45% in spent sheep under varying feeding studies has been achieved at CSWRI, Avikanagar (Karim and Mehta 2007). Meat from growing lambs has been converted into nuggets and salami, which has more acceptability by the consumers.

Live animal traits, carcass and non-carcass components yield, cut-ability, carcass composition, fat partitioning, meat composition of goat carcasses belonging to different breeds and age and the microbial and storage quality of goat meat have been studied at CIRG, Makhdoom. The effect of age, system of management and type of pulse straws on meat production, quality and composition has been studied.

Transportation, isolation, strange environment and animal density increase the pre-slaughter stress in goats as indicated by increase in the plasma cortisol concentration (Kanan *et al.* 2003, 2007). Consumers have become increasingly conscious about the drug residues in meat.

Recipe and processing technique for manufacture of value added products from spent goat meat such as pickle, sausages, cubes, shami kebab, samosa, patties, roll slices, cutlets, croquettes, meat balls, goat meat nimkee and chevonette have been standardized. The quality attributes of products and shelf-life have been evaluated.

5.2 Milk research

The effect of breed, season, parity, stage of lactation and month, time of milking on the major milk constituents and paneer yield has been investigated in goat at CIRG, Makhdoom. Keeping quality of Barbari and Jamunapari goat milk during summer, winter and rainy seasons at room temperature has been studied. Differences in major milk constituents of goat milk produced under farm and field conditions have been studied. Processing technique for preparation of paneer and fermented paneer whey have been developed and standardized. Quality and shelf-life of khoa, shrikhand, direct acid Mozzarella cheese, whey drink, dahi (curd) have been analysed.

5.3 Wool research

Native and crossbred sheep wools can be blended with coarse Indian wool in the ratio of 70:30 and 50:50 for development of value added products. These can be spun on woolen system and approximately 2.50±0.5 nanometer yarns can be prepared. After dying the yarns with natural colours extracted from various plants, the blankets of stripe and check designs can be prepared on handlooms and a standard weight of approximately 2.5 kg can be obtained.

Fibre from rabbits, camels, equines and goats can be blended with wool to produce customer attractive furnishing fabrics for medium to rich users. Low cost camel hair blankets can be prepared (approx. cost Rs. 15/kg) by blending with wool (approx cost Rs. 60/kg) for low and poor income users.

5.4 Marketing

Marketing of the livestock was a neglected area in earlier days and the market value was not dependent on market information. The nature of market varies with the type of livestock. The purchase of large livestock has been arranged through traditional animal fairs organized at particular place during a fixed period of time. However the marketing of small ruminants occurs at door step or on the route of migration (in case of migratory flock). Again marketing of livestock products is different than the sale of live animals. It has been ascertained that there is great potential in sheep and goat rearing provided the production and trade are organized properly. Generally, sheep and goat rearing is associated with small farmers and they do not understand the price trend and do not take advantage of market price. They sell the animal to fulfil their urgent family needs or to pay their loan.

Marketing of sheep and goat in India depends on the socioeconomic condition and religious factors. Male kids are sold at early age of 3-4 months to butchers or middlemen. The sale of male kids at early age depends on several factors such as to maintain the flock size according to farmer's space and feed resource, family need, better price during festive season. Some section of people also raise feed-lot male goat for their slaughter during festive seasons. The trade of sheep and goat in the market is in the hands of few traders/ butchers of nearby cities because they join hands in purchasing of good quality animals from farmers. There are specialized markets for livestock in the periphery but it is not always possible to transport the animals to market place, and again the middlemen also play significant role in fixing the price and selling the animal. The agents operating in the markets bring buyers and sellers together and negotiate the price for which they charge their commission depending on rate and number of animals. Some farmers also directly sell their animals to local butchers. The main marketing of the animals is based on bodyweight and males fetch better price than females. There is no value based marketing in village condition i.e type of animal, meat quality and other attributes.

Market slaughter data concerning sheep and goat reveal that 25 per cent animals slaughtered are below the 6 months age and about 50 per cent are in the age group of 6-12 months. The animals slaughtered before 9 months of age do not exhibit better dressing percentage and better skin quality. If we can adopt better slaughter strategy, we can produce additional amount of meat and large quantity of quality skin without additional inputs.

Wool is sheared at farmer's level and whole wool is put inside bags or bales and sold directly to middlemen from villages. Wool is not sold basing on fibre characteristics, fibre diameter, clean yield and average staple length.

Goats in India produce about 4% of total milk production in the country. There is no specific market for goat milk. The milk is being sold by adding to buffalo or cow milk. The families of goat keepers largely consume goat milk for feeding babies and for serving tea. The market for goat milk, which is considered to have high nutritive and therapeutic value, is yet to be developed. Goat milk has been successfully used for products like ghee, khoa, paneer, cheese and yoghurt. Goat cheese is a delicacy product world over, but has not been used in Indian market. There is a need to popularize goat milk for therapeutic value and cheese for its nutritive value for better income to farmers.

6. Climate Change and Small Ruminants

Livestock production is going to face heat stress, water scarcity, coastal flooding, disease onset and competition for feed with human beings. Therefore, it is necessary to evaluate different genotypes in location specific area for national and global application in future. It is necessary to analyse suitable livestock component for sustainable agriculture and analyze closely the consequence of climate change as it will cause problem to environment, subsequently affecting the animal productivity. Sheep and goat have evolved and adapted to all diverse environments and carry unique combinations of genes that define productive and adaptive capabilities. Sheep and goat have become important due to concern over sustainable development and for the upliftment of rural mass in terms of economic and nutritional stability. Goat has wider genetic base as it is distributed over varied geographical and climatic conditions with differential production capability. Due to wider genetic variability, goats can be manipulated to develop suitable adaptable animal in relation to different ecotypes. The livestock species or breeds will be remunerative if these have diverse gene pool to fit into desired climatic region, and are adaptable, ecologically stable, economically viable and energy efficient in a particular production environment.

7. Future Research Strategies

Small ruminants play an important role in rural based socio-economy development programme. This sector supplements family income and generates employments particularly for small, marginal and landless farmers. Improvement in the village flock by providing support service such as breeding bucks and healthcare should be taken up for nutritional security, providing employment and to alleviate poverty. Small ruminant sector will play a significant role in empowering rural women and will act as a triggering factor in transformation of socio-economic status of rural people. Small ruminant productivity in India varies greatly in all respects in different agro-climatic zones. For enhancing productivity, it is equally important to give greater attention to the biological attributes of indigenous breeds which need to be exploited for local advantage. The productivity of different sheep and goat breeds in different production systems gives a close look to their importance for conservation. So, it is necessary to characterize and evaluate the performance of different breeds in different production systems. We also have to develop strategy to maintain productivity of goats and sheep with reference to geographic shift of production system from temperate and dry areas to warmer, more humid and disease prone environment. We must give a close look to evaluate sheep and goat breeds as the best known gene pool for future global application for their greater use and conservation, their special characteristics should be noted and genetic origin of breeds should be established. It is necessary to identify the most diverse and distinctive population by analyzing genome and population diversity at various level in both descriptive and non-descriptive animals. Evaluation of the economic value of sheep and goat genetic resource by analyzing economics and demographic data (performance, management, product marketing) with respect to genetic distinctiveness should be carried out.

Our indigenous sheep and goat population has not been characterised and evaluated for genetic disease-resistance in natural population. Therefore, we must evaluate our stocks for the disease resistance parameter with respect to geographic, climatic and production system. Parasitic characterization of field condition as well as host response in kids upto one year age and in different physiological conditions should be carried out. Development of resistant line to parasitic nematode infection should be initiated in sheep breeds. Genetic selection for resistance to diseases should be analysed in goat in specific ecological conditions.

Moreover, adaptability to different kinds of stress, water requirement with respect to environmental condition and the endurance in desert and cold region should be analysed at molecular level. Molecular characterization with respect to DNA marker, epigenetic analysis and the role of different RNA in expression of these traits in different environmental condition should be carried out.

There is scope for improving sheep for mutton and carpet wool production in all parts of the country while fine wool production can be carried out in limited areas. The main thrust should be given to popularize dual purpose sheep breeds in collaboration with the state animal husbandry departments. Ram performance test is being used in the USA and other countries to evaluate the male. Ram performance test uses cutting-edge technology to evaluate residual feed intake as a measure of feed efficiency and to include the measures as an important part of selection Index. The techniques like near-infrared reflectance spectroscopic techniques have been developed to estimate the diet composition of free-ranging livestock by using faecal analysis. With this knowledge, deficiencies can be calculated as supplementation can be accurately tailored to meet the needs of the animal. Characterization of factors influencing and establishing simple means for predicting the grazing activity energy cost (GAEC) should be established. The intensive sheep and goat rearing system should be standardized with locally available feed resources. Appropriate management practices for intensive goat rearing are needed by providing economic feed stuff, adequate health management and maintaining product quality. Organic meat production will also be the system of choice for future to fulfil the consumer demand.

The major problem in small ruminant is kid mortality and we need to manage the stock upto 6 months age for getting optimum productivity and commercial viability. We need to address the problems like *E. coli* infection and coccidiosis to reduce the mortality and also getting better production in future life. Genetic epidemiological modeling should be established by developing simple producer-oriented model into which weather, animal, and pasture conditions could be considered to predict level of pasture infection and infection level in animals. This will solve the problem of disease control as well as the research required to handle the problem. As we are facing the problem of anthelmintic resistance, alternative approaches i.e. herbal formulations should be developed extensively. Development of vaccines and diagnostics needs to standardised for the effective control of disease in farmer's flock. Mechanisms of immune responses to internal parasites are not fully understood, and work is needed to demonstrate how the host reacts to parasite infection and whether parasites manipulate immune outcome of the host. Testing and screening for scrapie and other genetic abnormalities are carried out in the other part of the globe but not carried out in our country.

Transgenic research in sheep should be strengthened for enhancing prolificacy, reproductive efficiency, and for increasing disease resistance through various approaches. Embryo technology, particularly, juvenile *in vitro* embryo transfer technology (J/VET) should be explored for rapid multiplication of elite animals. Conservation of genetic material through cryopreservation of semen is essential for maintaining and future use of indigenous sheep breeds. It is necessary to establish a reference semen laboratory with all types of facilities and certification for future demand.

With the globalization of economy and regime of free trade for animal produce and products under the World Trade Organization, the scenario of animal genetic resource is likely to change by 2025. Sheep population may show decreasing trend and sheep would register a decline due to change in farming system. Goat population will be able to maintain its growth in the changing scenario. There is need to integrate meat quality component into breeding and genetic selection as well as nutrition and management studies. Developing a method to select animals for increased muscle mass is necessary for faster genetic progress on muscling attributes. It is necessary to analyse the effect of breed, diet, and geographical region on palatability, flavour, and tenderness attribute of meat and cheese quality and fatty acid composition of milk for evolving better quality goat for meat and milk. Developing a method to select live animals for increased muscle mass is necessary to form selection indices for faster genetic progress on muscling attributes. The application of genomics and proteomics in understanding the molecular basis of goat milk cheese, bioactive peptides and other neutraceuticals and therapeutic aspect should be explored. For the development of meat goat industry, performance testing and genetic evaluation will be necessary for the industry to make progress. For goats, assisted reproductive technologies are necessary for multiplication of elite animals for field application.

Besides better feeding, breeding and management of animals, animal welfare measures should be well managed during transportation of animals, kept in confinement or used for show purpose. Most importantly painless humane slaughter should be done in the slaughterhouse and the abattoir standards should be improved and efforts should be made to reduce unnecessary pain and suffering to the animals.

References

1. Acharya RM (1982). Sheep and goat breeds of India. FAO Animal Production and Health Paper 30, FAO of United Nations, Rome, Italy.

2. Acharya RM (1992). Goat genetic resources and their management. Research in Goats-Indian Experiences. p. 28-38. Central Institute for Research on Goats Makhdoom, Farah, Mathura, India.

3. AICRP (1985). All-India Coordinated Research Project on Goats. Terminal Report, Central Institute for Research on goats Makhdoom, Mathura, India.

4. Arora CL (1992). Organized goat breeding strategies. Research in Goats - Indian Experiences. Central Institute for Research on Goats Makhdoom, Farah, Mathura, India, p. 28-38.

5. Baker RL (1998). A review of genetic resistance to gastrointestinal nematode parasites in sheep and goats in the tropics and evidence for resistance in some sheep and goat breeds in sub humid coastal Kenya. AGRI 24:15-30.

6. Baumung R, Simianer H, Hoffmann I (2004). Genetic diversity studies in farm animals- A survey. J Anim Breed Genet 121:361-373.

7. Bishop SC, Morris CA (2007). Genetics of disease resistance in sheep and goats. Small Rumin Res 70:48-59.

8. Campbell KH, McWhir J, Ritchie V, Wilmut I (1996). Sheep cloned by nuclear transfer from a cultured cell line. Nature 380:64-66.

9. Chauhan KK, Rout PK, Singh PK, Mandal A, Singh SK, Roy R (2003). Genetic resistance of Barbari and Jamunapri kids to natural infection with gastrointestinal nematodes. Tropical Animal Health Prod 35 (5): 397-408.

10. CIRG (2007). Vision 2025. CIRG, Makhdoom, Mathura, India.

11. Cockett N, Beever J (2001). Screening for the molecular defect causing spider lamb syndrome in sheep. US Patent No. 6, 306, 591 BI.

12. Cockett NE, Shay TL, Beever JE, Nielsen D *et al.* (1999). Localization of the locus causing spider lamb syndrome to the distal end of ovine chromosome 6. Mamm Genome 10:35-38.

13. Crawford AM, Paterson KA, Dodds KG *et al.* (2006). Discovery of quantitative trait loci for resistance to parasitic nematode infection in sheep: 1. Analysis of outcross pedigrees BMC Genomics 7:178.

14. CSWRI (2007). Vision 2025. CSWRI, Avikanagar, India.

15. DAHD (2004). http://dahd.nic.in

16. DAHD (2008). http://dahd.nic.in

17. Dastagiri MB (2004). Policy Paper 21 Demand and Supply Projections for Livestock Products in India. National Centre for Agricultural Economics and Policy Research (ICAR), New Delhi, India.

18. Davies G, Stear MJ, Benothman M, Abuagob O, Kerr A, Mitchell S, Bishop SC (2006). Quantitative trait loci associated with parasitic infection in Scottish blackface sheep. Heredity 96 (3):252-258.

19. FAO (2007). FAOSTAT. http://faostat.fao.org

20. FAO (2008). FAOSTAT. http://faostat.fao.org

21. Feary ES, Juengel JL, Smith P, French MC *et al.* (2007). Patterns of expression of messenger RNAs encoding GDF9, BMP15, TGEBR1, BMPR1B, and BMPR2 during follicular development and characterization of ovarian follicular populations in ewes carrying the Woodlands Fec X2^{w} mutation. Biol Reprod 77:990-998.

22. Final Technical Report Pl-480 Research Project (1990). Studies on the combining ability of desirable characters of important goats breeds', RBS College Agra.

23. Foote WC (2004). History and accomplishments of the international goat association during the last 20 years Small Ruminant Research 51:115-121.

24. Fraps GS, Cory VL (1940). Composition and utilization of range vegetation of Sutton and Edwards counties. Bull 232. Texas Agric. Exp. Sta., College Station.

25. Gray GD, Woolaston R, Eaton BT (1995). Breeding for resistance to infectious diseases of small ruminants. ACIAR Monograph No. 34, Canberra, Australia.

26. Groot B, De Narayan, Somi RA *et al.* (1992). Performance of Sirohi goats under village conditions in Rajasthan, India. V International Conference on goats, 2-8 March, 1992, New Delhi, p. 534-544.

27. Haenlein GFW (1992). Advances in the nutrition of macro- and micro-elements in goats. In: Lokeshwar, RR (Eds.), Proceedings of the Fifth International conference on Goats, New Delhi, India, march 2-8, 1992, B.L. Kansal Pub., New Delhi, India, p. 933-950.

28. Haenlein GFW (2001). Past, present, and future perspectives of small ruminant research. J Dairy Sci 84:2097-2115.

29. Haenlein GFW, Devendra C (1983). Appropriate nutrition for goat production in the tropics, In: Proceedings of the Joint IFS/ILCA Conference on Small Ruminant Research in the tropics, Addis Ababa, Ethiopia, October, IFS Province Report No. 14, p. 79-109.

30. HAU (1983). Final Technical report of the Project-Evaluation of Genetic Potential of some Indigenous Breeds of Goats. Haryana Agricultural University, Hissar, India.

31. Hazel LN (1943). The genetic basis for constructing selection index. Genetics 28: 476-490.

32. Hole F (1996). The context of caprine domestication in the Zagros region. In: Harris, D.P. (Ed.), The origins and Spread of Agriculture. UCL Press Limited, University College, London, UK, 594 pp.

33. Jain A, Gupta SC, Nivsarkar AE (1998). Sheep and goat breeding research in India. Indian J Animal Sci 68:720-727.

34. Joshi MB, Rout PK, Mandal A, Thangaraj K, Singh L (2004). Phylogeography and origin of Indian domestic goats. Molecular Biology and Evolution 21 (3):454-462.

35. Kannan G, Jenkins AK, Eega KR *et al.* (2007). Preslaughter spray-washing effects on physiological stress responses and skin and carcass microbial counts in goats. Small Rumin Res 67:14-19.

36. Kannan G, Kouakou B, Terrill TH, Gelaye S (2003). Endocrine, blood metabolite, and meat quality changes in goatsas influenced by short-term, preslaughter stress. J Anim Sci 81:1499-1507.

37. Karim SA, Mehta BS (2007). Carcass traits in Bharat Merino male and female lambs maintained on grazing with concentrate supplementation. Indian J Anim Sci 77: 187-190.

38. Kassai T, Streeter T (1992). Genetic aspects of the host resistance to helminthic infection. Res Rev Parasit 53:67-74.

39. Kharche SD, Goel AK, Jindal SK and Sinha NK. (2008). Birth of a female kid from *in vitro* matured and fertilized goat oocytes. Indian J Anim Sci 78:680-685.

40. Kumar A, Rout PK, Mandal A, Roy R (2007). Identification of the CSN1S1 allele by PCR-RFLP method in Indian goats. Animal 8:1099-1104.

41. Lindahl II (1996). Detection of pregnancy in sheep by means of ultrasound. Nature 212:642-643.

42. Lush JL (1937). Animal Breeding Plans, 1st ed. Collegiate Press, Ames, IA.

43. Maddox JF (2008). Australian sheep gene mapping web site. http://rubens.its.unimelb.edu.au/~jillm/jill.htm

44. Mason IL. (Ed.), (1984). Evolution of domesticated Animals.Longman, London, UK, 452 pp.

45. McNatty KP, Hudson NL, Whiting L *et al.* (2007). The effects of immunizing sheep with different BMP15 or GDF9 peptide sequences on ovarian follicular activity and ovulation rate. Biol Reprod 76:552-560.

46. Mendel G (1985). Experiments in plant hybridization (English translation). http://www.mendelweb.org/mendel.html.

47. Meyer HH (1985). Breed differences in ovulation rate and uterine efficiency and their contribution to fecundity. In: Land RB, Robinson DW (eds) Genetics and Reproduction in Sheep. Butterworths, London, UK, p. 185-191.

48. Morand-Fehr P, Boutonnet JP, Devendra C *et al.* (2004). Strategy for goat Farming in the 21st Century. Small Rumin Res 51:175-183.

49. NCA (1976). National Commission on Agriculture, Government of India, New Delhi.

50. NRC (1957). Nutrient Requirements of Domestic Animals No. 5. Natl Acad Sci, Washington, DC.

51. NRC (2007). Nutrient Requirements of Small Ruminants. Sheep Goats, Cervids, and New World Camelids, Natl. Acad. Press, Washington, DC.

52. Rout PK, Joshi MB, Mandal A *et al.* (2008). Microsatellite-based phylogeny of Indian domestic goats. BMC Genetics 9:11.

53. Rout PK, Kumar A, Mandal A *et al.* (2010). Characterization of casein gene complex and genetic diversity analysis in Indian goats. Animal Biotech 21 (2):122-134.

54. Rout PK, Singh MK, Roy R, Sharma N, Haenlein GFW (2004). Jamunapari-a diary goat breed in India, Dairy Goat Journal (USA) 82 (3):37-39.

55. Ryan SM, Unruh JA, Corrigan ME *et al.* (2007). Effects of concentrate level on carcass traits of Boer crossbred goat. Small Rumin Res 73:67-76.

56. Schibler L, Vaiman D, Oustry A, Giraud-Delville C, Cribiu EP (1998). Comparative gene mapping: A fine-scale survey of chromosome rearrangements between ruminants and humans. Genome Res 1998 (8):901-915.

57. Sellner EM, Kim JW, McClure MC *et al.* (2007). Applications of genomic information in livestock. J Anim Sci 85:3148-3158.

58. Sharma GT, Kharche SD, Majumdar AC (2006). Vitrification of in-vitro matured goat oocytes and its effect on in-vitro fertilization. Small Rumin Res 64 (1-2):82-86.

59. Wilson TX, Wu Y, Juengelel JL *et al.* (2001). Highly prolific Booroola sheep have a mutation in the intracellular kinase domain of bone morphogenetic protein IB receptor (ALK-6) that is expressed in both oocytes and granulose cells. Biol Reprod 64:1225-1235.

60. Wright S1 (1921). Systems of mating I. The biometric relations between parent and offspring. Genetics 6:111-123.

□□□

Chapter 5

Action Plan for Capacity Building of Meat Sector

N. KONDAIAH
National Research Centre on Meat, Chengicherla, Hyderabad-500092

Contents

1. Introduction

Meat production is important because of the sustaining role of meat animals in providing livelihood, food and nutrition security to a large number of people involved in livestock production and utilization activities. Increased emphasis on animal production activities has been suggested to insulate the farmers from the miseries of crop production. Sustainable livestock production largely depends on production efficiency, feed supplies and costs and efficient utilization of the produce including marketing. Thus, pragmatic approaches for increased and efficient livestock production, processing and utilization have become more important for sustaining livestock production activities, particularly in the competitive environment of trade liberalization brought out by the WTO regime. Growth in demand for the product is an important criterion to sustain production which is generated by successful marketing. The essential principles of successful marketing are: good presentation and attractive appearance; diverse products suitable to taste and demand; competitive price per unit weight; quality assurance; reliable servicing; ethical aspects and effective advertising. Clean meat production, processing and utilization including marketing contribute for sustaining the role of meat animals in the society. The present meat production and utilization in the existing slaughterhouses in the country is largely unorganized with lack of basic facilities that compromise with the food safety, animal welfare and environmental aspects. Many consider it an undesirable activity due to the unsightly nature of the premises and unsanitary conditions. Improvement and modernization of abattoirs and meat plants, therefore, is important for development of meat sector in the country and for societal interest at large. Modernization of abattoirs and meat plants is also essential for fulfilling the constitutional obligations under Article 47 i.e. duty of the State to raise the level of nutrition and the standards of living and to improve public health.

2. Need for Development of Organized Meat Sector

The present meat sector is largely unorganized with respect to meat animal production, processing and utilization. As a result, it is neither efficient to fulfill the interests of stakeholders (producers, processors and consumers) nor providing a good public image as a contributor to the national economy. Thus there is need to improve its various facets to develop organized meat sector in the country. The characteristics of organized meat industry include:

- Sustainable production with efficient processing and marketing
- Protection of farmers' interests

- Protection of consumers' interests
- Fitting into national goals
- Ability to provide livelihood to many
- Less depletion of natural resources
- Socially more acceptable
- Ability to withstand competing situations
- Efficient utilization of meat and by-products
- Cost efficient and environment friendly effluent treatment and positive public image
- Provision to deal with surplus situation and ensure reasonable returns

The problem of improving the slaughterhouses and slaughter practices was realized as early as 1930 in the country. Over the years, slaughter facilities have deteriorated due to increase in the animal population and slaughter without corresponding increase in the number of authorized slaughterhouses and improvement of the existing ones. Slaughter takes place both in authorized premises (2702) and unauthorized places (more than 12000) and meat inspection is largely not feasible. Floor slaughter is practiced for large animals resulting in poor hygiene. Overcrowded slaughter in unaesthetic premises is commonly observed. Slaughterhouses are regulated by the local bodies which have been criticized for lack of interest for development. Sourcing of meat for export from domestic slaughterhouses has further compounded the hygiene problems. Developmental programmes for improvement of slaughterhouses and introduction of meat inspection practices have been initiated by the Government of India since 1950. Schemes for improvement of slaughterhouses were also initiated in the third Five Year Plan, however, the progress has not been satisfactory due to a number of constraints that are listed below.

- Difficulty in finding suitable location due to local resistance and vested interests
- Low priority given by the local bodies for investment in slaughterhouses
- Higher level of investments and inadequate funds
- Non-availability of consultants, equipments and machinery with in the country
- Resistance to increase in the slaughter fees

- Demand for quick slaughter by individual butchers and unwillingness for orderly line operations
- Continuing consumer willingness to buy meat from unauthorized slaughter places
- Lack of effective monitoring of abattoirs by the local bodies

3. Present Indian Perspective

Meat animals comprise sheep, goat, poultry (chicken and ducks), pigs, buffaloes, cattle and rabbits. India produces about 6322150 ton of meat annually comprising of buffalo meat 1500000 ton, beef (cattle) 1282350 ton, chicken 2200000 ton, duck meat 72800 ton, goat meat 527000 ton, sheep meat 243000 ton and pig meat 497000 ton (Table 1). Carcass yields are relatively low and need to be improved with appropriate feeding and slaughter practices to achieve better productivity. Indian meat production forms 2.21% of the world's total meat production and per capita meat consumption is about 5.2 kg per year compared to the world average of 39.8 kg. The annual meat consumption in the developed countries is 80.3 kg per person while it is 28.9 kg in the developing countries. Meat group contributed Rs.40399 crores (16.79%) to the total value of output from livestock sector at Rs. 240601 crores at current prices during 2007-08 (Table 2). The value of total exports from livestock products during 2006-07 was Rs. 5129.27 crores of which buffalo meat was of Rs. 3550 crores (69.7%) at 0.48 million ton. However, during 2009-10, the exports from meat and meat products increased by 60% to Rs. 6651 crores with the total livestock products rising to Rs. 7200 crores, recording an increase of 40.38% (Table 3). The rise was primarily due to increase in buffalo meat that suggests the necessity of backward linkages to produce quality buffalo meat to sustain the growth in meat exports.

3.1 Meat consumption among weaker sections

A large proportion of the weaker section communities comprise of non-vegetarians who prefer consuming meat and edible by-products. Meat consumption is important among the weaker sections to balance their marginal diets for better nutrition and health. Tribals are largely non-vegetarians and meat animals and meat contribute significantly to the nutrition of tribal and hill area people too.

Table 1 : Livestock population, slaughter rate and meat production - year 2008

Species	Population (million)	Contribution in world's total population (%)	Slaughtered (million)	Meat production (million ton)	Contribution in world's total meat production (%)
Buffaloes	98.70	48.77	10.86	1.50	46.88
Cattle	177.84	12.80	12.45	1.28	2.07
Sheep	64.27	5.78	19.54	0.24	2.70
Goat	125.46	14.76	54.30	0.53	10.30
Pigs	14.00	1.41	14.20	0.50	0.43
Chicken	505.00	2.93	2444	2.20	2.96
Ducks	35.00	3.27	56.00	0.07	1.77
Meat total	-	-	-	6.32	2.21

Source: FAOSTAT database 2008. www.faostat.fao.org

Table 2 : Contribution of livestock products to the value of output from livestock sector (at current prices)

Item	1990-91	2007-08	Increase (%)
Milk group	27508	162136	489.41
Meat group	7208	40399	460.46
-Beef and buffalo	686	3799	453.79
-Sheep and goat	2566	12920	403.51
-Pork	489	2694	450.92
Poultry meat	2528	14813	485.96
Meat products	243	1632	571.60
By-products	696	4541	552.44
-Hides	370	1625	339.19
-Skins	306	1652	439.87
-Other by-products	120	1264	953.33
Eggs	1307	8630	560.29
Wool and hair	142	361	154.23
-Wool	118	245	107.63
-Hair and bristles	24	116	383.33
Dung	4307	18498	329.47
Stock increment	703	9054	1187.91
Silk worm and honey	865	1523	76.07
Total	42040	240601	472.31

Source: FAOSTAT database 2008. www.faostat.fao.org

Table 3 : Animal products exported during 2009-10

Product category	Quantity (ton)	Value (Rs. crore)
Buffalo meat	495019.71	5480.60
Sheep/goat meat	52868.01	747.20
Poultry products	1016783.10	372.12
Processed meat	716.19	9.58
Swine meat	1117.96	10.34
Animal casings	2020.56	31.53
Dairy products	34379.97	402.68
Natural honey	13310.77	146.65
Total	1616216.27	7200.72

Source: APEDA (The Agricultural and Processed Food Products Export Development Authority), Ministry of Commerce, Government of India

3.2 Meat animal handling and slaughter

Meat animals are transported over long distances in the country and sometimes trekked to the urban centres for slaughter resulting in weight loss and deaths during transit. Regulation of animal transport is not effective for a variety of reasons. In urban areas, most of the animals are slaughtered inside the slaughterhouses but a sizeable number is slaughtered outside as well. The slaughterhouses constructed decades ago lack proper facilities and most of them are ill maintained. As a result, the meat produced and sold is far from satisfactory standards of hygiene. Hence, the slaughter practices as well as conditions of urban slaughterhouses need considerable improvement to produce hygienic meat, and also to minimize losses in the marketing chain of live animals as well as meat. Practice of meat hygiene regulations, prevention of cruelty to animals, prevention of contamination of carcasses and offal and economy in operations are essential features of improvement of slaughterhouses. This has become more important in view of the possibility of large scale imports after WTO liberalization. Rural meat production centres can be useful in meeting the urban meat demand due to the difficulties in establishing urban modern abattoirs. Urban slaughterhouses are generally old, constructed a few decades ago. These lack, basic amenities like sufficient water, lighting etc. Mostly located amidst residential areas, these are congested and inadequate, to meet the increasing slaughter. Unhygienic conditions lead to meat contamination while proper veterinary inspection is not feasible. Wastage of by-products and disposal of slaughterhouse waste are some other hurdles.

4. WTO and Livestock Sector

The uniqueness of Indian livestock sector is characterized as 'production by masses' as compared to 'mass production' by a few in developed countries, which needs to be kept in mind while deciding policies and approaches of the economic liberalization programme. A large number of livestock farmers need to be retained and sustained in livestock sector as no alternative is possible for their livelihood. World Trade Organization (WTO) can bring in benefits to Indian livestock sector provided the country's interests are defended well at the negotiation tables. The domestic animal product sector may, otherwise, meet severe competition from the imported products, consequently the farmers can lose their livelihood altogether. Important animal products that have reference to WTO are milk and milk products; meat and meat products; bone and bone products and leather and leather products. Among the livestock products, skim milk powder, butter oil, poultry meat, mutton (sheep meat), sausage products, and raw hides may find increased chance of being dumped to the detriment of domestic sector, if adequate attention is not paid. Buffalo meat, sheep and goat meat, poultry meat and some dairy products have better prospects for exports provided quality norms are achieved.

4.1 Advantages to Indian livestock sector

- Lower production cost of livestock products
- Lower labour cost as livestock sector is labour intensive
- Negligible subsidies in the pre-WTO period facilitating trade competition
- Large biodiversity and natural resources
- Rich traditional practices and technologies
- Absence of some diseases such as BSE (mad cow disease)
- Large scope of increasing livestock productivity and efficiency
- Lower infrastructure investments and less cost of adoption of changes
- Proximity to livestock products importing countries

4.2 Disadvantages to Indian livestock sector

- Livestock production in developed countries receives considerable subsidies which even after the WTO adoption may remain substantial to effectively compete with India.
- In the area of sanitary and phytosanitary measures, developed countries have adequate infrastructure to take advantage and put India in defence.
- Developed countries have sound statistics in livestock sector and can make precise estimates for initiating appropriate actions/programmes.

- Smaller numbers of units with large scale production facilities in developed countries have cost and quality benefits and they can adopt technological advances easily.
- Social and religious objections in India may affect adoption of programmes based on scientific and technical merit.
- There is unequal trade bargain.
- India has larger disease and residue monitoring costs due to larger livestock populations.
- Urbanization and fast changing cultural values in India may lead to increased demand for imported products.
- Labour and environment aspects have yet to be agreed at WTO which may have a bearing to India if not defended well.

The following aspects should be considered to take advantage of WTO and protect the livestock sector in the country.

1. Livestock producers should be enabled and empowered to produce better quality products with higher productivity and improved efficiency.
2. Stringent quality control measures and hygienic practices are required in production, processing and marketing of livestock products.
3. The economic interests of farmers with respect to sustainability and earning livelihood should be safeguarded through livestock production activities, particularly through analysis of implications of dumping in the area of livestock products.
4. Long term strategies should be developed for different livestock products based on analysis of impact/implications of WTO.
5. There is need to develop and evaluate newer processing technologies for improved efficiency of milk processing for adoption in the modernized milk processing and value addition for better competitiveness.
6. Technologies and strategies are required for promotion of meat exports particularly buffalo meat, taking advantage of reduction in subsidies by meat exporting countries.
7. Research on indigenous dairy products should be carried out to benefit the farmers, while the product technologies should be patented.
8. Chemical contaminants and residues should be monitored to formulate standards and develop quality assurance programmes to regulate imports and promote exports.

9. We should defend against imposition of irrational and inconsistent sanitary and phytosanitary (SPS) measures against Indian exports through scientific and technical evidence.
10. The country should provide information and actively participate in developing Codex standards.
11. Disease free zones should be established for promotion of exports.
12. Eradication of FMD and other livestock diseases should be given priority.
13. Developing competence for defending Indian interests in dispute settlement proceedings is important.
14. Livestock producers associations need to be formed and strengthened to defend their interests in the changing global trade and economic liberalization.
15. Farmers' ability to adopt new technologies should be strengthened for better competition.
16. Estimating and meeting the domestic requirements is essential to ward off large scale dumping of livestock products.
17. Conflict of interest between the livestock producers and consumers and commodity conflicts need to be addressed appropriately.
18. Steps should be taken to conserve and protect the genetic resources of different livestock breeds.

5. Comparative Scenario in Developed Nations

The scenario in the European countries, USA, and Australia is quite different from the developing nations. These have well organized meat animal production, processing and export as well as effective regulations to monitor the quality aspects. Promotional efforts for the growth of the meat industry in such countries have been supported by the government as well as other stake holders. In USA the Federal Meat Inspection Act came into existence in 1906 with a mandate of inspection of live animals, carcasses and processed products as well as improved sanitary conditions for slaughter and processing. On the other hand in India, though the Prevention of Food Adulteration Act was promulgated in 1955 covering meat as food, the Meat Food Products Order came into existence only in 1973 that covers only processed meat products but excludes fresh meat. The personnel and infrastructure are not adequate for effective implementation of regulatory aspects in meat sector in the country. The recent Food Safety Act, 2006 is an integrated Act incorporating a number of existing Acts and proposing adequate organization for effective implementation. The Act has to propose a number of rules and regulations along with implementing mechanism and resources.

Average animal protein intake in the developing countries is only 15 g compared to 60 g in developed countries, while for India it is 10.8 g as compared to world average of 29 g. Consumption of animal products is relatively much lower in India and is bound to increase at a rapid rate due to nutritional awareness for animal protein in diet and socioeconomic changes. In India, annual growth rates of 4.3%, 4.7% and 4.1% were achieved for milk, eggs and meat production during the last 10 years and 8-10% growth rate is desired for different animal products to provide 20 g animal protein per person per day by 2010 from the present 10.8 g. Livestock population dynamics of the recent years clearly indicates better prospects of buffaloes, sheep, goat and chicken. Meat production in India is largely described as a by- product system as the meat animals are not reared primarily for meat production. The data clearly indicate that average carcass yields are much lower in the country as compared to the world average (Table 4). These need to be increased by growing meat animals to larger weights.

Table 4 : Average carcass yield of meat animals

Animals	Carcass yield (kg)	
	India	World
Cattle	103	200
Buffaloes	138	138
Sheep	12	15.6
Goat	10	12.3
Pig	35	78.4
Chicken	0.95	1.45

Source: FAOSTAT database 2008. www.faostat.fao.org

6. Developmental Guidelines

National Meat and Poultry Processing Board (NMPPB) has been established recently. It is expected to contribute significantly in the development of meat sector. It has various short-term and long-term programmes with the following objectives.

Objectives of NMPPB

1. Fostering sustainable development of meat and poultry processing sector
2. Helping the industry in setting up/modernization of abattoirs by providing technical consultancy for production of hygienic meat and

meat products and for utilization of slaughterhouse waste to prepare animal by-products with value addition

3. Setting up quality control laboratories and analytical laboratories for meat and meat products to meet the required domestic and international market standards

4. Promoting and training of meat producers and entrepreneurs to adopt Good Manufacturing Practices (GMP), Hazard Analysis & Critical Control Points (HACCP) System, and ISO 22000 in meat production

5. Setting up a mechanism for implementation of the existing regulations and laws in India on meat and meat production, processing and marketing

6. To undertake market surveys and help the industry to create market intelligence, data base and its dissemination on regular basis for improvement of the meat sector.

7. To provide help for research and for setting up training institutions to train workers, technicians and managers in meat and meat processing industry

8. To help the industry to establish infrastructure for backward and forward linkages for traceability of meat in meat/ poultry meat processing sector

9. Work as a central/national hub to address the issues related to meat and poultry processing sector for its systematic and proper development

Department of Animal Husbandry and Dairying (Ministry of Agriculture, Government of India) and Ministry of Food Processing Industries (Government of India) are implementing schemes for modernization of abattoirs and meat processing plants.

6.1 Clean meat production

Improvement of slaughterhouses to produce hygienic meat is the most important requirement for developing organized meat industry. This has become more important in view of the possibility of large scale imports after WTO liberalization. Relevant approaches for production of hygienic meat and for providing a positive image to meat sector are important to sustain meat animal production and ensure livelihood to small farmers. Essential infrastructure facilities like water, shelter, dressing away from floor, waste removal to produce hygienic meat are important requirements and private entrepreneurs need to be facilitated to take up slaughter and meat production activities for domestic market. The cost of improvement and modernization of slaughterhouses of different capacities for the entire country has been estimated at more than Rs. 10000 crore (Table 5) that requires to be sourced by the developmental departments. While automation and heavy investments on machinery are required for large capacities, in a number of municipalities low cost slaughter facilities can be established that will be more relevant and feasible. Local bodies need to plan systematically for improving slaughterhouses, and more importantly, identifying appropriate place if the existing place is not adequate or suitable. Funds from developmental organizations should be utilized to establish facilities and sustainable management should be evolved to operate the facilities. Local bodies need to play effective role in the production of clean meat.

Table 5 : Estimated cost of improvement/modernization of abattoirs in India

Category	No.	Cost per city/ town/ village (Rs.)	Total cost (Rs. in crore)
I. Cities and Towns			
a) Class I cities with population of 1 lakh and above			
i) Cost of abattoirs for 20 large cities (above 10 lakh) except Mumbai and New Delhi	20		520.00
ii) Other 280 cities	280	6 crores	1680.00
b) Class II towns (population 50000-99999)	345	4 crores	1380.00
c) Class III towns (population 20000 to 49999)	947	2 crores	1994.00
d) Class IV towns (population 10000 to 19999)	1167	1 crore	1167.00
e) Class V towns (population 5000 to 9999)	740	50 lakh	370.00
f) Class VI towns (population less than 5000)	197	20 lakh	39.40
II. Villages			
a) Villages with 10000 and above population	1830	20 lakh	366.00
b) Villages with 5000 to 9999 population	7202	10 lakh	720.00
c) Villages with 2000 to 4999 population	46892	2 lakh	938.00
III. Export abattoirs in private sector	15		1000.00
Total			10174.00

6.2 Strategies for local bodies to ensure wholesome livestock products

- Preparation of master plan for meat and milk sectors
- Estimating the requirement for meat and milk

- Identifying the number and capacities of abattoirs to be established or improved
- Establishing abattoirs preferably in the peri-urban area where animals are received
- Promoting rural slaughterhouses
- Development of meat animal markets with essential facilities
- Developing wholesale/central markets for meat
- Programme for improving retail meat shops
- Monitoring transport of carcasses and cuts for hygiene and aesthetics
- Control on unhygienic poultry slaughter and waste disposal
- Effective waste disposal and effluent treatment at slaughterhouses
- Monitoring urban dairies for hygiene and waste disposal
- Awareness programmes on clean meat and milk production
- Active participation in the developmental schemes of state and central government

6.3 Important steps in establishing slaughterhouse

1. Identifying an appropriate official
2. Engaging a consultant
3. Determining capacity of abattoir based on requirement and consultation
4. Scrutiny of schemes available for development of slaughterhouses
5. Identifying suitable site
6. Project report preparation
7. Obtaining clearances
8. Submission of project for financial grants
9. Receiving grants and provision of balance grants
10. Detailed design, drawing and tenders preparation
11. Appointing committee for tenders floating and finalization
12. Inviting and finalizing tenders
13. Appointing agency for execution of project
14. Completion of project, trial runs and commissioning
15. Management committee for monitoring operations of slaughterhouses

7. Action Plans and Strategies

7.1 Augmenting production of animal products

The present production requires to be doubled to increase per capita animal protein consumption from 10 g to 20 g. It is necessary to increase milk, meat and egg production to meet the domestic requirement as well as export market demand. Some of the prospective measures to increase production potential of different species of livestock for increased milk, meat and egg production are:

1. Salvaging of buffalo calves from early death is required to increase buffalo calf crop. In particular, urban buffalo calves from city dairies need to be saved to conserve high value buffalo germplasm. In the present buffalo production system about 5-6 million buffalo calves can be salvaged allowing a 10 per cent mortality with low cost management practices and feed inputs to generate farmers' awareness and interest for undertaking large scale calf salvaging and growing activities.
2. Growth potential should be increased through adequate nutrition. Demonstrating appropriate feed processing technologies to produce low cost feeds from crop residues and biomass to achieve reasonable growth rates may find large scale adoption. Effective culling of surplus and unproductive buffaloes may contribute for increased production efficiency.
3. In case of cattle, all efforts to sustain cattle prosperity need to be promoted in view of the increasing mechanization and the uncertain adverse impacts affecting the farmers' economy and livelihood.
4. In case of sheep and goat, better production potential through appropriate nutritional intervention particularly in lean season by providing low cost feed inputs, complete feeds from crop residues and other supplements should be realized and demonstrated.
5. In case of poultry, broilers should be reared to larger weights (>2.5 kg) for better quality meat and processed products, because meat from higher weight broilers contains higher proportion of breast meat with higher protein and lower fat content.

Commissioning of model projects integrating farmers, animal husbandry departments, and meat, leather and feed industry will enhance buffalo production and quality buffalo meat export.

7.2 Rural meat production and processing

Rural abattoirs can be appropriate to meet the urban meat demand because of the difficulties in establishing urban modern abattoirs. Marketing of meat animals will be easier and costs and losses of transportation will be minimal. By-products can be gainfully utilized and effluent treatment costs will be minimal in view of land availability. Also, rural abattoirs will benefit livestock farmers with better returns due to elimination of middlemen and increased employment opportunities. Quality of animals will be better as animals will be subjected to less stress. These can be of smaller capacities to serve a village or group of villages or can be large to supply meat for urban demand.

As meat processing is labour intensive, the same can be sourced conveniently and at lower cost in the rural areas. Many times it can be a supplementary activity for some people to utilize their spare time to undertake processing activities such as deboning, product preparation etc. Rural farmers will thus have accessibility to meat products by producing choice products and ethnic tastes for better nutrition, convenience and satisfaction. It will generate employment and better utilization of local resources.

A rural meat processing facility can be established by a rural entrepreneur or collectively by the farmers of a village or group of villages as the viability demands. The center can have slaughtering facility or source dressed carcasses from rural abattoir and debone to produce meat emulsion as semi-convenience product or produce ready-to-eat or heat-and-serve products (nuggets, patties, kababs, sausages, meat balls, croquettes, vada, cutlets etc.). Simple machinery required will be a meat handling table, meat mincer, bowl chopper or food mixer, cooker, refrigerator, cooking vessels, trays, moulds, knives etc. The center will process quality carcasses from young animals for sale as fresh meat cuts and the aged or spent animals and poultry as ground meat, meat emulsion or mix for processed meat products or process into heat-and-serve products. Complimentarity of employment is an additional feature of rural meat processing as deboning of carcasses is an important step in value added meat products processing, particularly in chicken, and requires manual labour for small scale production. Underemployment is a common feature in Indian situation and complimentary utilization of such spare labour will go a long way in economizing cost of production of meat products. Deboned chicken frames, bones and other by-products can also be given towards payment for labour in kind. Housewives can utilize their spare time in these activities beneficially.

7.3 Complimentarity of meat and leather sectors

In order to realize higher growth rates and better returns, both meat and leather sectors are dependant on augmented buffalo production with better quality animals, thereby better quality products by following better handling and slaughter practices. A cooperative effort is required between meat and leather sectors so that animal welfare measures are adequately practised to contribute a positive image of these sectors and produce quality products of higher demand.

7.4 By-products utilization and waste disposal

The integrated meat export plants generally establish large scale modern rendering plants and effluent treatment plants. Thus, by-products are effectively utilized to a great extent and effluents are treated along with sanitary disposal of waste resulting in good environment in the plants. Facilities for bio-gas production using soft tissues for meeting energy requirements have also been established in some meat plants. More export plants need to go for establishing such facilities. However, in the slaughterhouses regulated by the local bodies, though by-products are collected by some agencies for processing but blood and rumenal contents remain accumulated in the premises, resulting in odour and pollution problems, spoiling the image of the meat sector. Local bodies need to facilitate proper disposal of waste without accumulation in order to maintain sanitary conditions in the slaughterhouses. Organised facilities for small scale processing of some of the by-products such as fat rendering, casings processing, bile processing etc. should be provided as the present facilities are not satisfactory.

By-products processing on cottage scale is also appropriate in Indian situation with limited quantities of by-products availability at any particular slaughterhouse. A number of by-products such as heads and legs, fatty trimmings (to provide cracklings), blood etc. are processed by individuals with very limited facilities and sold to local consumers. Though these units are unaesthetic, but these are relevant in practice. Simple interventions to improve such premises by providing implements for convenient operations will go a long way for the benefit of the society. These units are important to utilize the by-products in smaller quantities which cannot be processed in modern plants. The personnel engaged in this work need to be educated to prevent health risks associated with lack of hygiene and sanitation.

7.5 Role of simple and relevant technologies

A technology and strategy will find merit only when middle class households (which constitute larger proportion of population) are able to afford to buy meat and eggs and prepare products of their choice with ease and convenience to satisfy their unique requirements. While the centralized processing of high value products largely adopting complex machineries and processing can continue to provide products to the upper and elite urban consumers, it will be strategic to aim at simple technologies that can draw the attention of small scale entrepreneurs to fully exploit the Indian cookery to provide products of choice to masses. As the large scale modern technologies have equal number of demerits in the populous country with enough of food fads, it is only the small scale processing technologies that can satisfy the unsubstantiated preferences of the people with varying socioeconomic and ethnic implications in the vast country. Processing and supply of hygienic meat and chicken in fresh and frozen form will continue to grow both on large and small scale as per the demand. However, new strategies need to aim at frozen chicken primarily to absorb the market fluctuations and increase the demand for poultry products by increasing the number of consumers as well as per capita consumption, and by spreading the marketability over a wider area, unlike the present urban and peri-urban areas.

7.6 Some relevant processing technologies

7.6.1 Utilization of tough meats

A very large proportion of meat animals particularly buffaloes, sheep and goat are spent (aged/old) animals whose meat is generally tough and less palatable but more suitable for processing to derive products both on economic and quality considerations. With the rapid growth in poultry industry, the availability of layer and broiler hens as culls has also increased which can be beneficially utilized for products processing to the benefit of producer and consumer. Minced meat products such as meat balls, croquettes, kababs, meat vada, meat idli etc. are simple and more relevant for better utilization of tough meat that are rich in connective tissue, less palatable and unappealing as fresh meat to the consumers. Tenderization of tough meats for consumption as whole meat products such as curries, fries, boti kabas etc. is also relevant using marination with condiments such as ginger or treatment with papain or baking soda.

7.6.2 Developing emulsion based products

Production of emulsion based products not only facilitates the utilization of tough meats, less preferred cuts and by-products but also provides technological opportunity for incorporation of a number of other ingredients such as spices, condiments, fillers, vegetables etc. both for improving palatability and achieving economy. Use of different kinds of meat such as chicken and mutton; pork and beef; pork and chicken etc. to produce highly acceptable products is advantageous both technologically and economically. Emulsion technology also facilitates developing a number of value added products with better palatability, nutrition and convenience. Some edible by-products such as tripe, pig skin and chicken skin, gizzard and heart can be appropriately processed for gainful incorporation into meat products. Efficient use of by-products is necessary to contain meat processing costs and produce variety products of consumer choice. A typical meat emulsion formulation can have deboned meat 40-65%, by-products 5-15%, eggs 5-15%, vegetables 5-15%, soya nuggets wet mince 5-10%, salt 2%, polyphosphate 0.4%, spice mix 1.7%, wheat flour 3%, sugar 0.3%, condiments 3.5%, chilled water 9% and sodium nitrite 100 ppm. Proper mincing of meat, correct formulation and sequence of addition of ingredients, addition of polyphosphate and suitable binders and operation at lower temperatures adding chilled water or ice are important to produce better quality emulsion and achieve higher product yields. Emulsion is of good quality when cooked products yields are above 90%. Addition of polyphosphate has been found most relevant in Indian situation of meat handling for better yields and quality. Meat mincer and bowl chopper or food mixer or stone grinder are necessary to produce meat emulsion. Such meat emulsion/mix can be produced at strategic centralized places involving appropriate technologies and distributed to multiple numbers of secondary units which can process and market the value added products to consumers both in fresh and stored form. Emulsion/mix can also be produced at secondary units either from frozen meat items supplied from larger units or small scale processing of live animals or dressed carcasses. Third stage units which primarily function as retail units can also sell both value added products and consumer pack emulsion to consumers/households in the limited area with quality assurance. The households can further incorporate/mix ingredients before preparing products of their choice. Emulsion as semi-convenience product may find greater relevance in Indian situation. A number of simple technologies and appliances can be utilized to produce a number of convenience products such as nuggets, slices, pattis, kababs, balls, croquettes, spring rolls, samosa, vada etc.

7.6.3 Incorporation of eggs, vegetables and extenders

Eggs can be incorporated as whole eggs liquid or cooked eggs or in combination upto 20-30% level in the formulation with cost and nutrition advantage. Egg protein is superior to meat protein with higher biological value but cheaper in cost, hence advantageous. Eggs are also beneficial for incorporation of hard fats such as mutton or beef fat as pre-mix to minimize mouth coating of hard fats. Incorporation of a variety of seasonal vegetables found to be advantageous not only to produce lower cost nutritional products but also consumer choice products of wide variety. Blanching has been found advantageous for incorporation of some vegetables having strong raw flavour. Meat products with vegetables have been found to have good keeping quality on refrigerated and frozen storage. Several cereal flours, gram flour, bread crumbs, milk solids, whey proteins, soya products etc. can be incorporated upto 10% as binders, fillers, extenders to reduce cost and increase yield of edible product. Meat products with suitable extenders are more relevant in small holder situation for better nutrition.

7.6.4 Restructured products

The purpose of producing restructured products is to effectively market less valuable carcasses (from spent or aged animals and of poor conformation) and carcass components. The basic processes include chunking, flaking, tearing, grinding, chopping, mixing, tumbling, emulsification, forming, freezing, tempering, pressing, slicing, cooking etc. Tumbling, massaging and blade tenderization facilitate production of high quality restructured products. The products include bites, steaks, cutlets, chops, roasts, rolls and hams.

7.6.5 Enrobed products

Enrobing/ coating of meat products with edible materials in the form of batter using flours, whole egg liquid and other additives is a method of value addition which enhances the acceptability of meat products. Enrobing imparts the product a crispy texture and increases the pleasure of eating with more desirable colour. Products are juicier as natural juices are retained. Battered eggs is a novel enrobed product wherein boiled and peeled eggs can be enrobed with meat emulsion and cooked in water or fried in oil as a variety meat product.

7.6.6 Meat nuggets

Meat emulsion or mix prepared from a desired formulation is filled into moulds (15 cm x 10 cm x 4 cm) with tightly applied lid and cooked in a simple drum type cooker for 45 min to reach an internal temperature of 85°C. Moulds are taken out, cooled and the cooked meat blocks removed and cut into slices or nuggets of different sizes and shapes. Cooked blocks can also be chilled for further cutting. The products are fully cooked and can be packed and stored for 20 days at 4°C or 5 months at -18°C. The process facilitates using a number of formulations and varying consistency of the emulsion or mix unlike the modern forming machines which operate with mix of required consistency. Nuggets can be consumed as snack or nugget curry can be produced or pickled or smoked or used in rice pulav or biriyani.

7.6.7 Shelf-stable products

Pickles and dried meat products are appropriate in rural situation. They provide even smaller quantities for regular consumption which will be useful in balancing diets. Bone-in and bone-out meats of different species can be used to produce these products of excellent convenience and nutritional significance in rural areas.

7.6.8 Smoked products

Chicken cuts such as legs and breasts, mutton cuts, pork cuts, buffalo meat cuts can be suitably cured and lightly smoked to produce a variety of smoked meat products to meet the consumer choice. Some of the emulsion products such as slices, nuggets and idlis can also be smoked to add variety. Smoking enhances shelf life in addition to better flavour and taste.

8. Constraints and Remedies

There are many challenges for development of meat sector in India in terms of socioeconomic, technological and international happenings. A time has come to analyse the constraints and find effective remedies for development of this sector. Important considerations concerning meat and its products include their highly perishability, potential as a source of pathogens, high ambient temperature, aesthetic considerations, religious and social taboos and animal welfare.

8.1 Food safety aspects in meat sector

Ensuring safety of animal products has received greater attention in the recent years because of the fast changing consumer demands, socioeconomic changes, changes in agriculture and livestock production practices and the need for meeting the requirements of export trade. Food safety and quality assurance are also important due to the implications of liberalized trade regulations. While the prospects are large for introduction of quality assurance in Indian meat sector, the implications pose a challenge for all the stakeholders. Understanding different factors contributing to food safety in meat sector is important to propose and practice quality assurance of Indian meat and meat products towards developing an organized meat industry in the country. Production of safe animal products with quality assurance has become important concern in the recent years in view of the increased trade in animal products due to globalization, rapid and increased international travel, changes in agricultural practices, developments in processing technologies, changes in consumption patterns, resource constraints, cost effectiveness of sanitary production and distribution, emergence and reemergence of pathogens, evolution of antibiotic resistant pathogens, and potential of apparently healthy animals as reservoirs of pathogens.

8.2 Promotion of processed meats in Indian situation

Organized development of processed meat sector is important to realize full benefits from meat animal and contribute for sustained meat production. Also, it is necessary to produce quality value added meat products to meet the requirements in the post WTO period for effectively facing global competition both to check large scale imports to the detriment of domestic sector and to promote exports. The growth of processed meat sector assures the farmers a regular off take of their produce at reasonable prices and provides a variety to the consumer. This is more so in poultry sector, when the market prices fall due to excess supply. Poultry can be processed and stored to be released into market at an appropriate time and farmer's returns can be protected to sustain his operations. In addition, employment potential will be substantial.

Development of formulations and appropriate processes and technologies for a range of meat products that will find acceptability in Indian situation are important for achieving growth in meat sector. Relevant and low cost technologies for small scale production of meat products need to be developed to initiate a large number of entrepreneurs to processed meat sector. Value addition is an important avenue for efficient utilization of livestock resources with increased demand and higher returns. Small scale ventures of value added products will go a long way in improving the economics of livestock production and meeting the consumer demands. The major bottlenecks in the processed meat sector development are given below:

- Unavailability of good quality meat due to constraints in hygienic meat production
- Unavailability of good quality food additives due to their required import
- Unavailability of processing machinery due to limited demand
- Unavailability of appropriate packaging material to small scale ventures
- Difficulty in making best formulations for sausages due to restrictions on use of beef trimmings as lean and pork trimmings as fat source
- Suspicion of mixing of meats in processed meats which is taboo for consumption
- Inadequate cold chain facilities for sourcing inputs and marketing of processed meats

8.3 Economics of value added products

Availability of adequate raw materials at reasonable cost and distribution and marketing at minimum costs contribute favourably to the economics. Sale price depends on the economic status of consumers and the product aimed at. Low cost attracts wide range of consumers. All efforts have to be made to keep production cost at minimum with selection of appropriate formulation, processing conditions and infrastructure facilities. Addition of polyphosphates has been found to result in immense benefits such as higher product yield, better palatability and longer keeping quality in Indian situation of meat handling. Meat from spent (aged) animals is more suitable for products processing for improved economics. A project appraisal on different aspects of the value added products is necessary before planning a meat products venture.

9. Conclusion

Efficient meat animal production and clean meat production with good animal welfare and public image are important considerations of sustaining the role of meat animals for providing livelihood, nutrition and food security to a large proportion of the population. Relevant technologies that have applicability to Indian situation need priority consideration for developing organized meat sector in the country. The role of research and development departments to provide relevant technologies and bring awareness among the stakeholders for adoption is of greater importance in the present status of Indian meat sector.

Promotion of hygienic meat production can be done by the following measures.

- Improvement of existing slaughterhouses
- Adoption of semi-modern abattoir concept
- Establishment of modern abattoirs
- Establishment of rural meat production centres and rural abattoirs
- Minimization of unauthorized slaughter
- Regulation of export slaughter in abattoirs to maintain sanitary conditions

The following measures are envisaged to strengthen the meat sector.

- Promotion of small scale meat products centres
- Export promotion by providing level playing field to compete with developed countries
- Establishing cold storage to offset adverse impact of price fluctuations and promotion of processed meat

The National Meat and Poultry Processing Board should take concrete steps to promote development of organized meat sector to sustain animal production.

❑❑❑

Chapter 6

Rabbit Farming for Sustainable Development

VED PRAKASH
Central Sheep and Wool Research Institute, Avikanagar-304501

Contents

1. Introduction

The scarcity of food following the First and the Second World War paved the way for extensive rabbit rearing. Rabbit meat gained popularity due to its excellent quality. The Food and Agriculture Organization of the United Nations (FAO) through different package programmes also encouraged the farmers for rabbit farming. Thus, rabbit farming gradually became popular in many countries. The shrinking land holding, reduced grazing areas and changing climatic conditions are making the traditional livestock rearing difficult and uneconomical, as a result of which there is shift towards smaller animals like rabbits for steady and sustainable income and nutritional security. In developing countries where enormous meat shortages exist, the potential for rabbit production is the greatest.

2. Global Rabbit Production Scenario

Rabbit production is concentrated in two major areas (Europe and Asia). Europe accounts for about 50% and Asia about 40.5% of rabbit meat production. Production areas are also present in some regions of Africa and America. Rabbit meat is not produced in most of the countries of the Near East and Oceania. China accounts for 99% of Asian production (Szakály *et al.* 2006). China, Italy, Spain and France, the four biggest global producers, contribute almost three fourth of the world production. China accounts for approximately a quarter of world's exports, with Netherlands, Germany, Japan, Switzerland, United States and other European countries being the major importing nations. Global rabbit meat consumption in 2004 was 1.1 million ton.

Angora wool production is modest and ranked third largest animal fibre industry in the world. Currently, China is the dominant angora producing country. With about 50 million Angora rabbits, China produces about 10,000 ton rabbit fibre per year and exports about 50% of the fiber into the international market (Tang 2002). The main end-user countries of angora are Japan, United States, Germany and Italy. Most of the rabbits in China, Central Europe and South American countries are 70-90% German Angora and 5-10% French Angora type. The Chinese Angora rabbits, which contribute 90% of the Angora rabbit hair in the International trade, were developed by crossing German and French Angoras and the crossbred subsequently crossed with New Zealand White, a meat breed. It weighs 4.1-4.4 Kg at 11 month age and is dual purpose breed, good for fibre and meat both. According to conservative estimates, total angora production in India is about 25-30 ton per annum.

3. Rabbit Farming in India

Organized promotion of rabbit production in India took place during late seventies by the import of rabbits from the United Kingdom and the former Soviet Union (USSR), by the Indian Council of Agricultural Research (ICAR) at the North Temperate Regional Station (NTRS) of the Central Sheep and Wool Research Institute (CSWRI) at Garsa in Kullu district in Himachal Pradesh. In India, rabbit rearing has been attracting the farmers for the two decades. The ever growing demand for non-vegetarian proteins in the country is helping in the growth of rabbit. Though it has not yet made much impact in the meat industry, there is tremendous scope for popularizing rabbit meat in the country. Tamil Nadu and Kerala are known for broiler rabbit while Himachal Pradesh for Angora rabbit farming. Largely the crosses of New Zealand White, White Giant, Soviet Chinchilla and Dutch are reared for meat in India while Angora is raised for wool.

The late beginning of rabbit farming in India is mainly because rabbit meat was not much acceptable as a standard dietary item in the country. Because rabbits were seldom grown for meat, they were not grown for fur either. This view is now changing somewhat rapidly, though in most regions of the country rabbit farms are still being run mostly on an small, medium and backyard basis. The performance and adaptability studies in the temperate, sub-temperate and semi-arid regions of the CSWRI and its stations have demonstrated that rabbit can be reared successfully in all regions of the country.

4. Economic Sustainability of Rabbit Rearing

Rabbit rearing has certain inherent advantages over the traditional livestock rearing making it more economically sustainable proposition for farmers as shown below.

- Rabbits are herbivores and they can be fed almost anything vegetarian including waste or surplus vegetables from the market, tree leaves, grasses or even kitchen scrap. Hence, it is very easy and affordable to feed rabbits.
- Rate of reproduction of rabbits is high. They are prolific breeders with high fecundity rate of 6 to 8 kits in short gestation period. The doe can be mated to a buck after 15-20 days of delivery and a female can deliver babies every 45 days.

- Rabbits provide useful by-products. Rabbit skin can be used for several purposes (mat, rugs and clothes). Manure is very valuable organic fertilizer.
- Rabbit farming requires less space and it can be done as commercial or as backyard farming. Rabbits have small body size enabling efficient space utilization.
- Rabbits have limited competition with human food in contrast to poultry.
- Rabbits have early sexual maturity, 6 months in does and 7 months in bucks.
- Breeding is possible all round the year under appropriate management conditions.
- Rabbits have higher growth rate and feed conversion efficiency in comparison to pigs and poultry. The feed : gain ratio in rabbits is 1 : 2-3 on dry matter basis.
- Due to low nutrient requirement, rabbits produce 6 pounds of meat while on the same feed and water, a cow will produce only 1 pound of meat.
- Within 3 months a baby rabbit gains market weight of around 2 Kg.
- Rabbit meat is known to be among the most nutritious meats. It is white, pearly and highly delicious meat but comparatively low in fat and calorie and high in protein.
- Rabbits can utilize forage protein more efficiently as compared to other livestock.
- Due to short gestation, faster weight gains and early sexual maturity rabbits mature 30% faster as compared to other animals.
- Rabbits have higher biological productivity. A female rabbit produces 10-25 times her weight in offspring as compared to cow producing about 0.6 times and an ewe 0.8 times her weight in a year.

Rabbit rearing business is simple, easy, affordable where huge and quick returns are possible. Angora rabbit business is more profitable than broiler rabbit business. A unit comprising of 100 adult rabbits can generate an income of Rs. 2000-3000 per month (Sharma and Karim 2010).

5. Breeds of Rabbit

There are many breeds of domestic rabbits that have different qualities. About 38 breeds and 87 varieties are recognised worldwide. Some popular rabbit breeds have been shown in Fig. 1-7.

5.1 Breeds for wool production

Angora rabbit is reared for wool production. It is usually white and albino. Normally the main demand of angora wool is of white colour and long staple for uniform dying and processing. At present, the most common Angora reared by Indian farmers is 2-3 breed crosses between German, British and Russian which have been developed at NTRS of CSWRI at Garsa. The strain is well adapted to temperate region of the country and has better reproductive efficiency, exhibits more disease resistance and produces medium fine wool. A German Angora rabbit can produce 800 g wool annually. Wool production per Kg of live weight is almost 6 times higher in rabbits as compared to sheep (Mahajan 2002). Brief description of some popular wool rabbit breeds is given in Table 1.

Table 1 : Characteristics of wool producing rabbit breeds

Particulars	Russian Angora	British Angora	German Angora	French Angroa	Crossbred Angora
Origin	Russia	Britain	Germany	France	India
Bodyweight (Kg)	3.5-5.5	2.5-4.5	3.0-4.5	3.5-4.0	3.0-4.0
Wool yield (g per year)	250-400	400-600	800-1200	700-800	500-600
Quality of wool	Medium fine	Fine	Superior	Fine	Medium fine
Guard wool (percent)	>7	<7	<3	>5	>4

5.2 Breeds for meat and fur skin production

A brief description of some popular broiler rabbit breeds like Soviet Chinchilla, Grey Giant, New Zealand White, White Giant, and Black Brown has been given in Table 2. Several other breeds like White California, Flemish Giant, Havana etc. are also known for their meat producing ability. The adult bodyweight of these breeds ranges from 3.0 to 6.0 Kg in females and 2.5 to 5.5 Kg in males (Mahajan 2002).

Table 2 : Characteristics of meat producing rabbit breeds

Breeds	Origin	Adult weight (Kg)	Special feature
Soviet Chinchilla	USSR	3.0-5.0	Fur is a fancy in fur crafts.
Grey Giant	USSR	3.0-5.0	Due to the resemblance of its fur with that of hare, it is often mistaken as hare. It is also reared for skin.
New Zealand White	England	3.0-5.0	Fur is white and skin is albino. The eye colour is red due to the absence of melanin pigment.
White Giant	USSR	3.0-5.0	It is almost similar in appearance to New Zealand White. Colour of the fur is white while eyes and skin are red. The length of hind limbs as well as body size is larger than that of New Zealand White.
Crossbreds like Black brown	India	3.0-4.5	These are crosses between the above mentioned breeds and local types. They are highly adaptive to Indian conditions and breed all through the year. Colour of fur is not uniform.

Besides meat and wool production, rabbits are also used in biological research and in teaching laboratories. New Zealand White, California, Dutch and Black Brown breeds are generally used for this purpose. The breeds like Polish, Palmino, Havana, Bevran New Zealand Red are reared as hobby as they are lighter in weight and very fancy to look at.

6. Selection of Breeding Stock

The foundation stock should be true to breed. Breeding stock should be purchased from government farms or recognised rabbit breeders. Selection of one male and two females from same genetic line is desirable.

6.1 Selection of doe

Doe with good physical condition and health and having 2.5-3 Kg weight at 6-7 month of age should be selected. Doe should have eight functional teats.

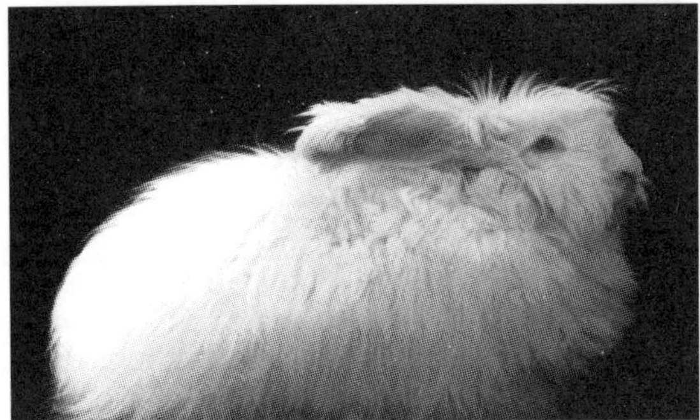

Fig. 1 : Angora rabbit

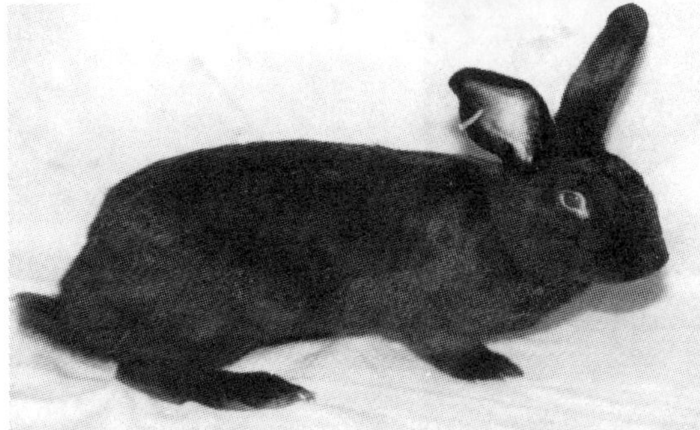

Fig. 2 : Black Brown rabbit

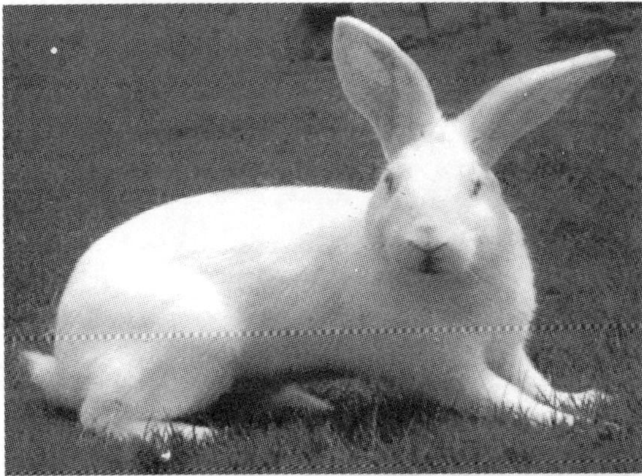

Fig. 3 : New Zealand White rabbit

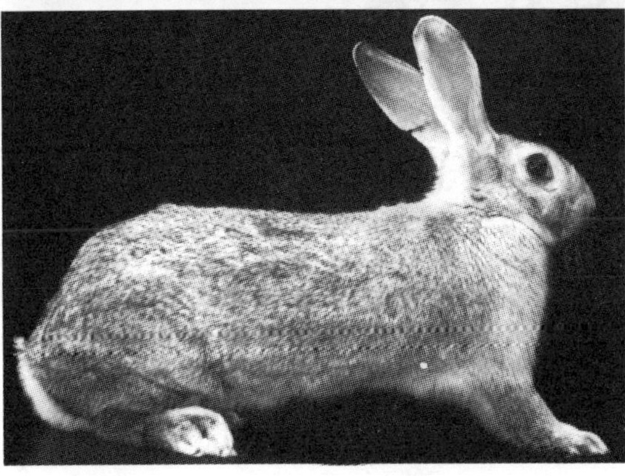

Fig. 4 : Soviet Chinchilla rabbit

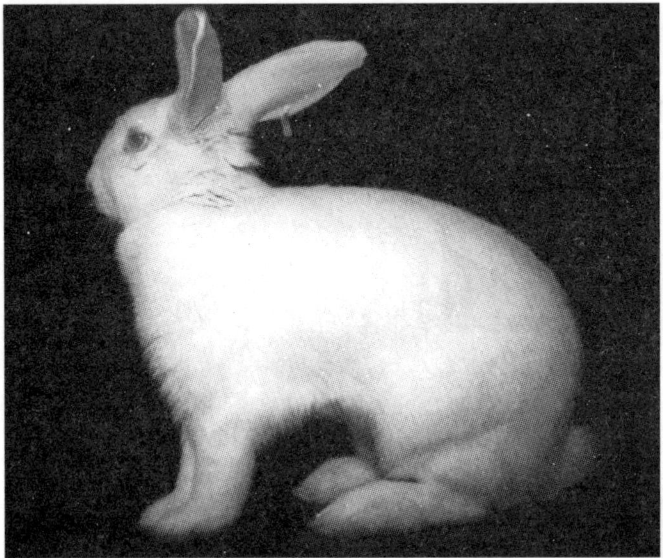

Fig. 5 : White Giant rabbit

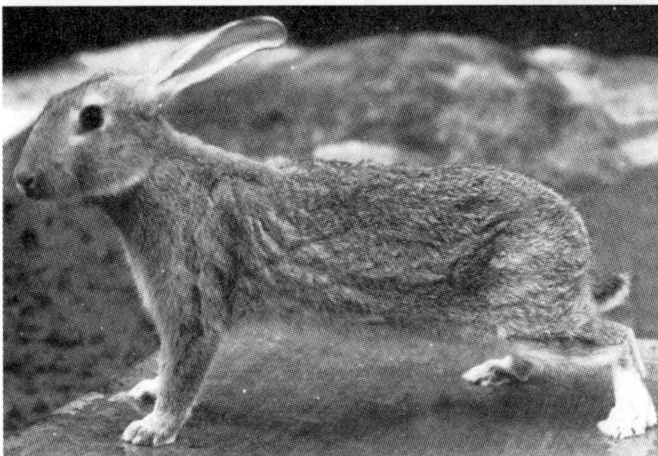

Fig. 6 : Grey Giant rabbit

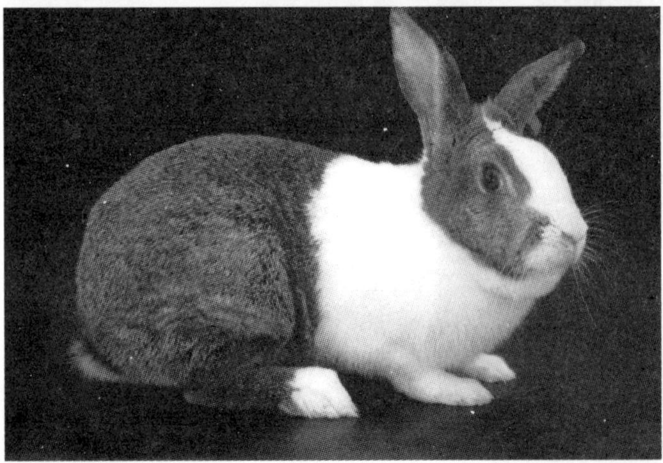

Fig. 7 : Dutch rabbit

6.2 Selection of bucks

A buck having good breeding record and pedigree should be selected. A virile and active buck having two well developed testicles should be selected.

6.3 Economic traits in rabbits used for selection

The traits of the animals resulting in financial gains to the farmers are called economic traits. The performance of rabbits in such traits, as given below, forms the basis for selecting breeding animals.

- *Litter size at birth*: The optimum value should be 6-8. Average birth weight of kits of a litter in broiler rabbits should be 40-50 g or more.
- *Litter weight at 21-days age (three weeks):* The young kits depend fully on their mother for the first 10-12 days of their life. The litter weight at three weeks age is taken as the criterion for measurement of mothering ability of the doe. The optimum value for the litter weight at 21 days age is 1.2 - 1.5 Kg.
- *Litter size at 21 days*: This trait is also equally important in measuring the mothering ability of doe. The doe selected for breeding must have at least six kits in the litter at 21 days.
- *Weaning weight of litter*: The young kits are weaned between 28 days and 42 days. At the time of weaning, the bodyweight of kits should be between 350-650 g depending upon the age of weaning. Litter weight at weaning must be more than 2 Kg.
- *Litter size at weaning*: At least 5-6 kits should be available from each litter at the time of weaning. More weaned kits are always advantageous for the farmer.
- *Number of kindling per year per doe*: The gestation period of doe is thirty days. If weaning is practised at thirty days, there should be five litters for weaning from each breeding doe. These can be increased by following intensive breeding by breeding the doe just after kindling (delivery).
- *Number of weaned bunnies per year per doe*: If five to six kits are available for weaning from each litter and if five litters are produced by the doe per year, the number of weaned bunnies from the doe per year should be 25-30.
- *Feed conversion efficiency*: The number of days taken to attain 2 Kg bodyweight is taken as a yardstick for feed conversion efficiency. Animals that achieve it at lower age are assumed to be better converters of feed and are selected as breeding animals.

7. Genetic Improvement

Genetic improvement in rabbits can be brought about by planned selection, planned breeding and proper record keeping. The genetic improvement programme should also be supported by proper environmental factors like housing, nutrition, disease control etc.

7.1 Record keeping

Planned breeding and selection can only be observed when proper records are maintained by a rabbit breeder. For this purpose, each rabbit born or brought in the farm should be identified with an individual number. Various records that need to be maintained include breeding record (doe record and buck record), wool record, growth record, slaughter record, feed record, medication record and financial records.

8. Feeding

Feed costs are the major expense in rabbit production as it accounts for 70-80 per cent of the cost of production. It is, therefore, extremely important to use a sound feeding programme. Under natural conditions, rabbits have the habit of coprophagy. Coprophagy is a unique phenomenon, which enhances the digestibility of feedstuffs and utilization of nutrients. Rabbit normally turns the head towards the anal region and sucks the soft faeces directly from anus during early morning everyday. The soft faeces are formed in the caecum and rapidly passes out through the large intestine. It appears as clusters and contains more moisture and looks like jelly. Caecotropes also called as night faeces or soft faeces provides microbial protein, vitamins and small quantity of volatile fatty acids. It has twice the protein and half of the fiber of the typical hard faecal pellet. They also contain high levels of vitamin K and vitamin B. The act of coprophagy takes place after three weeks of age. A dietary supply of vitamins A, D and E is necessary. Rabbits need to be given about 15% of fibre in diet for promoting intestinal motility, preventing fur chewing and minimizing intestinal disease. Rabbit prefer a pelleted diet to that in meal form.

Under commercial system, rabbits can be fed with concentrate feed pellets of 4-6 mm diameter and 10-15 mm length along with 200 g of greens per day. Generally, concentrate feeding precedes greens (grass + forages) feeding. Concentrate feed can be given in two divided doses. Rabbits generally eat more during night in summer. With the onset of winter, the requirement increases and the feeding shifts to daytime. However, regular timetable for feeding is advisable so that rabbits do not feel any stress due to the change in their daily routine. Sudden changes in feeds and feeding systems should be avoided. The rabbits must be fed at the same time everyday. While offering green grass, it should be preferably wilted.

Fur chewing can be controlled by increasing the fibre and protein contents of the ration. Further, addition of 200 g of magnesium oxide per quintal of feed helps control fur chewing. Since weaners are more sensitive to change of feed, care must be taken to avoid carbohydrate overload. Clean potable water must be provided throughout the day.

Rabbits under backyard system can be raised on grain free diets comprising of forages, grain by-products, tree leaves, vegetable wastes, culled vegetables and kitchen wastes. Daily nutrient requirements of rabbits as per ICAR standards are given in Table 3.

Table 3 : Daily nutrient requirements of rabbits (ICAR 1998)

Nutrients	Growth	Maintenance	Gestation	Lactation
Digestible energy (Kcal/Kg)	2500	2300	2500	2500
Crude protein (%)	18	16	17	19
Crude fibre (%)	10-12	12-14	10-12	10-12
Ether extract (%)	2	2	2	2

9. Watering

Water should be available round the clock particularly to a lactating doe. Always fresh and clean drinking water should be provided. Water pots should be cleaned thoroughly every week. Use of properly designed automatic watering equipment can also be made. A rabbit on average takes about 120 ml of water per kg bodyweight.

10. Breeding and Reproduction Management

Reproduction plays a vital role in profitable rabbit farming. Rabbits can be bred any time of the year. They are polyoestrous animals having 44 numbers of diploid chromosomes. The ideal age of buck and doe to start breeding is 7-8 months and 6-7 months, respectively. Rabbits do not ovulate on a regular cycle; as a result they do not actually go into heat. Common oestrous signs in the doe are restlessness, rubbing of chin on the cage, water trough and feed trough, and trying to join other rabbits in the nearby cages. When the doe is ready to breed, her vent area becomes dark pink, red or purple.

Mating should be done either early in the morning or in the evening. The doe is to be taken to the buck cage and never vice versa. When a successful mating occurs, the buck literally falls to its side, and usually lets out a grunt. The mating of the rabbit will cause the doe to produce eggs necessary for fertilization, usually 10-13 hours after breeding has occurred. This phenomenon is called as induced ovulation. The best way to determine if the doe is pregnant is to palpate the doe. Palpating the doe to determine pregnancy requires practice and should be done after 12 days from mating. The average pregnancy period is 30 days. Rebreeding of doe should be performed after weaning to achieve at least 5 kindlings in a year.

At least 14 hours of light daily has been found beneficial. Artificial light can be provided in winter when daylight hours are less than 14 hours. A 40 watt bulb every 10 feet works satisfactorily. Such a lighting programme provides better conception in winter. The conception rate decreases during winter which can be prevented by increasing the daily feed allotment to does by 25-50 per cent. A cyclic breeding programme (Table 4) is recommended in ideal broiler rabbit farming. The breeding should be planned in such a way that about 3 to 5 litters per doe are obtained per year during multiplicative stage.

Table 4 : Spread of annual cyclic breeding and growth activity

		Spread over of breeding and growth details			
Month	**Parameter**	**First batch**	**Second batch**	**Third batch**	**Fourth batch**
January	Breeding				
February	Kindling	Born, growth			
March	Breeding	Growth			
April	Kindling	Growth, sold	Born, growth		
May			Growth		
June	Breeding		Growth, sold		
July	Kindling			Born, growth	
August				Growth	
September	Breeding			Growth, sold	
October	Kindling				Born, growth
November					Growth
December					Growth, sold

Male rabbits can be used for mating until they are about 3-4 years old. In order to prevent inbreeding depression, rabbits from the same family should not be bred. Using bucks from different units and sire lines is always beneficial. Therefore, male rabbit should be replaced about once every year. After three to four years, the full grown female rabbits should be replaced either by new purchases or females of own farm. Care should be taken that bucks and does are always housed separately. Housing does together leads to 'pseudo pregnancy', keeping bucks and does together leads to castration of bucks by does and housing only bucks together leads to fight and injuries. The male to female ratio should be 1: 5 for efficient breeding of rabbits. A mature buck can successfully mate 4-6 does a week. Buck should not be overfed to avoid overweight and decreased libido. Productive and reproductive data of bucks and does should be maintained.

11. Housing

Housing system depends on the location of rabbitry, local climate and size of the enterprise. Neat design and comfort are essential (Fig. 8). There are three types of housings systems - shed cage system, hutch system and colony system.

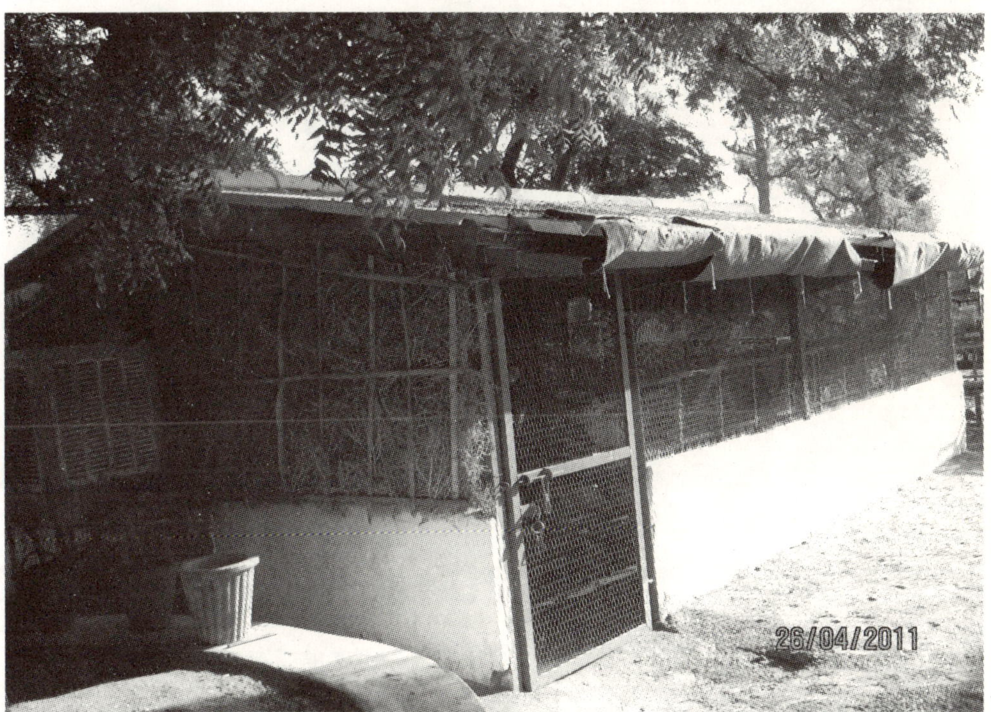

Fig. 8 : Rabbit shed

11.1 Shed cage system

In the shed cage system (indoor housing system), the cages are arranged inside the sheds in single, two or three tier system (Fig. 9). In single tier, they are either placed on wooden or metal stands or suspended by wire from the roof. In the two-tier system, they are placed in a staggered step system or a single rack with trays placed between the cages. The three-tier system is an extension of the two-tier system. Long and narrow buildings with single tier cages are easier to ventilate than wide buildings or the buildings with multiple tiers of cages. The floor should not be of solid concrete, mud floor is the best. Rabbitry must be equipped with lights to provide extra hours of lighting during night. The roofing should preferably be of asbestos, wood, thatch or other locally available material. The cages are commonly made with wire mesh and wood or iron angles (Fig. 10). The bottom of the cage should be made of galvanized welded 16 gauge wire mesh.

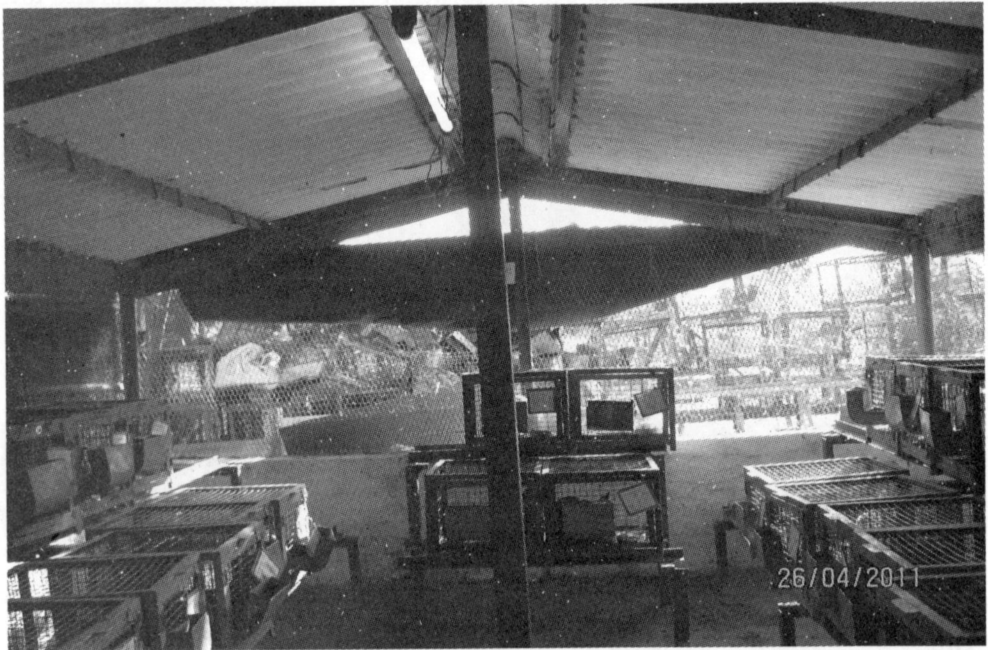

Fig. 9 : Cage arrangement in shed

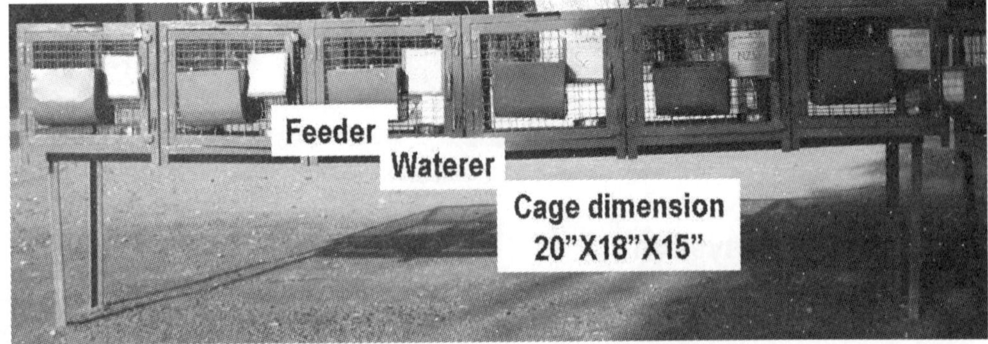

Fig. 10 : Construction design of cages

The nest box measures 50 cm x 30 cm in floor area with 30 cm height upto half the length of the box (Fig. 11). The bottom of the nest box should have a number of small holes to drain the urine. This can be used as a separate box or as an attachment with the single cage.

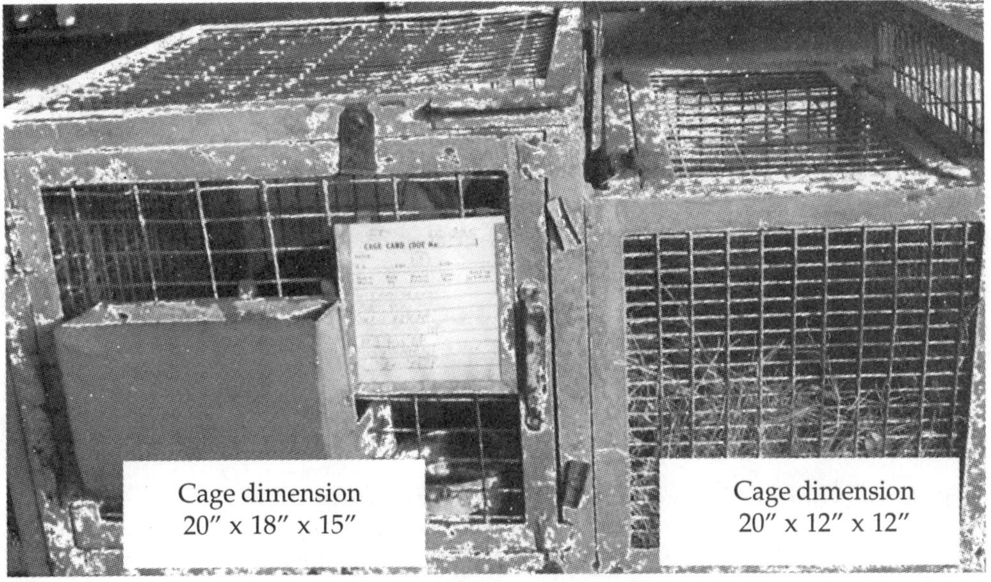

Fig. 11 : Rabbit cage with nest box

11.1.1 Feeders and waterers

The feeders are made of galvanized iron sheets. They are 'L' or 'J' shaped and are arranged such that feed can be poured from outside. The edges should be rounded off. The height of the feeders should be 5-7 cm above the cage floor to avoid contamination by urine, faeces and water. Hay feeders are attached to the outside of the cage. Aluminium bowl of 500 ml capacity or baked earthen bowls are used to contain drinking water.

11.2 Hutch system

The hutch system is a self-contained cage-cum-nest box, which can be moved around as the need arises. The hutches have their own foot and roofing. There can be 2-20 hutches in a row. This system is generally used if the numbers of rabbits are small and they are reared in the backyard or orchards. Generally 5- 6 rabbit can be kept in each compartment. This system is otherwise called 'outdoor housing system'. The hutch should have foot upto waist level. Floor area should be 60 cm x 80 cm with a built in nest box (60 cm x 30 cm) on the sides or at the back. A V-shaped partition is used for separating two hutches and also for feeding hay. The height should be 53 cm at the front and 37 cm at the back. The back of the hutch and the sides of the nest box are covered with wooden or asbestos sheets. Waterers and feeders are to be provided separately inside the hutches (Rajendran 2007).

11.3 Colony system

In colony system, more number of rabbits can be kept together from weaning to marketing age (90 days).The walls of the colony house system can be cemented to half the height and the remaining half is made with wire net. The floor is concrete and roof can be made using corrugated tin or bamboo. In a room of 10 x 10 x 10 ft size, 25 to 30 rabbits can be kept (Ghosh *et al.* 2008). The disadvantage with the system is that the rabbits develop soreness by digging the floor and fight among themselves leading to injuries.

11.4 Points to be considered before constructing a rabbit house

- Rabbit house must have adequate space otherwise stress and injury may occur.
- House must be rainproof as rabbits cannot tolerate wet conditions.
- Rooms should be well ventilated and free from dust.
- Preferable temperature is 10-25°C but meat breed can tolerate temperature as high as 35-40°C. Keeping indoor temperature 32°C with relative humidity of 66-70% is advantageous, so housing material which can cool the room should be used.
- Rabbitry should be at a quiet place as animals get frightened easily by sudden noise and presence of predators.
- Rooms should be clean and hygienic and a well drained site is important.
- House must be in east-west direction to give protection from the sun.

12. Management

Rabbits are very gentle and timid animals. They are scared of almost everything and can get easily disturbed by any sudden action or noise resulting in injuries. It is advisable to keep at the farm only the persons familiar to the animals and visitors should be avoided. Rabbits require regular attention and a fixed timetable. Cleanliness, ventilation and close observation of rabbits are important. One labour is sufficient to look after 500 caged rabbits.

12.1 Care of newborn

A pregnant doe should be shifted to the kindling cage at 28th day of pregnancy. Pregnant doe generally starts making nest by plucking her own hair one or two days before kindling (delivery). If she does not pluck hair, some fine quality straw should be provided in the cage (Fig. 12). The average fecundity rate is 6-8 kits (Fig. 13). The pups are 'altricial' i.e. deaf, dumb and blind at the time of birth. The kits should not be touched until some emergency comes and gloves should be used in such a case. The dead or defective kits from the cage should be removed. Sometimes does kills her own kits or does not give milk, especially after first kindling. If that particular doe repeats the same habit at the next kindling, it is advisable to cull that doe. Doe gives milk once or twice daily, so all the kits should be kept together for proper feeding. Care should be taken that *ad libitum* feed and water is available in the cages before and during the delivery period. Water and feed deficiency at the time of delivery can lead to cannibalism. In broiler rabbits, the survival rate of young ones till maturity or the age of slaughter is 85-90%. Eyes of the kits generally open at the age of 10 days. Hair start growing from two weeks of age. At three weeks of age, kits start taking feed along with mother's milk. If mother's milk is insufficient for the kits, they can be fed to a healthy foster mother with low litter size within the first 2-3 days of kindling. Appropriate material, mainly low grade cotton or soft hay, should be used for bedding in the nest box. Bedding material should be replaced at regular intervals. The best time to wean the kits is at 42 days. No sudden change in feed is advisable. While weaning, the doe should be removed and the kits should be left in the cage in which they were born.

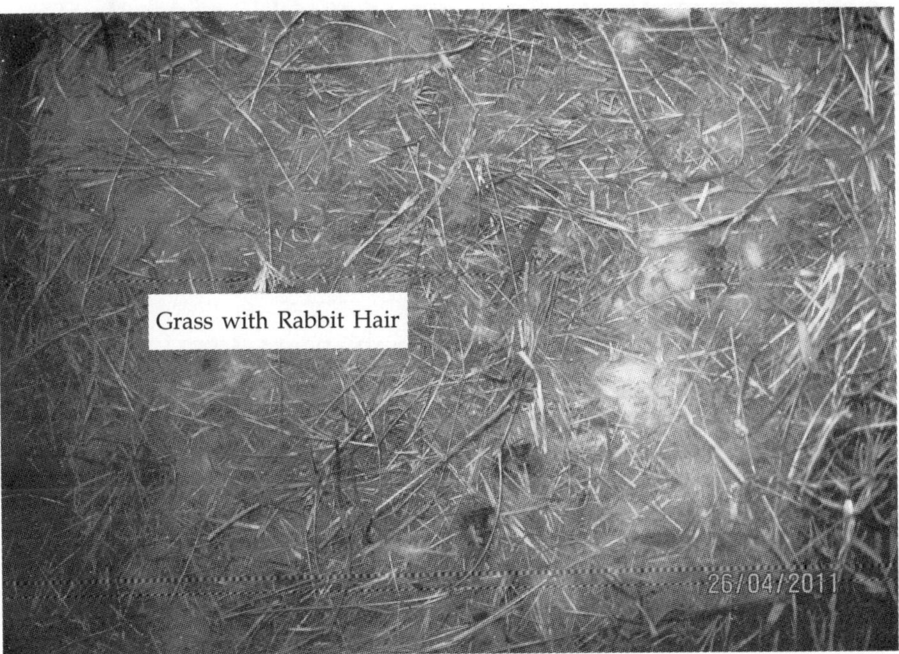

Fig. 12 : Bedding material in nest box

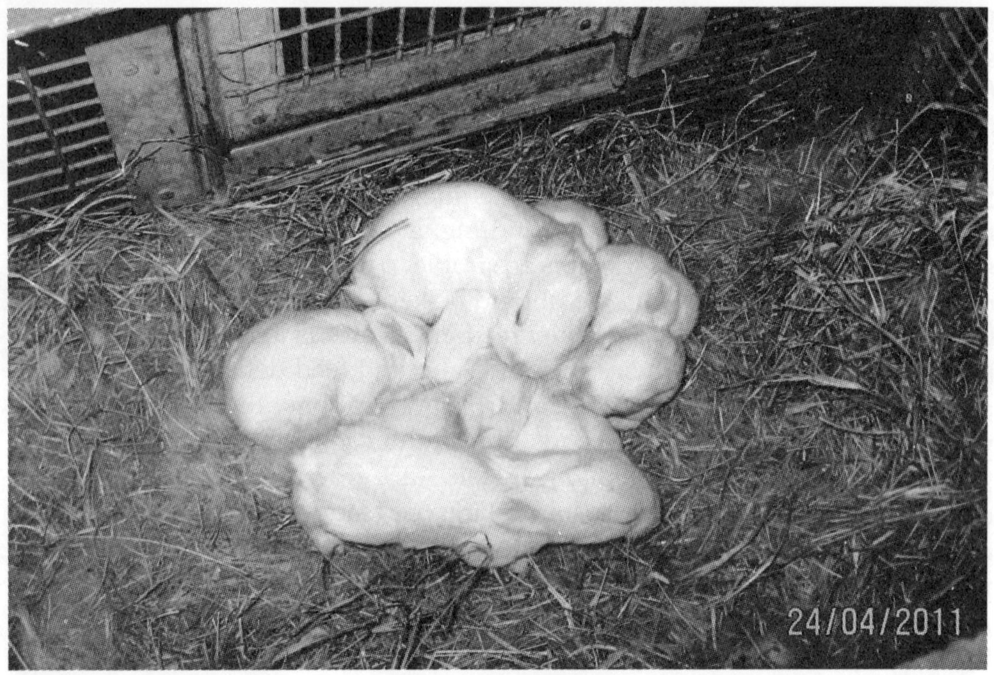

Fig. 13 : Rabbit kits

12.2 Handling

Rabbits should be lifted gently by the scruff of their neck and not by their legs or ears alone. Broiler rabbits can be handled by firm and gentle grasping of their loin region upto 15 weeks. Other rabbits may be handled by grasping a fold of skin over the shoulder with one hand and placing the other hand under the rump to support the weight of the animal. While carrying, rabbits need to be supported from the bottom. Care should be taken as not to startle the animals.

12.3 Identification

Tattooing in the rabbit's ear makes a permanent system for identification. The inner side of the ear is cleaned with alcohol and perforated with a tattooing instrument. Tattoo ink or Indian ink should be rubbed over the spot. Ear tags are now more popular for identification of animals.

12.4 Sexing

The sex of young rabbits may be determined a day or two following kindling. A kit can be restrained on its back in the palm with its head facing the person. The genitals should be pressed gently with fingers to expose the reddish mucous membrane; if it is a male kit the mucous membrane protrudes sufficiently to form a circle. If it is a female kit, the mucous membrane protrudes and forms a slit which has a slight depression at the end. Generally, the distance between the penis and anus is greater than the distance between the vulva and anus. Until the technique of sexing rabbits has been perfected, it may be good to sex the kits at weaning.

12.5 Herd replacement

One doe for every 12 does in production and one buck for every 5 bucks in service should be replaced per month.

12.6 Protection from heat stress

Rabbits are susceptible to heat stress as they don't have sweat glands. They respond differently to sudden acute exposure to high temperature than to chronic exposure to high temperatures. Shady trees around rabbit sheds help preventing heat stress. Exhaust fan, desert cooler and fogger can be provided in the rabbit shed for protection from heat stress (Fig. 14-16).

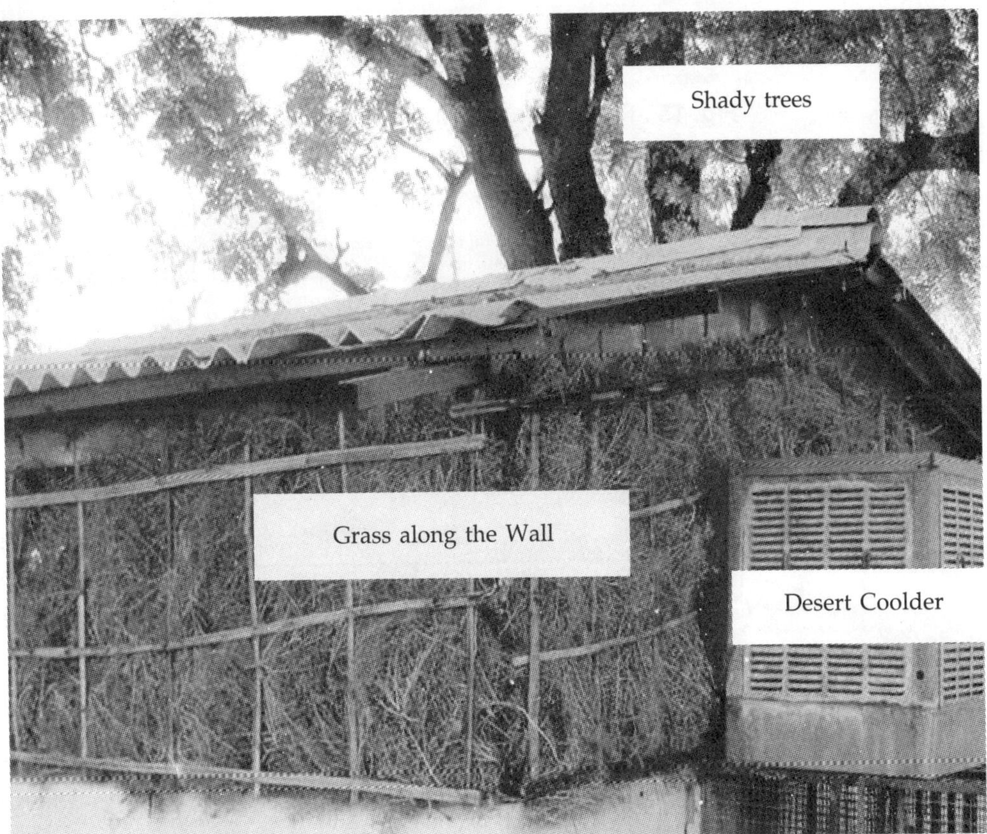

Fig. 14 : Heat protection arrangements in rabbit shed

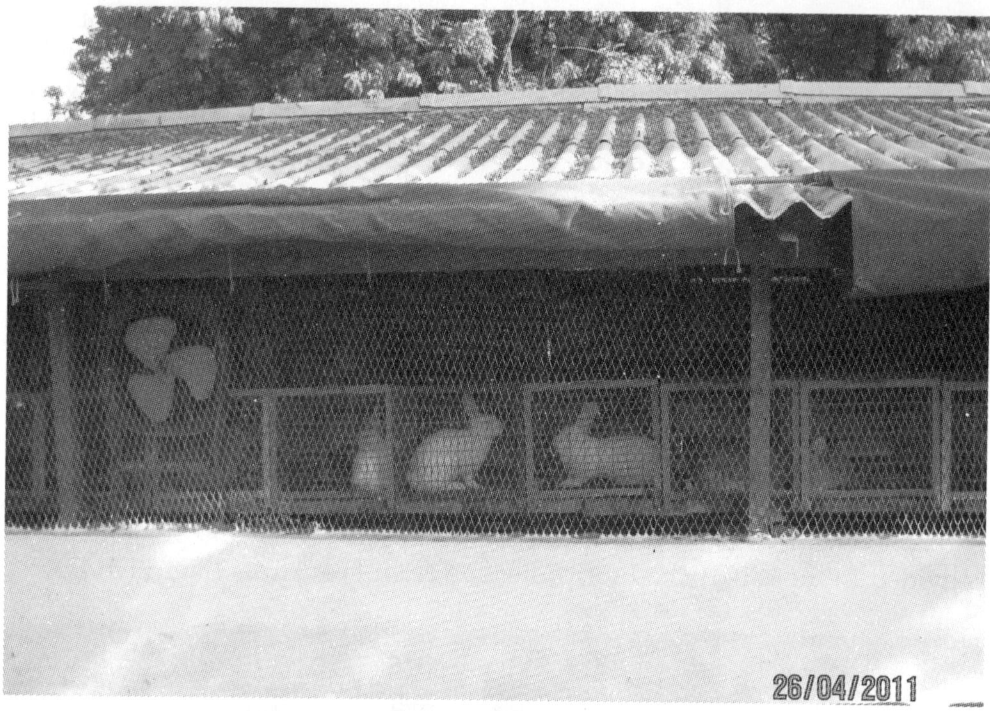

Fig. 15 : Rabbit shed fitted with exhaust fan

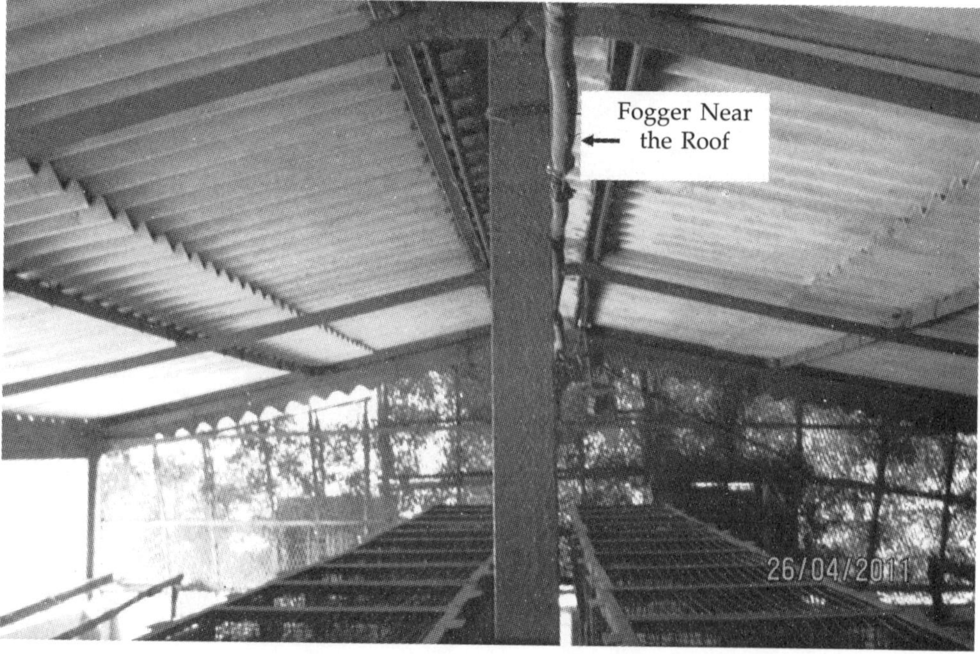

Fig. 16 : Fogger in the rabbit shed

12.7 Sanitation

Cages should be cleaned with wire brush daily. Cages can also be kept in direct sunlight (once a week) for disinfection. Ammonia production should be minimized. Lime powder has to be sprayed underneath the cages. Adequate ventilation and close observation of rabbits are important. Sick rabbits should be isolated immediately and the colony treatment should be started if required. The best way to disinfect the cages is to burn the inside of cages with a flame gun.

12.8 Health management

Clean sanitary conditions of rabbit cages, sheds and equipment, balanced feed and fresh clean water are essential to prevent chances of infection. The rabbits should be prevented from coming in contact with the faeces. Over crowding should be avoided. Proper ventilation should be provided. Flies which may act as carriers of the infection should be kept under control in the rabbitry. Rabbit cages should be disinfected with blow lamp after every shearing and the kindling cage before the doe is shifted and after weaning. The carcasses of the rabbits dying due to infectious diseases should be incinerated or buried to prevent the diseases from spreading. Rabbits suffer from many diseases; some important ones have been described in Table 5.

Table 5 : Some common diseases of rabbits

Disease	Major symptoms	Prevention and control measures
Pasteurellosis (Snuffles)	Discharges from nostrils, wiping of nose with paws, loss of appetite, high rise of temperature.	400000 IU of penicillin and 0.5 g streptomycin given I/M
Coccidiosis	Diarrhoea with blood smears, loss of appetite and dehydration. May cause death in 24-36 hours.	Coccidiostats like sulphaquinoxaline + sulphamerazine @ 0.02 to 0.10% in drinking water, strict hygienic measures
Body mange (Ear canker)	Intense pruritis, scratching, scaling of the skin, loss of fur and animal becomes weak	Application of ascabiol lotion, ivermectin injection 0.02 ml/ Kg body wt (S/C), strict hygienic measures
Mastitis	Mammary glands become painful with a change in colour and the doe will not let her litter to suck and kits will probably die.	Antibiotics, try to foster the kits if they are very young.

Heat stroke	Lie in lateral recumbency, panting, tip of ear may turn pink	Sprinkling of water, adequate cool drinking water, electrolyte and vitamin C
Myxomatosis	Oedema of head, conjunctivitis, milky discharge from eye, poor appetite,	Broad spectrum antibiotic, control of vector, vaccination
Wryneck	Permanent turning of neck to one side, unable to eat, weakness.	Affected animals should be slaughtered.
Enteritis complex	Subnormal temperature, crouched posture, roughned hair coat, gelatinous mucus with dry feaces and bloat	No successful treatment, tetracycline in feed @ 100 g/ ton feed, adequate amount of fibre should be given. Reduce soluble carbohydrate from diet.
Hair ball occlusion	Wool gets accumulated in stomach and blocks normal passage of food.	Treat the animal with mineral oil or neopeptin or fresh pineapple juice.
Hindquarter paralysis (Paraplegia)	Sudden jerk, excitement, paralysis, loss of control over urination and defecation	Affected animals should be slaughtered.
Shorehock	Inflamed areas or sores on the under surface of hind paws, weakness and dehydration	Sores should be opened and antiseptic dressing should be applied. Provide soft bedding during treatment period.
Conjunctivitis	Reddening of conjunctiva, mucopurulent discharge from eye	Wash eye with boric lotion, apply sulphacetamide ointment or eye drops.

13. Backyard Rabbitry

Rabbits are the only 'micro livestock' suitable for rearing by small farmers and landless agricultural labourers with simple housing in their backyards and can be fed with forages, agricultural by-products and kitchen wastes. In fact, backyard rabbitries are best suited for the country to increase the per capita income and animal protein availability.

Backyard rabbit rearing is a potential means of improving the nutritional status of low-income people. A unit of one male and three female rabbits can provide one slaughter per week round the year. The edible meat per slaughter will be about 1 Kg, which is sufficient for a small family for one time meal. The meat can also be allowed to store in the animal without slaughtering it (biological refrigeration) and when it is needed the animal can be slaughtered.

Villagers can keep few rabbits in their backyard to produce enough meat to satisfy the needs of a family. Weeds, tropical forages, vegetable tops and table scraps can be used as feed for them. Apart from meat, rabbit skins are used for various apparel items such as fur coats, fur garments, fur trimmings, toys, hats and fancy items.

14. Rabbit Products

14.1 Rabbit meat

Young rabbits can attain about 2 Kg live weight in 12-14 weeks on *ad lib* concentrate and high roughage diet. An adult animal may dress out at 50 to 55%. About 70% rabbit carcass is composed of edible meat as compared to 50% in chicken. Meat is very tender, highly delicious and juicy. Its flavour is not strong and it is comparable to the taste of turkey. Rabbit meat is white meat and constitutes healthy food. It is a lean meat rich in protein of high biological value with high level of essential amino acids, low purine contents and absence of uric acid (Hernandez 2008). Cholesterol is almost half of beef and chicken meat. The unsaturated fatty acid content in rabbit meat is 63% of total fatty acids and the ratio of n-6 and n-3 fatty acids is 7.4-7.5, which is advantageous from nutrition point of view. It has low bone to meat ratio, about 20-21% protein, 7-10% fat and produces about 800 calories per 450 g meat consumption. In comparison to the meat of other common species like poultry, cattle, turkey, sheep and goat, rabbit meat has more protein, less fat and less calorie content.

14.2 Rabbit manure

An adult rabbit on an average produces about 100-150 Kg manure per year. Rabbit manure is considered to be highest in nitrogen among all domesticated animal species. It has about 3.7% nitrogen, 1.3% phosphoric acid and 3.5% potash (Mahajan 2002). Thus, rabbit manure may constitute an additional source of income for the farmers.

14.3 Rabbit wool

Angora rabbit produces one of the finest fibres. Angora rabbit pelage has three types of fibres: (i) the bristle or guard hairs (longest, thick and tight hairs with 25-100μ diameter), (ii) the awn hairs (medium in length having a thick and tight top and a thin curly body with 16-30μ diameter, and (iii) the down hairs (shortest, thin and curly fibres lying under guard hairs with 6-18μ average fibre diameter). The bristle content varies among breeds and is normally within permissible limits and prevents felting of fleece on the body of the rabbit and provides fullness to the Angora rabbit yarn. All hairs have a hollow structure-medulla, characterized by tiny air spaces which makes them lighter due to low specific weight than wool and increases their insulating/heat penetration properties. Clean, pure and soft Angora rabbit hairs with an average fibre diameter of 13 μ, staple length > 6 cm and guard hairs < 5% is graded as A or first grade and is preferred by the industry (Sharma and Karim 2010). The wool from Angora rabbit is removed by depilation, plucking, combing or shearing. Shearing is the most common method of wool removal. Wool is clipped 4-5 times in a year.

14.4 Fur skins

Properly cured or processed skin fetches good price. Processed fur skin can be sold as skin or by making fur garments which may fetch better price to farmers. Salt alum method is the most common method of skin processing.

14.5 Rabbit milk

Milk production by rabbit is an important indicator of growth and health of young rabbits and slaughter weight achieved at 12 weeks of age. Mechanical or manual milking, though possible, is not a usual and practical method to measure milk production. An accurate indirect method is to weigh the female before and after the once a day nursing event or weighing the litter mates before and after suckling. Gulyani (2010) reported 4.37 Kg milk yield in Soviet Chinchilla, 4.33 Kg in White Giant and 4.18 Kg in Black Brown in a 35 days lactation period. He also reported sudden decline in milk yield if lactation continued beyond 28 days. Compared with cow and sow milk, rabbit milk is much more concentrated in fat (12.9 g/100 g), protein (12.3 g/100 g) and energy (8.4 MJ/Kg) which explains the extremely rapid growth of the young (within 3 weeks it attains body weight 6 time its birth weight). Near absence of lactose (< 2 g/100 g) is another characteristic of rabbit milk (Maertens 2008). Apart from nutrition, other factors that influence the milk yield of rabbits include the number of suckling kits, the parity order (primiparous vs multiparous), breed and the gestation overlapping degree (rapid decline after 17-20 days of gestation).

15. Constraints in Rabbit Farming

Rabbit farming has a great scope for economic development, but there are some bottleneck and limiting factors which hinder rabbit farming in big way.

1. Unavailability of quality parent stock of pure breed rabbits. Consequently, unhygienic, poor quality rabbits are sold at a high cost.
2. Capital cost is high for large scale and commercial rabbit farming as it requires costly infrastructure and cages.

3. Availability of balanced and compound pellet feed in the country is limited and expensive.
4. Since there is no vaccination for rabbits, improper and inadequate prophylaxis leads to severe mortality in young stock of rabbits (kits and weaners).
5. Animal husbandry department is not paying desirable level of attention to rabbit farming despite the importance of rabbit farming in rural economy.
6. Marketing channels are not well defined and demand, supply and prices are always fluctuating.
7. Rabbit farming needs definite skill. It is not like other livestock farming. One should be well trained on all aspects of rabbit husbandry
8. Caged rabbits need all the nutrients in a balanced form. Deficiency of nutrients (minerals and vitamins) adversely affects the overall performance of the rabbits.
9. Due to poor thermoregulatory mechanism, hot climate of tropics is a major constraint in production.

16. Research Initiatives to Improve Rabbit Production in India

The major research initiatives for raising rabbits for meat, fur skins and hair were undertaken by the CSWRI at NTRS in Himachal Pradesh. Four strains of broiler rabbits viz. White Giant (WG), Grey Giant (GG), New Zealand White (NZW) and Soviet Chinchilla (SC) were introduced in 1979 to study the performance of purebreds and their reciprocal crosses with respect to litter size at kindling, litter size at weaning, growth in litter live weight up to weaning, number of kindling per year, kit survival, bodyweight at slaughter, dressing percentage and percentage of different cuts. Later, Black Brown (BB) was developed by crossing SC and GG. Similar studies were also carried out at the main campus of CSWRI and at the Southern Regional Temperate Research Station at Mannavanur in Kodai Hills in Tamil Nadu. Studies on thermoregulatory responses to hot-semiarid environment were also carried out. In semi-arid hot environment at Avikanagar in Rajasthan, the number of kindling per doe per year ranged from 3.3-3.7 (average 3.5), with kits born ranging from 22.4-25.9 (average 23.9), and the kits weaned ranging from 15.5-17.3 (average 16.7) in WG, SC and BB. The highest performance was in WG. The litter size at birth ranged from 6.46 to 7.26, at weaning (6 weeks) from 4.92 to 6.17, litter weight at birth from 258 to 391 g and litter weight at weaning (6 weeks) from 3.02 Kg to 3.68 Kg in GG, WG, NZW, SC and BB (Gulyani 2010). Mortality ranged from 20-25%.

Over all conception rate in broiler rabbit has been reported as 50.25% and number of services per conception as 1.98 (Kumar *et al.* 1998). The highest conception rate has been seen in SC. Carcass yield and percentage of different cuts has also been studied in SC and GG. The pre-slaughter weight has been recorded as 2.13 to 2.21 Kg with 57% and 56% dressing percentage of pre-slaughter weight in the two breeds. The selection in German Angora for fibre production has shown a reasonable increase from 751 g to 956 g in breeding stock maintained at NTRS during 2001-05. They produced wool having staple length of about 6.1 cm, fiber diameter of 12.9-13.4μ and 2.5 to 4.1% guard hair (Sharma and Karim 2010). The British Angora had relatively poorer annual fibre production. The Russian Angora also had performance similar to British Angora. It has been shown that annual wool yield could be improved with the demarcation of separate wool production and reproduction flocks. The wool production in the wool production flock was higher by 10 to 30% as compared to the reproduction flock.

The physiological studies on rabbit semen carried out under the semi-arid conditions of CSWRI have shown that semen quality of RA and SC remains good from November to the first fortnight of April and declined from second fortnight of April. While in the temperate region the semen quality deteriorates during extreme winter. During summer, the semen quality of angora bucks is more affected because of its heavy fleece as compared to broiler rabbits. It has been shown that castration of Angora males results in 17-21% increase in their wool yield. Since 50% animals in rabbitry are males there is scope of substantially improving the wool yield in this way. Studies on the physiological responses of rabbits in semi-arid region have revealed that rabbits are most susceptible to heat stress (CSWRI Report 1998).

The NTRS at Garsa is now a National Germ Plasm Centre for Angora rabbits and is meeting the demand of research and development organizations. With the initiative and support of the United Nations Development Programme (UNDP) through the Central Wool Development Board (CWDB), Angora rabbit farming has increased self-employment and foreign exchange earnings through rabbit farming in hilly areas of Uttarakhand, Darjeeling and Sikkim. The Defence Research and Development Organization (DRDO) is propagating Angora rabbits in Pithoragarh district successfully. In Jammu and Kashmir, Angora rabbit farming is regaining after initial setback during 1990 due to sharp fall in Angora fibre prices and other input constraints. Angora fibre is being blended with Merino wool and pashmina to establish most versatile shawl industry in the state.

17. Future Strategy to Enhance Rabbit Farming in India

The following strategic steps can help in popularising and strengthening rabbit farming in the country.

1. Development of linkage between various stakeholders involved in broiler as well Angora rabbit production
2. Development of dual purpose breeds instead of having separate rabbit breeds for fibre and meat/fur skins, which may be used for fibre and meat production
3. Organization of marketing channel for rabbit meat, fibre and skin
4. Formation of self-help groups to improve production and marketing
5. Government support to rabbit farmers through subsidies and loans
6. Popularisation of Angora rabbit farming in hilly and temperate climatic areas and broiler rabbit farming in other parts of the country
7. Steps to take advantage of special quality of rabbit meat for getting premium price
8. Embryo import of animals in large scale to overcome the problem of breeding stock
9. Use of embryo transfer technology and artificial insemination for rapid multiplication of germplasm
10. Development of vaccines for common rabbit diseases
11. Strengthening of research and extension concerning rabbit production
12. Development and strengthening of facilities for utilization of by-products

18. Conclusion

Rabbit is considered to be one of the best among 'micro-livestocks' by the FAO and other national and international agencies. Rabbit production is of recent origin in India but it offers huge advantages over other livestock. Due to small size, high prolificacy and short generation interval, rabbit farming is poised to take great leap forwards through the length and breadth of the country. The fast changing scenario of climate change, decreasing pasture land and growing demand for meat is certain to help this industry to grow. It has been amply demonstrated that rabbits can be raised in any part of country and that rabbitry is economically viable both at small as well as large scale. A sustainable system of rabbit production can be developed by using renewable on-farm resources such as local breeds, feedstuffs from forage or kitchen wastes, local materials for hutches and equipments, and family labour. Small or medium rabbit farming plays great role in the supply of meat, lowering unemployment in urban and rural areas and in farmers' welfare in term of additional income and nutritious food. Rabbit farming can be made more beneficial by integrating it with other agricultural operations. Horticulture, food crops, forest plants nursery and fish farming can benefit from organic fertilizer from rabbits, while plenty of agricultural wastes can be fed to rabbits. Such integration may increase the production both from rabbits and crop farming, while it reduces agricultural residues into a zero-waste system. Considering huge scope of rabbit farming, it seeks better attention of policymakers. It is high time to do away with the constraints faced by rabbit farmers by providing better infrastructure support for germplasm, housing, feeding, healthcare, marketing, training, testing and processing of raw materials.

References

1. CSWRI Report (1998). 35 years of research. Central Sheep and Wool Research Institute, Avikanagar.
2. Ghosh SK, Datt C, Singh NP, Ngachan SV (2008). Broiler rabbit production in Tripura. Publication No. 30, ICAR Research Complex for NEH Region, Tripura Centre, Lembucherra, Tripura.
3. Gulyani R (2010). Broiler rabbit production under prevailing climate change. In: Karim SA *et al.* (Editors) Climate change and stress management: sheep and goat production. Satish Serial Publishing House, New Delhi. pp. 481-496.
4. Hernandez P (2008). Enhancement of nutritional quality and safety in rabbit meat. Proc. 9th World Rabbit Congress, June 10-13, 2008, Verona, Italy. pp. 1287-1299.
5. ICAR (1998). Nutrient requirements of domestic animals. Indian Council of Agricultural Research, New Delhi, India. p. 11.
6. Kumar S, Gulyani R, Singh G, Singh RN (1998). Reproductive efficiency and reproductive performance of broiler rabbit does in semiarid region. Proc. Golden Jubilee Seminar on Sheep, goat and rabbit production and utilization, 24-26 April 1998, Jaipur. p. 33.
7. Maertens L (2008). Milk production in rabbits: quantity and quality. World Rabbit Science 16:35-49.
8. Mahajan G M (2002). Rabbitry. In handbook of Animal Husbandry, Indian Council of Agricultural Research, New Delhi. pp. 326-348.
9. Rajendran AS (2007). Broiler rabbit production http://asrajendiran.blogspot.com/2007/03/commercial-rabbit-production.html. Accessed 10 April 2010.
10. Sharma SR, Karim SA (2010). Angora wool production in country under changing climate and market. In: Karim SA *et al.* (Editors) Climate change and stress management: sheep and goat production. Satish Serial Publishing House, New Delhi. pp. 497-512.

11. Szakály Z, Szigeti O, Berke Sz, Szente V (2006). The market analysis of branded, new generation hungaricums. 98th EAAE Seminar on Marketing dynamics within the global trading system: New perspectives, Chania, Crete, Greece, 29 June-2 July 2006.

12. Tang FK (2002). Current production and predicted future of rabbit industries in China Chinese J Rabbit Farming 1:3-7.

□□□

Chapter 7

Animal Genetic Resources : Conservation, Utilization and Sustainable Development

A. S. KHANNA
Department of Animal Genetics & Breeding, College of Veterinary Sciences,
Lala Lajpat Rai University of Veterinary and Animal Sciences, Hisar-125004

Contents

1. Introduction

Having passed through an era of green revolution, the growth in agricultural production has slowed down, while the growth in animal production is still keeping up an encouraging pace. The production of milk has shown a consistent growth rate of 5%, egg production of over 7% and meat production still higher, in addition to non-food benefits of livestock. The contribution of animal production is estimated at about 6% to GDP and about 25% to the over all agriculture production. India has pride possession of large livestock wealth both in terms of number as well as diversity, which is endeavored with the capacity to sustain under harsh climatic conditions and scarce resources.

Animal production is the backbone of agriculture sector in the economy and social development of our country. The range of products and services that are provided by Animal Genetic Resources (AnGRs) to the society in general and the farmers in particular include food, fibre, transport and fuel. In addition, important inputs are also provided to crop production as manure and draft power. Indigenous AnGRs also have great non-use values like adaptability to harsh climatic conditions, better disease resistance and survival on meager resources and agri-waste. *Panch gavya* utility of indigenous cattle to improve public health and immunity is their special value. This optional value of indigenous AnGRs increases the capacity of livestock production systems to withstand future challenges like emergence of epidemic diseases. Sustainable utilization of animal genetic resources for food and agriculture is recommended by FAO as the preferred avenue for safeguarding genetic diversity.

Sustainable development is defined by FAO as the management and conservation of the natural resource base and orientation of technological and institutional change so as to ensure the attainment and continued satisfaction of human needs for present and future generations. Such sustainable development in animal agriculture emphasizes upon conservation of land, water, plant and animal genetic resources in such a way that it is environmentally non-degrading, technically appropriate, economically viable and socially acceptable.

In respect of domesticated biological diversity, modern production systems heavily depend on few varieties, strains, breeds, crosses etc. of plants and animals. Farm AnGR are those animal species that are used for the production of food and agriculture and populations within each species, which can further be classified as wild and feral, landraces and primary populations, standard breeds, selected lines and any conserved material.

Management of AnGR includes the formation of technical policies and logistic operations involved in understanding (characterization), using and developing (utilization), maintaining (conservation) and assessing and sharing the benefits of AnGR.

Utilization of AnGR has been defined by FAO (1999) as the use and development of AnGR for the production of food and agriculture. The use in production systems of AnGRs that already possess high levels of adaptive fitness to the environment concerned and the deployment of sound genetic principles will facilitate sustainable development of AnGRs and the sustainable intensification of the production systems themselves. The wise use of AnGRs is possible without depleting domestic animal diversity.

Development of AnGRs includes a broad mix of ongoing activities that must be well planned and executed for success, and compounded over time, hence with high value. It requires careful definition of breeding objectives and the planning, establishment and maintenance of effective and efficient animal recording and breeding strategies.

Local livestock breeds have suffered neglect and degeneration due to changing needs and low economic viability, which has also contributed to endangerment of certain forms.

The resource conservation in its widest terms means judicious management of resources to improve quality of life of farmers and society of the present as well as the future generations. The modern conservation includes protection of ecology, habitat and genetic level conservation along with retaining and enhancing the production potential to meet the needs and aspirations of future generations. It is now accepted that conservation of animal genetic resources is essential but economic compulsions have overriding influence and often jeopardize the attempts to preserve them. Convention on Biological Diversity (CBD) has heightened the awareness about the need for conservation of biological diversity.

International agreement on Intellectual Property Rights (IPR) has also strengthened its regime in the areas of biodiversity conservation as well as in context to emerging biotechnologies. There is need to develop the awareness and understanding of IPR in the following contexts:

- To take an overview of the national responses to the international negotiations and legal developments
- To present in holistic perspective the issues involved specially in relation to protection and registration of breeds, varieties, strains etc. and technology transfer
- To raise some key points in the negotiating strategies to underline the need for legal and policy measures, taking into consideration the national and international dimensions

International Union for Protection of New Varieties of Plants (UPOV) Convention in 1991 decided that a variety can be protected or patented provided it is:

i. New and distinct from other existing known varieties
ii. Uniform and homogenous
iii. Stable in terms of its marked traits

It authorized a breeder of protected variety for production or reproduction; conditioning for the purpose of propagation; offering for sale, marketing, exporting, importing and stocking for any purpose.

2. Present Status of AnGRs and Strategies for their Conservation

AnGR Conservation in broader sense is inclusive of:

- Ensuring the maintenance of all relevant AnGRs and their sustainable utilization to achieve the breeding goals
- Planning and reviewing the state of current operational capacity
- Ensuring that genetic resources are available to farmers and breeders in the future

Utilization of livestock species began about 12,000 years ago, which led to their domestication gradually. Out of about 40 domesticated mammalian species, only 14 are important for livestock farming. India is the seventh largest country in the world with almost $3/4^{th}$ population dependent on agriculture and livestock farming as major occupation.

- The Indian subcontinent is rich in domestic animal resources having 64 breeds of cattle, 23 of buffaloes, 34 of goats, 62 breeds of sheep, 10 of camels, 7 of horses, 8 of pigs and about 28 of poultry.

- India in addition to almost all the breeds of water buffalo has a pride possession of about one-ninth breeds of cattle, one-fifth breeds of sheep and one-third breeds of goat available in the world.
- According to the FAO World Watch List 1995 estimate, three breeds are lost every two weeks all over the world due to one or the more reasons.
- Well-defined breeds constitute around 18% of the nations total population, while rest are nondescript.
- About 30% breeds out of about 5,000 identified breeds of livestock are at high risk of extinction.

FAO has identified following imperative actions by each country for conservation of domestic AnGRs.

- Each country must identify and understand the unique genetic resources so that the global gene pools for each of the important domestic animal species used for food and agriculture can be made sustainable.
- The livestock diversity should be made to increase production and productivity under the local sustainable agricultural systems that meet the demands for specific product types.
- There should be a sound arrangement with each country to monitor all the genetic resources, particularly where small populations have been left or are being replaced by one breed or the other.
- All the unique genetic resources must be preserved immediately even if they are poor in production as they may have other traits of value in animal adaptability or survivability under given ecological niche.
- More number of people involved in the management of these resources must be trained at national or global level.

2.1 Status of AnGRs

The Domestic Animal Diversity available for different livestock species in India is presented in Table 1 while the animal breeds facing extinction are listed in Box 1. Table 2 reveals the criteria for putting a breed in the endangered category.

Table 1 : Domestic Animal Diversity in India

Species	Local breeds	Regional transboundary	International transboundary
Buffalo (23)	Assamese, Banni. Bhadaw ari, Chilka, Diyara, Godavari, Jerangi, Manipuri, Kalahandi, Manda, Marrathwada, Nagpuri, Pandharpuri, Sambalpur, Parlekhemundi, South Kanara, Toda (17)	Mehsana, Surti, Nili-Ravi, Tarai (4)	Jaffarabadi, Murrah (2)
Cattle (64)	Alambadi, Amritmahal, Bachaur, Bargur, Binjha rpuri, Cutchi, Dangi, Deoni, Frieswal, Gangatiri, Gaolao, Ghumsuri, Gujamavu, Hallikar, Jersind, Kankrej, Kappilliyan, Karan Fries, Karan Swiss, Kenkatha, Khamala, Khasi, Kherigarh, Krishna Valley, Kumauni, Ladakhi, Malnad Gidda, Malvi, Mampati, Manapari, Mewati, Mhaswad, Motu, Nagami, Nagori, Nimari, Ponwar, Pullikulam, Punganur, Red Purnea, Ramgarhi, Rathi, Red Kandhari, Sanchori, Shahabadi, Son Valley, Tarai, Taylor, Tho Tho, Umblachery, Vechur, Zosial . (52)	Hariana, Hissar, Kangayam, Siri, Khillari. Sunandini (6)	Sahiwal. Ongole Red Sindhi, Gir, Nelore, Tharparkar (6)
Goat (34)	Andaman Feral Goat, Assamese Hill, Attapady Black, Baigani, Barren goat, Bidari, Changthangi, Chegu, Dalua, Ganjam, Gohilwadi, Himalayan ibex, Himalayan Tahr, Indian Mohair, Jhakrana, Kannai Adu, Kutchi, Malabari, Marwari, Mehsana, Nilgiri Tahr, Osmanabadi, Ramdhan, Sangamneri, Sirohi, Surti, Teressa, Zalawadi. (28)	Bengal, Gaddi, Tibetan (3)	Barbari, Beetal, Jamunapari (3)
Sheep (62)	Avikalin, Avimanns, Avivastra, Bagri, Balangir, Bellary, Berari, Bhakarwal, Bharat Merino, Biangi, Bonpala, Changthangi, Chokla, Chotanagpuri, Coimbatore, Dkshini, Deccani, Desi, Dhamda, Dumba, Gaddi, Ganjam, Garole, Godavari, Gurez, Hassan, Indian Karakul, Jaisalmeri, Jalauni,	Hissardale, Madras Red, Poonchi, Tibetan (4)	

	Karanah, Kashmir Meri no, Kashmir Valley, Kenguri, Kheri, Kilakarsal, Magra, Malpura, Mandya, Marathwada, Marwari, Mecheri, Munjal, Muzaffarnagri, Nali, Nellore, Nilgiri, Patanwadi, Pugal, Ramnad White, Rampur Bushair, Vembur. Sangamneri, Sardarsamand, Shahabadi, Shapo, Sonadi, Telengana, Tiruchy Black (58)		
Yak (5)	Arunachal, Chour -gau, Himachal, Ladakhi, Sikkim (5)		
Pig (8)	Andaman wild pig, Ankamali, Boer, Dashi, Doom, Ghungroo, Nicobari (7)	Ghori (1)	
Horse (7)	Deccani, Kathia wari, Spiti Pony, Manipuri Pony, Marwari, Zaniskari Pony (6)	Bhutia (1)	
Ass (3)	Indian, Indian wild, Kiang (3)		
Camel (10)	Bikaneri, Jaisalmeri, Kutchi, Malvi, Marwari, Mewari, Mewati, Sindhi, Shekhawati, Indian Bectrian (10)		
Rabbit (3)	British Angora, Grey Giant, Russian Angora (3)		
Chicken (28)	Cari Gold, Debendra, Dhanraja, Gramalakshmi, Gramapriya, Kadaknath, Kalinga Brown, Kashmir Faverolla, Krishna -J, Miri, Mrityunjay, Nicobari, Vanaraja, Yamuna, Ankleshwar, Bursa, Chittagong, Danki, Daothigi r, Ghagus, Haringhatta black, Kalasthi, Punjab brown (23)	Gir Raja (1)	Assel, Brahma, Indian Game, Cochin (4)
Duck (6)	Chemballi, Kuttanadu Chara, Nageshwari, Sythetemete (4)		Indian Runner, Khaki Campbell (2)

Figures in parentheses are number of breeds.

Source: Adopted from Ranchi Declaration on Conservation and Management of Farm Animal Genetic Resources 2009.

Box 1 : Breeds facing extinction

Cattle	Buffaloes	Goat	Sheep	Camel	Chicken
Red Sindhi	Nili-Ravi	Beetal	Bhakarwal	Bactrian	Kashmir
Tharparkar	Bhadawari	Jamnapari	Mandya	Sindhi	Faverolla
Sahiwal	Toda	Chegu	Muzaffarnagri	Jaisalmeri	Miri
Punganur		Surti	Changthangi		Nicobari
Siri		Jakhrana	Nilgiri		Ankleshwar
Kenketha		Barbari	Munjal		Bursa
Dangi		Changthangi	Poonchi		Chittagong
Vechur			Jaisalmeri		Danki
Kherigarh			Chokla		Daothigir
Bargur			Bonpala		Ghagus
Krishna Valley			Gurez		Kalasthi
Ponwar			Karanah		Punjab brown
Bachaur			Kilakarsal		Haringhata black

2.2 Reasons for extinction

1. Introduction of exotic breeds with high performance
2. Unplanned mating due to lack of breeding policies
3. Lack of knowledge among farmers regarding importance of a breed
4. Failure of most of the native breeds to meet people's demands due to incorrect production directions
5. Intermixing among breeds in the borderline areas
6. Lack of understanding and efforts among breeders/farmers in developing countries
7. Small population size and livestock diseases
8. Less profitability of animal farming than other industries

2.3 Challenges in sustainable conservation

- Low productivity
- Preponderance of diseases
- High population vis-à-vis available resources for upkeep

- Injudicious utilization of farm animals
- Unavailability of superior bulls for breeding
- Inadequate artificial insemination and field based services
- Lack of coordination
- Inadequate funding
- Loss of superior germplasm
- Over mechanization
- Human population pressure
- Pollution and environmental concerns
- Lack of export orientation to meet global challenges

Table 2 : Criteria for inclusion of a breed in endangered category

Reference	Cattle	Sheep	Goat	Pigs	Horses
Alderson (1981)	750	1500	500	150	1000
Simak (1991)	7500	15000	5000	-	5000
Maijala (1982)	1000	500	200	200	-
FAO	10000	10000	10000	10000	10000
Others	5000*	5000*	5000*	5000*	5000*

*Number of pure breeding females in the populations suggested by FAO.
Source: Sahai (1995)

2.4 Essential considerations for conservation (Sahai 1999)

- Judicious and scientific management of livestock breeds
- Strategies for preservation of less productive breeds with adequate genetic variability and distinct characteristics
- Alternate use/value addition of products of the breed
- Establishment of the *in situ* and *ex situ* gene banks
- Establishment of informatics and computation system with data banks and interactive networking with other global agencies
- Setting up of Livestock Conservation Boards
- Formulation of well defined breeding policies consistent both with conservation and economic situations of the farmers
- Formulation of livestock population policy consistent with the carrying capacity and environmental management

- People's participation through Breed societies, Associations, Breed survival trusts and NGOs
- Setting modalities for gene banks, data banks, genetic resource movement/transfer
- Development of financial and institutional mechanism for conservation programmes

2.5 Important rules for conservation

- Every breeding animal must be replaced by his/ her progeny.
- The percentage of the known or visible characteristics must be kept approximately around the foundation frequency.
- The immunogenetic characteristics should possibly also be used.
- The generation interval must be kept as long as possible according to breed or species.
- The number of males in consecutive years must be as many as possible.

2.6 Problems faced in conservation approaches

- General dearth of information on animal genetic resources
- Fragmentation of land holding and preponderance of small number of animals with location in remote rural areas
- Virtual nonexistence of breed registry societies for operation of pedigree/ performance recording programme and breed characterization work, Lack of maintenance and reliability of breed wise genus data
- No proper tie up of livestock development programmes with problems of conservation, management and evaluation of genetic resources and their utilization
- Lack of a balance between conservation goal and resource utilization
- Incredible pressure of human population leading to conflict situations and problems due to variety of interactions between people and our natural environment
- Monetary resource crunch

3. Methods of Conservation

In addition to the traditional methods of conservation wide ranges of new biotechnological tools have emerged and can effectively be utilized for conservation of native AnGRs and their germplasm.

3.1 *In situ* conservation

It means the conservation of ecosystems and natural habitats and the maintenance and recovery of viable populations of species in their natural surroundings and, in the case of domesticated or cultivated species, in the surroundings where they have developed their distinctive properties. It is the best method as it ensures the following.

1. Improvement of the breed continuously over the time through selective breeding
2. The breed gradually adapting to the changing environment conditions
3. Maintenance of true to breed characteristics through avoiding intermixing of breeds
4. Screening of lethal genes by elimination of unwanted traits
5. Ecosystem management and use for the sustainable production of food and agriculture
6. Availability of animals for immediate use with desirable characteristics
7. Involvement of stake holders and farmers

The major limiting factor is that, it is expensive because of large number of animals to be maintained. A minimum herd size of about 100 breedable animals per closed nucleus herd is necessary to keep tolerable inbreeding level of about 1% per generation. For *in situ* conservation of a breed beyond extinction level, a minimum of 5 such herds need to be located in the breeding tract. Following models of *in situ* conservation may be adopted depending upon the size of animal population and the available infrastructure facilities.

A. Model-I : An animal herd with *nucleus breeding system*, controlled management and all required facilities

B. Model-II : Animal herd with associated units to have required population with controlled management under *open nucleus breeding system*

C. Model-III : As in Model I or Model II with additional collaboration with farmers' herds under the monitoring and regular supervision of breeding institution.

3.2 *Ex situ* conservation

It means the conservation of components of biological diversity outside their natural habitats. It is the maintenance of representative population of breed *in vivo* or preservation of germplasm *in vitro*.

3.2.1 In vivo method

It involves the maintenance of the herd of sufficient size to avoid inbreeding at a place away from the main breeding tract or native environment of the breed, in the form of Zoo/Livestock Breeding Park on the pattern of wild animals, state owned livestock farm, bull mother farm or a research institutional herd. It will also ensure scientific breeding, efficient management and continuous production improvement over the years.

3.2.2 In vitro method

It is the storage and preservation of a wide variety of living cells (germ line or somatic) for long period of time. The following modes of *in vitro* conservation can now be utilized successfully:

- Cryopreservation of sperms and oocytes
- Splitting, cloning and cryopreservation of embryos
- Storage of DNA and creation of gene pool
- Establishment of embryonic stem cell lines
- Conservation and cloning of somatic cells

4. Livestock Breeding Strategies Supportive to Conservation

The development of breeding policy under existing farming structure is complex as it requires the following (Mangurkar 1998).

- Creation of employment
- Improvement of income distribution and alleviation of poverty
- Conservation of natural resources and biodiversity
- Avoiding environmental degradation and negative effect on ecosystem
- Balancing of international market i.e. reducing imports and increasing exports
- Satisfying sociocultural obligations

Important considerations for planning the breeding strategies for Indian farming situations are listed below.

- High livestock density leading to diminished availability of inputs, poor maintenance of livestock and degeneration of genetic worth
- Unavailability of authentic information on population documentation and status of various breeds of livestock

- Nondescript livestock constituting 60-80% of total livestock population
- Crossbreeding happening to be in casual factors responsible for endangerment of native germplasm
- Inadequate infrastructural and technical facilities at appropriate level
- Lack of coordination in policy formulation, funding and implementation
- Conservation of biological diversity and heritage of local livestock breeds along with their specialized potential to meet the future needs
- Extrapolation of information on productivity of breeds on organized farms for farmer's herds.
- Low input production system causing animals' failure to remain efficient producers; optimization of input efficiencies
- Herd Book registration of animals of a breed conforming to well-defined genetic attributes and production traits i.e. characterization and accreditation of cattle and buffalo breeds

The following livestock breeding strategies are proposed for effective and sustainable conservation.

4.1 Maximum coverage of livestock through artificial insemination and to increase the reproductive ability through embryo transfer

Existing infrastructure facilities for artificial insemination (AI) are sufficient to cover more than 50% of the cattle and buffalo population; whereas the present coverage is hardly available to 10-15% of the population. Sincere efforts are needed to properly utilize the existing facilities before creating the facilities for more coverage of livestock. Technical facilities to increase the reproductive ability through embryo transfer (ET) need to be created. Technology to attain satisfactory success rate have been standardized. At various centers of the National Dairy Development Board, the successful recovery of 14 embryos in single flush in field conditions and 11 calves from these embryos have been obtained. The targets for success are 6 to 12 offspring per donor per year or 30 to 60 offspring per donor lifetime.

4.2 Grading up of nondescript cattle and buffaloes

The low producing local nondescript livestock constitutes more than three-fourth of cattle and buffalo population, which is the target population to be improved upon. For the farmers with insufficient feed, fodder and other resources; inadequate infrastructure and poor marketing facilities, the nondescript livestock may be improved by grading up using elite proven bulls of regional pure breeds.

The well-defined breeds are maintained on several organized government and private farms and *gaushalas*. There is large genetic variation available within breeds and some of the animals have quite high milk yield per day during judging and milk competitions that indicates their high genetic potential. In addition, their potentials for draught, traction, tilling and power generation can also be better utilized simultaneously.

The bulls to be used for this purpose should be produced from superior dams, which have more than 3500 and 2000 kg lactation yield for Murrah buffaloes and Hariana cattle, respectively. This is expected to improve the milk yield substantially in the next generation. In a period of 5-6 generations of continuous grading up, the nondescript stock will be transformed into well-defined purebreds.

4.3 Crossbreeding programme for nondescript low producing animals

Another approach to improve nondescript low producing dairy cattle is through crossbreeding with exotic dairy cattle breeds of temperate origin. This is strictly recommended only for milk-shed areas around peri-urban areas where good market for milk and milk products is available and adequate quantity of quality feed and fodder resources exist.

Holstein Friesian is the breed of choice in the irrigated plains and Jersey in the hilly terrains and coastal areas for crossbreeding. Intensive management, high input and excellent resource availability are the basic requirements to attain early maturity, regular reproduction and faster increase in milk production of dairy cattle through crossbreeding.

The optimum level of exotic inheritance is 50-75%. To overcome the adverse effects of inter-se mating, it will be better to backcross or crisscross the crossbreds with high exotic inheritance with indigenous milch breeds like Sahiwal or Gir.

Success through crossbreeding also requires strong networking of infrastructure facilities including AI, ET, bull mother farms and semen and embryo freezing facilities, trained manpower, intensive health and prophylactic measures, and good market for milk and milk products.

4.4 Field progeny testing programme

A schematic representation of field progeny testing programme that can be followed in cattle and buffalo both is given in Fig. 1.

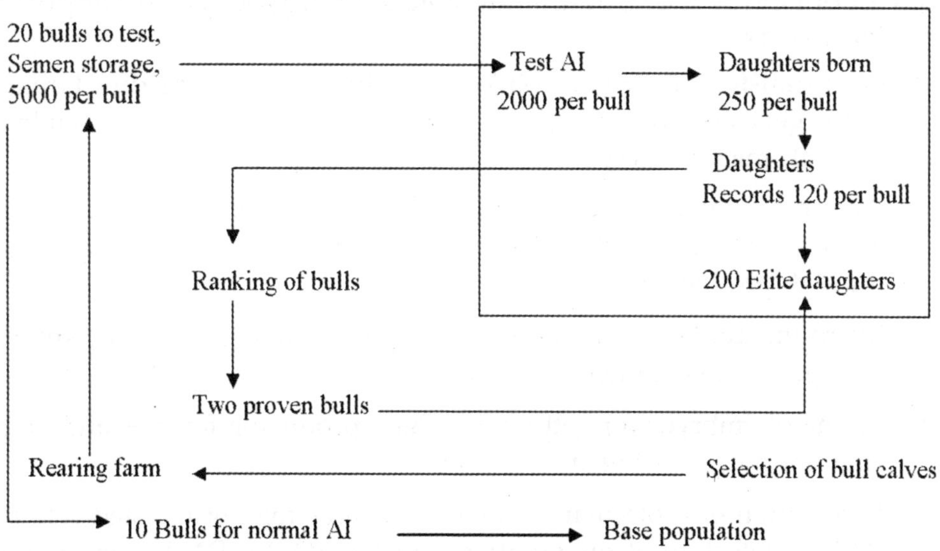

Fig. 1 : Schematic representation of field progeny testing programme (*Source:* Mishra *et al.* 1998)

4.5 Open Nucleus Breeding System

A schematic presentation of Open Nucleus Breeding System (Mishra et al. 1998) that can be followed in cattle and buffalo both is given in Fig. 2.

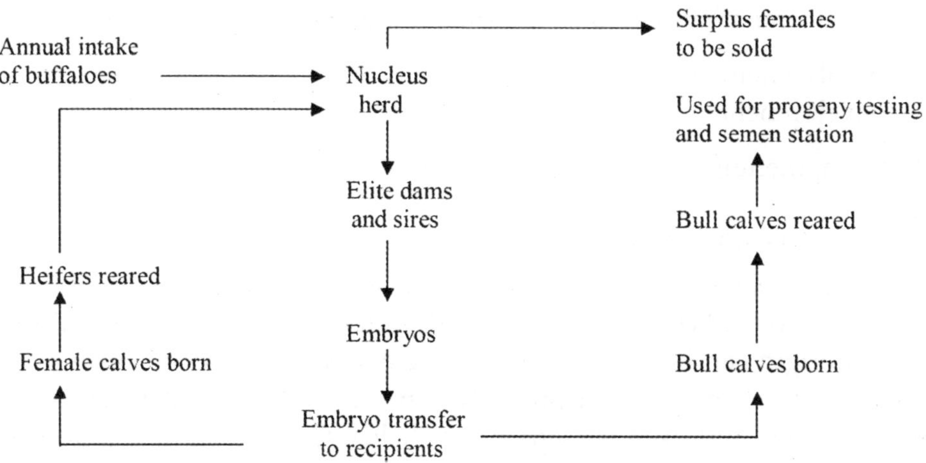

Fig. 2 : Schematic presentation of Open Nucleus Breeding System (*Source:* Mishra *et al.* 1998)

4.6 Recent innovations in animal biotechnology and other important considerations

- Gene transfer through microinjection technique involving direct transfer of the genes responsible for the high productive traits into the embryos through microsurgery
- Advancement to harvest elite germplasm to produce clones of the embryonic cells of highly elite cows and buffaloes and propagate them for high production ability
- Micro-manipulation of embryo of a high producing animal by splitting it surgically to get identical twins
- Sexing of embryos for getting only high producing females and highly superior males for breeding purpose
- Exploration of molecular techniques such as marker assisted selection (MAS), detection of quantitative trait loci (QTL), DNA level markers and mini- and micro-satellites explorations
- Upgrading infrastructure facilities at state agricultural universities (SAU) and national institutes for standardization of advance technologies indigenously.

Other important considerations

- Expansion and strengthening of central herd registration scheme; breeders' associations involving farmers; documentation and data base management system; and information management system
- Involvement of private sector, NGOs and *gaushalas* in research and development
- Strengthening of banker loan facilities

4.7 Strengthening of *gaushalas*

The *Gaushala* movement is synonymous with the protection of cows and cattle wealth of our country. Being practised for the last five thousand years or so, its origin can be traced in the Vedic period when social customs and rules laid great emphasis on protection, preservation and development of cows for home, and oxen for agriculture-fields. Cow being the backbone of rural life and economy in India, care was taken for their well-being and uplift. Grazing areas and grasslands (*Gochar bhumi*) were kept reserved in abundance everywhere. People used to donate their lands to gaushalas on auspicious occasions so that cows may have sufficient land for grazing. During the first five year plan, there were nearly 3,000 gaushalas spread over the whole country. These institutions maintained over six lac cattle at an annual cost of seven crore rupees. It has been realized that, in spite of their drawbacks, with better organization these institutions could very well serve as useful centres for the improvement of cattle and milk production, supplementing the government's efforts in this direction. At present there are more than 4000 gaushalas in the country, which have the following objectives:

1. Preserving Indian cows and their progeny and to breed and upgrading them for supplying plenty of unadulterated milk and milk products to the people and distribution of the best female calves to the villagers
2. Preparation of the best pedigree Indian bulls and supply to villagers for breeding and upgrading village nondescript cows
3. Production of best quality and healthy bullocks for draught work and preserving male calves for distribution to agriculturists

4.7.1 Concept of gaushalas *in present context*

Comparison of *gaushala* on the basis of the concepts of Datar Singh Committee in 1947 and National Commission on Cattle in 2002 is given in Box 2.

With the advancement of the concept of organic farming, the gaushalas are entering a new phase. Now there is awareness among them that they have lot of potential in terms of bio-fertilizers, biopesticides, bioenergy and panch-gavya medicines. They have also started thinking in this direction. Most of them are convinced that if this potential is harnessed, the gaushalas can be economically viable units. They can get rid of the long dependence of donations. The old and infirm cattle will no longer be a burden on them. In spite of all such ideas reaching them, most of the existing 4000 gaushalas are still the same as they used to be two decades ago. It is mainly because of the lack of technical know-how and marketing infrastructure.

In the light of the above facts, the National Commission on Cattle is confident that the proposed 'Village Gaushalas' will have very many more chances of succeeding than did the Gosadans envisaged by the Datar Singh Committee.

***Box 2* : Comparison of 'Gaushala' concepts of Datar Singh Committee and National Commission on Cattle**

	Datar Singh Committee (1947)	National Commission on Cattle (2002)
i)	Big size organization involving 4000 acres of land and 2000 cattle	A small village level institution having stray cattle of only Gram Panchayat area, and land of 100 acres or as per availability
ii)	A government-run institution	An institution run by community participation
iii)	Involved only expenditure	Increased income by way of biogas, biofertilizers, biopesticides, panch-gavya medicines, breed improvement, bull service and milk
iv)	Totally based on governmental funding	Community funding in the form of fodder and feed, no cash subsidy, governmental assistance in form of infrastructure and H.R.D.
v)	Functioning in isolation	Linkages with Krishi Go-vigyan Anusandhan Kendra, research organizations, agriculture and veterinary extension units
vi)	50 years back there was no use of cow urine, no thought for exploring avenues.	Organic farming popularisation, increased awareness of scientific use of cow dung, research on cow dung and cow urine to make them basis for economic viability of the so called 'useless' cattle
vii)	'Gosadan' then was a sectoral function.	Establishment of Gosadan will be part allotted to a particular department of the District Plan now.

4.7.2 Measures for strengthening gaushalas

1. The main drawbacks of gaushalas are the paucity of funds, unskilled workers and traditional outlook. To make them self-sustaining units, they have to be motivated to make the best use of their so far underutilized resources viz. cow dung and urine.
2. At least one gaushala in each District may be got developed into a 'Krishi-Govigyan Anusandhan Kendra' with demonstration units to show the making of Nadep compost, vermicompost, biopesticides and bioenergy.

3. The Animal Husbandry Department of the state should ensure that complete veterinary cover is provided to gaushalas.
4. The central and the state governments should have some mechanism of providing financial assistance to gaushalas, if not directly, then through village panchayat, Block Samities, MLA/MP development funds etc.
5. For good working arrangement between gaushalas, state governments and SAUs a project/cell should be funded by the Department of Animal Husbandry with technical control under the SAU.
6. The state government may consider organizing annual meetings at state level in which the persons-in-charge of all the gaushalas and state government and SAU functionaries meet to discuss problems of common interest and to take steps and decisions for improvement and maintenance of gaushalas.
7. SAUs should start vocational training courses on a regular basis to train technicians, who can work in Krishi Go-vigyan Anusandhan Kendras and gaushalas.
8. It should be made mandatory for gaushalas having land, to grow fodder crops, fodder trees and grasses. The states, Gram Panchayats and Panchayat Samitis should develop and maintain pasture and fodder patches along water reservoirs, canals and rivers.
9. It should be made mandatory for gaushalas to upgrade the nondescript animals to the true breed local to the area by keeping the bulls of that breed for breeding purposes so that gaushalas become the breed conservation centers of the state.
10. Bull mother farms for each indigenous breed should be located at SAUs or ICAR Institutes so that progeny tested bulls or their semen for AI is provided to the gaushalas for breed conservation programmes. Bull mother farms are funded either by State Animal Husbandry Department or ICAR.
11. Suitable sanitary and phytosanitary standards for clean milk production and export quality products may be adopted at gaushalas.
12. Gaushala management must lay emphasis on improving the quality of animals for higher milk production of cows and better draught capacity of bullocks.
13. Main emphasis of gaushalas should be to meet the local consumer demands of liquid milk, however, surplus milk may be diverted to processing of export quality milk products.
14. Gaushalas in order to become economically self-sustaining may operate the following units:

i. In farm units of local indigenous breeds and crossbred cattle, which have viable production to become income-generating units

ii. Stray and non-producing cattle units located in the vicinity of the Gochar/ community/panchayati pasture lands, forest grazing areas, waste lands to be developed as gochars etc. and generating income through utilization of dung, urine or biowastes

iii. Injured and physically disabled cattle units to be housed near the veterinary hospital/dispensary

5. Legal Framework, Issues and Requirements

The provision of legal coverage to indigenous domesticated animals is being raised for the last one to two decades in almost all the countries. Most of the legal coverage which is in existence is for control on slaughter of animals, prevention of cruelty to animals and on improvement of animals. The existing framework is presented in Annexure I and II. This legal coverage is not only very old but does not meet the present day requirement. No legal coverage exists for the conservation and preservation of domestic animal diversity (DAD). Similarly, there is hardly any law for sharing the benefits on the utilization of DAD and sovereignty over these resources. However, with the introduction of IPR, it is necessary now to provide better coverage for protecting our DAD. However, these laws should not be very stringent to make their implementation difficult.

It is, therefore, necessary to consider the important aspects on priority before framing laws for which an in-depth knowledge of DAD would only help in deciding about our requirements. The following points need to be considered in depth and for which necessary information should be generated before taking further action. It is also necessary to know for whom this legal frame work is being prepared and who are the beneficiaries and its long term consequences.

5.1 Important areas needing legal framework

1. The government policies, particularly organized farms or national breeding plans should not be frequently changed and not by one person.
2. Laws should be enacted for prohibiting businessmen/farmers keeping a bull for breeding purpose, and the necessity of providing a license for keeping a breeding bull.
3. Scrub bull should be castrated.
4. National breeding policies/programmes need to be prepared.

5. Revision of quarantine policies should be undertaken.
6. Regulation for livestock slaughter should be implemented.
7. Handling and conservation of genetic material should be regulated.

5.2 Requirements from legal standpoint

- Laws regarding trusteeship/ownership of animal genetic resources in gene banks, outside the country
- Laws prohibiting or permitting use of genetic resources or material including punitive measures for infringements
- Third party and further on transfer of genetic resources-terms, conditions, rights and obligation in such transactions
- Transfer of animal genetic resources for commercial use and for research-rights and obligations and benefit sharing
- Regulations on networking with global agencies
- Legal framework for the establishment and working of data banks
- Laws regarding benefit sharing by parties and local communities
- Rules and monetary obligations of non-government organizations handling animal genetic conservation programmes
- Laws covering breed registration societies and other similar organizations

5.3 Issues

Identification: It is necessary to identify the existing DAD and characterize them to know about their distribution, status and economic importance for considering them for legal coverage.

Protection in-situ : This is more appropriate for the existing livestock farms as under field conditions its implications are such that it may not be possible as for wild species. However, this may be extended to domesticated species to protect them from getting extinct.

Protection ex-situ : This is very important for genetic material used for conservation in the form of semen, embryo, ova, cell line etc.

Access/extraction : Legal provisions may be made for access/extraction of the genetic material.

Use : Utilization of bio-diversity for subsistence, scientific or commercial use.

Breeding : The methods used for breeding of animals are either natural mating or artificial insemination for multiplying or regeneration of populations should have full protection to prevent loss of genetic material.

Trade : Import or export of animals, genetic material from region to region or country to country needs to be regulated and strictly watched both for preventing loss or prevention of diseases.

Release : Though this is not critically defined but needs to be made very effective for identification of existing breeds, release of new breeds/strains or genetic groups.

IPR : Already lot of debating is being done at national and international level but the existing breeds need to be protected by giving the sovereignty rights over them by genetic characterization particularly for those breeds with important/unique characteristics.

However, so far very little has been done for providing legal protection to the existing genetic material/breeds of the country to protect them from disappearance and their exploitation.

5.4 Biological Diversity Act

The United Nations Environment Programme (UNEP) convened the Ad hoc Working Group of Experts on Biological Diversity in November 1988 to explore the need for an international convention on biological diversity. In May 1989, it established the ad hoc working group of technical and legal experts to prepare an international legal instrument for the conservation and sustainable use of biological diversity. In February 1991, the ad hoc working group had become known as Inter Governmental Negotiating Committee. Its work culminated on 22 May, 1992 with the Nairobi Conference for adoption of the agreed text of the Convention on Biological Diversity (CBD), which was signed by 168 countries including India. The main objectives of CBD are:

1. Conservation of Biological Diversity
2. Sustainable use of its components
3. Fair and equitable sharing of benefits arising out of utilization of genetic resources

India is one of the 12 mega biodiversity countries of the world. With only 2.5% of land area, India already accounts for 7-8% of the recorded species of the world. Recognizing the sovereign rights of states to use their own biological resources, the convention expects the parties as given below.

- Article 3 and 15 of the Convention facilitate access to genetic resources by other parties for environmentally sound purpose subject to national legislation on mutually agreed upon terms.
- Article 8j of the Convention recognizes contribution of local and indigenous communities to the conservation and sustainable utilization

of biological diversity through traditional knowledge, practices and innovations and provides for equitable sharing of benefits with such people arising from the utilization of their knowledge, practices and innovations.

- Article 8k of the Convention provides the provision to develop or maintain necessary legislation/or other regulatory provisions for the protection of threatened species and population.

5.5 The Addis Ababa Principles and Guidelines

These focus on biodiversity in general and on general principles and policies. The introduction to the Addis Ababa Principles and Guidelines states that:

- Sustainable use is a valuable tool to promote conservation of biological diversity.
- Sustainable use can not be achieved without effective conservation measures.
- The application of the practical principles and operational guidelines is set within the context of the ecosystem approach.

Thus, sustainable use is here understood as an option for conserving biodiversity, and conservation is seen as the long-term maintenance of biodiversity. This is different from the understanding of conservation in AnGR management, where conservation is used in the more narrow sense of activities needed when utilization of breeds is no longer guaranteed. In this view, sustainable use of AnGRs renders conservation measures superfluous. Hence, utilization of AnGRs and use and development of AnGRs refers to strategies for breeds that are currently not at risk.

The introductory statements of the Addis Ababa Principles and Guidelines are followed by seven underlying conditions for sustainable use.

a) The first underlying condition establishes the principle of long-term viability of the use of biodiversity that it is possible to use biodiversity components in a manner in which ecological processes, species and genetic variability remain above thresholds needed for long-term viability, and thus all resource managers and users have the responsibility to ensure that use does not exceed these capacities.

b) The second condition establishes dynamics of ecosystems as a principle. Ecosystems, ecological processes within them, species variability and genetic variation change over time whether or not they are used. Therefore, governments, resource managers and users should take into account the need to accommodate change, including stochastic events that may adversely affect biodiversity and influence the sustainability of a use.

c-e) The next three principles do not apply to AnGRs.

f) The sixth and seventh principles are relevant for AnGRs. To ameliorate any potential negative long-term effects of uses it is incumbent on all resource users to apply precaution in their management decisions and to opt for sustainable use management strategies and policies that favour uses that provide increased sustainable benefits while not adversely affecting biodiversity. Likewise, the governments should be certain that licensed or authorized sustainable uses of biological diversity are taking such precaution in their management.

g) In considering individual guidelines provided below, it is necessary to refer to and apply the provisions of Article 8(j), Article 10(c) and other related provisions and their development in relevant decisions of the Conference of the Parties in all matters that relate to indigenous and local communities.

Keeping the above in view, Government of India decided to bring legislation on biological diversity in 2002 with the following objectives:

1. To regulate access to biological resources of the country with the purpose of securing equitable share in benefits arising out of the use of biological resources; and associated knowledge relating to biological resources
2. To conserve and sustainable use of the biological diversity
3. To secure sharing of benefits with local people as conservers of biological resources and holders of knowledge and information relating to the use of biological resources
4. To respect and protect knowledge of local communities related to biodiversity
5. Conservation and development of areas important from the stand point of biological diversity by declaring them as biological heritage sites
6. Protection and rehabilitation of threatened species
7. Involvement of institutions of self government in the broad scheme of the implementation of the Act through consultation of committees

The duties, location, composition, constitution and functions of National and State Biodiversity Boards and Biodiversity Management Committee were also laid down (Appendix-III).

5.6 Futuristic actions

Some important points still needing their incorporation to ensure the conservation and sustainable utilization of domestic animal diversity are given below.

1. It is suggested that following representation in National Biodiversity Authority may also be made:
   - A representative from Department of Animal Husbandry and Dairying, Ministry of Agriculture, Government of India
   - A representative from Veterinary Council of India

   At least three meetings of National Biodiversity Authority should be convened in a year. In the Article 12 (1) of the Act, the number of meetings is not mentioned.
2. It is suggested that in State Biodiversity Board one representative each from the departments of Agriculture, Animal Husbandry/Veterinary services and Forest may be mandatory. Rest two representatives may be included as per the discretion of state government concerned.
3. In consideration of the clause 13(2), a committee on Domestic Animal Diversity is suggested and the role and functions of this committee may be defined.
4. It is suggested that like National Biodiversity Authority, the State Biodiversity Board may also constitute several committees for its smooth and efficient functioning. Such a committee is suggested for domestic animal diversity in each state. The functions of this committee may be defined.
5. As per provisions made in the chapter X (clause-42) Biodiversity Management Committee may be constituted within its area for the purpose of promoting conservation, sustainable use and documentation of biological diversity including preservation, conservation of land races, folk varieties, domestic stock and breed of animals and microorganisms and chronicling of knowledge relating to biological diversity.
6. For fulfilling the purpose of above clause in relation to domestic animal biodiversity a concept of establishment of Breed Societies for all the breeds at local level with in area of its origin and distribution is suggested. The functions of these societies may be defined.

India being a signatory to the Convention on Biological Diversity (CBD), the International Treaty on Plant Genetic Resources for Food and Agriculture (ITPGRFA) and the Interlaken Declaration as well as Global Plan of Action on Animal Genetic Resources adopted in 2007 urgent need was felt to have a National Plan of Action to manage, improve and conserve valuable farm animal genetic resources.

In this connection a Workshop on Strategy for Conservation of Farm Animal Genetic Resources was jointly organized by the Trust for Advancement of Agricultural Sciences (TAAS) and Birsa Agricultural University, Ranchi in April 2009 at Ranchi. The following Ranchi Declaration was unanimously adopted.

1. India should prepare a National Plan of Action on management and conservation of AnGR for its speedy implementation.
2. Cattle, buffalo, goat, sheep and chicken should be declared as Big Five species of India.
3. The current resources should be doubled for livestock research and development sector and a specific policy directive be given in favour of AnGR.
4. Maintenance and further improvement of pure breeds and retaining their valuable characteristics, including that adaptation to climate change becomes a national priority.
5. A strong legal instrument is needed to deal with the registration of livestock breeds, protection of animal keepers' rights and related issues, on the pattern of Protection of Plant Varieties and Farmers' Rights Act (2001).
6. The currently engaged staff at government livestock farms and specialized goshalas should be properly trained.
7. There is an urgency to initiate action to conserve our valuable livestock and poultry breeds that are currently at risk.
8. India may become a focal point for the management and conservation of AnGRs for South Asia.
9. There is need to strengthen research aimed at scientific management, genetic enhancement, sustainable use and conservation of farm AnGRs.

References

1. Alderson L (1981). Conservation of animal genetic resources in Great Britain. FAO – Rome. Animal Genetic Resources Information No. 24:53-76.
2. FAO (1996). Livestock - environment interactions: issues and options (H. Steinfeld, C. de Haan and H. Blackburn). FAO, Rome.

3. FAO (1999). The global strategy for the management of farm animal genetic resources. Executive Brief. FAO, Rome.

4. Maijala K, Devillard JM, Reklewaski Z, Rognoni G, Simon DL, Stene D (1984). Conservation of animal genetic resources in Europe. Report on EAAP working party. Livestock Production Science 11:3-22.

5. Mangurkar BR (1998). Breeding policy for sustainable milk production. Indian Dairyman 50(12):41-43.

6. Mishra AK, Kasi Raj R, Arun Prasad B (1998). Genetic development of the buffalo. Indian Dairyman 50(11):7-13.

7. Ranchi Declaration (2009). Conservation and management of farm animal genetic resources. TAAS, IARI, New Delhi.

8. Sahai R (1995). Livestock genetic resources productivity and conservation. Proceedings of National Symposium on Modern Trends in Animal Health and Production Research and its Impact on Rural Development. IAAVR pub. 303-308.

9. Sahai R (1999). Issues of intellectual property rights (IPRs) and legal concerns on bioresources. Summer course on characterization and conservation of domesticated livestock and poultry resources. NBAGR, Karnal.

10. Simak E (1991). The conservation of rare breeds in West Germany. In: Lawrence A (Ed) Genetic Conservation of Domestic Livestock, CAB International 1991:65-69.

Appendix-I : Central Acts relevant to domestic animals (Acts arranged chronologically)

Name of Act	Year
Import and Export (Control) Act	1947
Prevention of Cruelty to Animals Act	1960
Customs Act	1950
Marine Product Export Development Authority Act	1972
Wildlife Protection Act	1972, 1991
Marine Zone of India (Regulation of Fishing by Foreign Vessels) Act	1981
Environment (Protection) Act	1986
National Dairy Development Board Act	1987
Biological Diversity Act	2002

Appendix-II : Major relevant provisions of central acts relating to domestic animal bio-diversity

1. Custom Act, 1962

a) Regulation or prohibition of import and export of specified articles (21)

b) Regulation of import-export specifically for;
   i) The protection of human, animal or plant life or health (11t)
   ii) The conservation of exhaustible natural resources {II(m)}

c) Regulation of transportation and storage of notified items {II(j, k, l, m)

2. Environment (Protection) Act, 1986

a) General measures to protect environment {3(1)}

b) Restriction of Industrial and other processes/activities in specified areas {3(2)(v)}

c) Read with Rule 5 of Environment (Protection) Rules, 1986.

d) Prevention and Control of hazardous substances, including the manufacture, use, release and movement {3(2), 7,8}.

3. Import and Export (Control) Act, 1947

a) Prohibition or restriction on imports and exports of specified items {3}

b) Regulations of transportation of specified items {4c}

4. Marine Products Export Development Authority, 1972

a) Establishment of an authority for developing and controlling marine products {4.9(1)}

b) Developing and regulating off-shore and deep-sea fishing, taking measures for conservation, fixing standards for export and regulating exports {9(2a, c, 1)}.

c) Prohibition/restriction on export and import of marine products {20(1)}

5. Marine Zones of India (Regulation of fishing by Foreign Vessels) Act, 1981

a) Regulation of fishing in India's EEZ by people using foreign vessels {3}

b) Permits only to be granted within definition of public interest, and for scientific research experiments etc. {5(3), 8}

6. National Dairy Development Board Act, 1987

a) Establishment of a board which promotes dairy development and other agricultural based industries {4, 16 (1a)}.

b) Financing and facilitating animal husbandry, agriculture, high yielding cattle wealth 16(1).

7. Prevention of Cruelty to Animals Act, 1960

a) Restrictions on cruel treatment of animals, including transportation, and trade {chapter II, & Rules under Section 38}

b) Restrictions on use of animals for purpose of experimentation.

8. Wildlife (Protection) Act, 1972 and Wildlife (Protection) Amendment Act, 1991)

a) Restriction of prohibition on hunting of animals {chapter III)

b) Protection of specified plants (chapter IIIA)

c) Setting up and managing sanctuaries and National parks (chapter IV)

d) Setting up of zoo authority, control of zoos and captive breeding {chapter 1va}

e) Control of trade and commerce in wild animals, and animal articles {chapter V & VΛ).

Appendix-III : Regulation, duties, constitution and functions of the National and State Biodiversity Authority

Regulation of biological diversity

1. The following persons, without previous approval of the National Biodiversity Authority, shall not obtain any biological resources occurring in India or knowledge associate thereto for research or for commercial utilization or for bio-survey and bio-utilization:

a. A person who is not a citizen of India;

b. A citizen of India who is non-resident

c. A body corporate, association or organization not registered in India or registered in India under any law for the time being in force which has any non-Indian participation in its share capital or management.

2. No person shall, without the previous approval of National Biodiversity Authority, transfer the results of any research relating to any biological resources occurring or obtained from India for monetary consideration or otherwise to any person who is not a citizen of India or a body corporate or organization which is not registered or incorporated in India or which has any non-Indian participation in its share capital or management. Here transfer does not include publication of research paper or dissemination of knowledge in any seminar or workshop provided such publication is as per guidelines issued by the central government.

3. The above said provisions shall not apply to collaborative research projects involving transfer or exchange of biological resources or information relating thereto between institutions, including government sponsored institutions of India, and such institutions in other countries, if such collaborative research projects satisfy the conditions specified in SN 1 and shall conform to the policy guidelines issued by central government and be approved by the central government

4. No person shall apply for any intellectual property right by whatever name called in or outside India for any invention based on any research or information on a biological resource obtained from India without obtaining the prior approval of National Biodiversity Authority before making such application. The NBA may, while granting the approval under this section, impose benefit sharing fee or royalty or both or impose conditions including the sharing of financial benefits arising out of the commercial utilization of such rights. The provisions of above shall not apply to any person making an application for any right under any law relating to protection of plant varieties enacted by the Parliament.

5. No person who is a citizen of India or a body corporate, association or organization, which is registered in India, shall obtain any biological resource for commercial utilization or bio-survey and bio-utilization except after giving prior intimation to the State Biodiversity Board concerned.

Duties of the central and state governments

1. The central government shall development national strategies, plans, programmes for conservation and sustainable use of biological diversity including measures for identification and monitoring areas rich in biological resources, promotion of *in situ* conservation and *ex situ* conservation of biological resources, incentives for research, training, public education to increase awareness with respect to biodiversity.
2. The central government shall, as far as practicable wherever it deems appropriate, integrate the conservation and sustainable use of biological diversity into relevant sectoral or cross-sectoral plans, programmes and policies.
3. The central government shall undertake measures:

a. Wherever necessary, for assessment of environmental impact of that project which is likely to have adverse effect on biological diversity, with a view to avoid or minimize such effects and where appropriate provide for public participation in such assessment;
b. To regulate, manage or control the risks associated with the use and release of living modified organisms resulting from biotechnology likely to have adverse impact on the conservation and sustainable use of biological diversity and human health.

4. The central government shall endeavor to respect and protect the knowledge of local people relating to biological diversity, as recommended by the National Biodiversity Authority through such measures, which may include registration of such knowledge at the local, state or national levels, and other measures for protection, including sui generic system.
5. With prejudice to any other law for the time being in force, the state government may from time to time in consultation with the local bodies, notify in the Official Gazette, areas of biodiversity importance as biodiversity heritage sites under this Act.
6. The state government, in consultation with the central government, may frame rules for the management and conservation of all the heritage sites.

7. The state government shall frame schemes for compensating or rehabilitating any person or section of people economically affected by such notification.
8. Without prejudice to the provisions of any other law for the time being in force, the central government may from time to time notify, any species which is on the verge of extinction or likely to become extinct in the near future as a threatened species and prohibit or regulate collection thereof for any purpose and take appropriate steps to rehabilitate and preserve those species.
9. The central government may in consultation with the National Biodiversity Authority, designate institutions as repositories under this Act for different categories of biological resources.
10. The repositories shall keep in safe custody the biological material including voucher specimens deposited with them.
11. Any new tax should be notified to the repositories or any institution designated for this purpose and deposits the voucher specimens with such repository or institution.
12. Notwithstanding anything contained in this Act, the central government may in consultation with the National Biodiversity Authority, by notification in the Official Gazette, declare that the provisions of this Act shall not apply to any items, including biological resources normally traded as commodities.

National Biodiversity Authority

The National Biodiversity Authority shall be a body corporate by the name aforesaid, having perpetual succession and a common seal, with power to acquire, hold and dispose of property, both movable and immovable, and to contract, and shall by the said name sue and be sued.

Headquarter : Proposed at Chennai

Composition

i. Chairperson to be appointed by the central government.

ii. Three ex-officio members to be appointed by the central government, one representing Ministry of tribal affairs and two from Ministry of Environment and Forest, of which one should be Addl. I.G./I.G. of the Forests.

iii. Five ex-officio members to be appointed by the central government to represent the Agriculture Research and Education; Bio Technology; Ocean Development; Agriculture and Cooperation; Indian System of Medicine and Homeopathy.

iv. Five non-official members to be appointed from amongst specialist, Scientists, industry, conservers, creators and knowledge holders of biological resources.

Functions of National Biodiversity Authority

1. It shall be the duty of NBA to regulate activities referred to regulations, issue guidelines for access to and equitable benefit sharing.
2. The NBA may grant approval for undertaking any activity referred in guidelines regulations.
3. The NBA may advise the central government on matters relating to the conservation of biodiversity, sustainable use of its components and equitable sharing of benefits arising out of the utilization of biological resources.
4. The NBA may advise the state governments In the selection of areas of biodiversity importance to be notified as heritage sites and measures for the management of such heritage sites.
5. The NBA may perform other functions as may be necessary to carry out the provisions of this Act.
6. The NBA may, on behalf of the central government, take any measures necessary to oppose the grant of IPR in any country outside India on any biological resource obtained from India or knowledge associated with such biological resource which is derived from India.
7. The NBA may constitute a Committee to deal with agro-biodiversity (biological diversity of agriculture related species and their wild relatives). With prejudice to this, the NBA may constitute such number of committees as it deems fit for the efficient discharge of its duties and performance of its function under this Act.

State Biodiversity Board

The board shall be a body corporate by the name aforesaid, having perpetual succession and a common seal, with power to acquire, hold and dispose the property, both movable and immovable, and to contract, and shall by the said name sue and be sued.

Headquarter : At such a place as the state government may specify by notification in the Official Gazette.

Composition

i. A chairperson to be appointed by the state government.
ii. Note more than five ex-officio members to be appointed by the state government to represent the departments of the state government.

iii. Not more than five members to be appointed from amongst experts in matters relating to conservation of biological diversity, sustainable use of biological resources and equitable sharing of benefits arising out of the use of biological resources.

Functions of State Biodiversity Board

i. Advise the state government subject to any guidelines issued by the central government on matters relating to the conservation of biodiversity, sustainable use of its components and equitable sharing of the benefits arising out of the utilization of biological resources.

ii. Regulate by granting of approvals or otherwise request for commercial utilization or bio-survey and bio-utilization of any biological resources by Indians.

iii. Perform such other functions as may be necessary to carry out the provisions of this Act or as may be prescribed by the state government.

iv. No person who is a citizen of India or a body corporate, association or organization, which is registered in India, shall obtain any biological resource for commercial utilization or bio-survey and bio-utilization except after giving prior intimation to the State Biodiversity Board concerned.

Biodiversity Management Committee

1. Every local body shall constitute a Biodiversity Management Committee within its area for the purpose of promoting conservation, sustainable use and documentation of biological diversity including preservation of habitats, conservation of land races, folk varieties and cultivars, domesticated stocks and breeds of animals and microorganisms and chronicling of knowledge relating to biological diversity.

2. The NBA and the SBBs shall consult the Biodiversity Management Committees while taking any decision relating to use of biological resources and knowledge associated with such resources occurring within the territorial jurisdiction of the Biodiversity Management Committees.

3. The Biodiversity Management Committees may levy charges by way of collection fee from any person for accessing or collecting any biological resource from area falling within its territorial jurisdiction.

❑❑❑

Chapter 8

Nutritional Strategies for Raising Livestock Productivity

A. SAHOO
Animal Nutrition Division, Central Sheep & Wool Research Institute, Avikanagar-304501

Contents

1. Introduction

Domestic animals are an integral part of agriculture in India, and are likely to be the instruments of future growth and development of the agricultural sector. The importance of livestock in India goes beyond the function of food production. It is an important source of draught power, manure for crop production and fuel for domestic use. The livestock sector generates employment and earns foreign exchange besides improving food and nutritional security. It can benefit millions of landless and small landholders who constitute more than 60% of the total rural population and possess about three-fourths of the country's livestock wealth.

Livestock, particularly ruminants have served and will continue to serve a valuable role in sustainable agricultural systems. They are particularly useful in converting vast renewable resources from rangeland, pasture, and crop residues (CR) or other by-products into food edible for humans. The demand for livestock products is elastic and is expected to grow further where in India can derive substantial benefits from the emerging international economic order under WTO through export of livestock products. Planning the development of livestock in the tropical regions including India needs holistic interactions with plants and soil, involving TRM (Total Resources Management), this means optimum utilization of the available resources including the available biomass, through its recycling, which has a huge implication for sustainable food production and reduced environmental degradation. Feed is the main input factor for milk and meat production from livestock constituting 60-70% of the cost of livestock production and, therefore, needs to be strategically delivered for enhancing output of livestock products to fetch money and render remunerable economy to the larger population base. The concurrent demand of food for increasing human population and feed for its growing livestock population draws many challenges viz. to produce more foodstuffs in limited land for feed production, to upgrade feed ingredients through genetic modification and lastly to enhance the utilization of feed through innovative feed additives.

2. Livestock Productivity and Economic Importance

Livestock keeping is critical for many of the poor in the developing world, often contributing to multiple livelihood objectives and offering pathways out of poverty. Livestock keeping also affects an indispensable asset of the poor, their human capital, through its impact on their own nutrition and health. Although crops and livestock are interdependent to a large extent, the latter constitute an important mechanism for coping with the risks of crop failure. Limited data from a number of case-studies on mixed farming systems in Asia have indicated increased productivity and income and improved sustainability from the integration of crops and animals (Devendra and Thomas 2002). Since livestock wealth is mainly concentrated among the majority of marginal and small landholders, in land-scarce economies, livestock provides livelihood support in terms of income and employment generation to the millions of landless and small landholders. Technology-induced growth in the livestock subsector would thus improve food and nutritional security, alleviate poverty, and reduce interregional and interpersonal economic inequities.

India has approximately one billion animals for a billion humans, but our per capita animal production is much less. In spite of this weakness, our per unit cost of production of livestock products is not only less but is economical and our livestock farming thus exists without any subsidy and has great potential to be sustainable. The improvements in breeding and nutritional management have won us the first rank in the world milk production, but our grains are over shadowed by export restrictions to developed and developing countries except Bangladesh and Sri Lanka. As per ICMR (2008) recommendations, unlike per capita milk availability of 214 g which is more close to the recommended requirement of 250 g, per capita meat requirement is 25 g as against the availability of 9 g per person per day. This critical gap abridgement needs more emphasis on enhancing meat production. At 485 million, India has the world's largest livestock population - accounting for over 55 and 16% of the world's buffalo and cattle populations respectively (the world's largest bovine population). It ranks second in goats, third in sheep and camels, and seventh in poultry population in the world. Despite constraints like rearing of livestock under suboptimal conditions due to low economic status of livestock owners, India has now become the largest producer of milk in the world since 2004-05 with an annual production of 91 million tonnes (MT) that increased to 100.4 MT in 2007-08 (GOI report). The same year, the country recorded a production of 45.2 billion eggs (seventh in the world), 44.5 million kg of wool and 2.2 MT of meat, which ranked us eight in the world in meat exports. Taken together, the value of livestock output (2003-04) accounts for over six per cent of GDP, just a little under a third of the contribution of agriculture and allied sectors. By all accounts, it appears that India has an extremely fast growing livestock economy and there are avenues to exploit this potential resource through controlling animal diseases, scientific management and upgrading genetic resources, increasing availability of nutritious feeds and fodder etc.

3. Raising Livestock Production

Livestock is ubiquitous in poor communities across the developing world and an estimated two-thirds of resource-poor rural households keep some type of livestock and its development efforts in lower-income countries are primarily intended to generate income and meet the growing demand for animal products. These efforts often give priority to technologies that maximize the productivity of individual animals, which may not be appropriate in the developing-country context. Hoffman (2008) questioned the appropriateness of this strategy for Asia, noting examples of introduced animal breeds that were poorly adapted to the needs and constraints of poorer smallholder producers. There are several other misconceptions (mis-)guiding the design of livestock development interventions which should aim at describing the complexity of the livelihood strategies used by the poor, the role of livestock, and their linkages to nutritional and health status. Improving food supply from animals through higher livestock numbers (as in the past) is now severely constrained due to the feed-fodder deficit and declining per capita land availability. A large proportion of India's livestock, particularly in the arid and semi-arid environments, suffers from inadequate feeding. Most of the feed requirement is met from crop by-products and grazing on common lands, but the former is nutrient-deficit and the later have been dwindling quantitatively as well as qualitatively. Further, only 10 to 35% of the energy intake through fibrous forages is captured as net energy because of poor digestion of structural carbohydrates and thus underutilizing the only potential feed resources for ruminant livestock. In an ex-ante framework Kristjanson and Zerbini (1999) have estimated that a 1% improvement in digestibility of coarse cereal fodder through genetic manipulation would enhance production of different livestock outputs by 3-10%. This essentiality confers the importance of nutritional enhancement in augmenting livestock production.

According to the FAO statistics human population will increase from current about 6.5 to 9 billion people (about 40% more) on the earth in 2050 (Steinfeld *et al.* 2006) and the estimated need for meat (from 229 to 465 MT per year) and milk (from 580 to 1043 MT per year) will nearly double if we take into account the changing demand for high quality food of animal origin. Thus, the production of food of animal origin needs high amounts of resources and land (which is questionable?) for feed production because doubling of meat/milk output requires doubling of feed production or a dramatic improvement in the efficiency of conversion of feed into animal products. Due to rapid population growth in India, the situation is more demanding and raising the livestock production seems quite necessary to meet the reasonable demand.

4. Significance of Nutritional Input

The most important objective of animal nutrition is to meet the energy and nutrient requirements of animals in dependence on animal species/ categories and level of performance. There are many interlinking factors that influence animal nutrition and feed science to finally achieve the prime objective of livestock production (Fig. 1). Thus, animal nutrition has moved from a more natural science to a science of public interest along the total food chain soil-plant-animal-human.

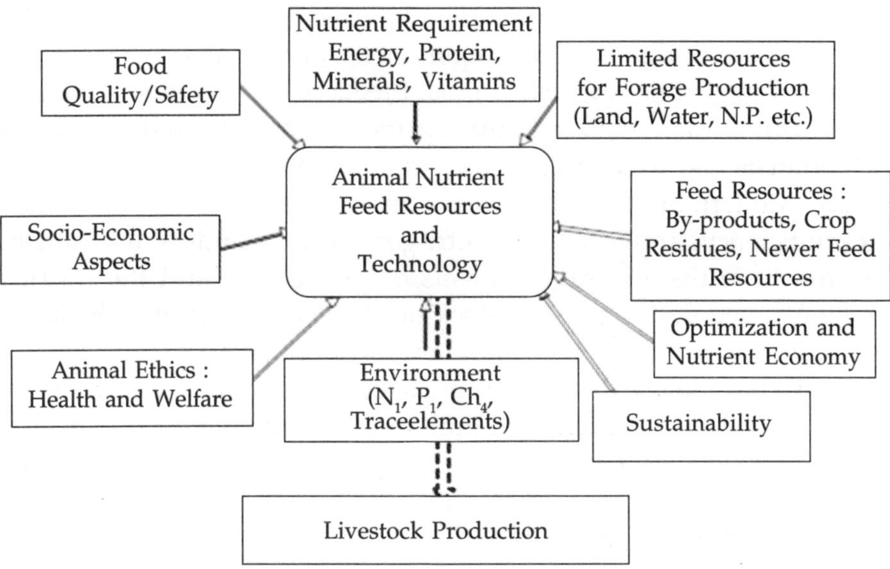

Fig. 1 : Factors influencing animal nutrition and feed science to achieve livestock production

The limited agricultural area and the higher demand of food of animal origin need a certain level of intensity of plant and animal production. In addition, the traditional competition of land use between production of vegetarian food for human consumption and feed production for animal production, and increase in use of land area for bio-energy/fuel production put pressure on animal nutritionists to find ways to i) optimize nutrient use to minimize wastage, ii) enhancing feed conversion, iii) increasing efficiency of nutrient utilization towards higher outputs (milk, meat, egg, wool, fibre), iv) economize feed cost to minimize input: output ratio, v) explore newer feed resources to widen feed resource base, vi) search for technology for feed delivery, storage and transportation, vii) sustain futuristic demand driven livestock production. Above all, a nutritionally healthy animal sustains higher level of production at minimized input and in most efficient manner. Therefore, the most important prerequisite for healthy animals, efficient feed conversion and sustenance of food producing animals is to meet their energy and nutrient requirements. Presently, National Research Council (NRC) and other statutory bodies analyse the current references and update the feeding standards. However, more research is necessary to study the requirements of all food producing animal species and categories of energy (metabolisable and/or net energy; ME/NE), protein/amino acids, major and trace elements and all vitamins in dependence on animal keeping and performances keeping in view trans-boundary genetic make-up of animals, feed resources and availability and level and state of production. The objective of the studies should be to avoid deficiencies and to meet the requirements of animals on the locale. With the advances in genetic research, animal breeders will develop animals with higher growth rates or yields and the nutritionists have to study the demands of such animals and to determine their energy and nutrient requirements in the future. Modern biotechnological and molecular tools to enhance nutrient use and efficiency, application of nutri-genomics to understand nutritional health and to withstand higher levels of production and the nutritional technology aimed at designer livestock products throw greater challenges in years to come. New challenges result in new developments/consequences in research. We have to use this chance and should communicate with the public in order to show the potentials and limitations of animal nutrition in efficient resource utilization, food quality and safety as well as environmental aspects.

4.1 Impact of feed on animal health

Role of nutrition in disease prevention, invasion of a disease process and amelioration of a disease condition is the resultant of nutrition-disease interactions in livestock. Thus, 'therapeutic nutrition' is aimed at correction of nutritional deficiencies or excesses, replacement of nutrients to ameliorate a disease or disorder which does not have a nutritional cause and feeding of drugs or nutrients to aid in the inhibition of diseases and 'preventative nutrition' is concerned with the adjustment of the amount of nutrients ingested for a primary deficiency or correcting the primary or secondary causes of the disease in the case of a secondary deficiency (Sahoo and Singh 2006).

There is increasing evidence that consumption of certain types of feed within a balanced diet may have a positive and even protective effect on health. The objective is to provide the scientific basis for improving health through diet. This will involve the use of dietary advice strategies, the development of new health promoting feeds, e.g. new products, products resulting from organic farming, functional foods, products containing genetically modified organisms and those arising from recent biotechnology developments. Disorders associated with an animal's inability to cope with the demands of high production include diseases such as milk fever and ketosis, which clearly are related to the cow's inability to maintain bodily functions in the face of negative calcium or energy balance. Improved nutrition of the late gestation cow can reduce the incidence of some of these disorders. Susceptibility to infectious disease is dependent on the integrity of the immune system, and recent studies have shed light on nutritional factors that affect leukocyte function. Other disorders, such as retained foetal membranes, udder oedema, and displacement of the abomasum are not easily categorized as to their cause, but nutritional strategies have been developed to help prevent these disorders as well (Goff 2006). Although advancements have been made in feeding practices to minimize the risk of metabolic diseases, the periparturient period continues to present some of the greatest challenges in animal health. The concepts of clinical/therapeutic nutrition, pharmaco-nutrition, orthomolecular nutrition, and dietetics and animal health are emerging to give a broad view of nutritional implications rendering animal health and sustaining optimum production. It will be achieved by means of an improved understanding of food metabolism and by harnessing the opportunities now available from proteomics and biotechnology.

5. Present Status and Future Requirements

India is having the highest density of bovine wealth (185 million cattle and 97 million buffaloes) and additionally, it possesses 124 million goats, 61 million sheep (GOI 2007-08). In similar pace, increasing human population, rapid urbanization and sustained rise in per capita income are fuelling rapid growth in the demand for animal food products. India has systematically quantified feed resources showing that CR were the most important single fodder source providing about 44% of the overall feed resources. Although the overall dry matter (DM) availability has increased from 348 MT in 1980-81 to 511 MT in 2002-2003, the present deficit with regard to dry fodder, green fodder and concentrate is to the tune of 19, 62 and 45% respectively (NIANP 2008). In this scenario, non-conventional feeds-fibrous CR and by-products; tree leaves and pods; industrial by-products (fruit and vegetable processing, vegetable oil industry, human food industry, alcohol fermentation industry); by-products of animal origin (poultry industry wastes, slaughterhouse and rendering industry, fish processing by-products) and others (aquatic weeds, algae, opentia etc.) are going to play important role in future. Ramachandra *et al.* (2007) predicted the contribution of CR to the Indian feed budget to reach almost 70% by the year 2020.

6. Feed and Fodder Availability

Crop-livestock integration is a common and efficient pathway for intensification of agriculture in developing countries, especially in tropical semi-arid and sub-humid environments prevalent in India. Both quantity and quality of feeds are required to support the efficient production of ruminants on a year-round basis. In India, the area under fodder cultivation has remained static for the last three decades at 4.5% of the total cultivable land, due to pressure of human population. The only way to increase fodder production is through intensive fodder production, especially using high yielding varieties of fodder crops. In view of the feed sources available at hand for feeding to livestock, poultry and aquatics, it is to be seen how India can focus attention in two areas, one is the development of genetically modified feed ingredients in order to nutritionally enhance and improve the production capabilities and the second is to improve certain feed ingredients which have inherently low nutritional capabilities like high fibre, anti-nutritive factors, low protein, deficiency of certain amino acids, and deficit micronutrients through the addition of feed additives/supplements.

The area under green fodder crops is squeezing day by day, presently constituting no more than 5% of the gross cropped area. The growth in area under fodder crops has been sluggish in most parts of the country, except in the irrigated regions, which is also a reflection of the rising competition between food and fodder crops for limited land and other resources. Common grazing lands comprise an important source of grasses, and there exists considerable scope to raise the production of grasses/ shrubs from these lands through technological and management interventions. Technological interventions such as reseeding with high-yielding grasses and watershed development, complemented with appropriate management interventions such as preventing encroachment, promotion of rotational grazing practices, and charging grazing fees have helped raise the productivity of common grazing resources and thereby improved animal performance. In cultivated land, intercropping of cereal and a forage legume can serve the dual purpose of increased grain yield and grazing between harvests and ploughing, in place of unproductive fallow. The integration of crop and animal production is well developed in the farming systems, particularly those in small-scale agriculture (Devendra and Thomas 2002). There is marked complementarity in resource use in these systems, with inputs from one sector being supplied to others. Integration of forage legumes in this cropping system improves soil fertility and soil structure and controls soil erosion and thus, helps in sustainable development of agriculture and at the same time continuity in forage resource. Due to the major rural-uphold on livestock population, small-scale, mixed crop–livestock systems has potential to remunerate and sustain the dwindling economy, thus contributing to the total output of animal products, especially meat and milk.

6.1 Food-feed-system

As much of the arable land is already under cultivation, increased productivity is most likely to come from improving productivity per unit area. Dual purpose crops that provide both food (grain) and feed (residues) are attractive options to meet household needs under this current and likely future scenario. Thus, in years to come, food-feed crops will become the most important feed source for ruminants (Thomas 2002). The system is intended at producing both foods for human and feeds for animal production. The International Crop Research Institute for Semi Arid Tropics (ICRISAT), in collaboration with the International Livestock Research Institute (ILRI) and the National Agricultural Research Systems (NARS) have been successful in jointly developing dual purpose crops of sorghum, pearl millet and groundnut that are capable of fulfilling the feed requirements of livestock, besides producing the grains for food through conventional breeding and biotechnological approaches. Estimates based on ex-ante impact assessments predict that improvement of stover quality through genetic enhancement can result in benefit cost ratios of 15:1 or higher (Kristjanson and Zerbini 1999). Resource-poor farmers are adopting and improving crop-livestock systems as they see clear benefits from food-feed crops: human food, livestock feed, manure and draft power. In addition, they also obtain cash income to purchase farm inputs, pay household expenses (food, health, education etc.) and making provision of insurance during times of crisis and uncertainty.

The importance of both feed quantity as well as feed quality (nutritive value) as key to improved livestock production has been emphasized and it indicates that small improvements in straws/stover digestibility could result in acceptable increases in ruminant productivity and impressive benefit: cost ratios. Thus, by improving the productivity and nutritive quality of food-feed crops and fostering the growth of delivery systems to improve access to research products, we can achieve improved utilization of such crops by resource-poor livestock keepers and their ruminant animals. Moreover, the CR based feeding systems can be improved by multidimensional crop improvement that includes nutritionally significant cultivar-dependent variation in CR fodder quality and sufficient independence between CR fodder traits and primary traits such as grain and pod yield besides addressing some of the important issues like breeding techniques for genetic enhancement of food-feed traits, technologies for quick and inexpensive phenotyping of large set of samples for simple fodder quality vis-à-vis livestock productivity, upgrading CR fodder in value chains through densification and fortification.

6.2 Feed technology, storage and feed/fodder bank

Technologies for improving the nutritive quality of CR by physical, chemical or biological treatments have not been widely adopted, because of inadequate technology demonstration and dissemination. Establishment of demonstration unit at village Panchayat/ Block level, accessibility to technology and the relevant resources, establishment of mini feed/fodder bank to meet immediate feed scarcity during natural calamity, ease in delivery of technologies and methodologies for a profit driven output will definitely encompass the bottlenecks and increase technology adoption. Apart from traditional techniques of fodder chopping and conservation, technologies such as urea treatment of fodder, strategic supplementation, urea molasses mineral blocks, and bypass protein use have the potential to alleviate feed and fodder scarcity. These technologies improve digestibility and palatability of feed, reduce feed requirements, avoid feed wastage, and contribute towards improving animal productivity.

7. Livestock Production and Economic Nutrient Use

Nutrient economy aims at efficient conversion of feeds/nutrients into food of animal origin with minimal wastage of input feed and nutrients. The conversion losses in food production from animal sources remain the principal concern of animal nutritionists. On one hand, these losses contribute to considerable resource consumption and on the other to the excretion of nutrients that pollute the environment. It is estimated that protein production via milk and eggs is more efficient and has a lower N and P excretion than via pork and beef (Flachowsky and Lebzien 2009). As the feed conversion into food improves, the excretion decreases with higher animal performance. The research in ruminant nutrition that are most applicable to the animal husbandry by small farmers in developing countries emphasises improving productivity of ruminants from mostly the fibrous feed resources and the primary constraint to ruminant production on these resources is the low efficiency of feed utilization. In practice improving the ratio of protein (amino acids) absorbed relative to energy nutrients (largely volatile fatty acids arising in fermentative digestion) is the primary factor that influences efficiency of product formation by ruminants. The energy density of a feed (often meaning only digestibility) only becomes a constraint after the nutrient balances of the animal have been corrected. Thus, improving the digestibility of poor quality forage allows increased intake, which can only be capitalised upon by the animal when the protein to energy ratio is appropriate. Efficiency of ruminal fermentation and digestibility of the dietary components are key factors in improving the efficiency of feed use. Therefore, it is possible to enhance feed efficiency and animal health by improving quality of feeds, increasing feedstuff and overall diet digestibility, better defining interactions among feedstuffs in diets, identifying alternative feed ingredients, better defining nutrient requirements, and improving efficiency of ruminal fermentation.

The primary feeding system today is the total mixed ration, with still considerable use of the pasture system. Cereal grains continue to be the primary contributors of starch to diets, and thus are very important in meeting the energy needs of dairy cattle and other meat producing livestock species including pigs and poultry in competition with human population. Processing of cereal grains has improved their use. Feeding by-products contributes valuable nutrients to diets and allows feedstuffs to be used that would otherwise be handled as wastes in landfills. Many of these by-products provide a considerable amount of protein, nonforage fibre, fat, and minerals (sometimes a detriment as in the case of P) to diets.

8. Scope of Nutritional Adequacy

The food requirement of animals can be estimated by calculating the amount of food needed to provide the requisite amount of ME for maintaining its state of production. An estimate of daily food intake depends primarily on data obtained from practical feeding trials. However, the recorded data needs scientific validation based on information from the local people, chemical composition of available pasture/fodder species, *in vitro* and *in sacco* study trials. Nutritional adequacy, on the other hand, needs assessment of the availability of feed and nutrients and sustainability for a particular state of production without affecting the productive life cycle of the animal. The time spent grazing, is dependent on the amount of forage consumed and the relative availability of herbage. Therefore, free ranging animals pay relatively higher costs of foraging for dispersed foods, avoiding or battling predators and parasites, dealing with more extreme climatic conditions, and interacting socially with other species competing for the same pasture or fodder resources (Sahoo 2005). In free ranging, if the food availability is scarce, the animals are forced to travel long distances in search of food to meet their energy requirements and this extra energy drain can be an important contributor to the ME need for maintenance. Thus the energy requirements in open range may increase several fold over values assessed for restrained animals. NRC considers that the increased muscular activity of the animal under grazing conditions accounts for a 25% increment in the case of light activity, a 50% increment on semi-arid rangeland pasture and on slightly hilly land and a 75% increment in case of long-distance travel on sparsely vegetated grassland or on mountainous transhumance pasture. Similarly, nutritional allowance during winter and high altitude temperate climatic condition is needed to maintain thermoregulation. In the same line there is a strong need to assess the nutrient requirements of migratory flock of sheep and goats which followed an annual cycle of upward (4000-5000 m above msl) and downward migration (plains) and exposed to a variable degree of under-nutrition.

8.1 Fibrous feed base - Understanding inefficiency and enhancing nutritional adequacy

The levels of ruminant production on roughage based diets are in general well below that is possible from the available resources and often between 10 and 30% of the genetic potential of the animal species. The utilization of agro-cellulosic residues is a major milestone in biotechnological generation for the production of valuable animal feed, food and energy. One approach is microbial treatment of straw and other CR to improve digestibility. The solid substrate/state fermentation (SSF) technology has a very wide scope for enriched animal feed production. The combination of SSF and silage making is a novel process that converts poor quality lignocellulosic materials into highly digestible animal feed. SSF with lignocellulolytic organisms increase the protein content of the product and partially degrade lignocellulose with enzymes produced during fermentation. The white rot fungi have the capacity to attack lignin polymers, open aromatic rings and release low molecular weight fragments (Zadrazil *et al.* 1996). On the other hand, silage making in the presence of such enzymes and lactic cultures preserves the nutritional value of the feed and increases its digestibility and palatability. Keeping the threat of population explosion and protein crisis in view, microbial biomass/single cell protein production from different organic residues may serve as good protein source and substrate in food or feed to meet the demands of protein requirements of the hunger and poverty-stricken nations.

9. Strategies for Optimal Use of Nutrients/Enhancing Nutrient Utilization

There are a number of nutritional technologies for improvement in rumen efficiency like, diet manipulation, direct inhibitors, feed additives, propionate enhancers, methane oxidisers, probiotics, defaunation and hormones and some of the issues are discussed below.

9.1 Manipulation of rumen ecosystem

Ruminant animals are exceptionally inefficient in their retention of nitrogen under conditions where the diet contains protein which can be fermented rapidly in the rumen. Protein is converted via peptides and amino acids to NH_3, which can be incorporated by ruminal microorganisms, but which, when present in excess, is absorbed rapidly across the ruminal wall. Proteolysis is carried out by many ruminal species, and large variation between individual animals occurs. The released amino acids are then deaminated by ciliate protozoa (Jouany 2008) and two categories of ruminal bacteria: the first category is comprised of many of the most numerous species of ruminal bacteria, which possess a low deaminative activity, and the second category is comprised of a much smaller population of so-called hyper-ammonia-producing (HAP) bacteria, which have much higher deaminative activity and which are believed to rely on amino acids rather than sugars for energy generation (Attwood *et al.* 1998). Inhibition of any of these catabolic steps would benefit nitrogen retention in ruminal fermentation. Wang *et al.* (2004) found that dipeptidyl peptidases inhibitors can influence the rate of NH_3 production in the rumen and may form the basis for developing protein-sparing feed additives for ruminants.

9.2 Defaunation

Protozoa account for upto 50% of the biomass of rumen microorganisms. Their elimination (i.e. defaunation) causes modification in the microbial population (increase in total number of bacteria with more small Gram-negative rods and *Selenomonas* and increase in fungal biomass). Protozoa host methanogenic bacteria that are closely associated with their surface and thus defaunation is aimed at reducing the feed energy loss via methane and augmenting efficiency of ME utilization. A more efficient use of diets in ciliate-free animals, especially when poor diets limiting growth are given, is noted and the enhancing effect is attributed to the higher amino acids supply to the host animal, more balanced VFAs and enhanced microbial fatty acids synthesis (Eugene *et al.* 2004). Part of the mechanism for improved N utilization in defaunated ruminants is an increase in the proportion of endogenous urea-N output that is recycled to the gastrointestinal tract, thus potentially providing additional N for microbial growth (Kiran and Mutsvangwa 2010) and may be considered to be an advantage only for animals fed low protein diets, in which bacterial nitrogen constitutes the main supply of intestinal proteins. Under conditions of defaunation, new strains of cellulolytic bacteria or genetically modified rumen bacteria could be developed to improve cell wall carbohydrate digestion.

9.3 Reducing emissions

Methane (CH_4) is the main electron sink in ruminal fermentation and its release to the atmosphere represents an energy loss between 2 and 15% of ingested gross energy (Van Nevel and Demeyer 1996) and therefore, various strategies are outlined to reduce methane emissions thereby reducing the energetic cost of feed utilization and thus increasing efficiency of energy use for productive purposes. Similarly, there will be increased excretion of N or P, if feed protein/N and dietary or supplemental P is improperly utilized or there is imbalance in C : N ratio or Ca : P ratio in the diet. The practices for reducing emissions from this source fall into three general categories: improving feeding practices, use of specific agents or dietary additives, and longer term management changes and animal breeding (Smith *et al.* 2008).

9.3.1 Improving feeding practices

Methane emissions can be reduced by feeding more concentrates, normally replacing forages. Although concentrates may increase daily methane emissions, emissions per kg feed intake and per kg product are almost invariably reduced. The net benefit, however, depends on reduced animal numbers or younger age at slaughter for beef animals. Other practices that can reduce CH_4 emissions include i) adding oils to the diet; ii) improving pasture quality, especially in less developed regions, because it improves animal productivity and reduces the proportion of energy lost as CH_4; and iii) optimizing protein intake to reduce N excretion and N_2O emissions.

9.3.2 Use of specific agents and dietary additives

A wide range of specific agents have been proposed as dietary additives to reduce CH_4 emissions as follows:

- Ionophores are antimicrobials that can reduce methane emissions, but their effect may be transitory and they have been banned in the EU.
- Halogenated compounds inhibit methanogenic bacteria but their effects are often transitory and they can have side effects such as reduced intake.
- Bioactive substances present in foods of plant origin significantly influence the bioavailability of minerals and requirements for vitamins and also modulate energy and protein metabolism in the rumen and body system.
- Probiotics such as yeast culture have shown only small, insignificant effects but selecting strains specifically for methane reducing ability could improve results.

- Propionate precursors such as fumarate or malate reduce methane formation by acting as alternative hydrogen acceptors, but they elicit response only at high doses and are therefore expensive.
- Vaccines against methanogenic bacteria are being developed but are not yet commercially available.
- Bovine somatotrophin (bST) and hormonal growth implants do not specifically suppress CH_4 formation, but by improving animal performance, they can reduce emissions per kg of animal product.

9.3.3 Nutritional intervention

Advancement in research and methodologies has outlined various approaches to reduce the excretions of N, P, CH_4 and trace elements (e.g. Cu, Zn) and the ones related to nutritional intervention are detailed below.

- Feeding systems, animal keeping, excrement management (avoid NH_3-losses etc.)
- More precise nutrient requirements of animals based on e.g. pre-caecal digestible amino acids and P in non-ruminants, better understanding of processes in rumen and utilization potential
- Avoiding excesses in nutrient supply (N, P, trace elements); meeting only the requirements of animals
- Use of rapid analyses for N, P and trace element determination in feed and native contents of feeds under consideration of bioavailability of nutrients
- Using knowledge on rumen metabolisms to optimize N-utilization in ruminants
- Adding crystalline amino acids to the diet if necessary, using phase-feeding depending on age; calculating amino acid requirements on the basis of pre-caecal digestible amino acids or on the basis of P (availability of P and trace elements in non-ruminants)
- Some activities (e.g. high propionate production by ration, fat supplementation, addition of propionate precursors or other feed additives) resulting in decreased methane emissions

9.4 Metabolic modifiers

Metabolism modifiers provide a potentially important means of altering both the extent to which amino acids are partitioned for protein deposition and the maximum rate of protein accretion. These are classified as compounds that alter metabolism in order to achieve an improvement in efficiency of a productive process. This may include improvements in growth rate, milk yield, body composition, or in nutrient utilization (Collier 2002). Metabolic modifiers can have more than one function (pleiotropy), and different metabolic modifiers may cause the same biologic effect (redundancy). Boyd and Bauman (1991) demonstrated that some compounds, like antibiotics, affect both growth and digestion because they influence microbial populations and digestive tract efficiency. Other compounds, such as anabolic steroids, á-adrenergic agonists, and somatotrophins, affect metabolism and utilization of absorbed nutrients and raise other considerations, such as effects on nutrient requirements.

9.5 Use of feed additives

Essential feed additives (e.g. amino acids, trace elements, vitamins) and nonessential substances (e.g. enzymes, prebiotics, phytogenic substances etc.) may contribute to a more efficient conversion of feed into food of animal origin. The feed additives are used in different animal feeding systems to i) enhance meeting the nutrient (amino acids, trace elements, vitamins) requirements of animals, ii) improve storage, transport and metabolism of food and nutrients, iii) regulate transfer of intended substances from feed to food (milk, meat, egg), iv) lower excretion of nutrients and enhance efficient conversion of feed, v) support high yield and animal health vi) improve quality of food of animal origin, vii) improve eco-balance by reducing methane and ammonia excretion. So, the developments/research activities in the field of feed additives needs to be directed at increased production through

- Supply of essential amino acids and analogues
- Rumen protected substances (amino acids, vitamins)
- More efficient trace elements and vitamins
- More efficient enzymes and probiotics
- Efficient phytogenic substances (essential oils)
- Detoxification of mycotoxins
- Influence on rumen metabolism
  - Efficient utilization of fibre fractions (lignin degradation)
  - Degradation/inactivation of antinutritive substances
  - Reduction of energy losses (methane) in the rumen (methane inhibitors)
  - Probably genetically modified microorganisms
- More efficient antioxidative substances, influence on food quality
- Antibodies, immunomodulators
- Products from nanotechnology

10. Nutritional Biotechnology for Raising Livestock Production

The principal targets of application of biotechnology in animal nutrition research are i) manipulation of the feed base, ii) manipulation of the metabolism and digestive physiology of the animal, iii) manipulation of the use of feed for production (partitioning of nutrients), iv) manipulation of the digestibility of feed prior to consumption, v) elimination or amelioration of diseases (Singh *et al.* 2008). In this line, the priorities for biotechnological application in nutritional research must be directed towards optimising protein: energy ratio in the nutrients absorbed by ruminants from poor quality forage based diets, digestibility of the basal feed resource, partitioning nutrients more effectively into the desired animal products and maintaining nutritional health and production of the animals.

The potential of genetically engineered (GE) crops is not limited to agronomic enhancement but may also serve as a means of enhancing the nutritional status of feed for livestock or food for humans. The greatest impact of biotechnology in livestock sector is in: i) improving the digestibility of CR by the release of glucose and other sugars from lignocellulose complexes, ii) increasing the nutrient content of forages/feeds, iii) decreasing the antinutritive factors, and iv) disease control of crops that also serve as animal feed. While most of the agricultural biotechnologies have primarily targeted towards improving the productivity of foods, the feed aspects have generally been overlooked. However, increased food production is generally accompanied by parallel improvement in residues and the availability of byproducts thereby strongly linking feed security to food security. It is expected that in the short-to medium-term, the largest impacts of biotechnologies on livestock production in the developing countries are likely to stem from increasing the quality of livestock feeds through improvements in the nutrient content of forages, the digestibility of low quality feeds and enhanced disease control (FAO 2007). Some of the ongoing successful biotechnological interventions involving molecular breeding with direct implication to livestock sector include developing dual purpose (food-feed) crops with higher biomass and digestibility of the CR, stay green and brown midrib traits in sorghum/maize, and high quality protein in maize/soybean.

10.1 Designer livestock production

Nutritional and genetic interventions to alter the milk composition for specific health and/or processing opportunities are gaining importance in dairy biotechnology. Less fat in milk, altered fatty acid profiles to include more healthy fatty acids such as conjugated linoleic acid (CLA) and ù-fats, improved amino acid profiles, more protein, less lactose, and absence of ß-lactoglobulin (ß-LG) are some opportunities of "designing" milk for human health benefits (Sabikhi 2007). Alteration of primary structure of casein and lipid profile, increased protein recovery, milk containing nutraceuticals and replacement for infant formula offer several advantages in the area of processing and all these have a definite impact on increased net return from dairy products. Similarly, the meat quality can be improved as per consumer choice, e.g. low fat, low cholesterol, more CLA etc. Lean red meat is a good source of protein, ù-3 fatty acids, vitamin B_{12}, niacin, zinc and iron and the meat, trimmed of visible fat, when consumed in a diet low in saturated fat does not increase cardiovascular risk factors e.g. plasma cholesterol levels or thrombotic risk factors (Li *et al.* 2005, Wagemakers *et al.* 2009). Various ethical, legal, and social aspects of biotechnological research would need to be addressed in the current economic and social climate before designer transgenic herds thrive along with the conventional counterpart. Animal welfare, demonstrable and sustained safety of the product, improved health properties of the product, and enhanced profitability vis-à-vis conventional practices would be the key factors that would eventually decide the future of designer foods.

A lot many areas in animal nutrition may encompass application of modern biotechnological tools which are detailed below.

- Balancing nutrition for reproduction/pregnancy, lactation, draught power. Ensuring balanced nutrition for ruminants and understanding its inefficiency on forage based diets
- Maximizing digestibility of fibrous feeds, improving the enzymatic ability of rumen microbes to degrade fibre and exploring potential targets for improving fibre digestion
- Physical, chemical, microbial treatments to increase digestibility, increasing the digestibility of poor quality roughage by manipulating the digestive physiology of the animal
- Altering the partitioning of nutrients within the animal
- Increasing fermentative efficiency in the rumen, meeting the requirements for efficient microbial growth in the rumen, optimizing microbial growth in the rumen
- Elimination of rumen protozoa (defaunation) and preservation of the fauna-free state
- Protein utilization by ruminants and requirements for amino acids/ peptides by rumen organisms especially microbes digesting fibre
- Adjusting P/E ratio in the nutrients absorbed by ruminants with protein supplements

- Alteration of protein and amino acid composition of rumen microbes - recombinant DNA technology
- Feed technology and development of supplements - bypass nutrient technologies
- Supplements and additives: micronutrient supplements, pre and probiotics, nutraceuticals, phytoadditives
- Green consumerism: Green livestock production and organic food supply
- Implication of parasite/disease nutrition interaction
- Orthomolecular nutrition: therapeutic nutrients aim at restoring the optimum environment of the body by correcting imbalances or deficiencies
- Bioengineering of rumen organisms - selection of anaerobic fungi for better fibre degradation in the rumen, selection of bacteria for fibrolytic activity, solubilisation of lignin, detoxification of anti-microbial, toxic and anti-quality factors in plants, developing detoxification mechanisms in rumen organisms
- Biotechnology and environment: maintaining healthy environment by reducing excretory metabolites and evolving efficient waste disposal management
- Nutrigenomics and nutrigenetics: interaction between diet and genes to unravel the complex relationship between nutritional molecules, genetic polymorphisms, and the biological system as a whole.
- *Transgenics*: Recombinant DNA technology with promise to improve livestock metabolism and possibility of modifying the digestive function through development of transgenic animals
- GM plants/animals and food safety: Animal and human health concern due to biotechnological applications need to be addressed in priority

11. Conclusion

Research strategies that are less capital intensive, with a low gestation period, a higher probability of success and acceptability by clientele, and that yield a good rate of return should be emphasized; and animal nutrition and health fall in this category. However, genetic research would be a key factor in growth and development of the livestock subsector in the long run. Nutrition being the major determinant of livestock production and shares more than half of the total cost, rationalization of input: output ratio by taking in to account the estimate of actual feed fodder consumption, contributions from grazing lands and forests will give an account of livestock production scenario, the contribution to national GDP and avenues of intervention for further enhancement. Besides, research input on newer feed resources, supplementation strategies, use of feed additives, manipulation of rumen fermentation, optimization of nutrients for efficient production, biotechnological application in feed and feed utilization process and economic livestock production will have a greater impact on future of livestock production. On the whole, issues of sustainability of livestock production systems, their environmental effects, and the role of technology in addressing these issues also merit attention for an in-depth empiricism in a resource economics perspective. Apart from the traditional animal nutrition, dealing with energy and nutrient requirements to produce enough and safe food of animal origin with healthy animals, the more efficient use of limited resources such as arable land or grassland, fuel, water and phosphorus, lower emissions of greenhouse gases (CO_2, CH_4, N_2O) and other pollutants (e.g. N, P, trace elements), the utilisation of agricultural and industrial by-products are new research fields of animal nutrition.

References

1. Attwood GT, Klieve AV, Ouwerkerk D, Patel BKC (1998). Ammonia-hyperproducing bacteria from New Zealand ruminants. Appl Env Microbiol 64:1796-1804.

2. Boyd RD, Bauman DE, Fox DG, Scanes CG (1991). Impact of metabolism modifiers on protein accretion and on protein and energy requirements of domestic animals. J Anim Sci 69 (Suppl 2):56-75.

3. Collier RJ (2002). Metabolic modifiers: advances in economic production of safe food. In: Bauman DE, Collier RJ (eds) Scientific Advances in Animal Nutrition: Promise for the New Century, Proceedings of a Symposium. National Academy Press, Washington DC.

4. Devendra C, Thomas D (2002). Crop-animal interactions in mixed farming systems. Agric Syst 71:27-40.

5. Eugene M, Archimede H, Sauvan D (2004). Quantitative meta-analysis on the effects of defaunation of the rumen on growth, intake and digestion in ruminants. Livest. Prod. Sci 85:81-97.

6. FAO (2007). Status of research and application of crop biotechnologies in developing countries. Food and Agriculture Organization, Rome.

7. Flachowsky G, Lebzien P (2009). Future in Animal Nutrition Research. In: Proceeding of Animal Nutrition Association World Conference, 14-17 February, 2009, New Delhi.

8. Flachowsky G, Chesson A, Aulrich K (2005). Animal nutrition with feeds from genetically modified plants. Arch Anim Nutr 59:1-40.

9. Goff JP (2006). Major advances in our understanding of nutritional influences on bovine health. J Dairy Sci 89:1292-1301.
10. GOI (2007-08). National Accounts and Statistics, Central Statistics Organisation, Ministry of Statistics and Programme Implementation, Government of India, New Delhi.
11. Hoffmann (2008). Livestock genetic diversity and Climate Change Adaptation. Livestock and Global Change conference proceeding. May 2008, Tunisia.
12. ICMR (2008). Guidelines for the Safety Assessment of Feeds Derived from Genetically Engineering Plants. Indian Council of Medical Research, New Delhi, pp 31.
13. Jouany JP (2008). Enteric methane production by ruminants and its control. Gut efficiency; the key ingredient in ruminants. Andrieu A, Wilde D (Ed.) Wageningen Academic Publ. p 35-59.
14. Kiran D, Mutsvangwa T (2010). Effects of partial ruminal defaunation on urea-nitrogen recycling, nitrogen metabolism, and microbial nitrogen supply in growing lambs fed low or high dietary crude protein concentrations. J Anim Sci. 88:1034-1047.
15. Kristjanson PM, Zerbini E (1999). Genetic enhancement of sorghum and millet residues fed to ruminants: an ex ante assessment of returns to research. ILRI Impact Assessment Series No. 3. ILRI, Nairobi, Kenya, pp 44.
16. Lenné JM, Fernandez-Rivera S, Blümmel M (2003). Approaches to improve the utilization of food-feed crops - synthesis. Field Crops Research 84:213-222.
17. Li D, Siriamornpun S, Wahlqvist ML, Mann NJ, Sinclair AJ (2005). Lean meat and heart health. Asia Pacific J Clin Nutr 14:113-119.
18. Moss AR (1994). Methane production by ruminants – literature review of I. Dietary manipulation to reduce methane production and II. Laboratory procedures for estimating methane potential of diets. Nutr Abstr Rev Ser B 64:786-806.
19. NIANP (2008). Feed Base. National Institute for Animal Nutrition and Physiology, Bangalore.
20. Ramachandra KS, Taneja RP, Sampath KT, Angadi UB, Anandan S (2007). Availability and requirement of feeds and fodders in India. National Institute of Animal Nutrition and Physiology, Bangalore.
21. Sabikhi L (2007). Designer milk. Adv Food Nutr Res 53:161-198.
22. Sahoo A (2005). Nutritional requirement of wild mammalian herbivores. In: Proceedings, National Symposium on Wildlife Health and Husbandry Constraints, 4th Annual Convention of Association of Indian Zoo and Wildlife Veterinarians. 25-26 Oct., 2005, College of Veterinary Science, AAU, Khanapara, Guwahati, Assam.
23. Sahoo A, Singh RK (2006). Therapeutic diets in clinical pet nutrition. In: Clinical Nutrition of Livestock and Pets, 3-23 Nov. 2006, CAS in Animal Nutrition, IVRI, Izatnagar. p 93-101.

24. Singh RK, Sahoo A, Chakravarti S (2008). Biotechnology in Animal Nutrition Research: Applications and opportunities. In: Compendium of Short Course on Nutritional strategies for sustainable and green livestock production September 10- 30, 2008, CAS in Animal Nutrition, IVRI, Izatnagar.

25. Smith P, Martino D *et al.* (2008). Greenhouse gas mitigation in agriculture. Philosophical Transactions The Royal Society B 363:789-813.

26. Steinfeld H, Gerber P, Wassenaar T, Castel V, Rosales M, deHaan C (2006). Livestock's long shadow: Environmental issues and options. FAO, Rome.

27. Thomas D (2002). Crop-animal systems in Asia. Agricultural System 71:1-4.

28. Van Nevel CJ, Demeyer DI (1996). Control of rumen methanogenesis. Environmental Monitoring Assessment 42:73-97.

29. Wagemakers JJ, Prynne CJ, Stephen AM, Wadsworth ME. (2009). Consumption of red or processed meat does not predict risk factors for coronary heart disease; results from a cohort of British adults in 1989 and 1999. Eur J Clin Nutr 63:303-311.

30. Wang H, McKain N, Walker ND, Wallace RJ. (2004). Influence of dipeptidyl peptidase inhibitors on growth, peptidase activity, and ammonia production by ruminal microorganisms. Curr Microbiol 49:115-122.

31. Zadrazil F, Kamra DN, Isikhnemhen OS, Schuchardt F, Flachowsky G (1996). Bioconversion feed with white rot fungi - Review of work done at FAL Braunschweig. J Appl Animal Res 10:105-124.

❑❑❑

Chapter 9

Tackling Drug Residues in Animal Products

R. C. PATRA
College of Veterinary Science and Animal Husbandry,
Orissa University of Agriculture and Technology, Bhubaneswar-751003

Contents

1. Introduction

Veterinary drug residues refer to the traces of chemicals or drugs that remain in the animal products, and include the breakdown products of the drugs or components of certain chemicals used in animals. These residues make their way into the human food chain and may cause hazards to food safety and public health. The surveillance and monitoring of residues in meat and their products were relatively a neglected area until the last decade. Due to the advances in technological intervention on livestock rearing, disease control and intensive crop production system, chances of residues in animal products have increased tremendously. The issue of drug residues in animal-derived food products is a major concern in many developing countries including India. The potential health problems associated with drug residues include allergic reactions, direct toxic effects, and a change in the resistance pattern of bacteria exposed to antibiotics.

The catastrophic decline in vulture population in India in the last one decade has been attributed, at least in part, to the drug residue problem. Diclofenac, a non-steroidal anti-inflammatory drug, has been banned by the Drug Controller of India in the year 2006 following the reports that diclofenac residues in the tissues of livestock treated with this drug before death is the major cause of visceral gout in vultures leading to massive death of the scavenging birds in Indian subcontinent. Such an overt scenario is the tip of the iceberg of drug residues-associated problems.

Drugs are being increasingly used in food producing animals to treat, prevent and diagnose diseases; to promote growth; to affect structure and function of the animal body; to improve quality of meat; to improve feed efficiency; and even to tranquilize animals for shipment, handling and surgical intervention. These drugs are administered either orally, parentrally (intramuscular, intravenous, subcutaneous route), through intramammary infusion or per rectally. These drugs are not completely eliminated from the body short while after administration nor are always metabolized to harmless end products. Human consumption of the animal tissues before the drug is completely eliminated from the body, or its level sufficiently falls below the permissible limit results in drug residue associated health problem for consumers.

2. Classification of Drug Residues

Drugs or chemicals are classified into three basic groups from residue stand point: (1) Medicated feeds, (2) insecticides, pesticides, and agricultural chemicals; and (3) therapeutic agents. The use of medicated feed is not an uncommon practice in organized system of livestock rearing. A large number of animals are fed with medicated feed at one time or the other to reduce the cost and labour. The drugs frequently incorporated in the animals' diet include antibiotics, arsenicals, anthelmentics, tranquilizer and hormone like substances. Antibiotics and nitrofurans are added to the feed to provide treatment against a specific infectious problem, to increase rate of growth and feed conversion ratio, and to enhance livestock production by reducing mortality and production losses. Dietary level considered safe for animals cannot be assumed to be safe for human consumption as cumulative accumulation of the drug increases its level in the target organ. Small doses of residues in foods of animal origin at times elicit allergic reactions or may lead to drug resistance.

Use of insecticides, pesticides and agricultural chemicals in livestock practice is not uncommon, and some insecticides are the major concern from residue point of view as these chemicals accumulate in adipose tissue. Pesticides have the unique status as these compounds are routinely used to increase the food production to meet the food demand. It is estimated that world food production shall reduce by 20% without the use of pesticides. Occasional misuse of such chemicals has resulted in intoxication of the animals and accumulation of residues in meat and meat products. Amongst all pesticides, organochlorine (OC) compounds such as DDT, lindane or hexachlorobenzene, heptachlor, heptachlor epoxide, aldrin and dieldrin are mostly persistent in the environment and cause major health hazards. Topical application of chemicals for parasite control, or consumption of feed and forage which has been sprayed or dusted with pesticides may result in residue accumulation in animal body through dermal absorption or inhalation.

A wide range of veterinary medicinal products are being used in animal husbandry practices. But residues problem due to veterinary drugs can be well avoided or minimized with proper use of the drugs and observing sufficient withdrawal period of time. About 42% of all veterinary pharmaceuticals used worldwide are used as feed additives, 19% as anti-infective, 13% as pesticides, 11% as biologicals and 15% as other pharmaceuticals (Mitchell *et al.* 1998).

Some of the therapeutic agents administered through oral route or in the form of injections by parenteral route produce harmful residues in meat and milk, particularly when these commodities are used for human consumption before completing the withdrawal period after the drug administration. Some anthelmentics, antibiotics and tranquilizers are included in this group. Regardless of the withdrawal period specified to assure residue elimination, no animal should be under the effect of tranquilizer at the time of ante-mortem inspection since the effects of the drug may mask the clinical signs of a disease. The most important concern in the use of therapeutic agents is the possibility of persistence of antibacterial agents in the milk. Three major public health hazard associated with antibiotic residues in milk are hypersensitivity to antibiotics like penicillin, development of resistance to antibiotics, and the spread of antibiotic resistant strains of infectious bacteria through food.

In some countries, the addition of medicinal compounds to animal feeds is a lawful and low-cost tool used to promote growth. Antimicrobials, anti-inflammatories and hormones are the pharmacologically active substances most commonly used for these purposes, but an illegal or improper use increases the risk of introducing harmful residues into the human food chain.

3. Indian Perspective

The drug residues associated problem in developing countries is not surprising due to the absence or ineffective implementation of the regulatory mechanisms and legislation for drug approval, sale and use, or for residues monitoring. Unapproved and unregulated drugs with no ADI (Average Daily Intake) can often be easily purchased from village shops and informal vendors. There may be no quality control of the substances supplied and, thus, concentrations and dose rates may be incorrectly recorded. There is often a lack of veterinary advice regarding withdrawal periods. Illiteracy of the animal owners does not permit proper reading of labels and printed instructions. Unqualified farmers, para-veterinary field staffs, and unskilled animal-handlers are frequently administering drugs, even without consultation with the veterinarians. Extended usage and excessive or multiple dosage of the compounds are not uncommon. Treatment records are hardly maintained or non-existent, and individual animal identification and traceability is often impossible. The fear of economic loss coupled with scarcity of meat may prompt the resource-poor farmers to slaughter sick or unhealthy animals for food. Many of the less developed countries lack the resources to assure food safety, so the issues like drug residues have a very low priority. Educational programmes and awareness campaigns targeted at farmers and field workers on the correct and appropriate use of veterinary drugs can help avoiding many of these scenarios. Such campaigns must take into account the socioeconomic status of the farmers and the level of veterinary advice available to them in the field and should be included in the design of residue programmes.

Antibiotics are widely used in developing countries, partly due to the high incidence of infectious diseases and partly because of indiscriminate use of drugs by the unskilled non-professionals. Anthelmintics are also commonly used and there is widespread use of drugs that may not be relevant in the developed world. The per capita consumption of meat and dairy products, especially poultry products has been increasing in developed countries including India. It is estimated that the *per capita* consumption of livestock products in developing countries could rise to as high as 144% by 2030. So, the use of antibiotics, coccidiostats and growth promoting hormones is expected to rise further with the growth of commercial enterprises and intensive or semi-intensive production systems that are supposed to play major role in pushing the production to meet the future demand. This will certainly lead to drug residue problem and increased drug resistance. As public awareness of food safety and quality aspect grows, there is increased pressure on the governments to address these issues even in low-income countries. Many middle or high income developing countries already have accredited control systems in place, or are working towards that goal. Since the late 1990s, the Joint Food and Agriculture Organisation and International Atomic Energy Agency (FAO/IAEA) Division of Nuclear Techniques in Food and Agriculture has been active in assisting capacity-building for drug residue monitoring in developing countries, through technical cooperation, technology transfer, coordinated research and other awareness-building and training activities.

Besides food safety and possibility of the development of antibiotic resistant pathogens, the main impetus behind the increased interest on tackling drug residues in developed countries is the need to meet the requirements for international trade. Failure to do so can have serious economic consequences. A glaring example is the EU suspension of imports of products of animal origin from China in March 2002, a market worth Rs 22.6 billion.

4. Food Safety and Drug Residue Scenario in the Developed Nations

The Codex Alimentarius Commission was created in 1963 by FAO and WHO to develop food standards, guidelines and related texts such as codes of practice under the Joint FAO/WHO Food Standards Programme. The main purposes of this Programme include protecting health of the consumers and ensuring fair trade practices in the food trade, and promoting coordination of all food standards work undertaken by the international governmental and nongovernmental organizations. The recent trade problems caused by food commodities containing substances that have no defined acceptable daily intake (ADI) or maximum residue limit (MRL) was highlighted in the meeting of the Joint FAO/WHO Expert Committee on Food Additives (JECFA) held in Rome. A committee was formed with the purpose to provide guidance to the FAO and WHO Member States and to the Codex Alimentarius Commission on public health issues pertaining to residues of veterinary drugs in foods of animal origin. The specific task before the committee was to elaborate further principles for evaluating the safety of residues of veterinary drugs in food, for establishing ADIs, and for recommending MRLs for such chemicals when the drugs under consideration are administered to food-producing animals in accordance with good practices in the use of veterinary drugs, and to evaluate the safety of residues of certain veterinary drugs (FAO/WHO 2009). MRLs of some commonly used drugs/chemicals in food animal tissues as per Codex Alimentarius Commission guidelines are given in Table 1.

Table 1 : Maximum Residues Limits (MRL) of some commonly used drugs/chemicals in veterinary practice

Drugs/chemical s	Species	MRL (µg/kg) in tissues/milk/egg			
		Muscles	Liver	Fat	Milk/eggs
Antibiotics/antibacterials					
Penicillin	Cattle	50	50	-	4
	Pig	50	50	-	-
	Chicken	50	50	-	-
Ceftiofur	Cattle	1000	2000	2000	100
	Pig	1000	2000	2000	-
Tetraclycline/	Cattle	200	600	-	100
oxytetracycline/	Sheep	200	600	-	100
chlortetracyclin	Pig	200	600	-	
	Chicken	200	600	-	400
Streptomycin/	Cattle	600	600	600	200
dihydrostreptomycin	Sheep	600	600	600	200
	Pig	600	600	600	-
	Chicken	600	600	600	-
Gentamycin	Cattle	100	2000	100	200
	Pig	100	2000	100	-
Lincomycin	Cattle	-	-	-	150
	Pig	200	500	100	-
	Chicken	200	500	100	-
Neomycin	Cattle	500	500	500	1500
	Sheep/goat	500	500	500	-
	Pig	500	500	500	-
	Chicken	500	500	500	500
Sulfadimidine	Cattle	100	100	100	25

Anthelmentics/antiprotozoals					
Albendazole	Cattle	100	5000	100	-
Thiabendazole	Cattle	100	100	100	100
	Sheep/goat	100	100	100	100
	Pig	100	100	100	-
Fenbendazole/	Cattle	100	500	100	100
febantel/	Sheep/goat	100	500	100	100
oxfenbendazole	Pig	100	500	100	-
Closantel	Cattle	1000	1000	3000	-
	Sheep	1500	1500	2000	-
Diminazene (Berenil®)	Cattle	500	12000	-	150
Doramectin	Cattle	10	100	150	15
	Pig	5	100	150	-
Imidocarb	Cattle	300	1500	50	50
Ivermectin	Cattle	-	100	40	10
	Sheep	-	15	20	-
	Pig	-	15	20	-
Levamisole	Cattle	10	100	10	-
	Sheep	10	100	10	-
	Pig	10	100	10	-
	Chicken	10	100	10	-
Pesticides/insecticides/agrochemicals					
Cypermethrin/	Cattle	50	50	1000	100
α-cypermethrin	Sheep	50	50	1000	-
Deltamethrin	Cattle	30	50	500	30
	Sheep	30	50	500	
	Chicken	30	50	500	30

Source: FAO/WHO (2009)

There has been no increase in drug residues in animal food products, and in fact, the rate of violation of food safety rules has steadily decreased in developed countries. Outbreak of illness, allergic reactions or deaths due to drug residues has not been reported in Utah State in USA in the last 20 years, nor has there been a decrease in the quality of food animal products (Bagley 2009). On the contrary, consumers have shown increased concern about antibiotic and other drug or chemical residues. The regulatory agencies are giving more emphasis on monitoring and preventing residues. Improved tests for sensitive detection of drug residue and enforcement of regulatory measures and penalties for violations by regulator agencies have made these changes possible.

There are a number of safeguard measures in the developed nations to reduce the risk of the problems, both in the animals and in the food processing system. Even with increased surveillance, the rate of detection of residues is low and the actual rate of violation of the permissible levels is very low there. Food animal industries in developed countries have responded to consumer and regulatory concerns by establishing quality assurance programmes to help their producers ensure improved quality of food products. Producers have recognized that they can do a better job in preventing residues. The mistakes detected in the future will be so costly that they will put some producers out of business because of one minor error. Contaminated milk from one cow could result in residue detection and cause the condemnation of mixed milk from 1,000 to 60,000 other cows. The regulations could force a producer to pay for the contaminated, discarded milk. Few producers could afford it or they would be forced out of business.

The Food and Drug Administration (FDA) in USA has primary responsibility for regulating most foods, including milk, transported between the states. FDA's milk safety programme relies on participation by state regulatory agencies. This participation is described in a 1977 Memorandum of Understanding (MOU) between the National Conference on Interstate Milk Shipments (NCIMS) and the FDA is designed to provide assurance of clean and safe national milk supply. The FDA, with the support of the NCIMS initiated the National Drug Residue Milk Monitoring Programme (NDRMMP) in February 1991. The NDRMMP is designed to assist and supplement the longstanding NCIMS programme. The NDRMMP is designed to provide an indication of animal drug residues that may be present in milk and the extent that farmers, distributors, and veterinarians comply with the Federal Food, Drug, and Cosmetic Act, implementing regulations and applicable policies.

5. Detection of Residues

5.1 Veterinary drugs

Microbial growth inhibition assay, microbial receptor assay, enzymatic colourimetric assay, receptor binding assays, chromatographic methods and immunoassays are being employed as conventional methods for detection of veterinary drug resides in food of animal origin. These are commonly used for monitoring of antimicrobial residues in meat and meat products. Biosensors have been developed to determine veterinary drug residues in biological and food samples. The Surface Plasmon Resonance (SPR) technique is used for online and at-line detection of veterinary drug residues in milk, porcine bile and bovine urine. This sensor operates real time and detect up to 8 different veterinary drugs simultaneously with a thoroughput of upto 600 samples per day.

5.2 Pesticides

Colourimetric methods, thin layer chromatography (TLC), high performance liquid chromatography (HPLC), gas liquid chromatography (GLC), gas chromatography-mass spectroscopy (GC-MS), liquid chromatography-mass spectroscopy-mass photometry (LC-MS-MS) are the conventional methods used for detection of pesticide residues in animal products. Colorimetric methods and TLC are relatively less sensitive, whereas GLC or GC-MS are normally used for determination of non-volatile compounds and thermolabile compounds such as synthetic pyrethroid and N-methyl carbamate pesticides. HPLC, MS and GC-MS give satisfactory results for analysis of pesticide residues.

New assay techniques including sensors have been developed for faster and on-site detection of pesticide residues. Enzymatic biosensors based on inhibition of a selected enzyme are the most extended biosensors used for determination of these compounds. These technique is very sensitive but may not be selective, thus their use for quantitative analysis of individual pesticide or class of pesticides are not possible. Recombinant enzyme for biosensor application and River analyser (RIANA) immunosensor has been developed for detection of pesticides. However, these techniques have limited application in detection of pesticide compound in meat system.

Sample preparation for the isolation of veterinary drugs and growth promoters from foods is very important. A review by Kinsella (2009) focuses on sample preparation techniques, new techniques and technologies to improve efficiency and coverage of residues, multi-residue detection methods.

6. Residues Associated Health Risk

About 2 million poisoning and 10,000 deaths occur each year from pesticides with about 75% of this occurring in developing countries. The acute and malicious consumption involving higher dose results in death whereas chronic insidious intakes lead to elevated cancer risk and disruption of body's reproductive, immune, endocrine, and nervous system etc. The organochlorines such as DDT increase the incidence of lung tumour and lymphoma in mice, liver tumours in rats and adenomas in hamster.

Health risks associated with veterinary drug residues are quite common. The indirect and long term hazards include microbiological effects, carcinogenicity, reproductive effects and teratogenicity. Microbiological effects are one of the major health hazards in human beings. Antibiotic residues consumed along with edible tissues like milk, meat and eggs can produce resistance in bacterial populations in the consumers. This is one of the major reasons of therapeutic failures amongst such people. Nitroimidiazoles and 3-nitrofurans can cause cancer in human population. Some drugs produce reproductive and teratogenic effects at very low doses consumed for a prolonged period of time.

The overuse of antimicrobials such as tetracycline, sulfonamides, aminoglycosides, ß-lactam derivatives etc. in animal production or their residues in food of animal origin pose potential allergic reactions in sensitized individuals. Use of hormonal compounds like diethylestilbestrol in meat production is known to have strong carcinogenic effects and thus, is banned for use in food producing animals. The adverse effects of the residues of ß-adrenergic agonistic due to its excess administration for lean meat production are less tolerable and require hospital treatment. Thus, health risk of veterinary medicinal products and their metabolites are very difficult to define and their presence above the violative level is illegal and subject to financial penalties in many countries.

7. Handling Drug Residue Issues

Risk assessment, risk management and risk communication are to be taken into consideration to resolve the residues problem. Risk assessment is a systematic scientific characterization of potential adverse health effects following exposure to hazardous agents. Results from the risk assessment can be used to inform risk management, who work with factors like social importance of risk, social acceptability of the risk, economic impacts etc. Finally, risk communication involves making the risk assessment and risk management information comprehensible to lawyers, politicians, judges, environmentalists and community groups. These will help to build a foundation for determining residue levels in our foods. The edible products from the animal source should be collected and verified for legal requirement and to ensure that drug concentrations in these products are not at levels higher than those established as safe by the relevant regulatory authority in the country of origin. In many countries of the world, this upper level is referred to as MRL, while in the United States it is termed as tolerance (Riviere 1999). MRLs or tolerances are established by regulatory authorities based on many factors primarily relating to the safety of the animal product to the consumer, the usage pattern of the compound (pesticide in the field), and analytical methodology. The food safety is evaluated based on the length of time after discontinuation of drug administration or chemical exposure required to allow a tissue to deplete to a concentration below the MRL, called pre-slaughter meat withdrawal time. The tissue tolerances or MRLs are generally established in animal source edible tissues such as fat, milk, muscle, liver, kidney, skin, or sometime meat by-products. So, sufficient withdrawal time should be given to reduce the residue level below the tolerance level. The recommended withdrawal periods of some important veterinary drugs in dairy cows are given in Table 2.

Table 2 : Withdrawal periods of some important drugs used in veterinary practice

Drugs	Route of administration	Pre-slaughter withdrawal (days)	Milk discard (days)
Antibiotics			
Amoxicillin	Intramammary	12	2.5
Amoxicillin trihydrate	Parental	25	4
Erythromycin	Intramammary	14	1.5
Erythromycin	Parental	14	4
Novobiocin + procaine penicillin G	Intramammary	15	3
Pirlimycin	Intramammary	28	1.5
Procaine penicillin G	Intramammary	3	2.5
Procaine penicillin G	Parental	10	2
Sodium cloxacillin	Intramammary	10	2
Ampicillin trihydrate	Parental	6	2
Ceftiofur hydrochloride	Parental	2	0
Ceftiofur sodium	Parental	0	0
Oxytetracycline	Parental	28	4
Antibacterial			
Sulfadimethoxine	Parental	5	2.5
Anthelemetics			
Fenbendazole (suspension/paste)	oral	8	0
Fenbendazole	oral	13	0
Organochlorine/ Organophosphates			
Fenthion	Oral	35	28
Coumaphos	Oral	0	14
Other drugs			
Furosemide	Parental	2	2

Source: Adopted from Muhammad *et al.* (2009)

The first step in calculating the tolerance is to determine the safe concentration of drug that could be consumed by individuals eating the animal products. The safe concentration is determined by taking the ratio of ADI x bodyweight and food consumption factor (Muhammad *et al.* 2009). The food consumption factor is the amount of edible product estimated to be consumed daily by an individual. The food consumption factor is based upon the average individual's daily intake of different types of foods.

8. Residue Control Programme and Limitations

Developing countries face many difficulties when planning to implement a residue control programme. However, with the assistance from the developed world, several of the projects implemented by the IAEA have resulted in accredited (ISO/IEC 17025) screening laboratories and National Plans being put in place, with a consequent positive impact on food quality and the ability to participate in international trade. The ultimate outcome is an increase in foreign exchange and a contribution to the alleviation of poverty. The IAEA has recently completed veterinary drug residue projects in various countries, including Cyprus, The Dominican Republic, Jamaica, Malaysia, Malta, Mongolia, Morocco, Namibia, South Africa, Sri Lanka and Yemen. The continuing development of international networks and collaboration between developed and developing countries must be actively promoted to progress towards the goal of a safe food supply.

One basic limitation to conduct residue analysis is the detection of chemical residues in edible animal products. The exact risk is impossible to assess without accurate detection. This process needs highly qualified expertise, sensitive instruments and modern analytical techniques. With limited infrastructural resources and personnel, it is very difficult task for the laboratories in many countries to meet the criteria set out for confirmatory analysis. The goal is often to set up a quality-assured screening laboratory using techniques such as microbial inhibition tests and immunoassays. Certain countries like Thailand, where the export market is very important, have invested in LC-MS-MS instrumentation and personnel. In certain countries in Latin America commercial laboratories are contracted by government to perform confirmatory analyses. There is a need for the provision of affordable confirmatory services from advanced laboratories in the developed world.

The implementation of screening methods can also be problematic. Such problems are being addressed under a FAO/IAEA research project in which several groups will study the problem and investigate reagent stabilisation. Immunoassay reagents have also been produced in several countries to develop in-house methods and ensure regional reagent supply. The specific technical problems such as difficulties with supply of laboratory materials, analytical standards and reference materials, sourcing of analytical equipment and availability of local servicing and consumables in the laboratories in developing country can also impede the implementation of quality systems. Scientific literature may and methodologies may not be readily available in the local language. Poor laboratory conditions such as high temperatures, unstable power supplies and inadequate safety facilities can adversely affect performance.

There is also confusion concerning the lack of harmonisation with respect to aspects such as maximum residue limits (MRLs). Developing countries exporting to the EU are required under the Commission Decision 2001/487/EC to comply with the Directive 96/23/EC for residue plans and Council Regulation (EEC) No 2377/90 for MRLs. However, the EU sampling strategy and MRLs may differ from those set by Codex (Ellis 2008), which is intended to be used as a point of reference in trade disputes under the Sanitary and Phytosanitary Standards (SPS) Agreement of the World Trade Organization. These differences can have a significant effect on developing country trade; for example, it is estimated that if Codex MRLs were adopted for tetracyclines, global trade in beef would increase by over Rs. 150 billion. The implementation of sampling regimes as outlined in Codex guidelines CAC/GL/16 1993 or the European Directive 96/23/EC can be difficult given the problems with animal identification and traceability and the lack of resources and infrastructure for sample collection and transport.

9. Future Scope and Challenges

The developing countries have to focus on good management practices and implement sanitary and phytosanitary measures if they wish to compete in the global market for trade of animal produce. This is certainly a big challenge for developing countries like India where food security is a major issue for food security of human population. The documentation of the production procedures has to be more stringent for traceability of the produce. Emphasis has to be given on quality produce where periodical quality checking at different collection points is required to survive in the international market.

The problem associated with drug residues is a major concern in domestic market too with increasing awareness among the consumers. The Standards and Conformity Assessment Bodies of India such as BIS (Bureau of Indian Standards), QCI (Quality Council of India), NCC (National Codex Committee) and CCA (Controller of Certifying Authorities) should work hand in hand to ensure food safety and regulate the drug residue limits, and food safety regulation have to be implemented with more force.

The Drug Controller of India and the State Drug Control bodies are required to create more awareness among the consumers and the livestock owners regarding the rules and regulations governing the use, sale and administration of drugs including vaccines for disease control. This will bring out altogether a different scenario where the drugs could be administered only under the supervision of trained persons who have adequate knowledge about the administered drug including its safety, residues problem and withdrawal period etc., thus minimizing veterinary drugs entering into human food chain.

10. Conclusion

With the implementation of World Trade Organization treaty for import and export of food of animal origin, the concern in developing countries with respect to monitoring and controlling drug residues has become more visible. Some of the developing countries with the support from developed countries and international bodies have set up quality control laboratories to ensure food safety. Increasing the awareness amongst the producers and consumers could minimize the drug residues problem. The future of livestock industry should witness that the veterinary drugs are used by a skilled person having sufficient knowledge about the veterinary formulations, their safety, withdrawal period, and the toxic consequences upon entering into food chain. Stringent steps are required to reduce the abuse of drugs and the magnitude of the residue problem.

References

1. Bagley CV (2009). Drug resides and food safety, Fact Sheet. Utah State Agricultural University Bulletin.
2. Ellis RL (2008). Development of veterinary drug residue controls by the Codex Alimentarius Commission: a review. Food Addit Contam Part A Chem Anal Control Expo Risk Assess 25(12):1432-1438.
3. FAO/WHO (2009). Joint FAO/WHO expert committee on food additives. Seventieth meeting (Residues of veterinary drugs), Geneva, (21-29 October 2008). Summary & conclusions-Corrected, Issued 10 March 2009. www.fao.org/ag/agn/agns/jecfa/JECFA70_Summary_report_final_corr.pdf
4. Kinsella B, Mahony JO, Malone E, Moloney M, Cantwell H, Furey A, Martin Danaher M (2009). Current trends in sample preparation for growth promoter and veterinary drug residue analysis. J Chromatography A 1216:7977-8015.
5. Mitchell JM, Griffiths MW, McEwen SA, ScNab WB, Yee AE (1998). Anitmicrobial drug residues in milk and meat: Causes, concerns, prevalence, regulations, tests and test performance: A review. J Food Protect 61:742-756.
6. Muhammad F, Akhtar M, Rahman ZU, Javed I, Irfan Anwar M (2009). Role of veterinarians in providing residue-free animal food. Pakistan Vet J 29(1):42-46.
7. Riviere JE (1999). Comparative Pharmacokinetics, Principles, Techniques and Applications. Iowa State Univ. Press, Ames, Iowa, USA.

❑❑❑

Chapter 10

Modernization of Veterinary Healthcare Services

P. DHANAPALAN AND P. SELVARAJ
Madras Veterinary College, Tamil Nadu Veterinary and Animal Sciences University, Chennai-600007

Contents

1. Introduction

India has the unique distinction of establishing and running the world's first animal hospitals during the period of the great Emperor Ashoka. Organized communities had been providing animal healthcare services even prior to that in ancient India. India is a home to several records or treatises on animal healthcare. Animal husbandry plays a major role in the economic and industrial growth of the country. More than 70% of rural people depend upon animal husbandry activity for their daily income and the livestock farming forms the backbone of rural economy especially when there is failure of monsoon. The government's efforts for poverty alleviation and creation of self employment opportunities among the rural masses are successfully channelised through animal husbandry activities in villages. Moreover, growing human population, rapid urbanization, increasing domestic income and changing lifestyles of the people have led to the demand for better healthcare for the farm and companion animals.

While the major thrust of animal husbandry department is currently towards augmenting animal production through innovative breeding and feeding strategies, health cover and patient care usually take the back seat in planning and implementation. The livestock production has been steadily growing, faster than any other agricultural sub-sector, and it is foreseen that by 2020, livestock will account for more than half of total global agricultural output in economic terms. The increasing production levels put enormous stress on farm animals, predisposing them to diseases. Increased trans-border movement of animals and animal products is also creating risk of newer diseases, which at times may even have public health consequences.

It is, therefore, imperative that a robust animal healthcare system should be put in place throughout the country to meet the enormous challenge posed by the emerging and reemerging livestock diseases, a large number of which may influence human health and/or food security.

2. Current Status of Animal Husbandry Departments

Augmentation of the production potentialities of livestock and poultry; increasing the production of milk, egg and meat; providing necessary and timely modern veterinary assistance and health cover to the livestock and poultry; implementation of various central and state government schemes for the uplift of rural poor; providing information and training on basic and the latest animal husbandry practices; and protection of human health by preventing major zoonotic diseases of animals are the usual major objectives of animal husbandry departments in India. However, as such kind of multitasking is usually entrusted to the veterinarians working in the government veterinary dispensaries, it becomes naturally impracticable for a single person to give adequate attention to all these activities. It is particularly so because the veterinary institutions all over the country are generally running short of adequate human resources. Consequently, the results are poor or unsatisfactory. The animal husbandry departments all over the country need to evolve strategies to upgrade and modernize the human as well as infrastructural resources to improve upon the quality of veterinary services.

3. Strategies for Modernization of Veterinary Services

Modernization of animal health services may involve several spheres of activities. The following thrust areas require high priority.

1. Establishment of modern veterinary hospitals
2. Establishment of referral veterinary hospitals
3. Establishment of superspeciality veterinary hospitals
4. Establishment of local, regional and central veterinary laboratories
5. Establishment of referral veterinary laboratories of international standards
6. Establishment of professional and technician cadre programmes in veterinary care support for effective service delivery
7. Strengthening of animal quarantine and certification services
8. Establishment of national level species specific special clinical research centers
9. Establishment of national boards of veterinary hospitals and laboratories accreditation
10. Establishment of national surveillance centre and programmes for animal diseases and zoonotic diseases
11. Strengthening of animal disease investigation and control programmes
12. Establishment of national animal disaster and rescue management agency
13. Strengthening of wildlife veterinary services
14. Establishment of aquatic animal medicine facilities

4. Establishment of Modern Veterinary Hospitals

The organized veterinary dispensaries and hospitals though exist throughout the country, the infrastructure and services available in these are abysmally inadequate and technically of poor quality. Besides the infrastructure, the human resource in such institutions too needs to be augmented both in terms of quality and quantity. Utilizing the existing space, efforts must be made to establish modern veterinary hospitals at least at block levels in each district. As the veterinary hospitals in the country generally have a major case load of farm animals, these hospitals should have well equipped large animal services. These should provide individual animal care as well as herd healthcare to cattle, buffalo, sheep, goats, horses and other animals depending on the local requirement at each location.

Facilities should be provided for integrated livestock health management. The veterinary practitioners should be provided access to state-of-the-art equipments and should use the latest diagnostic and therapeutic techniques. Large animal emergency services should also be made available at all times and round the clock in such establishments.

A modern veterinary hospital should be able to provide the following facilities:

- Complete vaccination service for all animal species with quality vaccine storage facilities
- Ectoparasite and endoparasite diagnostics and therapeutic service for all species
- Modern restraint facilities for physical examination of farm and pet animals
- Set of basic diagnostic equipments for complete physical examination
- Clinical sample collection, processing and storage facility for basic clinical pathology protocols
- Bedside testing facilities such as microscope and dry chemistry test kits for common diseases
- Bedside urinalysis kits
- Fluid therapy facility with multiple trevis support for simultaneous care of more animals
- Oral rehydration therapy facility
- Complete set of stomach tubes and speculums for all species
- Downer cow support slings and aqua floatation tanks
- Mastitis trevis and mastitis bedside testing kits

5. Establishment of Referral Veterinary Hospitals

A referral veterinary hospital with specialised equipments and facilities for advanced food animal medicine and surgical services should be provided at each block or *tehsil* (*taluka*) level in a district. Specialists and adequate supportive staff should be posted to man the hospital and to provide the required advanced care for the entire region. Round the clock services should be the mandate of such hospitals.

5.1 Food animal medical services

Facilities shall be made available for detailed examination and treatment of infectious diseases, metabolic disorders, gastrointestinal disorders, respiratory problems, urinary tract problems, trace mineral deficiencies, poisonings and other disorders. Advanced diagnostic procedures such as ultrasound, endoscopy and radiography should be made available for accurate diagnosis and intensive care management. Such facilities will be helpful in protecting valuable animals, for example, a valuable calf with diarrhoea can be given intravenous fluid therapy under specialist's supervision by the round the clock nursing staff. Continuous laboratory monitoring can help in making the changes and immediate adjustments in therapy in critical cases.

Animals representing a herd problem can often yield valuable information when they are given a thorough diagnostic workup at such services, leading to a solution for the herd. The food animal medicine section should also take up routine activities like vaccinations and health examinations.

5.2 Modern equipments requirement of a referral veterinary hospital

Some major equipment required in a referral veterinary hospital are depicted in Table 1.

Table 1 : Major equipment requirement in a referral veterinary hospital

S. No	Name of the equipment	Approximate cost as in 2010 (Rs. in lacs)
1.	Ultrasound scanner	6.5
2.	Doppler echo ultrasound	18.0
3.	Fresenius haemodialyzer	7.5
4.	Reverse osmosis plant	0.5
5.	Mechanical ventilator	5.5
6.	Centralised oxygen supply system	4.5
7.	Infusion pumps	0.5
8.	Suction apparatus	0.25
9.	Vital signs monitor	3.75
10.	Doppler BP apparatus	0.50
11.	Blood gas analyzer	4.0
12.	Semi-automated biochemistry analyzer	2.5

13.	Emergency crash cart	0.5
14.	ECG machine	1.25
15.	PCG machine and analysis system	1.50
16.	Holter ECG and analysis system	3.75
17.	Cardiac defibrillator	4.25
18.	Video endoscopy system for small animals	25.0
19.	Video endoscopy system for large animals	30.0
20.	Video otoendoscopy and digital suction systems	7.5
21.	Treadmill and ECG system	5.0
22.	Small animal bronchoscopy system	15.0
23.	Milk checker, Ferroscopy and Rumen fluid microscopy	3.5

5.3 Food animal surgical services

A team of food animal veterinarians with expertise in routine surgical procedures should be available. The facilities should exist for rumenotomy, correction of displaced abomasum and other abdominal surgeries, castration, dehorning, removal of tumours associated with cancer eye, caesarean sections, and fracture repair. For complex fractures, the expertise of orthopedic surgeons should be utilized. A trained anaesthesiologist should be available in such referral hospitals to provide anaesthesia and for effective monitoring of the anaesthetized animals.

5.4 Food animal reproduction services

Specialist veterinarians should attend to the animals with complex issues of fertility and reproduction at the district level hospitals. Beginning from the vaccination against brucellosis to testing for trichomoniasis and testing for male fertility evaluation, the reproductive services should provide state-of-the-art preventive care and diagnostics. Semen testing and fertility evaluation facility should be made available as it is the key to a good conception rate. The other services should include oestrous synchronization, hormone treatments, male fertility testing, nutrition counseling, pregnancy testing including use of reproductive ultrasound, and the treatment for anoestrus, cystic follicles and other problems.

6. Establishment of Superspeciality Veterinary Hospitals

Each district should have a state of the art superspeciality veterinary hospital (Fig. 1-19). It should be under the administrative and operational control of the nearby veterinary college or veterinary university. The state animal husbandry departments should ensure to provide adequate financial support to these superspeciality hospitals so as to run these services free of cost for the farming community. Such hospitals should provide the services for the following.

- Complete healthcare
- Critical and intensive care
- Emergency care
- Eye disorders
- Farm visits for herd problems
- Fertility evaluation
- Fracture repair
- Lameness
- Mastitis
- Metabolic health problems
- Neonatal services
- Pharmaceutical services
- Pregnancy testing
- Reproductive services
- Surgery consultations

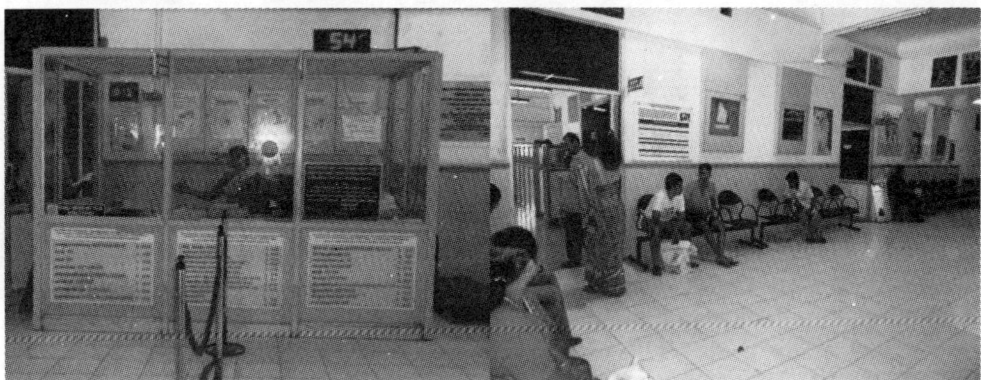

Fig. 1 : Reception and client waiting area

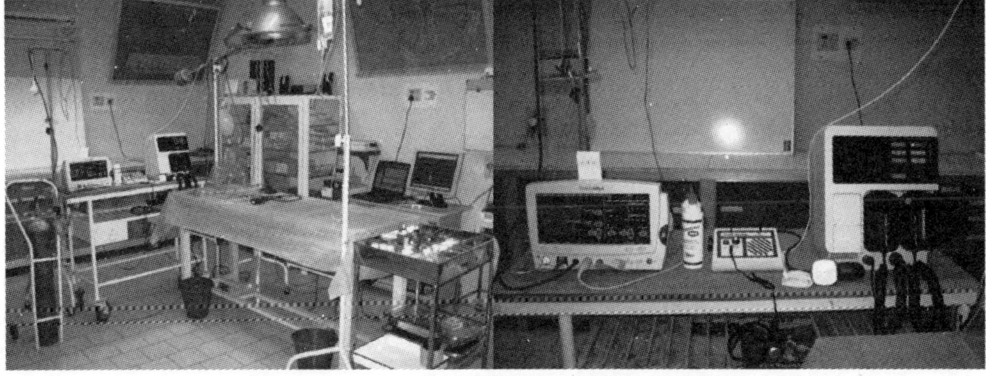

Fig. 2 : Small animal ICU and CCU facilities

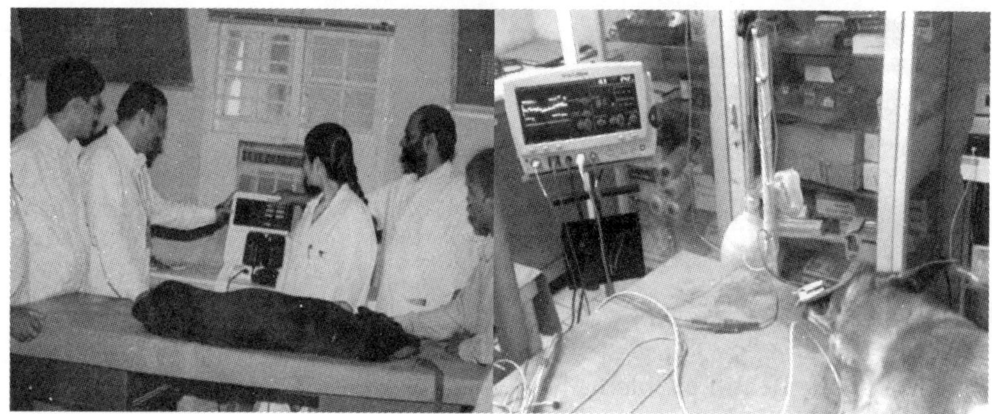

Fig. 3 : ECG and vital signs monitoring

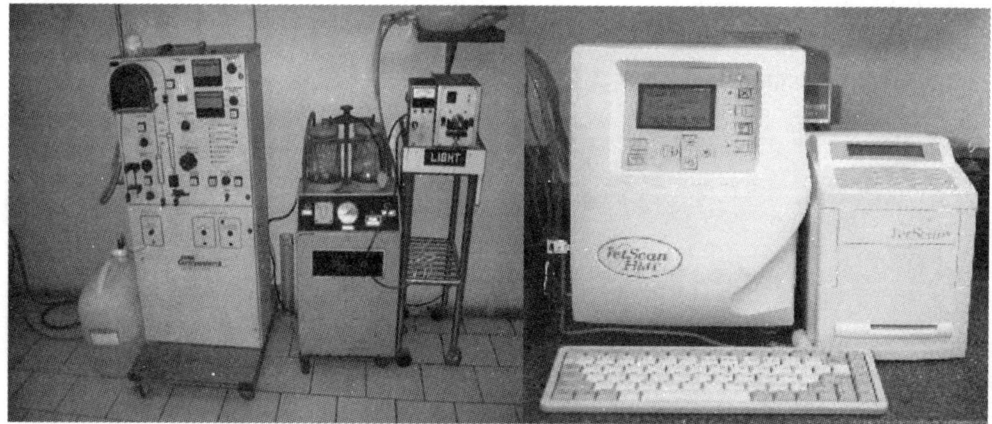

Fig. 4 : Haemodialysis and haematology analyser

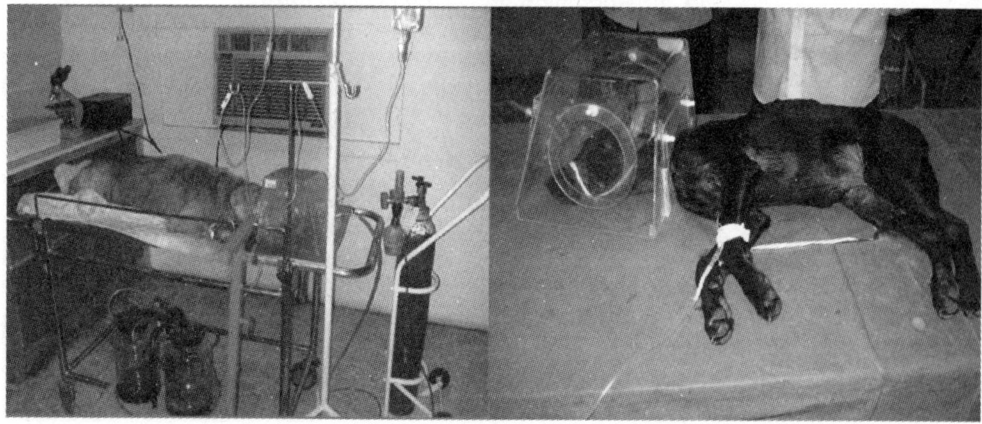

Fig. 5 : Oxygen therapy facilities

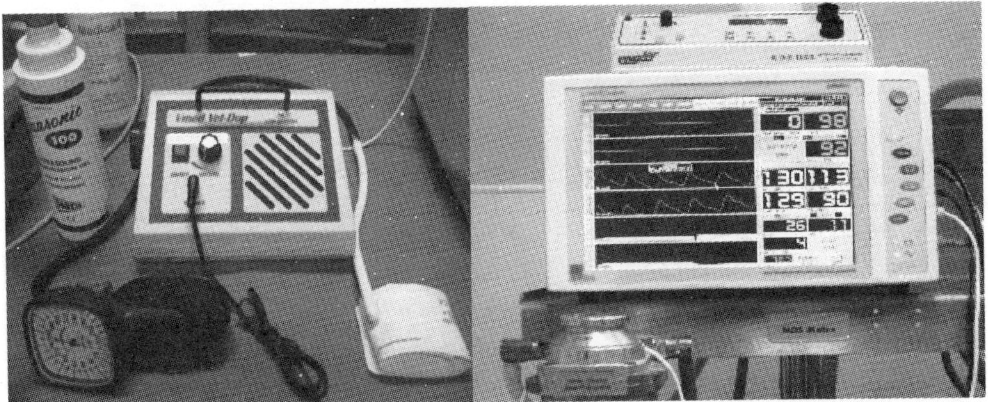

Fig. 6 : Doppler blood pressure apparatus and haemodynamic monitor

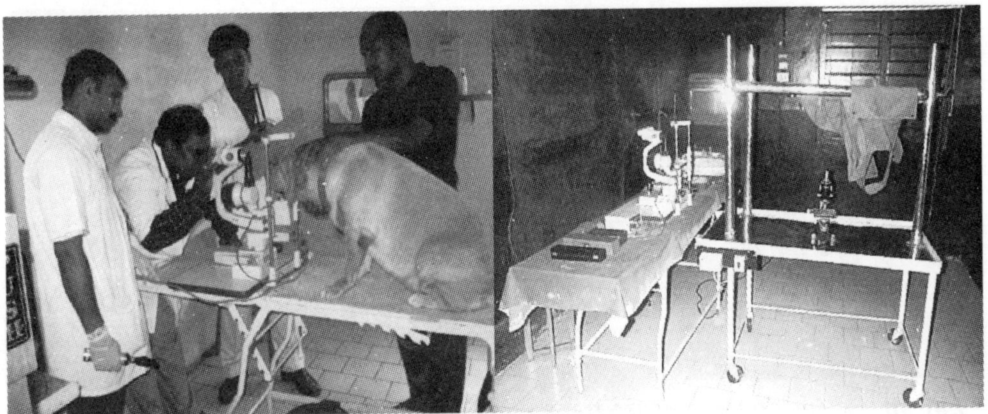

Fig. 7 : Ophthalmoscopy

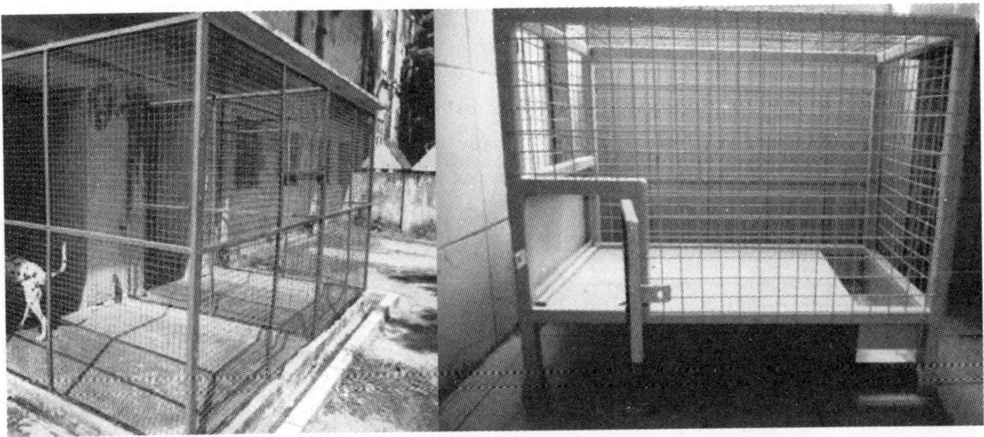

Fig. 8 : Small animal inpatient and feline cage facilities

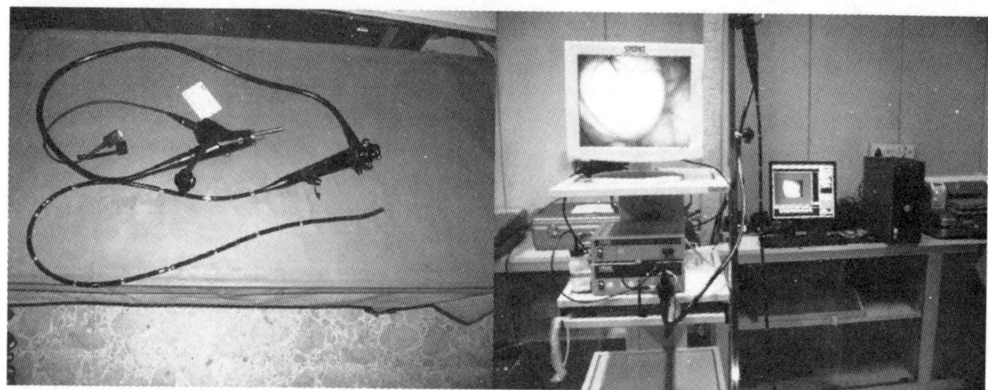

Fig. 9 : Endoscopy

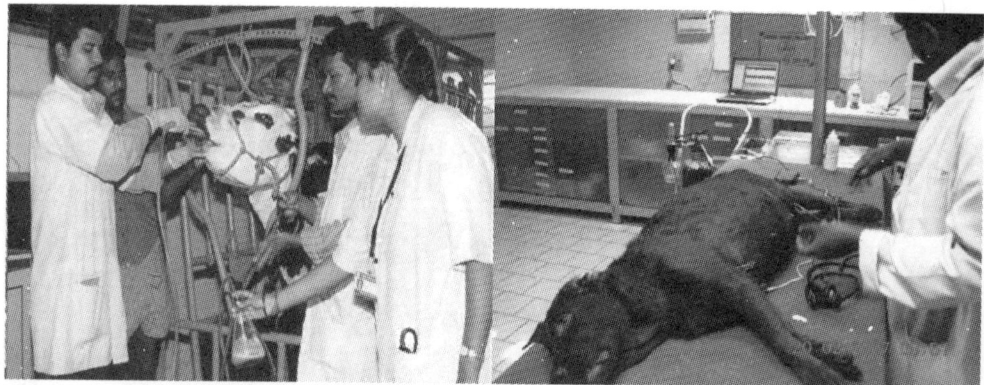

Fig. 10 : Bovine endoscopy and rumen fluid collection facilities

Fig. 11 : Computerised phonocardiography

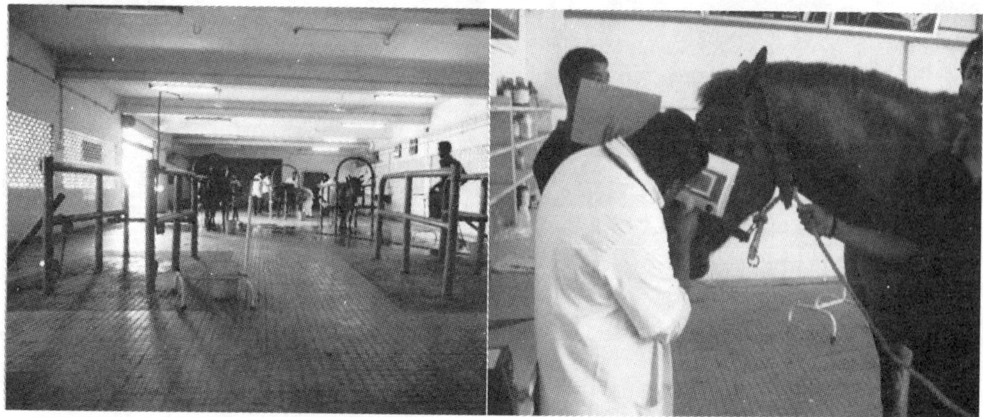

Fig. 12 : Large animal examination

Fig. 13 : Wood's lamp examination

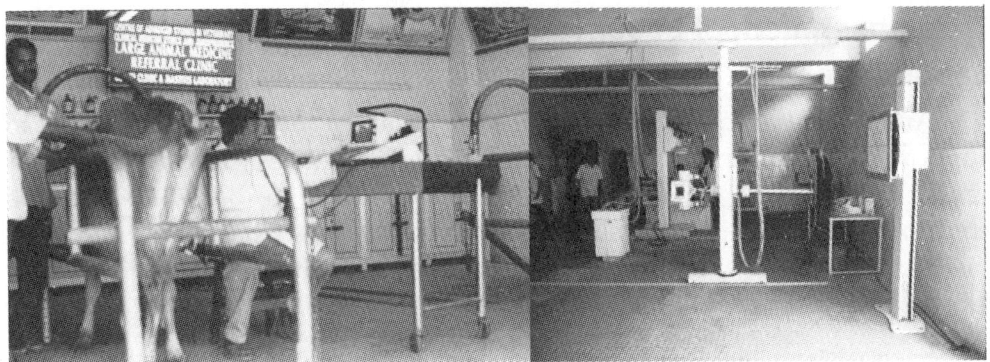

Fig. 14 : Ultrasonography facilities

Fig. 15 : Radiography suite

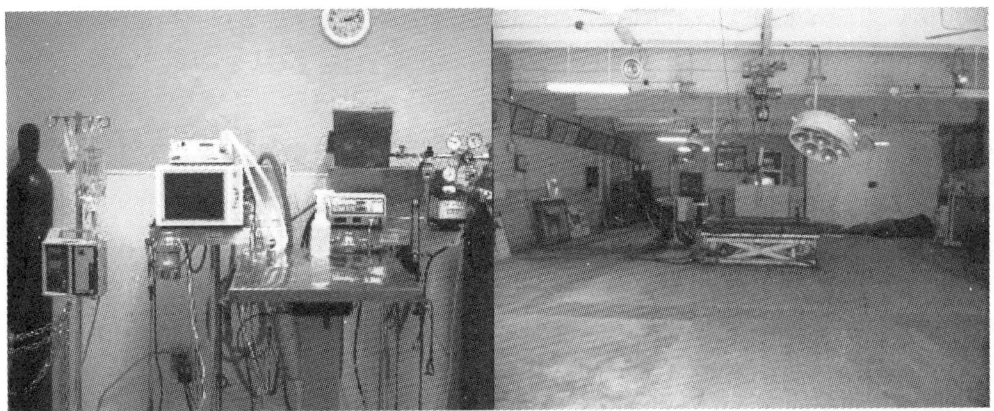

Fig. 16 : Anaesthetic equipment

Fig. 17 : Large animal surgery suite

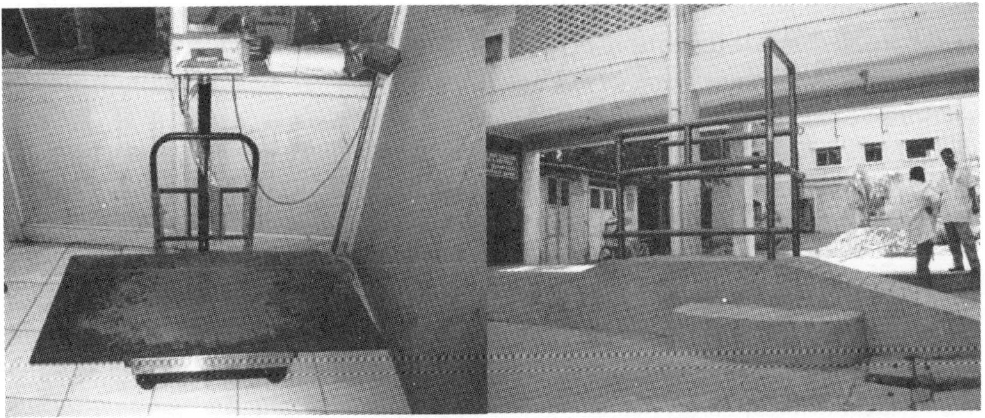

Fig. 18 : Animal weighing balance

Fig. 19 : Mastitis trevis

7. Establishment of Local, Regional and Central Veterinary Laboratories

An efficient animal disease diagnostic organizational setup is needed to support various activities of the animal health services, both for the state services and for the private sector. The veterinarians in the field should be equipped to collect specimens from live animals suspected of being diseased, or at postmortem examination, and to dispatch them to the diagnostic laboratories.

Each district needs a well-equipped centralized diagnostic laboratory. Depending on the livestock population and the efficiency of the communication system, satellite laboratories may be established and may be specialized in their scope according to the priorities of the particular area e.g. poultry diagnostic laboratories, small ruminant diagnostic laboratories, and dairy animal disease diagnostic laboratories etc.

7.1 Central veterinary laboratory

Central veterinary laboratory should be established as an executive agency of the Department of Animal Husbandry, Government of India. It should be a well known Centre of Scientific Excellence, delivering research, surveillance and laboratory services for animal and public health for the entire country.

The prime function of the central diagnostic laboratory should be the provision of field veterinarians with specialized services. It may also be required to investigate identified disease problems in depth in order to assist the state and central governments in defining proper control strategies. The central diagnostic laboratory should have technical links with international reference laboratories, WHO/FAO/OIE collaborating centres and other related diagnostic laboratories in the region and throughout the world in order to obtain confirmation of diagnosis of diseases for which it does not have sufficient experience or technical capability. It should have different sections covering major disciplines.

The services of central veterinary laboratory should include a wide range of interrelated core functions and capabilities described below.

7.1.1 Disease diagnostic studies

1. Reference microbiology and surveillance for bacteria, viruses, fungi, parasites and prions
2. International reference services support
3. Support in investigation of disease outbreaks

4. Detection and monitoring of emerging and imported infectious diseases and antimicrobial resistances
5. Search for new pathogens
6. Vector-borne diseases
7. Zoonoses
8. General and on-call support and expert advice
9. Vaccine production and introduction of immunization programmes, monitoring of vaccine efficacy and vaccine coverage
10. Evaluation of new antimicrobials against 'problem' isolates

7.1.2 Epidemiological and animal health research studies

1. National and international surveillance
2. Detection of national and transnational outbreaks
3. Syndromic surveillance for new and emerging diseases
4. Seroepidemiology and risk assessment
5. Evaluation and development of diagnostic and reference technologies
6. Search for new pathogens and antimicrobial resistances and mechanisms
7. Undertaking research, and support to the work of others, in animal infections
8. Vaccine development and evaluation
9. Epidemiology of rare and common pathogens
10. Seroepidemiology and seroprevalence studies
11. Mathematical models of the spread of infectious diseases
12. Economic evaluation of control programmes
13. Pathological investigations

7.1.3 Environmental health assessment

1. Assessment of zoonoses
2. Vector-borne infections
3. Environmental monitoring: Radiation, chemicals, animal feedstuff
4. Risk assessment
5. Food safety
6. Disinfectant testing
7. Decontamination confirmation
8. Effects of climate change

7.1.4 Reference and specialised testing of samples

1. Typing of organisms
2. Confirmation of laboratory test results (including atypical results)
3. Serodiagnosis and molecular assays
4. Identification of unusual or difficult and dangerous (containment level 4) pathogens
5. Antimicrobial resistance confirmation and mechanism determination
6. National and international officially designated reference services
7. National and international reference collection
8. Detection of pathogenicity and virulence determinants (including biotoxins)
9. Specialist *in vivo* and *ex vivo* assays
10. Forensic pathology, esoteric assays otherwise unavailable elsewhere

7.1.5 Quality control studies and quality improvement

1. Contribution to national and international guidelines and policy development
2. National and international quality assurance schemes
3. Establishment of quality systems
4. Provision of specialist biological reagents
5. Development of standards
6. Development of testing algorithms
7. Evaluation of diagnostic kits/tests/methods
8. Development of new kits/tests
9. Provision of assay controls and performance panels
10. Assessment of new technologies
11. Development of standard operating procedures
12. Animal and animal feed compliance with import controls and export compliance certification testing

7.1.6 Expert advice, enabling partnership and communication

1. Development of partnerships among animal health professionals, academia, industry, food manufacturers and public health services.
2. Contribution in national strategic policy planning and development

3. Maintenance and development of further international networks, and interactions with organizations like World Organization for Animal Health (OIE), World Trade Organization, European Food Safety Authority (EFSA)
4. Providing expert advice to farming industry, specialist and general press
5. Interactions with agencies and government departments e.g. devolved administrations, environment agencies, Departments of Health, Food Standards Agency, Ministry of Defence etc.
6. International interactions with European Commission, EFSA, OIE etc.

7.1.7 Special pathology service

The following services should be made available at the central veterinary laboratories.

1. Clinical and anatomic pathology research and diagnostic consultancy services
2. High sensitivity detection of host-pathogen interactions using modern immunological and molecular techniques
3. Immunohistochemistry and immunocytochemistry
4. Lectin histochemistry
5. In situ hybridisation
6. Immunofluorescence
7. Negative contrast and immunogold staining for electron microscopy
8. Specialist tissue fixation and cryopreservation
9. High resolution bio-imaging
10. Confocal laser scanning microscopy
11. Fluorescence microscopy
12. Laser capture microdissection
13. Transmission and scanning electron microscopy and image analysis

7.1.8 Support for emergency preparedness and response

1. Animal intoxication and chemical safety of food
2. Infectious disease emergencies
3. High volume testing
4. Deliberate release response
5. Mathematical models, risk assessment and scenario planning

6. Analytical and predictive epidemiology
7. All hours emergency call
8. Service continuity provision to public health

7.2 State veterinary laboratories

Well-equipped diagnostic laboratory should be established at the state level to carryout diagnostic procedures. Close cooperation between central and state laboratories is necessary for the success of animal health programmes. Financially and administratively, the state laboratories should be under the state veterinary authority. Technically and scientifically, they should come under the authority of the central veterinary laboratory.

State veterinary laboratories should have sufficient scientific expertise, high quality service, innovative methods and, in many cases, unique products and services to meet the existing demand as described below.

7.2.1 Diagnostic laboratory services

1. Animal feed testing
2. Antimicrobial testing
3. Clinical chemistry and haematological tests
4. Microbiological and virological investigations
5. Parasitological tests
6. Pet travel scheme
7. Serological tests
8. Testing service for veterinary practitioners
9. Imaging and histopathology service
10. Specialist laboratory reagents and diagnostic kits
11. A world-leading range of proficiency testing schemes
12. Testing and development services to the pharmaceutical industry
13. Disinfectant efficacy and product testing
14. Veterinary research and development projects
15. Risk analysis and data science services
16. Cell characterization services

7.3 Hospital based clinical laboratory

Veterinary hospitals should have a clinical laboratory with the facilities for the following diagnostic tests.

1. Haematological profiling
2. Blood biochemical profiling
3. Tissue and environmental sample biochemical profiling
4. Complete urine analysis
5. Clinical parasitological examination
6. Clinical microbiological and virological investigation
7. Histopathological examination
8. Serology and molecular diagnostics

8. Strengthening of Animal Quarantine and Certification Services

While efforts are made to ensure better livestock health, simultaneous efforts are equally necessary to prevent entry of any disease from outside into the country through import of livestock and livestock products. With this objective, Animal Quarantine and Certification Service Stations, one each at Mumbai, Kolkata, Delhi and Chennai have been established. These Stations are well equipped for the job. Keeping in mind the growth in animal population and transboundary movement of people and animals, it is necessary that these Quarantine Centres are strengthened to have capabilities to test and diagnose diseases of international origin and these should have infrastructure and manpower comparable to the most developed nations and should be accredited by international agencies and policymakers.

9. Modernization of Companion Animal Veterinary Care

Decades of research and technology developments have revolutionized the companion animal healthcare worldwide. The clinical developments in this area in developed nations are at par with developments in human medicine. However, the developments in the companion animal medicine in India are rather slow and passive. On a reasonable estimate, we might be two decades behind the developed nations in the delivery of companion animal healthcare.

Besides the increase in companion animal populations, the diseases are also on the rise, especially the geriatric and pediatric diseases. Many of these diseases are life threatening and require emergency medical care. Diseases such as cardiac failure, renal failure and other organ failures require not only conservative therapy but also critical care to prolong and enhance the quality of life. Further, due to the increasing urbanization, reduction of living spaces and increase in high-rise buildings, there is sizable number of cases with "high rise syndrome" throughout the year. There is also increase in the road traffic accidents and related complications round the year. For management of such disorders and to prolong the quality of life of such cases, Critical Care Medicine is the absolute need of the hour.

The companion animal healthcare services presently are not commensurate with the growing demand in the present day. Thus, to reduce the mortality and to improve the quality of life of companion animals, the country needs to develop Small Animal Medicine and Emergency and Critical Care Medicine as specialised areas in veterinary medicine.

10. Development of Emergency and Critical Care Medicine

Except a very few Teaching Veterinary Hospitals in the academic institutions, there are largely no organized Emergency and Critical Care setups in the country. Even in the Teaching Veterinary Hospitals, the capability to manage emergency and critical care cases is very limited, which ultimately leads to failures in the mortality reduction strategies. The unavailability of organized Veterinary Blood Bank Systems or Component Therapy Products in the country makes it difficult to arrange emergency transfusions. The search for donors causes delay, increasing the patient mortality. Further, any emergency patient after its successful revival, needs to be kept under continuous critical care and monitoring, requiring "Inpatient facilities" with round the clock veterinary services. Such facilities are very few in numbers and are usually not equipped with sufficient medical and support service infrastructure and manpower.

The practice of emergency and critical care requires a vast array of drugs and disposables, which may be expensive too. Largely, the material is not readily available even in the Teaching Veterinary Hospitals in sufficient quantum. Even the oxygen cylinders, which are hallmarks of emergency care, are many times not available in the veterinary care centers.

Client awareness and education about the need for timely institution of emergency therapy is abysmally very low in the country. The first aid advisory service for pets via telephone or electronic media is also very limited. All these factors need to be addressed efficiently in order to reduce high mortality rates associated with the emergency and critical care cases.

10.1 Short term strategies for development

10.1.1 Client education

Companion animal owners need to be advised about the common emergency conditions in day to day life, their recognition and timely presentation of even suspicious cases to the veterinarians. Print and electronic media should be used for this purpose. Organizations dealing with animal healthcare and animal welfare should take the responsibility of client education in consultation with experts in the field.

10.1.2 First aid services

The first aid facilities should be made available in all the animal welfare institutions and in the common service areas in the villages, for example, milk cooperative societies or government offices in the villages. Round the clock first aid advisory services should be made available in every part of the country. At least the district level veterinary hospital should house such facilities so as to cater to the need in the concerned district. Such facilities would ultimately form a Network of First Aid Centers which may act as the stepping stone for Emergency Medicine development.

10.1.3 Infrastructure at block level veterinary hospitals

Basic level emergency care infrastructure such as oxygen cylinders, emergency crash cart, minimal level life support equipments and trained human resource should be made available in all the taluk/tehsil/block headquarter veterinary hospitals.

10.1.4 Emergency veterinary service (EVS) at district veterinary hospitals

The district headquarter veterinary hospital should be equipped with all infrastructure facilities and human resource for delivery of round the clock emergency and critical care services. Such hospitals should have triage area, ICU, X-ray, basic ultrasound, oxygen therapy, blood transfusion facilities and round the clock laboratory services. Trained veterinary technicians should be available round the clock in such centers. Veterinarians should be available to attend the emergency cases immediately.

10.1.5 State level Veterinary Emergency Referral Hospital and Network Emergency Advisory Service

A state of the art Veterinary Emergency Referral Hospital (VERH) should be developed at the state capital with modern infrastructure inclusive of advanced life support and advanced critical care facilities. Specialist veterinary human resource should be made available in such centers round the clock. VERH should be networked with the district EVS hospitals to enable real time consultancy services. Networked EVS will enable timely reach of expert consultancy service to save patients in distress. This will ultimately improve the clients' confidence in the veterinary services.

10.1.6 Setting up of an emergency and critical care unit

A variety of diseases prompt admission of the animals to the critical care facility. Such animals can generally be grouped into three categories: animals requiring extensive nursing care, animals that are physiologically stable but require intense monitoring or observation, and physiologically unstable animals that require constant veterinary critical care.

Increased public awareness of the necessity and availability of critical care service obliges veterinarians to provide these services to them. The critical care facility should be designed to handle acute emergency situations efficiently and to provide continuous care for the critically ill. Intensive care facilities and the practice of critical care medicine should no longer be confined to larger institutions as these are now becoming available in veterinary private practice.

10.1.6.1 Physical plan

A critical care facility ideally should be located central to the veterinary hospitals or area that it services, with easy access from major roadways. The hospitals should be clearly identified and the entrance to the reception area easily noticeable. An inclined ramp to the reception area is often necessary. Examination rooms should be situated between the reception area and the treatment and ICU area.

An area within the ICU should be set up to enable rapid treatment of acute life threatening situations such as cardiac arrest. Direct access from the reception area to the ICU in such situations is critical. The necessary emergency equipments e.g. laryngeoscope, endotracheal tubes etc. should be readily accessible in this area at all times. A complete checklist of drugs and equipments in the emergency section should be reviewed daily and restocked after each use.

The functions of critical care/emergency unit revolve around the ICU. The ICU should be highly visible and easily accessible ward. Critical care facility is dependent on ancillary services too, hence complete laboratory capabilities and radiographic support should be available within this facility. The surgical suite should be located close to the ICU, minimizing transport time of post-surgery patients to the ICU. If space within the facility is available, a special procedures area can be set up for advanced diagnostic and therapeutic interventions, endoscopy, ultrasonography etc. An isolation ward should be close to but distinctly separate from the ICU and other hospital areas. A closed circuit television linkage and a viewing window connected to the ICU are useful to observe the patients in isolation.

Floor plan of the ICU should allow for constant visualization of all patients from a central work area. In the pre-existing buildings, the use of wide angle mirrors in the ICU may be useful to achieve this goal. Multiple sources of oxygen and suction are necessary for easy access when treating more than one animal. In addition, ample lighting and electrical outlets should be available. Ceiling track mounts may be used to suspend intravenous fluids administration sets. The intensive care unit should have an emergency generator for backup in the event of power failure.

10.1.6.2 Emergency care infrastructural facility requirements

All emergency and critical care units should have the capacity to provide the following facilities.

A. Diagnosis and management of life-threatening emergencies

- Cardiopulmonary resuscitation including electrical defibrillation
- Placement and maintenance of thoracostomy tubes
- Emergency tracheostomy and tracheostomy tube care
- Oxygen supplementation
- Assisted ventilation

B. Monitoring capabilities

- Electrocardiogram
- Arterial blood pressure
- Central venous pressure
- Pulse oximetry
- Oesophageal stethoscope

C. Emergency surgery

- Surgical haemostasis, wound debridement and application of wound dressings
- Stabilization of musculo-skeletal injuries
- Aseptic thoracic, abdominal, and neurosurgery
- Referral service to a facility that can perform these procedures in a timely manner

D. Treatment of circulatory shock

- Crystalloids, colloids and blood products
- Equipment such as calibrated burettes or infusion pumps for accurate delivery of fluids
- Natural and/or artificial blood products
- Capacity to type and cross match donor and patient blood

E. Anaesthetic and analgesic therapy

- Opiates, non-steroidal medication, and inhalational anaesthesia
- Intra-operative monitoring equipment - electrocardiogram, oesophageal stethoscope, blood pressure monitor and pulse oximetry when appropriate

F. Laboratory

- The laboratory should be able to provide support in a timely manner. It should be equipped for tests like a complete blood count, BUN, refractometric total solids, blood glucose, urinalysis, activated clotting time, electrolyte measurements (Na, K, Cl), FIV/FeLV serology, cytology, heartworm testing and faecal examination (flotation, cytology and parvovirus antigen test).
- Additionally, an emergency facility must have laboratory service to collect, prepare, and preserve samples for a complete serum biochemical profile, blood gas analysis, complete coagulation profiles, microbiological culture and histopathology.

G. Imaging facility

- Radiographic machine of at least 300 mA – ensuring good quality images and safety of patient and staff
- Automatic film processor
- On-site ultrasonography equipment

10.1.6.3 Drug requirements

Essential drugs that should be available in a critical care facility are listed in Table 2. Provision of a double-locked storage cabinet or safe should be made to keep the narcotic drugs and other classified drugs. An accompanying log should specify patient's name and identification number, date and time of usage, amount of drug used, amount of drug remaining, and signature of the clinician requiring these drugs. A listing of common drug interactions should be available in the critical care unit. In addition, poison control telephone numbers should be posted in an accessible place.

Table 2 : Essential drugs in a veterinary critical care unit

Acepromazine	Calcium gluconate	Heparin
Activated charcoal	Chlorpromazine	Inhalation anaesthetic
Aminophylline	Dexamethasone	Ketamine
Amrinone	Digoxin	Lactulose
Antibiotics	Dimercaprol	Lidocaine
Antihistamines	Dobutamine	Metoclopramide
Ascorbic acid	Epinephrine	Nitroglycerin ointment
Assorted eye and ear medications	Flunixin meglumine	Oxytocin
Atropine	Frusemide	Phenobarbital
Prednisolone succinate	Propanolol	Valium
Vitamins A,B,D and E injectable		

10.1.6.4 Staffing

The success of a critical care facility is largely dependent on the personnel staffing the facility and their willingness to work towards the common goal of coordinated veterinary care. The staff is often composed of a relatively small number of people where each member of the team has a set of individual tasks to perform to ensure continual smooth operation of the facility. The minimum number of team members necessary for optimal operation of a critical care facility at any given time should include a receptionist, two nurses, a primary care veterinary clinician, and a surgeon available on call. Some additional trained personnel should be available when necessary to reduce the stress of the staff.

The receptionist must be adept at recognizing and prioritizing emergencies and skillful client communication. Pet owners with critically ill animals are extremely anxious, hence it is the receptionist's responsibility to calm down the owners and keep them updated on their pet's status. The receptionist should be skilled in recognising life threatening emergencies of cardiopulmonary resuscitation as he/she is the first staff member to make contact with the patient and the owner. The receptionist should be responsible for discussing financial requirements with the animal owners, allowing the veterinarian to give quick attention to the patient.

The ICU nurses are responsible for direct patient care, such as monitoring of vital signs, attending to the patient's physiologic and psychologic needs, administering medications and keeping clear and concise records. Additional responsibilities delegated to the ICU nurses include maintenance of equipments and training of new critical care personnel. All the personnel should be skilled in aseptic techniques as higher infection rates in the critically ill are directly related to poor hygienic practices.

Responsibilities of the critical care veterinary clinician include treatment of patients, coordination of the critical care facility and counseling the client. Clinician should be efficient and competent in the diagnosis and treatment of trauma patients, which constitute the majority of critical care cases brought in emergency. It is for the clinician to make critical decisions governing patient care and changes in the treatment. Good communicative skills are extremely important in a critical care facility where tension and stress are high.

The need of an emergency surgeon at a critical care facility is often sporadic; however a surgeon should be available on call to handle the conditions requiring immediate surgical intervention.

10.2 Long term strategies for development

10.2.1 Higher education and training in emergency and critical care medicine

Trained human resource is essential to cater to the technically demanding needs of emergency cases. As specialized training in emergency medicine is lacking in the curriculum, it is the need of the hour to develop higher education and training capabilities in this field throughout the country. Short term certificate programmes and postgraduate degree programmes in emergency medicine should be introduced.

10.2.2 Professional capacity building

All the field veterinarians should be trained periodically to update their knowledge and skills in emergency medicine. Besides the residential training programmes, on-line e-courses can be developed and introduced.

10.2.3 Development of critical care cardiology

Since cardiovascular disorders remain the major silent killer, effort needs to be made to save cases with decomponsated heart failure and to prolong their life span. In the modern civilized world today, the pet owner clients are very compassionate. To save their pets, they look for the same kind of treatment which is provided in human hospitals. This necessitates deployment of certain possible clinical practices in critical care cardiology.

10.2.4 Development of Palliative Medicine

Incidence of cancer and related complications is high among canines. Because of the unlimited compassion for their pets, owners nowadays request for state of the art treatment facilities for cancer afflicted canine patients with an aim to prolong their life span. To the least possible, they want their pets not to suffer from cancer pain and adverse effects. Appropriate pharmacological and certain clinical interventions are required to relieve such cancer-associated distress. For these reasons, the field of Palliative Medicine needs to the nurtured and developed for the benefit of companion animal clients.

10.2.5 Development of Interventional Therapeutics

Internal bleeding is a major life threatening disorder of animals. Conventional surgical procedures generally fail to provide relief. Internal bleeding is challenging both diagnostically and therapeutically. For management of such clinical challenges, interventional therapeutics is the gold standard strategy. Through vascular access, a catheter armed with therapeutic agents travels via the vascular roads of arteries and veins and reaches the site of damage and plugs the bleeding sites and saves the patient.

Such non-invasive procedures are the need of the hour in critical care practice in the country.

11. Development of Aquatic Animal Medicine

Veterinarians need to provide healthcare to aquatic animals also (i.e. diagnose disease, perform surgery, evaluate and recommend management procedures and prescribe treatment). Due to their educational background, veterinarians are familiar with biosecurity, disease prevention and control, use of pharmaceuticals, biologics, pesticides and their potential for adverse effects. The principles acquired in this education also apply to aquatic species and their environments.

Veterinarians are licensed as animal healthcare providers who prescribe and dispense drugs for treatment of all animal species to relieve animal suffering and assure target animal safety, efficacy of treatment, and public health protection. The concern for maintaining a safe food supply and avoiding potential risks of drug residues and environmental contamination are parallel in terrestrial and aquatic environments.

Most countries in the world community recognize and require a veterinarian's examination and signed certificates for shipment and importation of aquatic species. To begin with, the management of aquatic animal health should be the part of professional practice of veterinary surgeons employed in coastal districts of the country. The state veterinary services should create dedicated professional cadres and conservation agencies for control over aquatic animal health issues, including those of the private aquaculture industries. Aquatic animal health authorities should be created to bear the responsibility of inspecting and certifying the health of aquatic animals.

12. Conclusion

Veterinary services have made explosive progress over the past two decades. This has been fuelled by an extensive research and technological innovations in both diagnostic and therapeutic procedures. The country's animal healthcare and veterinary service delivery requires to keep evolving to meet the emerging challenges by aggressively pursuing the modernization of healthcare delivery system, infrastructure and services. Veterinary practice standards and guidelines have to be evolved and implemented to raise the quality of animal patient care and veterinary service delivery.

Besides this, veterinary human resource needs to be upgraded. Veterinary professionals should be trained in modern clinical practice and patient care. A cadre of paraveterinary technicians needs to be developed for maintenance of veterinary hospital and laboratory infrastructures and to aid the veterinary professionals in upgrading the quality of service delivery. Veterinary curriculum also needs to be frequently updated and modernized for providing world class animal health services.

Lastly, the utmost commitment of veterinary professionals is paramount to address the emerging problems in a befitting manner. Capacity building in emergency and critical care medicine will be of great consequence to increase the societal trust and confidence on the veterinary services.

❏❏❏

Chapter 11

Application of Veterinary Surgical Procedures in Rural Settings

NARINDER SINGH SAINI AND JITENDER MOHINDROO
Department of Veterinary Surgery and Radiology, College of Veterinary Science,
Guru Angad Dev Veterinary & Animal Sciences University, Ludhiana-141004

Contents

1. Introduction

There is a considerable gap between the education and practice of veterinary surgery, particularly in the field conditions. Many times, the veterinarians are sufficiently competent but they face practical difficulties in terms of logistics. There are a number of conditions that can be surgically treated under rural settings that include upward fixation of patella, congenital flexor deformities, acute bloat, urinary obstruction, intestinal obstruction, accidental lacerations, fractures, testicular tumors, teat fistula etc. However, due to lack of adequate infrastructure and practical oriented training, the optimum utility of surgical techniques is not attained for the benefit of the dairy farmers.

The conditions that can be cured surgically in the rural areas and their preoperative, anesthetic and post-operative considerations are described below.

2. Preoperative Considerations

Before taking up any elective, routine or emergency surgery, a complete history and thorough physical examination of the animal in question is indicated. This is needed to assess the health status of the animal and to detect any other abnormality to avoid any complication at the time of operation. Emergency problems that arise during anesthesia or surgery are always stressful. Blood tests like packed cell volume (PCV) or total protein estimation or complete blood count (CBC) should be performed routinely before any surgical procedure. Other specific tests may also be performed as needed. If any abnormality is present, it should be further explored and corrected before surgery, except in emergency situations where it may not always be feasible to correct it. Even elective surgery is not free of risk and the veterinarian must convey the risks to the owner. The 'Risk Form' must always be filled up and signed by the owner before undertaking any anesthesia and operative procedure. It is advisable to always keep record of the patients that have been anesthetized or operated.

Use of face mask, cap, gown and gloves is recommended during all types of surgery. For surgical site and surgeon's preparation, chlorhexidine, povidone-iodine and savlon (1:30) solution (chlorhexidine gluconate 7.5% w/v, isopropyl alcohol 6-8% v/v, cetrimide 15% w/v) can be used (Singh *et al.* 1988, 1989). Efficient preparation of the surgical site and meticulous surgeon's preparation are mandatory for successful surgical outcome. Scrubbing of hands and arms with chlorhexidine scrubbing solution four times is recommended after soap wash (Singh *et al.* 1988). Surgical site should be prepared by hair clipping or shaving of adequate area around the site. Surgical site must be scrubbed at least four times with antiseptic scrub solution (Singh *et al.* 1989). Finally, the site should be mopped with povidone iodine solution or rinsed with 70% alcohol.

Surgeons must select the surgical instruments required for surgical procedure well in advance and prepare these by autoclaving or by other methods of sterilization like cold kit sterilization i.e. dipping the instruments in sterilizing fluid. Surgeon must prepare (clean and disinfect) the operative area well in advance as it also plays role in development of post-operative wound infection in animals (Saini *et al.* 1992a). Surgeons must also take into consideration the type of suture material. Most common absorbable suture materials include plain or chromic catgut, polyglycolic acid (Dexon), polyglactin-910 (Vicryl) and polydiaxanone whereas the non-absorbable suture materials include silk, polypropylene (Prolene), polyamide, nylon, stainless steel, cotton etc.

3. Anesthetic Considerations

For chemical restraint and anesthesia many alternatives are available but the personal preference depends upon the veterinarian's knowledge, competence and experience besides the availability and cost effectiveness of different anesthetic agents.

Adult patients undergoing chemical restraint should be kept off feed for 12-24 hours and off water for 12 hours. Calves may be kept off feed for 8-10 hours before the procedure.

For local infiltration, regional and intravenous regional limb anesthesia, lignocaine hydrochloride (2%) injection is the most commonly used local anesthetic agent in India. Local infiltration anesthesia in bovines can be used in the form of line infiltration, T-, inverted-L and ring block depending upon the type and site of surgery. One can also use paravertebral nerve block by blocking T_{13}, L_1 and L_2 nerve branches for flank surgery in ruminants. Auriclo-palpebral and retro-bulbar nerve blocks are useful for eye surgery. Cornual nerve block and ring block are used for horn amputation surgery. Intravenous limb anesthesia for limb surgery or limb amputation is a reliable technique. Intravenous limb anesthesia is achieved by administering 2% lignocaine (local anesthetic) after the application of tourniquet to limb proximal to the operation site. In ruminant practice, one may not need sedation in procedures like rumenotomy, cystorrhaphy or other minor surgery. However, sedation may be required in vicious or fractious animals. For chemical restraint, diazepam, midazolam, acepromazine and xylazine can be used as sole agents (Muir *et al.* 2007) (Table 1).

Table 1 : Drugs for chemical restraint in ruminants

Species	Drug	Dose (mg/kg bodyweight)	Concerns, reversal dose (mg/ kg bodyweight)
Cattle and buffalo	Diazepam	0.2 - 0.5 mg IV	• Bradycardia and hypotension if given IV, rapidly • Increased appetite in ruminants • Reversal by Flumazenil (0.01 to 0.1 mg IV)
	Xylazine	0.11 - 0.22 mg IM	• Pregnancy (End term) - oxytocin like effect • Hyperglycemia
		0.05 - 0.11 mg IV	• Bradycardia • Respiratory depression • Hypotension • Reversal by Yohimbine (0.12 mg IV) • Reversal by Atipamezole (0.02 to 0.05 mg IV)
	Midazolam	0.2 - 0.4 mg IV	• Reversal same as for diazepam
	Butorphenol	0.02 - 0.1 mg IM	• Ataxia, vocalization • Stimulate appetite • Also works as a good analgesic
	Acepromazine	0.03 - 0.1 mg IM 0.01 - 0.05 mg IV	• Hypotension • Regurgitation • Penile protrusion • Milk withdrawal for 2 days period • IM extremely painful
Goat and sheep	Diazepam	0.25 - 0.5 mg IV	• Same as in cattle
	Xylazine	0.25 - 0.5 mg IV/IM	• Avoid Xylazine due to high risk of hypoxia • Use low concentration 20 mg/ml • More sensitive than cattle • Reversal by Yohimbine (1 mg IV) • Reversal by Atipamezol (0.02 to 0.05 mg IV)
	Acepromazine	0.05 - 0.1 mg IM	• Same as in cattle

* All doses are expressed in mg/kg bodyweight, IV - intravenous, IM - Intramuscular

In bovines, to perform surgery of anus, vulva, pelvic limb, flank and udder, the anesthesia obtained by depositing local anesthetic (lignocain 2%) between first and second coccygeal vertebrae or sacrococcygeal site in the epidural space works well. Epidural anesthesia may be low (caudal) or high (cranial) according to the dose of the local anesthetic used. In low epidural anesthesia 0.5 to 1 ml/45 kg body weight of lignocain (2%) is injected in epidural space. By this technique, sensation will be lost from anus, vulva, perineum and caudal aspect of thighs but motor control of hind legs is not lost. For high (cranial) epidural anesthesia 1 ml/4.5 kg body weight of lignocain (2%) is given and surgical procedures like flank laparotomy, hind limb and udder surgery can be performed successfully (Turner and McIlwarith 1989).

4. Surgical Procedures Applicable in Rural Setting

Following surgical procedures can be applied for the treatment of various affections of dairy animals in rural settings.

4.1 Head and neck surgery

4.1.1 Irregular molars

Animals with irregular molars are mostly presented with symptoms of accumulation of feed in the mouth, quidding, hypersalivation and passing of undigested feed in the faeces. Exploration of oral cavity in such cases reveals the presence of irregular molar teeth. The treatment remains the same irrespective of the configuration of the irregularity and includes grinding/ rasping of the cheek tooth/molars using a long handled tooth rasp. Occasionally, molar tooth cutters may be required in the animals with excessively overshot molars. Nowadays, motorized grinders are also commercially available which increase the efficiency and significantly reduce the operative time and labour. The procedure may need sedation or general anaesthesia.

4.1.2 Disbudding

Disbudding is carried out in calves at the age of 2-3 weeks. The horn bud is burnt and scooped out from the base by chemical or electric method. Chemical disbudding is done by rubbing caustic paste (sodium or calcium hydroxide pH 14 or silver nitrate stick or caustic potash stick) over the horn bud till the bud is completely burnt. Vaseline is applied around the horn bud prior to application of the caustic agent. Care is taken to avoid the chemical trickling down into the eyes and keeping the calves away from pools or ponds for some time to avoid accidental entry of the chemical into the eyes. In electric disbudding, an electrically heated disbudder is used to burn and scoop out the horn bud (the disbudder can alternately be heated over flame). Other methods include cryosurgery and scoop disbudding methods.

4.1.3 Horn fractures/avulsions

In case the tip of the horn is broken it does not require any surgical intervention. However, if there is an incomplete fracture of the horn, application of plaster of paris in an '8' fashion involving the intact horn is sufficient to stabilize the fracture. In case of complete fracture of horn, it is always wise to amputate the horn from the base under cornual nerve and ring block. If amputation is not performed in such cases, there is a possibility of infection spreading into the frontal sinus. Sedation may be needed in vicious animals. For amputation of horn the animal is restrained in lateral recumbency with the affected horn uppermost. The skin is incised around the base of horn so that two flaps are formed exposing the frontal bone along with base of the horn. After ligating the cornual artery and vein, the horn is amputated from the base using a bone saw. The skin flaps are sutured using horizontal mattress non absorbable sutures. Post operatively antibiotics and anti-inflammatory analgesics are administered for 3-5 days. Horn avulsions do not need surgical intervention unless the horn core gets infected. Daily dressing of the avulsed horn with antiseptics is sufficient to treat the avulsion. It may take upto 6 months for the new horn to form which will be of poor quality and irregular in shape. Squamous cell carcinoma of horn (horn cancer) is commonly encountered in long horned bullocks in India. The horn becomes loose and deformed and produces variable swelling at the base of horn. Foul smelling discharge may be present. The cancer tissue invades the frontal sinus and horn amputation is performed along with curetting of the frontal sinus.

4.1.4 Salivary cyst or fistula

It may be a result of sialoliths and trauma. In case of salivary fistula, there will be drooling of saliva from the fistulous tract near the horizontal rami of the mandible. The salivary gland must be destroyed by injecting tincture of iodine or any irritant through the Stensons (salivary) duct after surgically isolating it.

4.1.5 Intermandibular fistula

When feed is seen coming out from the ventral aspect of the intermandibular space, it is diagnosed as a case of intermandibular fistula. It mostly occurs after the rupture of mature abscess at this location. Occasionally, tongue may protrude out through the fistula (Fig. 1). The fistula can be repaired under sedation after freshening the wound edges and suturing the wound in 2-3 layers starting from mucosa outwards using Vicryl No. 1 or 2 (Saini *et al.* 2005a).

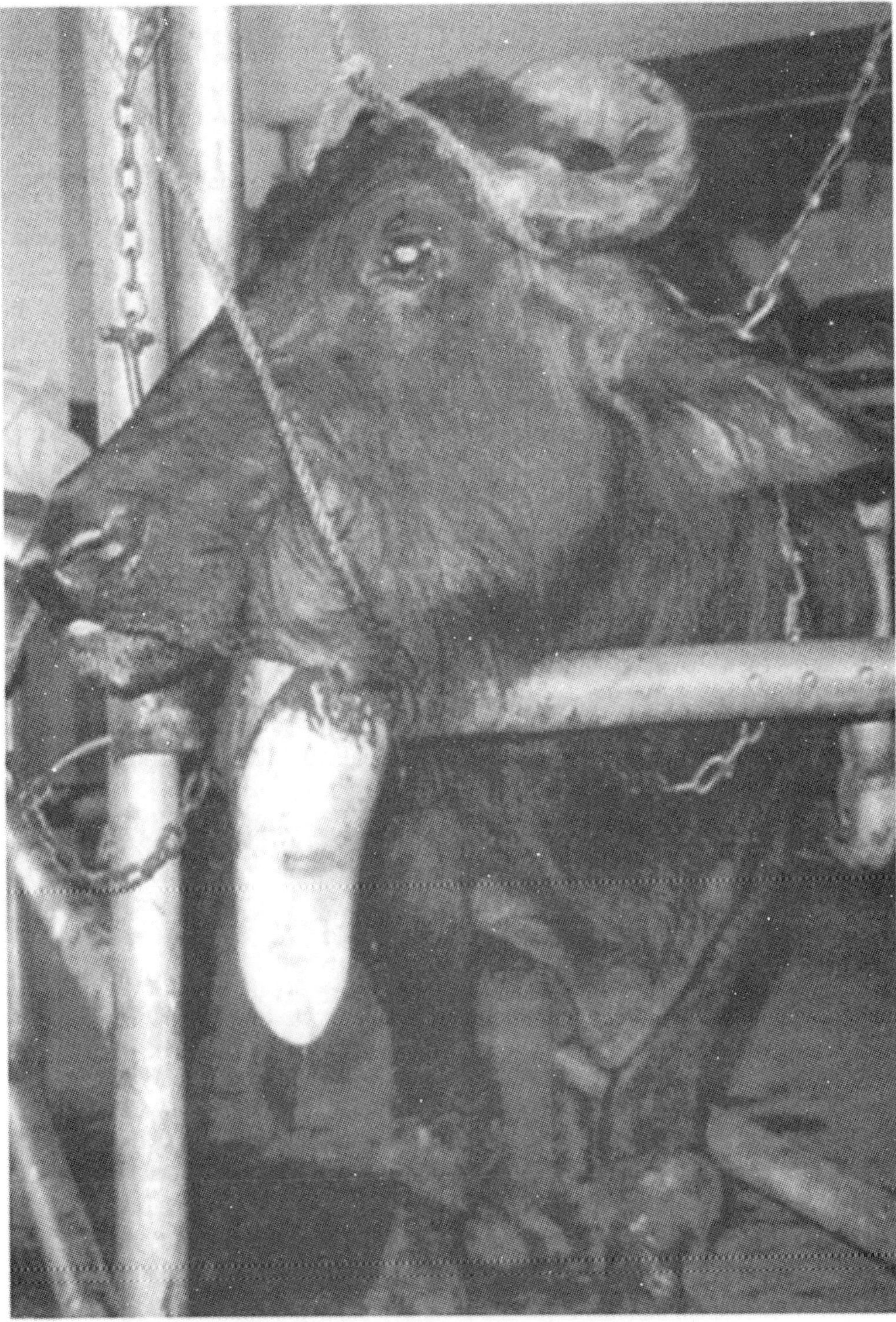

Fig. 1 : Buffalo with intermandibular fistula showing protrusion of tongue through fistula

4.1.6 Oesophageal obstruction

Generally it is known as 'choke' and is encountered in bovines due to swallowing of potatoes, onions, turnips, mango kernels etc. The foreign body gets obstructed in the cervical or thoracic esophagus and results in acute tympany (free gas bloat) due to failure in eructation (Sobti *et al.* 1995). Diagnosis may be confirmed by manual palpation. The first line of treatment is to relieve tympany by inserting a trocar and cannula or a large bore needle at the left para lumbar fossa. Any delay in relieving the bloat may be fatal for the animal. Our experience shows that trocarisation for long periods may result in spontaneous relief of the obstruction. If obstruction is close to the thoracic inlet attempt may be made to gently push the foreign body into the rumen using a probang/stomach tube. Oesophagotomy may be required to relieve the obstruction in exceptional cases. Oesophagotomy is done under local infiltration anesthesia with the animal in lateral recumbency. The subcuticular fascia is separated to locate the oesophagus. Incision is given on the oesophagus and the obstruction is gently relieved. The oesophagus is then sutured with inversion sutures using absorbable suture material. Animal is kept on I/V fluids for 2-3 days.

4.1.7 Eye tumor and trauma

Tumorous growth (ocular ganglioneuroma) at the corneoscleral junction is commonly encountered in buffaloes which can be easily removed under local eye nerve blocks (Saini *et al.* 1992b). In case of squamous cell carcinoma (Fig. 2) or trauma to eye, extirpation of eye ball may be required. It is done

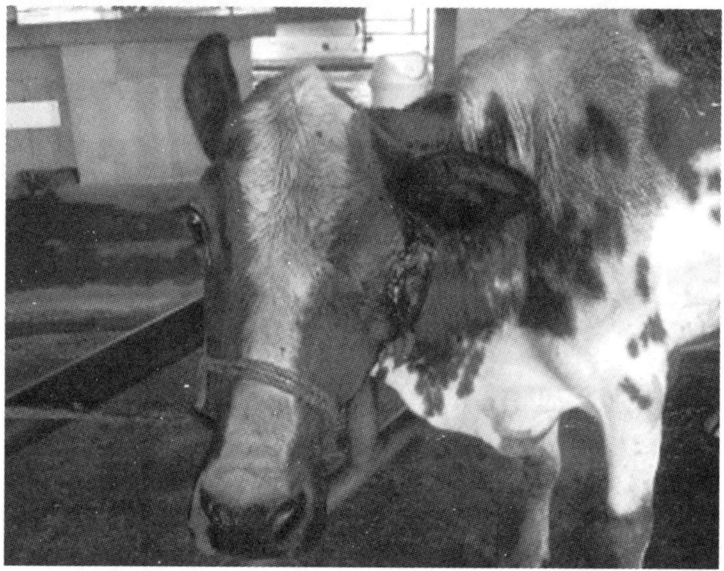

Fig. 2 : Cow with eye tumor (Squamous cell carcinoma, confirmed by histopathology)

using local blocks combined with sedation. In this procedure eye along with adjoining musculature is removed completely along with cancerous tissue. After the surgery, cotton bandage soaked in betadine is stuffed into the eye socket and changed everyday till complete healing.

4.2 Gastrointestinal surgery

4.2.1 Disorders of forestomach and abomasum

Disorders of the forestomach and abomasum are on a rise in cattle and buffaloes due to the changing agroclimatic scenario and feeding practices. The disorders include bloat, rumen impaction, foreign body syndrome, reticular abscess, reticular diaphragmatic hernia, traumatic reticuloperitonitis, omasal and abomasal impaction etc. Rumen impaction is mainly encountered during the months of feed scarcity when dry feed like wheat and paddy straw form a substantial part of the ration of the animals which develop inappetance and reduced milk yield. The digestibility of straw is less owing to high lignin content. Impaction may also occur subsequent to ingestion of polythene bags, ropes or poor quality mouldy and decomposed feed. Rectal and left flank palpation is the most reliable method for diagnosing rumen impaction in cattle. The lack of dietary discrimination in cattle and buffaloes leads to the ingestion of foreign materials causing traumatic reticulitis. Foreign bodies in the reticulum result in traumatic reticuloperitonitis, reticular abscess, reticulophrenic adhesions, traumatic pericarditis, vagal indigestion and reticular diaphragmatic hernia depending upon the site of reticular perforation and lesions caused by them (Saini *et al.* 2000, 2005, Athar *et al.* 2010). These conditions often lead to loss in production and sometimes may be fatal. Ingested foreign bodies are of major economic concern due to severe loss of production and sometimes may lead to the death of animals. Omasal impaction is a rare condition and is usually diagnosed at necropsy. In bovines, it is reported to occur secondary to rumen impaction as a result of poor quality feed. Omasal impaction can also occur due to dehydrated coarse feed such as shrubs, blady grass together with sand and constant confinement of animals in small barns with little exercise. Machine made wheat straw feeding is incriminated as risk factor for development of omasal impaction (Toor and Saini 2008). Clinically, the animals are presented with anorexia, scanty faeces, dullness, ruminal distension, dehydration, congested mucous membrane, and reduced milk yield. Inaccessibility of omasum for clinical examination makes omasal impaction a diagnostic challenge for the clinician. Abomasal impaction, left abomasal displacement and right abomasal displacement are infrequently encountered conditions of adult cattle and buffalo in Indian Scenario.

The symptoms presented by the animals suffering from all these conditions are so vague that at times it becomes difficult to identify the exact condition. Rumenotomy is required to confirm and treat many of these disorders including omasal impaction (Toor and Saini 2008). Rumenotomy is a simple procedure which can be done by any practicing veterinarian in a rural setting. Surgery is performed in a standing animal under local infiltration anesthesia.

For rumenotomy, the animals are restrained in a crate in standing position. The left flank area is prepared for aseptic surgery. Linear infiltration anesthesia or an inverted 'L' block is given in the left flank, four fingers caudal to the last rib for a length of 10 inches. Abdomen is opened by incising skin, subcutaneous fascia, muscle and peritoneum from left paralumbar fossa, caudal and parallel to the last rib. Weingarths rumenotomy frame is applied at the incision site by fixing it on the skin. Rumen is exteriorized and rumenotomy clamps are applied on the dorsal and ventral aspect of the exteriorized rumen. The abdominal cavity is packed with sterile drapes before incising the rumen. Rumen is opened by incising and rumenotomy hooks are applied on the rumen wall to fix it from all sides with the frame to prevent leakage of ruminal contents into the abdominal cavity (Fig. 3). The impacted contents in rumen are removed by

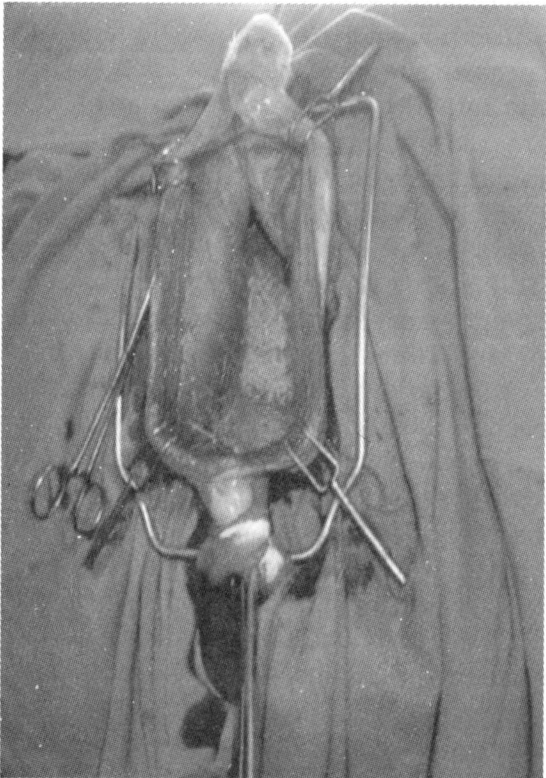

Fig. 3 : Rumenotomy operation site showing fixation of Weingarths rumenotomy frame and rumen hooks (Rumen content also visible)

diluting and mixing with water, and then by siphoning out. Sometimes the contents may require manual removal. Churned masses of polythene bags, ropes, and leather pieces, if any, may be broken down into small pieces and removed. Rumen contents are siphoned out to empty the rumen up to about $3/4^{th}$ of its capacity. The penetrating and non-penetrating foreign bodies in the reticulum are carefully removed. Search for any remaining metallic foreign bodies should also be done in the rumen and reticulum using a magnet. If any swelling is palpated in the reticulum or perireticular area, needle aspiration is performed from within the lumen and if pus is aspirated, it is drained within the lumen of reticulum by giving a 1-1.5 inch long stab incision on the base/ dependent part or belly of the abscess from within the reticular wall to drain content/pus into the reticulum (Saini *et al.* 2005b, Kumar *et al.* 2008). This is followed by flushing of abscess with water and then with 10-20 mL of povidone iodine. Any foreign bodies within the abscess are removed manually. The tone of reticulo-omasal orifice may be recorded by placing two fingers into the orifice (Toor and Saini 2008). This gives a fair indication of the reticulo-omasal transport of the contents. Omasal and abomasal impaction is determined by ascertaining the size and consistency (doughy to hard) of these organs on palpation through rumen wall during rumenotomy. In such cases, a long pipe of 0.5 inch diameter is inserted into the omasum/abomasum through reticulo-omasal-abomasal orifice. It is connected to a water supply pipe with larger bore. Omasum and abomasum are thoroughly flushed with water under moderate pressure, kneaded and most of the impacted contents are retrieved back into rumen (Toor and Saini 2008). About 2 liter of mineral oil may be poured directly into the omasum through the same pipe after complete resolution of the impaction. After completion of the required procedure(s) the rumen is closed.

Before closure, rumen is filled up to one third with water and 6-8 boluses of Yeasacc. Liquid potassium chloride (100 mL) and ruminotorics can be administered except in case of diaphragmatic hernia where rumen must be evacuated completely (leaving 1-2 liter of cud inside) and the case is referred to the appropriate institution for diaphragmatic herniorrhaphy which requires general anaesthesia intermittent positive pressure ventilation during surgery. The rumen is closed by double layer of inversion sutures i.e. Lambert followed by Cushing sutures using chromic catgut No. 2. The peritoneum and muscles are sutured in a continuous lock stitch pattern using chromic catgut No. 2. Skin is sutured using cross mattress or horizontal mattress suture pattern with silk No. 2 or 3.

4.2.2 Intestinal obstruction

In this condition, animal stops passing feaces. Diagnosis of intestinal obstruction is made on the basis of symptoms, clinical signs and per-rectal examination. Right flank laparotomy is performed under local infiltration/ paravertebral nerve block anesthesia to find the cause and surgical treatment of the obstruction. Faecolith and intussusception can be surgically removed and intestinal anastomosis is performed using catgut or Vicryl sutures.

4.2.3 Atresia-ani

This is congenital condition where natural opening for passing stools is not present. After preparation of the site in anal area, a cross shaped incision is made on the skin and it is reflected after dissection. Stay sutures are applied on the rectal wall and it is opened and sutured with skin to reconstruct the anal opening. About 2-4 cm diameter plastic pipe is placed with the help of stay sutures in the anal opening for ten days to prevent formation of anal stricture.

4.3 Musculoskeletal surgery

4.3.1. Upward fixation of patella

It is unilateral or bilateral functional disorder of femoropatellar articulation and exhibited by jerky movement to complete the flexion of limb during movement. There are three patellar ligaments i.e. lateral, middle (anterior) and medial. It is the medial patellar ligament which is severed surgically after local infiltration anesthesia in recumbent or standing animal. There are two surgical methods. One is the blind method in which ligament is severed by using No.12 B.P. blade at a site between middle and medial patellar ligament, keeping the sharp side of blade away from middle (anterior) patellar ligament. Going towards medial side from middle patellar ligament, the medial patellar ligament is severed. In the second method, 3-4 inch long skin incision is made. After dissecting fascia, the medial patellar ligament is identified and isolated by passing curved scissors underneath and thereafter severed surgically. In majority of the cases, walk of animal becomes normal immediately after the operation.

4.3.2 Contracted tendons or flexor deformities

The condition can be congenital or acquired. If treated early, in first week of life, it gives excellent results. There are various forms of treatment for this condition. The most common and easily available method under the rural setting is the application of plaster of Paris cast. After forceful extension of joint, the limb is immobilized with plaster of Paris cast by keeping the contracted part of the limb in extension. Plaster cast is changed every 5-7 days and forced extension is done every time till limb reaches near normal posture. If the contraction is more and limbs are flexed (Fig. 4), it may not be possible to bring the limb to normal position with forced extension and then surgery is indicated. There are two surgical methods which can be employed viz. tendon lengthening and tenotomy. For the tendon lengthening technique, partial accordion tenotomy and Z-tenotomy can be employed.

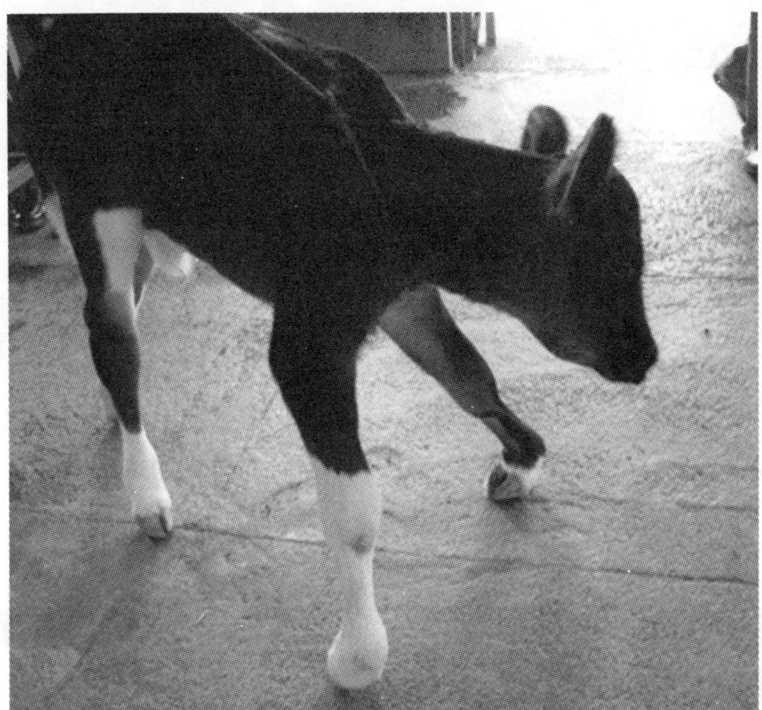

Fig. 4 : Cow calf with contracted tendon in forelimb (Note the abnormal posture)

Partial accordion technique does not involve severing of tendon and it should be preferred over Z-tenotomy. However, tenotomy is needed in severe cases most of the time. All these techniques, whether application of cast alone coupled with forced extension or surgery, work well and the animal is able to walk normally in 2-3 weeks.

4.3.3 Severed tendons

Severed superficial digital flexor (SDF) tendon, deep digital flexor (DDF) tendon, Achilles tendon can be sutured using double or triple locking loop or three loop pully sutures (Saini *et al.* 1998, 2002). If the gap is more, tendon grafting can be used and rigid immobilization is required after the tendon repair (Saini *et al.* 2002). In case of severed or ruptured SDF tendon, the pastern joint goes down while in case of severed DDF tendon, the fetlock drops down and toe is lifted upwards (Fig. 5). However, in case of severed or ruptured Achilles tendon, the hock joint sags down or may touch the ground (Fig. 6).

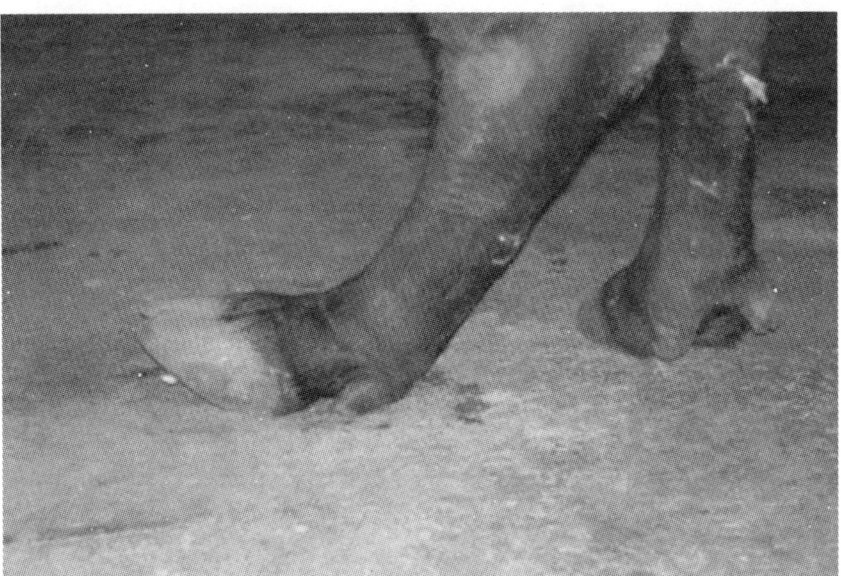

Fig. 5 : Severed superficial digital flexor and deep digital flexor (DDF) tendons in a buffalo (Note the raised toe which is characteristic of DDF tendon rapture/severed DDF tendon, wound on the plantar surface of metacarpal is the site of injury)

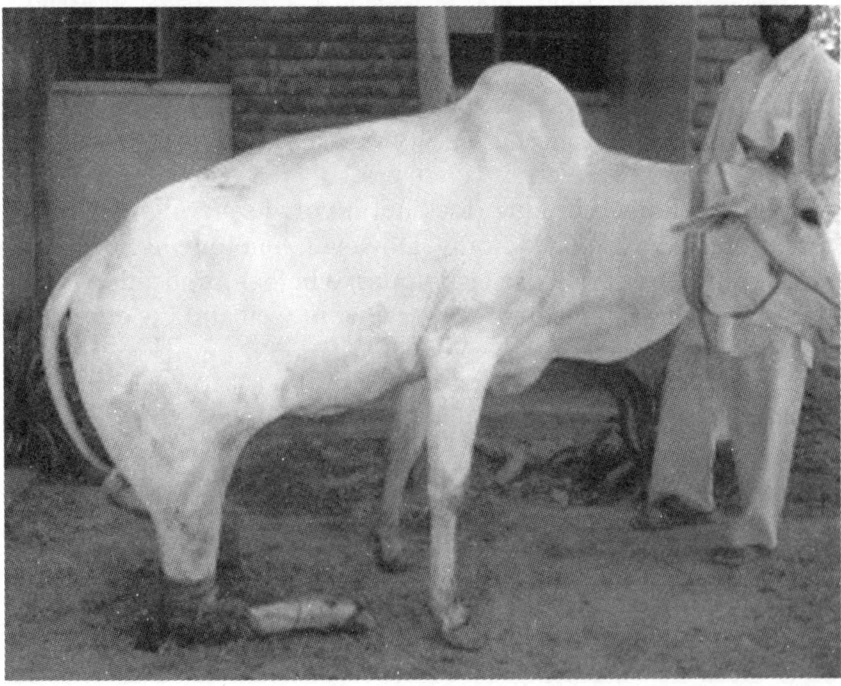

Fig. 6 : Bullock with severed Achilles tendon (Note the typical stance of animal with sagged/dropped hock to the ground level which is characteristic of Achilles tendon rupture)

4.3.4 Umbilical abscess and hernia and other hernias

Local infiltration anesthesia may be given along the margins of hernial ring. Sedation may be required in many animals. Diazepam works well in calves. Umbilical hernia (Fig. 7) and abscess are present together many times. Abscess can be treated by draining, douching and flushing daily with antiseptic solution like betadine or tincture of iodine. If abscess is present along with hernia, it is resected out after giving circular incision around the abscess and the hernial ring is closed by overlapping suture pattern using nonabsorbable or Vicryl suture material. Abdominal hernia is treated in similar manner. For hernial repair, all the sutures should be applied first and tied later. Sutures are tied after pulling next two sutures to bring the opposite margins of the ring together or in an overlapping fashion so that there is minimum tension on the suture when knots are being placed. However, diaphragmatic hernia is a form of internal hernia where continuous lock stitch sutures are preferred over any other type of suture pattern and it is repaired under general anesthesia making the procedure not feasible under field setting (Saini *et al.* 2000, 2007). Perineal hernia repair (Fig. 8) is carried under epidural anesthesia in standing animal (Sobti *et al.* 1994). Suturing is done between external anal sphincter muscle to one side, sacrococcygeal muscle on lateral side and internal obturator muscle on ventromedial side.

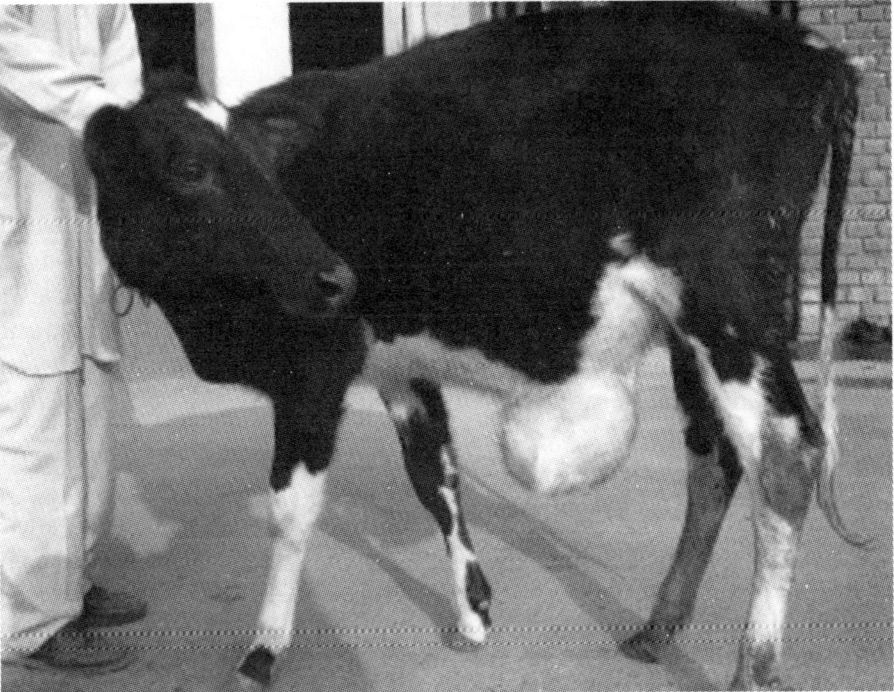

Fig. 7 : Calf with swelling at umbilicus showing umbilical hernia

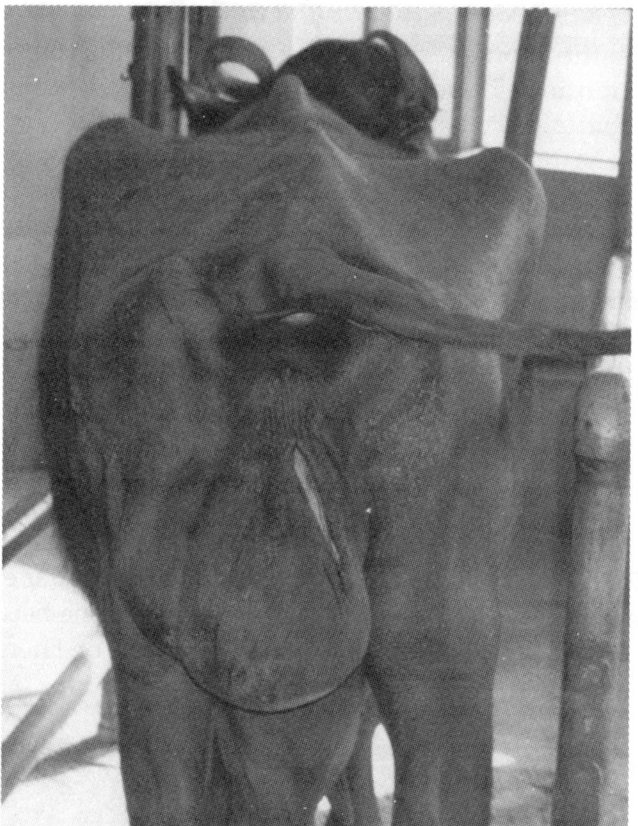

Fig. 8 : Perineal hernia in a buffalo

4.3.5 Teat fistula

It is common problem in cows and buffaloes (Fig. 9) which results from injury to the teat. Milk starts oozing out through the abnormal opening in the animals which are in lactation. Teat fistula is repaired under local anesthesia in standing or recumbent animals. Two or three tier closure is done for repairing the mucosa and muscle layers by using catgut or Vicryl. Finally, skin is closed in routine manner. A catheter needs to be kept intact into the teat canal for 7-10 days.

4.3.6 Dislocation and fracture management

Dislocations and fractures that do not have any external wound can be cured with application of plaster of Paris and splint. Basic principle is to bring the part to its normal position. Under chemical restraint or general anesthesia, the dislocations or fractures are manipulated by application of traction and counter traction to bring it to normal position by means of reduction. Then, immobilization is performed using plaster of Paris coupled with application of aluminum splint (2-3 mm thick) to maintain the part to near normal position and posture so that it heals in 6-8 weeks time. Temporary immobilization is recommended if permanent immobilization is to be performed after 1-2 days to avoid fracture or dislocation becoming compound.

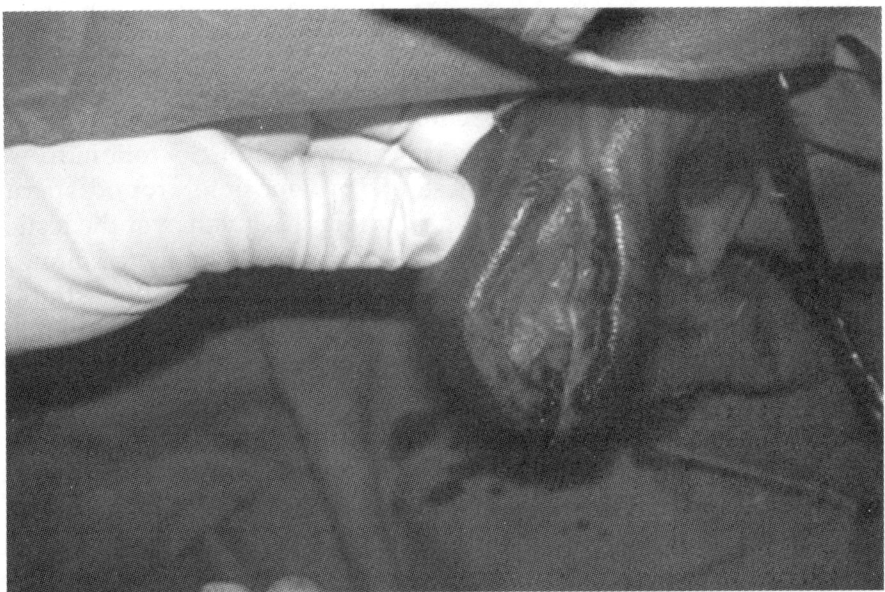

Fig. 9 : Teat laceration leading to teat fistula in a buffalo

4.3.7 Overgrown hoof

Overgrown hoofs are generally seen in cases of laminitis which is very prevalent in Indian scenario. The hoof can be trimmed using a hoof trimmer or hoof knife once every six months.

4.3.8 Amputations

Amputations include leg or digit amputation which can be performed under intravenous limb anaesthetic technique. Amputation of limb includes preparation of skin and muscle flap to cover the bone end projections. After the skin and muscle incision, all the major vessels are ligated. Muscles and ligaments are severed and the amputated part is removed. Flap of muscles is sutured over the projected end of bone and then skin flap is sutured.

For tail amputation, epidural anesthesia is used. In a similar manner, two flaps of skin one on dorsal and other on ventral side, are made and the vessels are ligated. Tail is then amputated between two coccygeal vertebrae and the wound is covered with skin flap by suturing with interrupted mattress sutures.

4.4 Urogenital surgery

4.4.1 Castration

This is a routine procedure which has been reported in early veterinary literature. It is done to make animal infertile and docile. It can also be performed in an animal suffering from testicular tumour (Fig. 10). It can be done by different methods. In the bloodless method, animal is restrained and after securing spermatic cord through palpation, each cord is crushed separately by application of single action (crushing) Burdizo emasculator or emasculatome. The other method is surgical method of castration, in which after restraining the animal, local anesthetic is deposited around spermatic cord and into the testicular tissue. Surgical incision is given over the testicle to expose tunica vaginalis. The contents of spermatic cord are ligated along with intact tunica vaginalis. It is called covered surgical method of castration. If tunica is incised, testicles and spermatic cord are further exposed and then ligated, The method is called uncovered method of castration. Ligation of the cord is carried by using chromic catgut or vicryl sutures at two adjoining locations and each suture is transfixed. Testicles are removed after severing the cord. Leftover part of the cord may be sutured with tunica using a single suture so that the cord does not slip into the abdomen after ligation and can be traced in case of emergency if the cord starts bleeding after the operation. Bleeding cord can be one of the complications of surgery. Dual action emasculator meant for cutting and crushing of individual spermatic cord can also be used instead of ligation. Vasectomy is another procedure which can

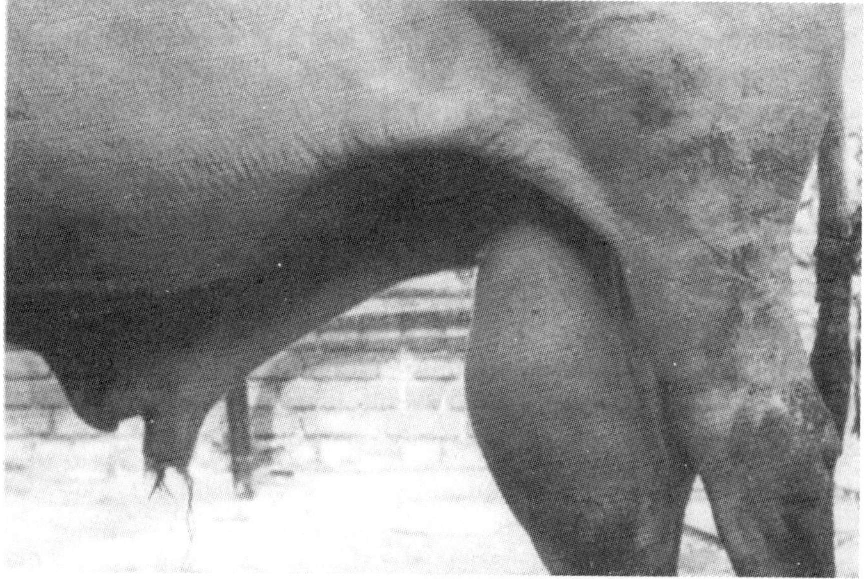

Fig. 10 : Bullock with testicular tumor (diagnosed as seminoma on histopathology)

also be done under local infiltration anesthesia under rural settings where only vas deferens is separated, ligated and 2-3 cm part of the vas is removed after severing between two ligatures.

4.4.2 Urinary obstruction

Urinary obstruction is most commonly reported in bullocks. The most common site of lodgement of calculi is at sigmoid flexure. Other sites of calculi location are ischeal and prescrotal parts of urethra. Less common causes of obstruction include urethritis, foreign bodies, urethral rupture etc. Struvite, silica and calcium carbonate uroliths are commonly seen in ruminants depending upon the type of diet given to the animal. It is an emergency situation where veterinarian needs to act fast. If surgery is not done within 24-48 hour, the rupture of urinary bladder becomes evident further complicating the prognosis and outcome of surgery. For relieving the obstruction, skin incision is given at post scrotal site on midline under local infiltration anesthesia after restraining the animal in lateral recumbency. After separation of facia, urethra is exposed and sigmoid flexure is straightened. Taking two retractor penii muscles as a guide, stone is located in urethra. The incision is given on the urethra and stone (s) is removed. Snugly-fitting polythene catheter is passed first caudally then cranially into the urethra. It is then transfixed with prepuce to prevent the downward migration of catheter. Skin is sutured by interrupted skin sutures using silk or polyamide. Catheter is kept intact for 2-3 weeks. Similarly, urethrotomy can also be performed at post scorotal, ischeal or prescrotal sites depending on the location of urolith.

4.4.3 Urinary bladder rupture

If urinary bladder ruptures, it collapses. Veterinarian need to palpate the urinary bladder per-rectally. Urethrotomy is followed by cystorrhaphy. Cystorrhaphy is performed in standing animal through left paralumbar incision under local infiltration anesthesia. Through left paralumbar laparotomy (Fig. 11) urinary bladder is approached and repaired blindly by application of continuous lock stitch suture pattern using chromic catgut. Intracystic catheterization may be performed by passing catheter through the rupture site and then directing though the neck of bladder by using a stout stilet through the sigmoid flexure. Simultaneously one needs to open the post secrotal urethrotomy site to guide the stilet. Urine accumulated in the abdomen after bladder rupture is drained by application of trocar and canula and/or at the time of cystorrhaphy operation by siphoning the urine through sterilized tube. Laparotomy incision is closed in 2-3 layers. Continuous lock stitches are applied on muscles using chromic catgut No. 2 or 3 in one or two layers and subcutaneous facia is apposed by continuous sutures. Skin is closed by interrupted cross mattress or horizontal mattress sutures. Per-rectal massage may be required intermittently to stimulate the bladder tone.

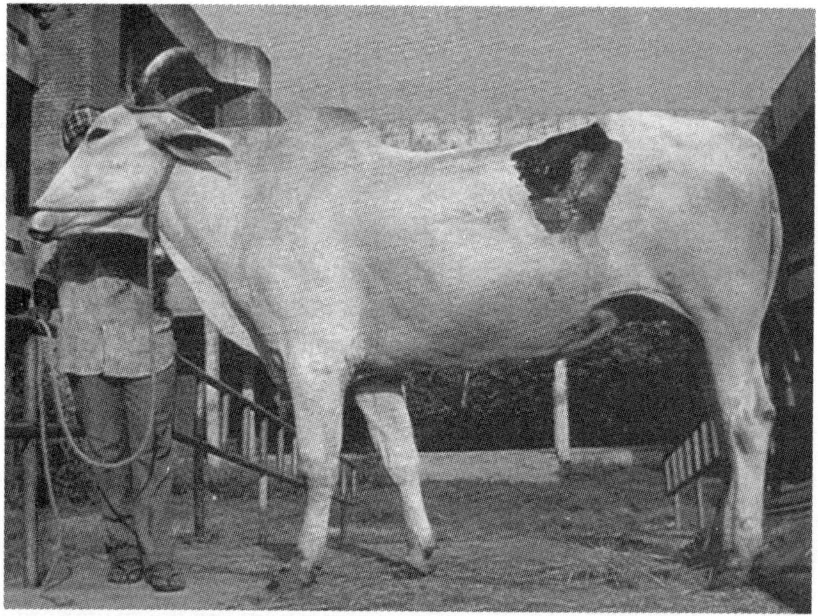

Fig. 11 : Bullock after cystorrhaphy (urinary bladder repair) showing site of operation at the left paralumbar fossa

4.4.4 Rupture of urethra

It occurs due to accidental injury or in cases where penis is accidently crushed during castration. The damage to urethra is managed as in urethrotomy by passing the catheter and retaining it for 2-3 weeks. If damage is more, partial penectomy may have to be performed. Multiple stab incisions may be needed to drain the subcutaneously accumulated urine.

4.4.5 Caesarean section

It can be performed in standing or more commonly through right lateral recumbency under local infiltration or epidural anesthesia in cattle or buffaloes. Standing flank approach is also used. In lateral recumbency, paramedian incision parallel and lateral or median to left milk vein is commonly used (Khar *et al.* 1993). For caesarean section, all layers of abdominal wall are incised one by one. Uterus is exposed by reflecting the omentum to the cranial side. Uterus is exteriorized and incision is made on greater curvature by avoiding caruncles. Foetus is grasped after opening the foetal membrane and removed. Umbilical cord is severed about 10 cm from umbilicus when the foetal respiration is established. It is recommended that placenta is kept intact for spontaneous expulsion after injecting 50 units of oxytocin into the wall of uterus for enhancing its involution. Uterus is closed using inversion sutures and muscles and skin are closed in routine manner.

4.4.6 Rectovaginal tear

Rectal or rectovaginal tear are repaired under epidural anesthesia. By applying stay sutures at the deep and superficial end of tear, the torn part can be exposed to outside and continuous or interrupted sutures can be applied with absorbable suture materials like catgut or Vicryl No. 1 thread. Suturing is done blindly or by pulling the rectum out to repair such defects (Saini and Mohindroo 2007). If it is a third degree perineal laceration in mares, it is advisable to repair after 4-5 weeks of injury in one or two stages. Incision is given at the healed junction of perineal laceration in mares, the vaginal and rectal walls are separated and sutured separately by interrupted sutures preferably using Vicryl or catgut. The skin can be repaired by using non-absorbable suture material like polyamide.

4.5 Wound management

Wounds are commonly encountered due to accidental lacerations in cattle and buffaloes (Fig. 12) and may be broadly classified into clean and contaminated wounds. A clean wound may be sutured if felt necessary after thorough lavage with antiseptic solution. A contaminated wound must be douched with potassium permanganate solution (1:1000) and scrubbed with

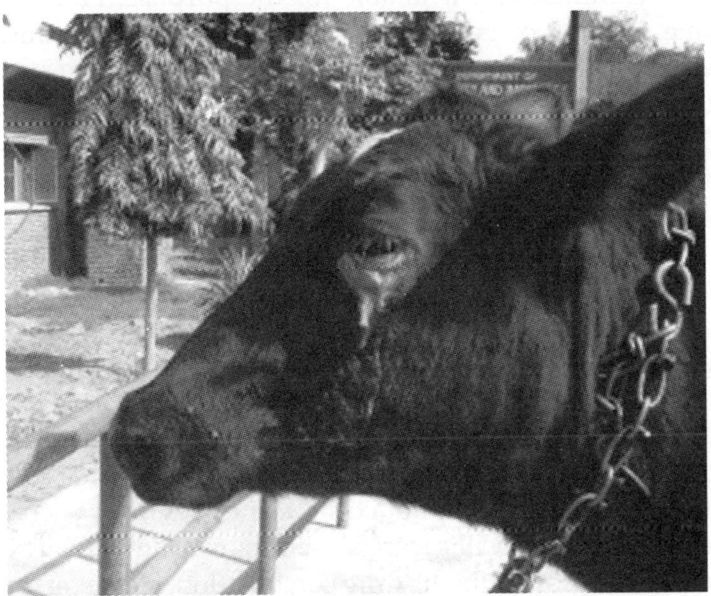

Fig. 12 : A cow with accidental lacerated wound near left eye

chlorhexidine solution. Such wounds are dressed with povidone iodine and left open to heal by second intention. In cases where it is mandatory to suture a contaminated wound (e.g. evisceration), adequate drainage must be provided by use of a penrose drain or fenestrated catheter or leaving one or two sutures open at the dependent part so that the discharge may drain properly. Dog bite wounds which are deep are not sutured and cleaning of such wounds must be done using latex gloves and should be followed by post bite vaccination of the animal. Gunshot, perforated and penetrating wounds must first be evaluated for injury to other vital organs. The wounds must then be treated as a contaminated wound as per the requirement of the case. Radiographs must be taken to locate the bullets etc. Maggot wounds are frequently encountered in the tropical climate of India. The maggots may be removed manually or by application of topical maggicidal preparations and then treated as open wound. Turpentine oil must not be used on mucosal surfaces and in ear or eye. Fly repellant sprays are also available which prevent flies sitting on the wounds. Punctured wounds on the sole due to sharp metal nails must be treated with caution. The nail must be removed manually and the punctured tract must be widened and flushed with antiseptic solutions. Chemical burns must immediately be neutralized by thorough lavage with tap water. Scalds or burns must be immediately subjected to cold water application to prevent burning of deeper tissues. Superficial burns which form blisters must be treated by rupturing the blisters (never peel off the blister) and applying astringent lotions over the burns. Ointments like burnol, silverex cream etc. are commercially available for the purpose. Fluid therapy with normal saline solution or lactated ringers solution must be initiated as per need. If the area of skin damage is large, skin grafting may be required in due course of time, for which the case can be referred to a specialized facility in the area. Antibiotic cover must be provided to prevent secondary infection along with antihistamines and pain killers. Steroid must be avoided unless it is felt absolutely necessary, especially in severe cases of burns. Patient must be evaluated for urine output, renal function and liver function along with complete blood work.

5. Postoperative Care

Post operative control of infection is of utmost importance to the surgeon. Any broad spectrum antibiotic can be used. Antibiotic should not be considered as substitute for poor asepsis. Antibiotics like ampiclox, streptopenicillin, gentamycin, enrofloxacin, cephotaxime are commonly used in bovines. Penicillin, ampicillin, amoxicillin, cephalosporins can individually be combined with aminoglycoside for antibiotic drug combination. However, penicillin and tetracyclin are antagonistic and should not be used in combination.

The surgical wound is dressed daily with povidone-iodine solution. Fly repellent spray or cream can be used depending upon fly season because flies are a major source of infection and maggots in bovines. If possible, wounds should be kept covered with clean cloth which must be changed every 12-24 hours. Animals with plaster of Paris should be kept on dry floor. The plaster should be changed immediately if it gets wet.

6. Present Indian Perspective

In Indian scenario, the veterinary services are mostly provided or controlled by government institutions. Bovine surgery under rural settings still needs lot of effort to gain momentum in terms of knowledge, practice and dedication of veterinary surgeons working in rural areas. Bovine surgery is still a distant dream in some parts of the country where bovine general anesthesia is considered a great risk or adequate facilities are not available. To the authors' knowledge surgical procedures that were undertaken few years back at field level were only limited to wound management, medial patellar desmotomy and castration by use of Burdizo emasculator.

It is only recently that some of the procedures like rumenotomy, caesarian section and application of plaster of Paris for fracture repair in bovine became popular in some parts of the country. Veterinarians under rural settings are generally concentrating more on medicine and obstetrical procedures. When the need of some surgical procedure is felt, cases are mostly referred to more specialized facilities like university hospitals rather than attempting at field level. Moreover, the economic feasibility of the surgical procedure is also a major consideration for the Indian farmers under rural settings.

7. Scenario in the Developed Nations

In the developed countries, veterinary services are mostly provided or controlled by private institutions. Bovine animal surgeons abroad are basically concentrating on abdominal disorders. The development of bovine abdominal surgery abroad is because bovines are well suited to successful surgical repair of commonly occurring abdominal diseases as compared to orthopedic and reproductive surgery. Bovine surgery is a reality at farm level in the developed nations and the number of surgical procedures like treatment of left displacement of abomasum (LDA), right displacement of abomasum (RDA), management of bloat (by rumenotomy), intestinal obstruction etc. are manageable at farm level. However, when the treatment is uneconomical, it is preferred to recommend slaughter of the animal for meat purpose to avoid economic loss to the farmer.

8. Comparative Analysis

Farm animal surgery is not much developed as hardly any surgery is done at farm level in most part of India. In advanced countries, on the contrary, abdominal surgery at farm level has taken a lead especially for treatment of LDA, RDA and reproductive problems. In India, due to religious and sentimental attachment to animals, the farmers prefer to bear the production loss and extra maintenance cost of diseased and nonproducing animals rather than sending them for slaughter. Due to financial constraints, surgery is out of reach of marginal or poor farmers. This is not the case in developed countries where accidentally injured or fractured (untreatable) animals are generally sent for slaughter keeping in view the economic criteria to limit the losses to the farmer. Farmers' education and veterinarians' training and practical skills are other factors that make the difference between the developing and developed nations.

9. Challenges and Constraints

In the present day scenario, bovine surgery has a lot of scope but is not considered as monetarily rewarding, which probably is the biggest challenge for the system. Another raging problem in the rural scenario is the intervention of quacks who mislead the farmers and compound the problem by delaying the availability of rational treatment. The inadequacy of veterinarians and frequent changes in their place of posting also indirectly promote quackery. It is at this point that the role of extension specialists/contact person becomes important. The extension experts can make sure that the farmers approach the right person for getting medical aid for their livestock. The hospitals in rural areas seldom have adequate facilities for surgical procedures and the lack of technical support makes the situation even worse in the rural areas. A particular rural veterinary hospital should have minimum facilities as mentioned in Table 2.

Rural veterinary hospitals are usually in a dilapidated state. The major reason behind the poor state of affairs is lack of funds and attention towards the precious livestock. The government has now started giving more emphasis to the livestock sector but lots of efforts still need to be done in terms of infrastructure development, manpower employment and working facilities. There is also a lack of expertise among the veterinarians who need to develop skills to perform surgical procedures at field level. India being a vast country has different agro-climatic zones and consequently region specific problems are encountered in the animals. Many times there is lack of expertise regarding the area specific diseases. The heavy built of the animal is another challenge, especially in cases where the cattle and buffaloes become recumbent. Although not much can be done about the weight of the animal, facilities should be made available to hoist the recumbent animal. The poor management practices and lack of know-how on raising clean and healthy animals are other causes of concern. The value of animal, sentiment of an owner, cost of treatment are other factors that decide surgical intervention and the outcome.

Table 2 : Minimum surgical facilities requirement for a rural veterinary hospital

Equipment/Instrument	Quantity
Travis	One
Autoclave (2-3 KW)	One
Sterilizer	One
Stainless steel kidney tray and instrument tray	Two each
8 ft x 8 ft padded mattress (6" thick)	One
5 ft x 3ft padded mattress (4" thick)	Two
Instrument trolley	One
Instrument cabinet	One
Dressing and sterilizing drum (Large)	One
Enamelled tray (15" x 18")	Two
Dressing scissors	Two
Cheatle forceps	Two
I.V. Stand	One
Mouth gag (Butler)	One
Dental rasps/ Float	Two
Burdizo castrator / Emasculator (for cattle and sheep/goat)	One each
Electric disbudder	One
Polythene catheters of different sizes (2, 3, 4, 5 mm)	50 meter each
Stainless steel urinary catheter (mare catheter)	One
Vaginal speculum (small and large)	One each
Flexible metallic stilet for intracystic catheterization	Ten
Trocar and cannula	One
Aluminum splints (2- 4 mm thick)	As per need
Teat instruments	Two sets
Weingarth rumenotomy set (hooks, frame and clamps)	Two sets
Magnet for retrieving metallic foreign bodies during rumenotomy	Two
Intestinal forceps (9") - straight and curved	Two each
Mechanical/electric tooth rasp(s)	One set
Molar tooth cutter	One
Tooth chisel and hammer	One each
Probang (stomach tube)	One

Hoof instruments (hoof knife, hoof tester, trimmer)	One set
Plaster saw (electric/manual)	One
Power drill with drill bits	One
Pin cutter	One
Extension board with at least 30 m wire for power supply	One
Chain pulley	One
Surgical Pack	
B.P. handle No. 3, 4 (1 each), groove director(1), Allis tissue forceps (4), Metzenbaum scissors (2), Mayo scissors (curved and straight - 1 each), artery forceps straight (4), artery forceps curved (4), Mayo Hegar needle holder (2), rat-toothed thumb forceps (1), Adsons tissue forceps (1), Backhaus towel clamps (4), drapes 1m x1m (5), shroud 1.5m x1.5m (1), base cloth 0.5 m x 0.5 m (1), towel (1), instrument hangar (1)	Two sets
Others (ropes, cotton, bandages, surgical gloves, scrub solutions, betadine, tincture iodine, zinc oxide, magnesium sulphate, copper sulphate, liquid paraffin, potassium permanganate, syringes (different sizes), B.P. blades (No. 11, 12, 23, 24, 26), biopsy instruments, penrose drains, Foleys catheters, I.V. set, cannula, suturing needles-cutting and non-cutting different sizes, hypodermic needles (4", 6"), razor, shaving blades, plaster of Paris, different types of suture material (Vicryl, silk, polyamide, catgut etc), lignocaine 2% and other medicines	As per need

10. Strategies for Future Development

A number of steps can be taken to improve the present situation of farm animal surgery in the country. These include:

1. Education and training of the farmers
2. Providing surgical facilities at the farmers' doorstep wherever possible
3. Easy access to veterinary help
4. Improving the knowledge and expertise of veterinarians
5. Commitment of the veterinary surgeons
6. Developing facilities for surgical procedures in rural hospitals and farms
7. Involvement of private sector in providing veterinary services

The farmers should be educated, how to recognize the disease problem and where to find a solution. Some basic knowledge should be imparted to the farmer to provide first aid to the animal before getting help of a veterinarian. Farmers should have an easy access to veterinary help. The veterinarians must be trained to address basic surgical procedures at their hospitals or in the livestock farms. For this, it is imperative to develop the facilities for it. The veterinarians must also know when to go in for surgery and when to refer the case to a specialized institution for further surgical intervention. A veterinarian must also be aware about the economic viability of a surgical procedure vis-à-vis the cost of the animal and should effectively convey proper message to the farmer. The expected surgical outcome and the usefulness of the animal after surgery (draught/milch/breeding) must be considered and discussed with the farmer. The surgeon must take into account all these factors before deciding to operate on a cattle or a buffalo.

India needs highly committed and dedicated veterinarians who are always ready to accept the challenge faced by the livestock industry in terms of providing healthcare in rural hospitals and at farm level. Special incentives should be extended to the bovine practitioners in rural areas and facilities must be created at the rural veterinary hospitals so that the veterinarian can perform surgery on the ailing animal at the hospital or at farm level. Technical support should be generated in the form of qualified technicians who can render help to the surgeon. Confidence building measures must be taken up so that the farmers gain confidence in the veterinarian. The first step in this direction should be to provide permanent postings to doctors for a period of at least ten years and their performance must be judged over this period. This will significantly reduce the quackery as well as promote the livestock health in the area.

The rural dispensaries must be attached to district level satellite hospitals operated by the specialized institutions in the state. This will provide adequate technical and expert support to the rural veterinarians. The veterinarians must be updated with recent advances in disease management and this may help them in taking appropriate steps in prevention of certain emerging problems. For example, a recent study revealed that feeding of machine made wheat straw may act as a risk factor for development of omasal impaction in bovines (Toor and Saini 2008). Such type of information needs to be conveyed to the farmers so that they can prevent the disease. The veterinarian must also have thorough knowledge of the diseases that exist in a particular area and must be well equipped and trained to address the problems. This only will be possible through strengthening extension activities at national, state and grassroots levels. Special lectures, demonstrations, TV shows, radio talks, newspaper articles, contact programmes etc. need to be organized for the farmers to keep them abreast with the emerging diseases and their preventions.

Some minimum surgical facilities to all the hospitals under rural settings should be provided and the training of the rural veterinary surgeons must be accomplished in the following stages:

Stage 1: Training of veterinarian resource persons in the university

Stage 2: Training of veterinarians working at district and sub-division level

Stage 3: Training of veterinarians working at rural settings by Stage 1 and 2 veterinarians

The veterinarians must get refresher trainings once every 2-3 years. A system of continuing education can be evolved in which field veterinarians must put in 20-30 hours of learning every year at specialized institutions. The veterinary hospitals or veterinarians must have continual links with the specialized institutions so that expert advice is readily available to them.

Lastly, the government should encourage the participation of private sector and individuals for setting up private hospitals for better livestock health coverage.

11. Conclusion

Bovine surgery is evolving as a major challenge in the rural settings where the surgical help is seldom available to the farmer at farm level. The farmer is usually unable to get veterinary help at the earliest. Most of the time, the farmer has to transport his animal over long distances to avail the surgical facilities from experts at the veterinary institutions. Many procedures like castration, disbudding, rumenotomy, herniorrhaphy, rasping of irregular molars, management of congenital abnormalities like tendon contractures and atrasia-ani, amputations, management of urolithiasis, fracture, fistulas, wounds etc can be easily performed at the farm level under rural settings. However, lack of infrastructure, facilities and expertise, make it difficult to perform these surgical procedures at the farm or in rural veterinary hospital. To provide the best surgical facilities to the livestock in remote places, it is imperative to develop the infrastructure and confidence of the veterinarians for basic and advanced surgical interventions. The veterinarians in the rural areas should be linked to the specialized institutions and must be encouraged to update their knowledge through regular continuing education programmes.

References

1. Athar Hakim, Mohindroo J, Singh K *et al.* (2010). Clinical, haematobiochemical, radiographic and ultrasonographic features of traumatic reticuloperitonitis in bovines. Indian J Anim Sci 80:608-612.
2. Hull BL (2004). History of farm animal surgery. In: Fubini SL and Ducharme NC (eds) Farm Animal Surgery, 1st edn. Saunders, Missouri, USA.
3. Khar SK, Mannari MN, Singh J (1993). The genital system. Section B. Female. In: Tyagi RPS, Singh J (eds) Ruminant Surgery 1st edn. CBS Publishers and Distributors, Delhi.

4. Kumar A, Sangwan V, Mohindroo J *et al.* (2008). Diagnostic and prognostic indicators, antibacterial sensitivity pattern and surgical treatment of perireticular abscess in cows and buffaloes. Indian J Anim Sci 78:1329-1332.

5. Muir WW, Hubbell JAE, Bednarshi RM *et al.* (2007). Handbook of veterinary anesthesia. 4th edn. Mosby Elsevier, USA.

6. Saini NS, Anand A, Bansal PS *et al.* (2005a). Surgical repair of inter-mandibular fistula with protrusion of tongue in a buffalo. Vet Record 150:638-639.

7. Saini NS, Mohindroo J (2007). Rectal tear leading to intestinal evisceration through anus in a calf. Canadian Vet J 48:1297-1298.

8. Saini NS, Kumar A, Mahajan SK *et al.* (2007). The use of ultrasonography, radiography and surgery in the successful recovery from diaphragmatic hernia in a cow. Canadian Vet J 48:757-759.

9. Saini NS, Kumar A, Mohindroo J *et al.* (2005b). Clinical features and survival in reticular abscessation in buffaloes. Buffalo J 65:167-173

10. Saini NS, Mirakhur KK, Singh M *et al.* (1998). Homologous plasma-stored tendon grafting in equids-gross and histomorphological observations. Res Vet Sci 64: 85-90.

11. Saini NS, Sanghera JS, Bishnoi P (2002). Immobilization using transfixation after allo-grafting of Achilles and flexor tendons in bovines. Indian Vet J 79:831-834.

12. Saini NS, Sharma SN, Oberoi MS *et al.* (1992a). Effect of operation theatre environment on laparotomy wound infection in bovines. J Vet Med Series A 39:258-363.

13. Saini NS, Singh KI, Sobti VK *et al.* (1992b). Surgical management of ocular ganglioneuroma in buffaloes. Indian Vet J 69:642.

14. Saini NS, Sobti VK, Mirakhur KK *et al.* (2000). Retrospective evaluation of 80 non surviving buffaloes with diaphragmatic hernia. Vet Record 147:275-276.

15. Singh N, Sharma SN, Oberoi MS (1988). Evaluation of surgeon's scrub during laparotomy in bovines. Indian Vet J 65:1035-1038.

16. Singh N, Sharma SN, Oberoi MS (1989). Skin scrubbing procedures for laparotomy in calves: A microbial evaluation. Indian J Vet Surg 10:42-45.

17. Sobti VK, Saini N S, Singh KI *et al.* (1995). Esophageal diverticulum due to foreign body in a buffalo. Indian Vet J 72:541-542.

18. Sobti VK, Singh KI, Bansal PS *et al.* (1994). Surgical repair of perineal hernia in buffaloes - review of five cases. Indian J Vet Surg 15:43.

19. Toor AS, Saini NS (2008). Diagnostic and prognostic indicators of omasal impaction in buffaloes (*Bubalus bubalis*). Vet Record 162:275-278.

20. Turner AS, McIlwarith CW (1989). Techniques in Large animal surgery. 2nd edn. Lea & Febiger, Philadelphia, USA.

□□□

Chapter 12

Mitigation of Infertility in Dairy Animals

R. K. CHANDOLIA
Department of Veterinary Gynaecology and Obstetrics, College of Veterinary Sciences, Lala Lajpat Rai University of Veterinary and Animal Sciences, Hisar-125004

Contents

1. Introduction

Infertility in dairy animals is a challenging problem. While it is prevalent all over the world, its incidence is comparatively higher in tropical than temperate climate. In the tropical conditions like in India, there is long summer period, where temperature rises over 40°C. Under such conditions, either some animals do not show oestrus signs or the manifestation is quite weak. The deficiency of green fodder aggravates the livestock infertility. The lack of education about proper heat detection and management of dairy animals further compounds the problem in the developing countries.

Dairymen frequently approach the veterinarians to seek remedy for this problem, however, with the available treatment regimen and lack of proper understanding of causes of infertility, success is variable. The dairy farmers, thus, get frustrated over the lack of response of animals even after expensive treatments. It gives rise to the presumption that infertility may not be cured and many a times they wait till natural normal recovery and conception. This practice leads to loss of valuable time in terms of production and next gestation. Dairymen also suffer economic losses on account of sale of such animals at lower price in the absence of pregnancy. The failure of treatment also influences the farmers' trust on the veterinarians, further aggravating the problem.

2. Indian Perspective

Infertility is a leading cause of economic setback due to loss of calf crop and overall milk production. The incidence of anoestrus and other forms of infertility varies from place to place and has been put at 9 to 60% in buffaloes and cows in different part of India (Rao and Sremannarayana 1982, Hussain and Maniraju 1984, Banerjee *et al.* 1992, Kumar and Kumar 1993, Singla and Verma 1994, Singh and Sahni 1995, Singh *et al.* 2003, Pandit 2004, Selvaraju *et al.* 2005, Srinivas *et al.* 2007). Infertility is seen in both heifers and adult females. The livestock owners particularly complain about the absence of oestrus even after the age of 4 or 5 years in buffalo heifers. On examination of such heifers, the genital organs are found to be small and underdeveloped. The ovaries lack follicular activity. Ultrasonography of such ovaries shows follicles smaller than 5 mm. Infertility in adult buffaloes is either due to the absence of oestrus or due to lack of proper signs of oestrus. Most of these adult females are lactating ones. Enquiry from the livestock owners reveals that generally such animals do not get mineral mixture. The animals are fed on wheat bhusa (straw) mixed with some kind of green. In the evening and morning, the animals are also given mustard cake or cottonseed cake. The animals receive almost same or similar kind of ration every day. There is no provision of pastures for grazing of these animals. The problem is further aggravated when the animals are kept away from males. In Indian conditions, many dairymen keep 5 to 6 buffaloes without a male. These animals are checked visually for heat or oestrus signs during day time. As the cycle of a cow or buffalo is of 20 to 22 days, one missed heat puts an animal almost one month late for conception. Three or four missed observations may extend infertility period for several months. In this way the causes of infertility are not only related to female but are also manmade.

3. Causes of Infertility

According to Singh *et al.* (2009), the major reasons of conception failure include faulty genital manipulations (7%), deficiency of circulating hormones (28%), infections (18%), poor management (15%) and combination of these factors (31%). Many other studies also agree for high prevalence of anoestrus and delayed puberty under Indian conditions (Tomar and Tripathi 1994, Bhattacharyya *et al.* 2009) and in other developing countries (El-Wishy 2009). Several factors that lead to such high infertility rate are mentioned below.

3.1 Nutritional deficiency

From the analysis of various factors, first and the foremost reason for infertility is the deficiency of phosphorus or improper ratio of calcium and phosphorus in heifers and energy deficiency in adult milch animals (Bhattacharyya *et al.* 2009). More than 70% of adult population of milking animals is not maintaining proper body score. In dairy animals, it has been reported that proper bodyweight and proper energy level are important for proper ovarian functions (Beam and Butler 1999). In Indian cities and villages, the dairymen generally follow hand-feed practices and purchase of feed and fodder is in limited quantity for milking animals, which fails to maintain proper energy level, body score and fertility of the animals.

3.2 High environmental temperature

The second factor that is currently affecting fertility of our animals is high summer temperature. During summer, it has been seen that most of animals do not maintain proper cyclicity (Agarwal *et al.* 2005). It has been reported through experiments that fertility is improved if the animals are given better management through maintaining a moderate temperature (Perera 1999). The dairymen, however, usually fail to implement it because they cannot provide adequate space and management for thermal regulation.

3.3 Lack of knowledge

Lack of knowledge about infertility management seems to be another reason of infertility in our animals. The literature about management of infertility is usually in English language while only limited information is available in local languages. Most of the dairymen are not in regular contact with the animal scientists and extension workers. They hardly take precautionary advice from local veterinarians.

3.4 Inadequate heat detection methods and faulty insemination

Deficient heat detection facilities and faulty insemination are other major reasons for high incidence of infertility in our animals (Jadon *et al.* 2005, Khan *et al.* 2009). Inadequate training of field staff in management of infertility adds to the problem (Kutty and Ramchandran 2003, Naidu and Rao 2004). Recently, introduction of layman inseminators in India has been considered as another factor towards more infertile cases.

3.5 Genital infections

Subclinical and clinical genital infections under field conditions are also on the suggestive list of the reasons of infertility (Prajapati *et al.* 2005, Ali *et al.* 2009).

3.6 Lack of contact of male and female animals

Lack of contact of male and female animals is considered another factor for higher incidence of infertility. Our dairymen keep five to ten buffaloes without a male. Therefore, the entire responsibility of detection of heat lies on the dairymen themselves, who may miss the signs of heat in the animals and may not have adequate knowledge about the abnormal discharge from the genital organs of postpartum animals (Singh *et al.* 2003).

4. Scenario in Developed Nations

The problem of livestock infertility exists in the developed countries too but the incidence is much lower than in the developing countries. The system of animal rearing is quite different in the developed nations where they have large pastures or grazing land for the animals. The herd size is quite large where male and females are kept together. The incidence of infertility increases in those herds, where artificial insemination (AI) is followed and detection of heat is done by the farm personnel themselves. It has been shown that even in well managed ranches; there may be at least 25% less detection of heat and the incidence of infertility can be reduced with simple physiological means (Short *et al.* 1990, Royal *et al.* 2000). Nutritional infertility in such farms is not common; however incidence of low body score during postpartum period and its negative effect on fertility has been reported (Lents *et al.* 2008). It has been opined that the fertility has declined over the generations due to the selection procedures for better milk yield (Lopaz-Gatius 2003). The infectious form of infertility is generally taken care of immediately due to proper management and treatment of affected animals. It is due to a quick contact between veterinarians, animal scientists and the dairymen. The dairymen are well trained in AI, handling of retained foetal membranes and intrauterine administration of antimicrobials. The dairymen are also given education regarding proper feeding to avoid infertility (Roche 1986). They are imparted knowledge and literature in their mother tongue, so that they follow proper procedure for the control of infertility (Hutchinson 2007).

Most of the dairymen own large agricultural farms and they usually have good financial resources. These dairymen benefit from the sale of milk as well as from sale of meat. Culling of the animals suffering from chronic infertility problems is done at regular intervals. The veterinarians in developed countries have adequate diagnostic and therapeutic facilities. The veterinarians also undergo periodic updating of their knowledge in various clinical and paraclinical fields.

The dairymen of developed countries get benefit from strong currency of their nation too. It enables them to buy the necessary equipments and facilities for their animals from national and international market for minimizing infertility problem. These days, many dairymen are regularly utilizing ultrasonography to assess the health status of uterus and ovaries of their livestock (Cavalieri 2010). Apart from this, most of the developed countries have temperate climate or they are able to reduce heat and humidity stress at their farms for better production and reproduction.

5. Comparative Analysis in Developing Countries

Analytic comparison between developed and developing nations is important. There are several practices in the developed nations that if adopted in developing countries might be beneficial. Some developing countries have already benefitted from such policies. An important policy is the liaison between the corporate sector and dairy industry. Several multinational companies are interested to finance private dairies. These companies help in providing modern diagnostic equipments and tools to minimize infertilities. They also support modernization of animal management system, minimizing the climatic stress on production and reproduction (Hutchinson 2007).

Infertility in developed nations is low due to large pastures and stress free roaming of animals, while developing countries lack this. Country like India, where land holding is decreasing every year, emphasis on animal husbandry is increasing with stall fed system, leading to inadequate exercise of the animal and nutritional deficiencies. Apart from this, the problem of infertility in developed nations is related mostly to high milk yield, while in developing countries it is usually infectious type of infertility. The developed nations prepare animal health worker and farmers to handle the problem of infertility, while such technical trainings, particularly diagnostics, are generally deficient in the developing countries (Noakes *et al.* 2009).

As far as infertility due to improper heat detection and manmade errors is concerned, it is higher in developing nations. Generally, a fixed time insemination approach is adopted after synchronization of oestrus in farm animals to minimize infertility due to failed heat detection. Such protocols have also been tried in India; however, looking into the high import cost of the hormones involved in it and only about 50% success rate, this programme is not popular among dairymen in the country.

Infertility due to sub-oestrus or silent-oestrus is on higher side in India and other tropical countries. The analysis of stress related infertility reveals that it is comparatively higher in developing nations (Abeygunawardena and Dematawewab 2004). The incidence of infectious infertility is also higher in developing countries as compared to developed countries (Noakes *et al.* 2009).

The literacy rate among farmers and the availability of scientific literature to them on production and reproduction in their local languages is far superior in the developed countries. Further, there are strong linkages between universities and dairymen. The lack of these in the developing nations results in difficulties in mitigation of infertility.

The vaccination programmes against various diseases that affect the health and fertility of animals are quite inadequate in developing countries in comparison to the developed ones. Adoption of regular vaccination e.g. against bovine viral diarrhoea, infectious bronchorhinitis (IBR), vibriosis, brucellosis etc. can be helpful in mitigating infertility in livestock to some extent.

6. Constraints in Infertility Mitigation

Mitigation of infertility faces several challenges and constraints outlined below.

6.1 Mineral deficiency

Indian soil has become deficient in several mineral contents. This has resulted into problem of infertility. Improvement in agricultural practices to improve soil deficiency is a big challenge. The assessment of minerals supplementation in soil and their transfer to plants and then animals need intensive efforts and coordinated research to mitigate infertility in animals. It has been generally agreed that animals in developing countries need feed supplementation either as oral calcium-phosphorus liquid preparations or as mineral mixture powders. The unavailability of adequate feed supplementation is a major constraint in resource poor countries in mitigating nutritional form of infertility.

6.2 Poor animal husbandry practices

The practice of keeping a single animal to meet the family milk requirements contributes to infertility problem in these animals. It is a challenge to encourage the people to establish mini dairies so that animals are kept in a group along with a teaser or normal male. Provision of regular exercise to the animals kept in small areas, particularly in cities or suburban areas, is another challenge.

6.3 Silent heat and subclinical infections

Silent heat in tropical environment is a big challenge. Moreover, undiagnosed subclinical infections of genital tract are other woes of fertility.

6.4 Proficiency of inseminators

In India, every year several thousand personnel are being trained for AI services. These are known as laymen inseminators. Since the procedure of AI requires good skill of passing AI guns and insemination at proper time of heat, an error on the part of inseminator may be a hindrance in mitigation of infertility.

6.5 Maintenance of veterinary teaching herds

Lack of teaching animal herds in many veterinary colleges is a common constraint. Therefore, the training of veterinary graduates in mitigation of infertility is not of required level.

6.6 Early diagnosis of pregnancy

Very early diagnosis of pregnancy can avoid delay in treatment of infertile animals; however, ultrasonography equipments needed for it are very expensive and usually remain out of reach in field practice.

6.7 High cost of animal medicines

The cost of animal medicines is high as compared to the milk price. The dairymen, therefore, tend to neglect minor health problems of the animals, which later turn into serious ones. Most of such health problems affect the reproductive process of the animals resulting in infertility.

6.8 Environmental temperature and humidity

Most of the developing countries are facing problem of high summer temperatures. Due to the limited space with most of dairymen, animals have to face the summer stress. This situation becomes worse in monsoon season when high temperature is accompanied by high humidity. The combination of these two stress factors affects the fertility of animals.

6.9 Early diagnosis of causes of infertility

The causes of infertility remain undiagnosed most of the times resulting in hit and trial methods of treatment. Though imaging technologies are available to differentiate the normal and abnormal genital tracts, these are not in common use. The manual palpation fails to diagnose the infertility problem fairly.

6.10 Good quality males

The availability of good quality males in developing countries is a problem. Moreover, the ratio of male and female animals is not proper. The lack of regular check up of breeding bulls in rural areas is another constraint. The street bulls in suburban areas are, thus, bound to spread infertility due to infectious diseases.

6.11 Poor training of veterinarians for breeding soundness evaluation of bulls

The veterinarians are generally good in female animal practice; however, they are generally not good at the breeding soundness evaluation of bulls.

6.12 Faulty vaccination of animals

Irregular vaccination and break in the cold chain lead to infections and diseases affecting fertility.

7. Strategies for Infertility Mitigation

Some major steps that can be helpful to reduce the problem of infertility in the livestock are discussed below.

7.1 Maintenance of proper energy, minerals and vitamins levels

It should be ensured that the animal feeds available in the market contain adequate levels of minerals and vitamins. These should also be able to maintain proper energy level in the livestock. Soil survey helps in evaluating the necessity of extra feed supplementation. Among minerals, attention should be given to proper ratio of calcium and phosphorus along with trace minerals. Among vitamins, vitamin E, B_{12} and D_3 should be in adequate quantity in all animal feed supplements. Vitamin A should also be given during summer days, when availability of green fodder is less. Dairy farmers should have a feeding chart for animals for production and maintenance of reproduction.

7.2 Efficient heat detection mechanism

Detection of oestrus based on external heat symptoms by the farmers may not be reliable, as such signs may not be pronounced during hotter months of the year. Dairymen should be advised to attempt heat detection during cooler hours i.e. during late night and early mornings. It might be helpful to use teaser bulls for heat detection. Modern dairy farmers may be equipped with some mechanical means of heat detection. In the developed countries, equipments are available to detect heat by analyzing the conductivity of oestrus mucus.

7.3 Stress management

The role of stress in infertility is well known. The stress factors can be environmental, managemental, nutritional, or lactational. Lactational stress is difficult to manage, but early weaning and proper calcium supplementation might be helpful in such cases. Under Indian conditions nutritional stress is widespread. Soil has been found deficient in many macro and micronutrients. Therefore, some animal nutritionists advise supplementation of mineral mixtures based on soil analysis reports. Phosphorus deficiency or wider ratio of Ca:P has been implicated as a factor in infertility in several reports. Usually the feed has less phosphorus content. There are few such feeds that contain higher phosphorus content viz. millet and cottonseeds. These days many researchers advocate supplementation of mineral mixtures that also contain vitamins. Summer stress can be managed by proper spacing of animals and timely watering and feeding. In India, long summer season is a challenge for dairymen and scientists. The incidence of infertility during these months is the highest. Maintaining cooler environment with water sprinkler, adequate ventilation and humidity control helps to reduce infertility.

7.4 Control of postpartum infertility

Postpartum infertility is generally related to ignorance on the part of animal owners. It can be controlled through education of dairymen regarding management of clean and infection free peri-parturient period, maintenance of proper energy level of the animal during two months after calving, supplementation of balanced ration and maintenance of proper bodyweight of the animal. Supplementation of calcium and phosphorus during postpartum period prevents this problem. It can be reduced through proper heat detection system.

7.5 Keeping male and female animals in the herd in proper ratio

The dairymen must keep males in the vicinity or company of females. Keeping males along with females will be helpful as a stimulant for proper cyclicity, heat detection and mating in time.

7.6 Regular check up of reproductive tract for control of infections

Regular check up of reproductive tract can help in assessing the etiology and remedy of infertility problem in animals. The check up is quite essential for postpartum animals to assess the involution of uterus. Any problem in involution should be corrected through the use of ecbolics, calcium supplementation or antimicrobial therapy based on the suspected etiology.

7.7 Regular deworming of adult animals

Regular deworming is important to prevent health problems and infertility. Deworming of pregnant animals is suggested to avoid body deficiencies that might affect postpartum interval from calving to oestrus.

7.8 Maintenance of bodyweight of the animal

It has been suggested that bodyweight is more important than age in animals particularly in heifers for proper reproductive process. All efforts should be made to maintain bodyweight of both, growing heifers and adult animals. To avoid infertility in heifers the bodyweight should be more than 250 kg. Underweight animals may not conceive.

7.9 Ultrasonographic imaging for early pregnancy detection

Early pregnancy detection can save the dairymen from keeping unproductive animals. The availability of ultrasonographic procedures for dairy animals can now detect pregnant and infertile animals. Detection of early pregnancy helps in proper feeding of the animal and birth of a healthy calf. In case the animal is not pregnant, the dairymen may try to induce cyclicity.

7.10 Regular evaluation of breeding bulls

There should be a regular check up programme of breeding bulls. This will be helpful in mitigation of infertility.

7.11 Continuing veterinary education

The veterinarians must be able to diagnose efficiently the factors responsible for infertility. Inadequate laboratory support in the field makes their task particularly difficult. Regular updating of their knowledge and skill through continuing education will certainly make them more proficient in tackling the problem of infertility.

8. Conclusion

Infertility in animals, particularly in developing countries is the leading cause of losses of production and reproduction. Infertility can be due to the factors associated with female animal, male animal and management. The female factors can be controlled through better management of animals, check on infectious causes and care about the health of reproductive tract. Infertility due to male factors is manageable through regular evaluation of breeding soundness of the bull. Better training of personnel helps in controlling human factors. Apart from these, there are certain environmental factors that are a challenge in the mitigation of infertility. High temperature and humidity, deficiencies in soil, and nutritional inadequacies also hinder the maintenance of optimum fertility levels. Resource constraints in the developing countries further aggravate the problem. Grazing lands and diagnostic services are also quite unsatisfactory in developing countries as compared to the developed nations. Better programmes and planning can definitely be helpful in mitigation of infertility in developing countries. The measures that can be helpful in mitigating infertility include improved deworming, proper vaccinations, high nutritional plane, knowledge about heat detection, and better communication among the animal health workers, scientists and dairymen.

References

1. Abeygunawardena H, Dematawewab CMB (2004). Pre-pubertal and postpartum anestrus in tropical Zebu cattle. Animal Reprod Sci 82:373-384.
2. Agarwal SK, Singh SK, Rajkumar R (2005). Reproductive disorders and their management in cattle and buffaloes: A Review. Indian J Anim Sci 75(7):858-873.
3. Ali A, Abdel-Razek AKh, Derar R, Abdel-Rheem HA, Shehata SH (2009). Forms of reproductive disorders in cattle and buffaloes in Middle east. Reproduction in Domestic Animals 44:580-586.
4. Banerjee AK, Roychoudury R, Bandyopadhya SK (1992). Incidence of anoestrus in Murrah grade buffaloes (*Bubalus bubalis*) of Calcutta Khatals. Indian J Anim Reprod 13(1):61-62.
5. Beam SW, Butler WR (1999). Effects of energy balance on follicular development and first ovulation in postpartum dairy cows. J Reprod Fertil Suppl. 54:411-424.
6. Bhattacharyya HK, Makhdoomi DM, Hafiz A (2009). Prevalence of true anoestrus and delayed puberty in cattle. Indian J Vet Res 18:27-30.
7. Cavalieri J (2010). Veterinary Reproduction & Obstetrics. Australian Veterinary Journal 88:404. doi: 10.1111/j.1751-0813.2010.00618.
8. El-Wishy AB (2009). The postpartum buffalo II. Acyclicity and anestrus. A Review. Anim Reprod Sci 97:216-236.
9. Hussain PM, Maniraju L (1984). Study on the incidence of reproductive disorders of bovines in a part of Southern Karnataka. Livestock Advisor 9:13-26.
10. Hutchison LJ (2007). Troubleshooting infertility problems in dairy cattle. IRM-19. http://www.wvu.edu/~exten/infores/pubs/livepoul/dirm19.pdf

11. Jadon RS, Dhaliwal GS, Jand SK (2005). Prevalence of aerobic and anaerobic uterine bacteria during peripartum period in normal and dystocia affected buffaloes. Anim Reprod Sci 88:215-224

12. Khan HM, Bhakat M, Mohanty TK, Gupta AK, Raina VS, Mir MS (2009). Peripartum reproductive disorders in buffaloes - An overview. Vet Scan 4 (2): Article 38.

13. Kumar S, Kumar H (1993). Clinical analysis of anoestrus in rural bovines. Indian J Dairy Sci 46(2):80-81.

14. Kutty IC, Ramchandran K (2003). Bovine infertility- a field oriented categorization based on investigation among cross-bred cattle in a district of Kerala. Indian J Anim Sci 73:155-157.

15. Lents CA, White FJ, Ciccioli NH, Wettemann RP, Spicer LJ, Lalman DL (2008). Effects of body condition score at parturition and postpartum protein supplementation on estrous behavior and size of the dominant follicle in beef cows. J Anim Sci 86 (10):2549-2556.

16. López-Gatius F (2003). Is fertility declining in dairy cattle? A retrospective study in northeastern Spain. Theriogenology 60 (1):89-99.

17. Naidu GV, Rao KB (2004). A note on the incidence of reproductive disorders in buffaloes in Guntur district of Andhra Pradesh. Indian J Anim Reprod 25(1):37-38.

18. Noakes DE, Parkinson TJ, England GCW, Arthur GH (2009). Veterinary Reproduction & Obstetrics. 9th edition. Saunders Ltd.

19. Pandit RK (2004). Incidence of different kinds of reproductive disorders in livestock. Indian J Anim Reprod 25:35-36.

20. Perera BMAO (1999). Reproduction in water buffalo: Comparative aspects and implications for management. J Reprod Fertil 45 (Suppl 1):157-168.

21. Prajapati SB, Ghodasara DJ, Joshi BP, Prajapati KS, Jani VR (2005). Etio-pathological study of endometritis in repeat breeder buffaloes. Buffalo J 2:145-165.

22. Rao AVN, Sremannarayana O (1982). Clinical analysis of reproductive failure among female buffaloes (*Bubalus bubalis*) under village management in Andhra Pradesh. Theriogenology 18:403-411.

23. Roche JF (1986). The effect of nutritional management of the dairy cow on reproductive efficiency. Anim Reprod Sci 96:282-296.

24. Royal M, Mann GE, Flint APE (2000). Strategies for reversing the trend towards sub-fertility in dairy cattle. Vet J 160:53-60.

25. Selvaraju M, Veerapandian C, Kathiresan D, Chandrahasan C (2005). Incidence of bovine reproductive disorders. Indian Vet J 82:556.

26. Short RE, Bellows RA, Staigmiller RB, Berardinelli JG, Custer EE (1990). Physiological mechanisms controlling anestrus and infertility in postpartum beef cattle. J Anim Sci 68(3):799-816.

27. Singh B, Sahni KL (1995). Causes of infertility in cattle and buffaloes under field conditions. Indian J Anim Sci 65(10):1119-1121.

28. Singh G, Sidhu SS, Verma H (2003). Incidences of reproductive disorders of buffaloes in different zones of Punjab state. J Research, Punjab Agricultural University 2003: 79-81.

29. Singh J, Dadarwal D, Honparkhe M, Kumar A (2009). Incidences of various etiological factors responsible for repeat breeding syndrome in cattle and buffaloes. Internet Journal of Veterinary Medicine 6: No. 1.

30. Singla VK, Verma HK (1994). Analysis of reproductive disorders of buffaloes. Livestock Adviser 19 (1):14-15.

31. Srinivas M, Subramanyam N, Naidu GV (2007). Incidence of reproductive disorders in rural buffaloes in Andhra Pradesh. Indian Vet J 84:865-866.

32. Tomar SS, Tripathi VN (1994). Incidence and association among certain reproductive problems in Murrah buffaloes. Indian J Dairy Sci 47(12):1050-1052.

□□□

Chapter 13

Strategies for Elimination of Rabies

SUDHI RANJAN GARG
Department of Veterinary Public Health and Epidemiology, College of Veterinary Sciences, Lala Lajpat Rai University of Veterinary and Animal Sciences, Hisar-125004

Contents

1. Introduction

Rabies, also known as hydrophobia in man, is a dreadful zoonotic disease caused by a neurotropic virus in the genus *Lyssavirus* belonging to family Rhabdoviridae (Fig.1). Once the symptoms of the disease develop, the disease is almost invariably fatal to both animals and humans. The disease is known to be present on all continents except Antarctica. The virus infects domestic and wild animals, and is transmitted to people through close contact with infected saliva via bites or scratches, mainly of dogs. Although rabies is a vaccine preventable disease, it still poses a serious public health problem in many countries in Asia and Africa which carry 95% of human rabies death burden. Even though safe, effective vaccines for both human and veterinary use exist, it is estimated that rabies kills more than 55000 people worldwide every year besides causing huge loss of domestic animals.

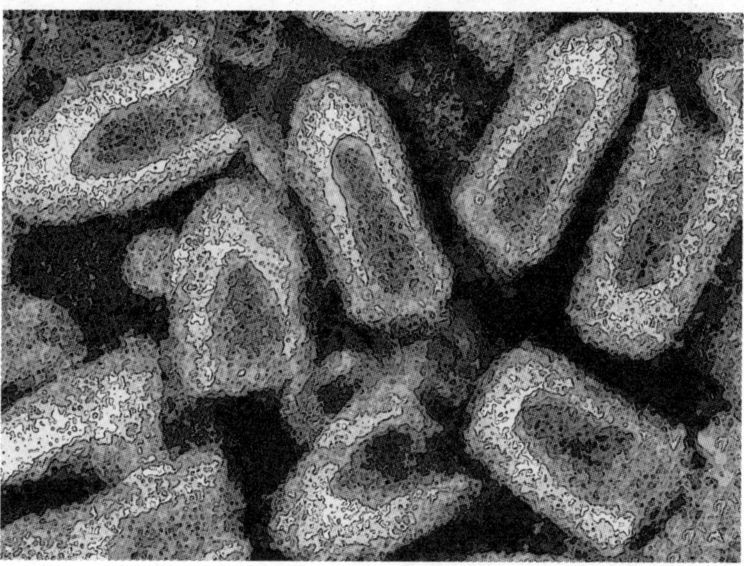

Fig. 1 : Bullet-shaped rabies virus (Magnification approx x70,000. Micrograph courtesy: F. A. Murphy, University of Texas Medical Branch, Galveston, Texas)

2. Rabies Burden

Rabies is prevalent worldwide and is known to be endemic in at least 150 countries. The number and size of rabies-free countries, territories or areas are small in comparison to those of rabies-affected areas. Some countries including the United Kingdom, Ireland, Sweden, Norway, Iceland, Japan, Australia, New Zealand, Singapore, most of Malaysia, Papua New Guinea, the Pacific Islands and some islands in Indonesia have been free of the classical rabies virus for many years (CFSPH 2009). Adequate surveillance, import regulations and vaccination programmes may prevent occurrence of cases of rabies in man and animals but the rabies-free status of any countries and area may change due to reintroduction of virus. For example, recently in the year 2008, rabies was introduced into the island of Bali (Indonesia), which had been free of rabies for many years. A lack of surveillance allowed the import of an unvaccinated rabid dog to Bali from Flores, a distant island where canine rabies was similarly introduced in 1997 and has since become endemic (Clifton 2010).

According to the World Health Organization estimates, out of the 55,000 human deaths due to rabies every year, mostly occur in the rural areas of Africa and Asia. The estimate for deaths due to rabies in Asia is more than 31,000 per year. In India alone, there are more than 20,000 human deaths due to rabies annually, which accounts for 36% of the global human rabies burden.

In India, rabies is endemic except in Andaman and Nicobar and Lakshadweep islands, which are historically known to be rabies-free. In a survey conducted in the year 2003 by the Association for the Prevention and Control of Rabies in India (APCRI), the annual incidence of human deaths due to rabies was estimated to be 20565 which is about 2 per 100,000 population (Sudarshan *et al.* 2007). The majority of the victims were male, adult, from rural areas and unvaccinated persons. According to the study, dogs were mainly responsible (96.2%) for human rabies deaths. Cats and other animals accounted for 1.7% and 2.1% of deaths, respectively. Two deaths due to the bites from jackals were also recorded. Among the dogs, 75.2% were stray dogs.

The extent of rabies burden among animals is not exactly known, but the incidence of the disease in India is quite high and the disease is frequently encountered in different parts of the country. The description of the outbreaks of rabies in animals during the years 1996 to 2004 reported to the World Organisation for Animal Health (OIE) is given in Table 1. The country reported 586 outbreaks among different species of animals leading to the death of 2463 animals during the period of 9 years. During the period 2005 to June 2010, the country reported 273 outbreaks of rabies in animals to OIE, the area-wise details of which are shown in Table 2. A quick look at the data reveals that many areas of the country did not report any case from 2005 to June 2010 despite rabies having an endemic status there. The actual numbers, therefore, may be considerably more because of the possibility of underreporting due to weak rabies surveillance as well as inadequate reporting mechanism in the country.

Table 1 : Rabies outbreaks in animals in India reported to OIE (1996 to 2004)

Year	Species	Number of		
		outbreaks	cases	deaths
2004	cattle	29	85	85
	buffaloes	1	1	1
	dogs	4	12	12
	sheep/goats	2	54	54
2003	cattle	51	130	130
	buffaloes	3	15	15
	dogs	7	20	20
	equidae	2	3	3
	sheep/goats	4	9	9
2002	cattle	126	420	420
	buffaloes	2	16	16
	dogs	14	214	214
	sheep/goats	5	7	7
2001	cattle	89	297	297
	buffaloes	5	41	41
	dogs	20	75	75
	sheep/goats	15	74	74
2000	cattle	23	62	62
	dogs	11	32	32
1999	cattle	21	55	55
	buffaloes	Information not available		
	dogs	13	29	29
1998	cattle	10	137	137
	buffaloes	Information not available		
	dogs	40	200	200
	cats	0	0	0
	sheep/goats	0	0	0
1997	cattle	12	70	70
	dogs	25	35	35
	sheep/goats	1	Information not available	
1996	cattle	16	286	286
	dogs	35	84	84
1996 to 2004	**Total**	**586**	**2463**	**2463**

Source: World Organisation for Animal Health (OIE 2011a), HANDISTATUS II. Accessed 15 March 2011.

Table 2 : Number of outbreaks of rabies in animals reported from India to OIE (2005 to June 2010)

Administrative divisions	2005	2006	2007	2008	2009	2010 (till June)	Total
Andhra Pradesh	3		7	1			**11**
Goa	1	1					**2**
Gujarat	1	1	1		5		**8**
Himachal Pradesh	1					1	**2**
Jammu and Kashmir	2	5	6	6	6		**25**
Karnataka			6	15	9	2	**32**
Kerala	3				1		**4**
Madhya Pradesh				1			**1**
Maharashtra					7	1	**8**
Manipur				1		3	**4**
Meghalaya				2	42	20	**64**
Mizoram					3		**3**
Nagaland	2		3	10	8	7	**30**
Orissa			4	5	9		**18**
Pondicherry	2				1		**3**
Rajasthan					2		**2**
Tamil Nadu					1		**1**
Tripura				2	2	2	**6**
West Bengal	16	10	16	4	1	1	**48**
Jharkhand						1	**1**
Total	**31**	**17**	**43**	**47**	**97**	**38**	**273**

Source: World Organisation for Animal Health (OIE 2011b), World Animal Health Information Database (WAHID) Interface. Accessed 15 March 2011.

3. Reservoirs and Host Range

Dogs are the main reservoirs and transmitters of rabies in developing countries. A wide range of wild animals including foxes, coyotes, skunks, jackals, wolves, bats, raccoons, mongooses etc. act as host or reservoir of the virus. Domesticated animals like cattle, sheep, goat, horses, and swine are also susceptible, so different animal species may contribute in maintaining rabies in nature.

In India, dog is a major reservoir. Red foxes are important in Western Europe; skunks, raccoons, coyotes and gray foxes in the United States; and mongooses, dogs, bat-eared foxes and jackals in South Africa. Dogs and wolves are major reservoirs in Iran, and dogs and foxes in Israel.

4. Rabies Transmission Pathways

Rabies is maintained in two epidemiological cycles, urban cycle and sylvatic cycle. In the urban rabies cycle, dogs are the main reservoir host. This cycle predominates in India and many other developing countries in Africa, Asia, and Central and South America with large population of stray and unvaccinated dogs. Such type of rabies transmission cycle has been virtually eliminated in North America and Europe, although sporadic cases occur in dogs infected by wild animals. Due to strict surveillance and control measures in these countries, the urban cycle is not perpetuated in the dog population usually. Developed countries generally have controlled rabies in dogs, but wildlife reservoirs have become increasingly important in rabies transmission in such areas. The sylvatic (or wildlife) cycle is, therefore, the predominant cycle in Europe and North America. More dangerously, in some parts of the world, the sylvatic cycle operates simultaneously with the urban cycle making the epidemiology more complex.

The pathways of rabies virus transmission are depicted in Fig. 2. The rabies virus is readily transmitted between mammals, whether they are the same or different species. The virus is usually transmitted through saliva, when an infected animal bites another. Less often, an animal or person is infected by contact with infectious saliva or neurological tissues, through mucous membranes or breaks in the skin. Licking of abraded or broken skin by an infected animal may thus cause infection but the rabies virus is not transmitted through intact skin.

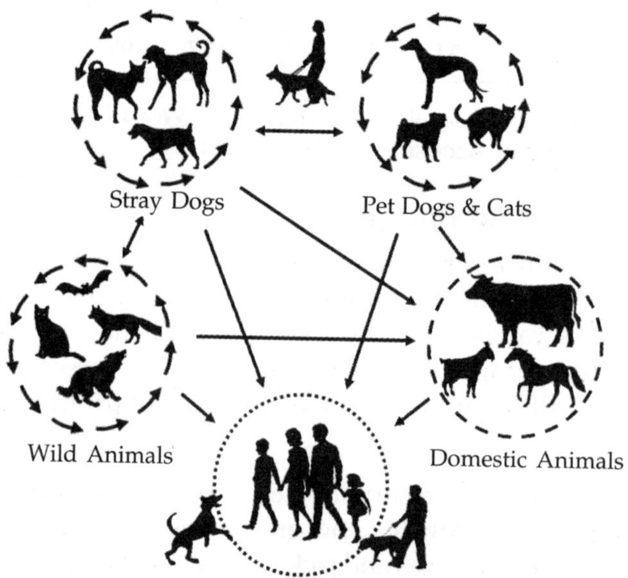

Fig. 2 : Rabies transmission pathways

In developed countries, rabies is present mainly in wild animal hosts, from which the disease spills over to domestic animals and humans. Bite of infected dogs and cats, wild carnivorous animals like foxes, raccoons, skunks, jackals and wolves, and insectivorous and vampire bats is the most frequent way of transmission of rabies infection to humans there. Cattle, horses, deer and other herbivorous animals can become infected and can be potential source of transmission of the virus but it is not common.

In Asia and Africa, dogs are the main hosts that are responsible for most of the human cases. In India, disease transmission is known to involve domestic animals (urban cycle) as well as wild animals (sylvatic cycle), the former being more common source. Wild animals in India are rarely implicated in the spread of disease to man.

Apart from the contact with saliva, there are rare reports of transmission by other routes too. A few cases have been reported after organ transplantation like cornea, pancreas, kidney and liver. Aerosol transmission has also been documented in laboratories and bat caves. Rabies viruses have been transmitted by ingestion in experimentally infected animals, and there is anecdotal evidence of transmission in milk to a lamb and a human infant (CFSPH 2009). Rabies virus is killed by heating, therefore consuming pasteurized milk or cooked meat is not an exposure. However, drinking unpasteurized milk from a rabid cow/goat is considered an exposure (Blueprint for Rabies Prevention and Control 2010). In two incidents investigated by the U.S. Centers for Disease Control and Prevention (CDC), people who drank unpasteurized milk from rabid cows were given post-exposure prophylaxis against rabies (CFSPH 2009).

5. Dissemination of Virus in the Body

Immediately after infection through cut, broken or abraded skin or through mucous membrane, the rabies virus enters an eclipse phase during which it is not easily detected. During this phase, it replicates in non-nervous tissue such as muscle. It does not usually stimulate an immune response at this time, but it is susceptible to neutralization if antibodies are present. The virus is neurotropic, so the uptake of virus into the peripheral nerves is important for progressive infection. After several days or months, the virus enters the peripheral nerves and is transported to the central nervous system (CNS) by retrograde flow in the axons and results in the onset of clinical signs of the disease. After dissemination within the CNS, the virus is distributed to highly innervated tissues via the peripheral nerves.

Most of the virus is found in nervous tissue, salivary glands, saliva and cerebrospinal fluid (CSF), which should all be handled with extreme caution. Some virus has also been detected in other tissues and organs.

6. Disease in Animals

All mammals are susceptible to rabies. The incubation period varies with the amount of virus transmitted, virus strain, site of inoculation, host immunity and the severity of the bite. The incubation period is shorter in the cases where the site of bite is near to the head and where the site has more nerves as compared to that in the cases of bites on the extremities. Similarly, deep and multiple wounds infected with higher concentration of rabies virus may result in a more severe and rapid onset of disease. In dogs and cats, the incubation period is 10 days to 6 months; most cases become apparent between 2 weeks and 3 months. In cattle, an incubation period from 25 days to more than 5 months has been reported in vampire bat-transmitted rabies (CFSPH 2009).

Rabies virus causes acute encephalitis in all warm-blooded hosts and the outcome is almost always fatal. The first symptoms of rabies may be nonspecific (prodromal phase) and may include apprehension, restlessness, anorexia or an increased appetite, vomiting, a slight fever, dilation of the pupils, hyperreactivity to stimuli and excessive salivation. There may be change in the behaviour and temperament of the animals, and they may either become unusually aggressive or uncharacteristically affectionate. The prodromal signs usually last for 2 to 5 days, and then may either lead to furious form of rabies or paralytic (dumb) rabies (CFSPH 2009).

The furious form of rabies is characterized by restlessness, wandering, howling, polypnea, drooling and attacks on animals, people or inanimate objects. Animals often swallow foreign objects such as sticks, stones, straw or faeces. Furious form of rabies is quite common in dogs and the dogs become quite excited and restless. A rabid dog becomes dangerously aggressive and bites objects like its own chain, stones, paper, wood and metal and even may show snapping at imaginary objects. There may be unusual bark and aimless wandering. Later, there is drooling of saliva due to paralysis of muscles of deglutition (Fig. 3). Partial paralysis of vocal cords leads to change in tone of barks to howl. Dog may not recognize its owner. In the terminal stage, there is muscular incoordination, paralysis of limbs and trunk and death that occurs mostly due to respiratory paralysis and convulsions.

In cat, the disease is usually of furious type. The cat may strike at the air with its forepaws as if it were catching mice. Paralysis of the hind part begins 2-4 days after the symptoms of excitement and the animal generally dies in 3-5 days due to convulsions and respiratory paralysis. Cattle may appear unusually alert. Convulsions can occur, particularly in the terminal stages. In the final stages, there is incoordination and ascending paralysis. The animal usually dies 4 to 8 days after the onset of the clinical signs (CFSPH 2009). Rabid wild animals lose fear of man; nocturnal animals are seen during daytime and may attack man.

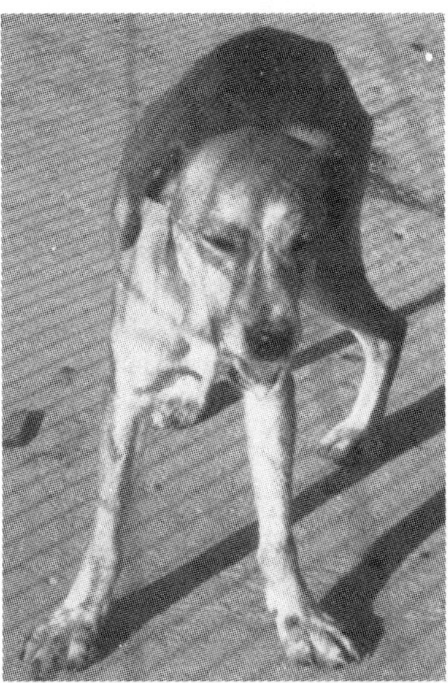

Fig. 3 : Rabies dog with saliva dripping from the mouth (Photo courtesy: CDC)

The paralytic form of rabies is characterized by progressive paralysis. In some cases it may develop without any noticeable signs of the furious form of the diseases. Throat and masseter muscles become paralyzed and the animal may be unable to swallow and it can salivate profusely. There may be facial paralysis or the lower jaw may drop. Dumb form of rabies is less common in dog. The phase of excitement is short or absent in the dumb form of rabies. The dog has vacant look and sits in a corner (Fig. 4). It may respond to its owner's call but there is tendency of forgetfulness. Paralysis begins with the muscles of head and neck region. The animal has difficulty in swallowing. This is often mistaken as bone stuck in the mouth and the owner out of ignorance tries to help the dog and gets exposed to infection. General paralysis results in the death of the animal generally in 3-5 days.

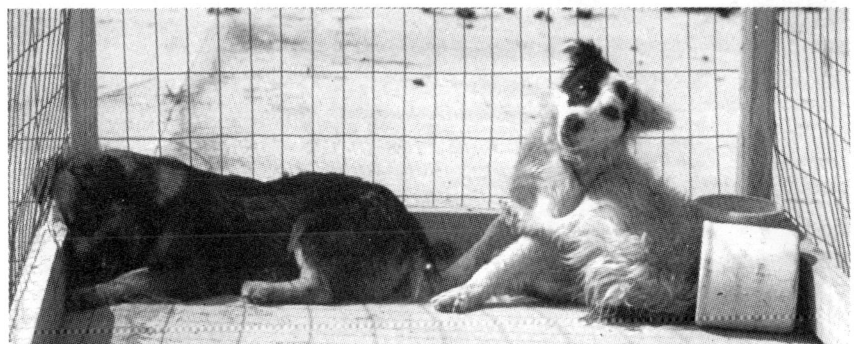

Fig. 4 : Dogs afflicted with dumb rabies, manifested as depression and self-imposed isolation (Photo courtesy: CDC)

Ruminants may separate from the herd and stop ruminating. Subsequently, there is ataxia, incoordination and ascending spinal paresis or paralysis. The paralytic form of rabies may be preceded by a brief excitatory phase or none at all. Biting is uncommon. Cattle affected with rabies show profuse salivation, excitation and paralysis. Laryngeal paralysis causes abnormal bellow in cattle. Horses may demonstrate excitation or aggression and sometimes may attack others. As a result of respiratory failure, death usually occurs within 2 to 6 days. The signs of rabies may not always be definitive and it becomes difficult to distinguish the two forms of rabies (CFSPH 2009).

7. Disease in Humans

In humans, the incubation period is a few days to several years. Most cases become apparent after 1 to 3 months. The disease in the beginning appears with non-specific symptoms. This stage is characterized with headache, anxiety, restlessness, and fever and itching at the site of bite. Subsequently, either an encephalitic (furious) form or a paralytic (dumb) form may predominate. Neural symptoms of the disease include excessive salivation, excitation, agitation, aggression and abnormal behaviour (Fig. 5, 6). Violent spasm of gullet, pharynx and larynx causes difficulty in swallowing of water and other fluids which leads to hydrophobia. The patient also becomes highly sensitive to noise and fearful of light (photophobia). These symptoms usually progress towards paralysis, coma and death. In the terminal stages, there is respiratory paralysis, cardiac arrest and death. Paralytic (dumb) form is less common which is characterized by generalized paralysis (CFSPH 2009).

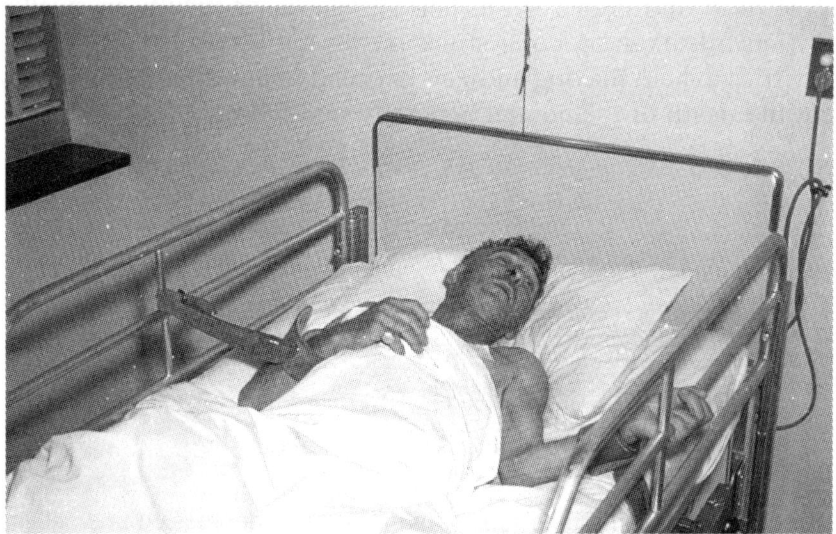

Fig. 5 : A patient with early progressive symptoms of rabies (Photo courtesy: CDC)

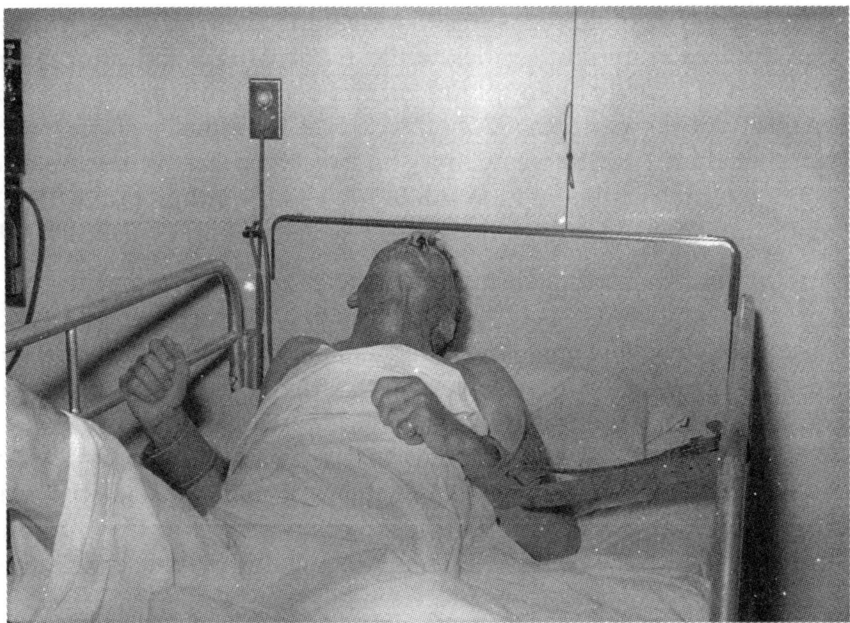

Fig. 6 : A hospitalized rabies victim in restraints (Photo courtesy: CDC)

8. Obstacles in Rabies Control

A number of developed countries have been successful in controlling dog rabies and eliminating human deaths due to rabies through extensive efforts. Highly successful rabies elimination programmes have also been carried out or are underway in many developing countries in Asia, South America and Africa. However, the situation in India remains grim. Despite the production and availability of safe and effective modern rabies vaccines, the country continues to be saddled with the greatest burden of rabies in the world. It is quite essential to examine the reasons for such a situation before attempting strategic actions for rabies control and elimination.

Several research studies and analytical documents reveal that there are a number of reasons responsible for the slow progress in rabies control. Some of these are discussed below.

8.1 Lack of community awareness about rabies

A number of studies quite clearly show that the people's general perception about rabies and animal bite wound management is quite low. A study of 2377 animal bite cases who attended the Anti-Rabies Clinic to seek post-exposure advice and treatment in Gwalior revealed that though 58.8% persons reported to the clinic within 3 days of exposure, others were late and 13.9% patients reported even after one week. Of these, only 23.9% of cases had taken some form of first aid measures like cleaning the wound with soap and water and applied some antiseptics while many (46%) had adopted some traditional kind of remedy like applying oil and pepper mixture on the wound. A vast majority of the patients (57.7%), who had previously taken treatment at places other than Anti-Rabies Clinic, had received the antirabies vaccine (ARV) shots over the gluteal region while rabies immunoglobulin (RIG) had not been administered in any of these cases (Agarwal and Mishra 2009).

In another study conducted to assess the knowledge regarding various aspects of rabies among 1434 college students of Maddur town in Karnataka state, it was revealed that only 46.4% students knew that rabies was caused by a virus, though 97.6% students were aware that it is transmitted by dogs. Only 52.6% students were positive about the transmission of rabies by cats. Only 42.6% students knew that rabies is 100% fatal and only 44% were knowledgeable about the requirement of 5 doses of rabies vaccine by IM route in case of an animal bite. Only 53.1% persons knew that the bite wound should immediately be washed with soap and water (Vinay and Mahendra 2009).

An electronic survey of 100 persons from all over India pointed to the ignorance about rabies prevention measures even among the computer-literate persons (Garg 2009). It was quite revealing that 52% of the respondents themselves or a member of their family had suffered dog bites sometime in life. Ninety per cent of the respondents agreed that the bite wound should be washed with soap and water. Seven per cent persons advocated the application of pepper (red chilli powder) on the bite wound. Regarding the requirement of ARV after a street dog bite, 96% persons thought it necessary. There was ignorance about the vaccination schedule as well. Only 68% persons knew that a minimum of three ARV injections were required. While 15% people thought that a single injection would be sufficient, the remaining 17% felt the need of 14 injections in such cases. Only 32% persons were aware that ARV is given on the arm while the others indicated hip (32%) or belly (36%) as the sites of injection.

The awareness among the pet dog owners about the antirabies vaccination schedule in pet dogs is also remarkably low. A recent survey carried out in Chandigarh in north India revealed that 18% pet owners did not know the vaccination status of their dogs while 66% persons had got the initial immunization done but subsequent annual boosters were not given (Singh *et al.* 2011).

8.2 Inadequate knowledge of physicians

Studies reveal that a large number of medical personnel are also deficient in their knowledge about administration of ARV and RIG. In many cases, the

ARV is administered in a wrong site (gluteal muscle) while RIG is not administered at all though it is indicated (Agarwal and Mishra 2009). Pratap *et al.* (2009) observed that out of 945 children (< 15 years) requiring post-exposure prophylaxis, 875 (92%) children had category III exposure but their local medical professionals had not administered RIG to any of them. Moreover, majority of the children had been given ARV injections over gluteal region.

8.3 Insufficient vaccine and other resources

According to a survey, the annual incidence of animal bites in India is estimated at 17.4 million (APCRI 2004), however, the vaccine utilization data indicate that only about 5 million people receive post exposure prophylaxis (Mittal 2009). This clearly indicates that a large number of people suffering animal bites do not get post-exposure treatment which is the key to prevention of rabies. Apart from ignorance, several reasons may be responsible for this gap. Financial resource constraints of the people and the health departments may be the major hurdle. The unavailability of adequate medical facilities, particularly in remote areas, may also make the people helpless. Experience shows that the post-exposure vaccines may be available in big towns and cities, but RIG is not readily available even at such places.

8.4 Deficient intersectoral coordination

Human beings and animals, including domestic animal species and wildlife species, are inextricably linked in the transmission cycle of rabies. Therefore, participation of multiple sectors with complete coordination is essential for rabies control. However, such coordination among the public health agencies, veterinary organisations, wildlife department and civic bodies is generally deficient, particularly in the developing countries.

8.5 Lack of stray animal management programme

Dog is the principal reservoir of rabies in developing countries and dog bites are the most common cause of human rabies infection. Today, Asia and Africa are the regions of the world that are most affected by canine rabies and that have the highest rates of human infection and human and animal deaths due to rabies. The increase in human cases is linked to the proliferation of roaming dogs, which include not only stray dogs but also the dogs having owners. According to estimates, the pet, owned and household dog population in India is around 28 million (APCRI 2004).

8.5.1 Categories of dogs

In Indian perspective, dogs can be distributed into four categories based on their dependence on humans and their movements.

1. Restricted or supervised pet dogs - These are wholly dependent on owners and the movements of these dogs are restricted by the pet owners.
2. Family dogs - These are wholly dependent on humans but their movements are only partially restricted by the owners.
3. Neighborhood or community dogs - These are partially dependent on humans (community) but their movements are wholly unrestricted.
4. Feral dogs - These are independent or depend on human waste/garbage alone. Their movements are completely unrestricted.

A vast majority of the dogs belong to the last three categories in India. The unrestricted movements of dogs not only make them vulnerable to infection but also increase the transmission of rabies to humans. Control of the stray dog population makes a significant contribution to preventing human rabies cases, however, it is not receiving the desired level of attention in the country.

8.6 Deficiency of resources for dog rabies control

Rabies control in dogs, livestock and wild animals constitutes an integral part of rabies control programme. Extensive efforts in developed countries have largely controlled dog rabies but it remains enzootic in much of the world. Highly successful rabies elimination programmes in dogs have been carried out or are underway in many developing countries but the situation in India despite the greatest rabies burden is not very satisfactory. Some efforts are going on to control stray dog population and vaccinate the dogs but these are to few areas. In a recent study on 100 street dogs and 50 household dogs in Chandigarh, a state capital modern city in India, the protective titre of antirabies antibodies in serum (0.5 IU/ml) was detected only in 1% of street dogs and 16% of pet dogs (Singh *et al.* 2011). The unavailability of sufficient resources (vaccine, funds, manpower) and lack of organized programmes and strict legislation are the reasons for such a grim situation.

8.7 Inadequate disease surveillance and laboratory facilities

Inadequate systematic disease surveillance in developing countries leads to difficulty in collecting factual epidemiological data concerning rabies and rabies reservoirs. Poor diagnostic aids and sparsely existing rabies diagnostic laboratories pose difficulty in rabies diagnosis. Similarly, the surveillance of vaccine efficacy and facilities for quality assurance of vaccines and immunoglobulins are practically nonexistent in developing countries giving rise to the problem of post-exposure prophylaxis failure.

8.8 Lack of public cooperation

In the developing countries, the cooperation of the people in public health programmes is generally low due to illiteracy, ignorance and financial constraints. For example, in India, irresponsible pet ownership is quite common resulting in unrestricted movements and unvaccinated status of even the pet dogs. People engage themselves in feeding stray animals and disposing garbage in open which attracts the stray dogs and brings them near to the residential colonies. Inadequate public support in the government programmes is quite common, resulting in poor outcome of any public health programme.

8.9 Prevalence of myths and religious factors among the community

Due to the widespread prevalence of myths, blind faith and certain religious factors, particularly in rural and remote areas, many victims of animal bites do not seek medical advice promptly. They lose precious time and put their lives to risk by depending on home remedies alone. In animal bite cases, the recourse to indigenous treatment (45.3%) and application of local remedies to wound (36.8%) is quite prevalent (Sudarshan *et al.* 2006). It is a common practice in the rural household to apply chilli powder on the bite wounds (Agarwal and Mishra 2009). Some bite victims also apply salt, turmeric powder, lime, snuff powder, paste of leaves, acid, and holy ash given by some local saints etc. These practices may vary from one region to another (Ichhpujani *et al.* 2008).

9. Success Stories in Rabies Control

Over the past three decades, marked success in canine rabies control has been demonstrated in many parts of the world. As a result, not only has dog rabies declined, but human rabies deaths have also been markedly reduced or eliminated. Such highly successful programmes have been carried out in several tropical countries including developing countries in Asia and South America. The success of these programmes demonstrates that the elimination of canine rabies and prevention of human rabies deaths is quite feasible.

9.1 Latin America

The elimination of human rabies transmitted by dogs in the Region of the Americas by 2005 was a decision made by all Pan American Health Organization (PAHO) Member States in the 1980s. Since then, these countries have made major efforts to eliminate this disease with marked success. The enormous efforts made by the countries are reflected from the results. The analysis of the trend in rabies cases during the period 1982-2003 reveals 91% decline in the number of human cases from 355 to 35. Rabies in dogs declined by 93% from 15,686 cases to 1,131 during this period. From 1990 to 2003, dogs were the source of infection in 65% of reported human cases, which fell from 152 to 27. This sharp reduction is attributable mainly to the control measures implemented by the countries of the Region, such as the mass vaccination of dogs and prophylactic treatment for people who have been exposed. In Latin America, about 44 million dogs are vaccinated every year and approximately 1 million people at risk of contracting the disease are tended to, 25% of them receiving post-exposure treatment (Schneider *et al.* 2005, Belotto *et al.* 2005).

9.2 Mexico

Among the Latin American countries, the remarkable success in Mexico requires special mention. In Mexico, the national rabies control programme using mass parenteral vaccination of dogs started in 1990 with about seven million dogs vaccinated the same year. The number of vaccinated dogs exceeded 10 and 15 million in 1995 and 2005, respectively. Between 1990 and 2005, more than 150 million vaccine doses of modern cell culture-based inactivated rabies virus vaccines were administered. As a result of the mass dog vaccination campaigns, human rabies cases due to dog-mediated rabies decreased from 60 in 1990 to 0 in 2000. The number of rabies cases in dogs decreased from 3,049 in 1990 to 70 cases (Lucas *et al.* 2008).

9.3 United States of America

Over the last 100 years, rabies in the United States has changed dramatically. More than 90% of all animal cases reported annually to the Centers for Disease Control and Prevention (CDC) now occur in wildlife; before 1960 the majority was in domestic animals. The principal rabies hosts today are wild carnivores and bats. According to the recent report on Rabies Surveillance in the United States during 2009, wild animals accounted for 92% of the reported cases of rabies in 2009. Raccoons continued to be the most frequently reported rabid wildlife species (34.8% of all animal cases during 2009), followed by bats (24.3%), skunks (23.9%), foxes (7.5%), and other wild animals, including rodents and lagomorphs (1.9%). Domestic species accounted for 8% of all rabid animals reported in the United States in 2009. During that year, 6,690 cases of rabies in animals and 4 human cases were reported in the US to CDC (CDC 2011a).

The number of rabies-related human deaths in the United States has declined from more than 100 annually at the turn of the twentieth century to one or two per year in the 1990s. Two programmes have been responsible for this decline. First, animal control and vaccination programmes started in the 1940s and oral rabies vaccination programmes in the 2000s have eliminated domestic dogs as reservoirs of rabies in the United States. Second, effective human rabies vaccines and immunoglobulins have been developed. In the United States, human fatalities associated with rabies occur in people who fail to seek medical assistance, usually because they were unaware of their exposure (CDC 2011a).

9.4 Sri Lanka

Sri Lanka has registered a sharp decline in the number of human rabies deaths through mass dog vaccination campaigns, improved accessibility to human post-exposure prophylaxis and an effective vaccine delivery system. Mass vaccination of dogs has shown great impact on human rabies cases in Sri Lanka. The number of dogs that were vaccinated each year was increased rapidly from few thousand in the year 1975 to more than 8,00,000 in 2005 and 1,000,000 in 2008. With the result, the human rabies incidence per 1,000,000 persons, which was more than 2 in the year 1975, declined to less than 1 in 1985 and less than 0.5 in the year 2005 onwards. The country has adopted cost-effective intradermal rabies vaccination to control human rabies (WHO 2008).

9.5 Bali

Bali, while fighting recent severe outbreaks of rabies, completed the first phase of antirabies vaccination campaign. Approximately 210,000 dogs (70% of the estimated total dog population) were vaccinated during the past one year period in 4126 villages across Bali. According to the latest statistics, the months December 2010 to March 2011 showed a 48% decrease in human rabies cases and a 45% decrease in canine rabies compared to the same period a year earlier. Programmes are also being conducted to educate the people about rabies, including prevention measures and post-bite procedures (Global Alliance for Rabies Control 2011).

9.6 Jaipur city, India

A programme to sterilise and vaccinate neighbourhood dogs against rabies established in Jaipur has shown very promising results. Neighbourhood dogs were captured humanely, sterilised surgically, vaccinated against rabies and, when they had recovered, released where they had been caught. Between November 1994 and December 2002, 24986 dogs were treated in this way. Direct observational surveys of the local dog population indicated that 65% of the females were sterilised and vaccinated, and that the population declined by 28%. The records of human cases of rabies seen in the main government hospital of the city between January 1992 and December 2002 showed that the number of cases had declined to zero in the programme area but increased in other areas (Reece and Chawla 2006).

10. Strategies for Rabies Prevention and Control

Rabies is largely a neglected zoonotic disease in developing countries. By far the most common cause of human rabies infections in the world is dog bites, though many other animal reservoirs are known to transmit rabies to human beings. In developing countries, dog is the principal reservoir of rabies. Eliminating rabies in dogs is, therefore, the optimal control method for preventing spread of the disease in the developing countries. It is quite evident that the rabies transmission cycle can be broken only through prevention and control of rabies in animal source. Multiplex strategies are required for successful and sustainable rabies control in animals and humans as shown below.

10.1 Develop a comprehensive national rabies control programme

Several countries and areas in the world have successfully eliminated or controlled rabies through rabies prevention and control programmes. Their operational strategies and the experiences should be used for evolving national plans for rabies control suitable for the developing countries. An Interregional Consultation organized by the World Health Organization in Geneva in 2001 (WHO 2001) recommended the inclusion of the following components in the national plans:

- Access to modern human vaccines and application of new economical post-exposure treatments
- Rabies surveillance and the collection and processing of data at the national, regional and global levels
- Intersectoral collaborative efforts for the control of rabies in dogs at the national and regional levels
- Plan to increase public and healthcare workers awareness regarding rabies control and prevention
- A detailed budget covering a 3 to 5 year period
- A time frame and targets for each year

It was recommended that the political commitment and leadership for the national plan should be through the Ministry of Health, with additional partnerships that are appropriate to implement the programme within each country. While the Health Department is mainly responsible for prevention of rabies in human beings, Veterinary Services are responsible for regulation of rabies control programmes in dogs and other animals. The support of many other relevant national departments and agencies is also inevitable in the rabies prevention and control programmes. These include departments of finance, education, internal home affairs, law and justice, municipalities, village *panchayats*, municipal councils, district councils, and academic and research institutions (e.g. Faculties of Veterinary Sciences and Human Medicine). Besides these, participation of non-governmental organisations (NGOs), private sector and media is also essential for the success of the programme. International agencies such as World Health Organization (WHO), World Organisation for Animal Health (OIE), Food and Agriculture Organization of the United Nations (FAO), Pan American Health Organization (PAHO) and worldwide veterinary associations provide guidelines for the provision and supply of appropriate biologicals and can help support national and regional planning of rabies control programmes (Blueprint for Rabies Prevention and Control 2010).

Recently, a rabies elimination programme funded by the Gates Foundation and coordinated by WHO has been launched in the Richards Bay/Uthungulu area of KwaZulu-Natal province in South Africa on 22 April 2011. Two similar programmes funded by Gates Foundation are running in Tanzania and the Philippines. However, India despite carrying the maximum burden of rabies still does not have a National Rabies Control Programme.

India has vast medical, paramedical and veterinary professional human resource. The country has also the capability to produce enough modern antirabies vaccines and immunoglobulins. A large number of dedicated scientific societies and NGOs are working for rabies control. There is need to bring all of them to a common platform, build consensus, establish intersectoral coordination and make a National Rabies Control Programme in India a reality. The Government of India has taken a step forward in this direction by approving a Pilot Project on Prevention and Control of Human Rabies in five cities across the country viz. Ahmedabad, Bangalore, Pune, Delhi and Madurai. It focuses on training health professionals about rabies and animal bite management, timely and adequate post-exposure treatment to all animal bite victims, implementation of intradermal route for vaccination, creating awareness about timely and adequate post-exposure treatment in the community and sensitization of veterinarians. This would be prelude to a National Rabies Control Programme (Mittal 2009).

The Association for Prevention and Control of Rabies in India (APCRI) has recommended launching of National Rabies Control Programme by the Government of India using the following approaches (APCRI 2006).

Prevention of Human Rabies

1. Post-exposure prophylaxis
2. Pre exposure prophylaxis
3. Diagnostics

Rabies-free areas

1. To keep rabies-free areas free
2. Monitoring and surveillance

Control of Animal reservoir

1. Control of community dog population
2. Compulsory vaccination and licensing of pet dogs
3. Mass parenteral annual vaccination of community dogs

10.2 Promote prompt appropriate care of animal bite wounds

The annual animal bite incidence rate in India has been estimated at 17.4 per 1000 population, which translates into 17.4 million bite cases in a year for 1 billion population (APCRI 2004). Avoiding bites from mammals (mainly dogs, monkeys, bats, cats and wild animals), naturally, is the best way of prevention of possible exposures to rabies virus. Licks from animals to fresh wounds or mucus membranes should also be avoided to ward off the possibility of exposure.

In case of animal bite exposures, bite wound care can substantially reduce the risk of infection. Animal bite or scratch should receive prompt local first aid by thorough cleansing of the wound with copious amounts of soap and water and disinfection with povidone iodine, if available, and then should be followed by proper post-exposure immunization. Thus, immediate and adequate medical care after an animal bite is critical to preventing rabies. The rabies virus can be inactivated by soap solutions, 45-75% ethanol, iodine preparations, quaternary ammonium compounds, or a low pH. Being susceptible to ultraviolet radiation, the virus is rapidly inactivated in sunlight.

It is, therefore, quite important to educate the public about immediate and thorough cleansing and flushing of dog-bite wounds with simple soap and water and application of an appropriate disinfectant. The bite wounds should be left open without suturing for a few days. However, if suturing is necessary to control bleeding or for functional or cosmetic reasons, RIG should be administered into the wound before closing the wound. The use of local anaesthetic is not contraindicated in wound management.

10.3 Increase access to modern cell-culture vaccines

Prompt immunization of humans following exposure significantly reduces the number of human deaths from rabies. It is estimated that in the absence of post-exposure prophylaxis, about 3,27,000 persons would die from rabies in Africa and Asia each year (Knobel *et al.* 2005). Modern purified cell-culture and embryonated egg-based rabies vaccines are safe and effective in pre-exposure prophylaxis as well as post-exposure prophylaxis against rabies (WHO 2010). These are quite better than the nerve tissue vaccines which induce more severe adverse reactions and are less immunogenic. The production and use of nerve tissue vaccines is, therefore, not recommended by WHO (WHO 2005). India has already stopped producing and using nerve tissue vaccine (Semple vaccine produced in sheep) since 2005 and has replaced it with modern vaccines. However, few countries, mainly in Asia and Latin America, still depend on rabies vaccines derived from animal nerve tissues for post-exposure prophylaxis (WHO 2010).

Earlier in India, Semple (sheep brain) vaccine was freely available in government hospitals but the availability of the cell culture vaccines is not as good due to budgetary constraints. The cost of one dose of cell culture rabies vaccine is about Rs. 300, so a full course of 5 doses by intramuscular route costs around Rs. 1500 which becomes quite expensive for the animal bite victims who are generally poor. Further, the unavailability of these vaccines in rural and remote areas may pose grave challenge to timely immunization.

10.4 Promote timely and adequate immunization

Post-exposure treatment should start immediately wherever recommended according to the guidelines. Factors that should be taken into consideration when deciding whether to initiate post-exposure prophylaxis include the epidemiological likelihood of the implicated animal being rabid, the category of exposure, clinical features of the animal, as well as its availability for observation and laboratory testing. Many times, particularly in developing countries, the information about the pre-exposure prophylactic vaccination status of the implicated animal may not be reliable; hence it may not be advisable to withhold post-exposure vaccination even if the animal is vaccinated (WHO 2010).

The World Health Organization has laid down guidelines for post-exposure immunization. Depending upon the type of exposure, the cases are differentiated into Category I, II and III. The post-exposure antirabies immunization involves administration of antirabies vaccine and application of antirabies serum/immunoglobulin based on the Category of the exposure as shown in Table 3.

For categories II and III, thorough washing and flushing (for about 15 minutes, if possible) with soap or detergent and copious amounts of water of all bite wounds and scratches should be done immediately, or as early as possible. Where available, an iodine-containing, or similarly viricidal, topical preparation should be applied to the wound (WHO 2010). It may also be noted that vaccination alone may not be sufficient for protection against rabies. Rabies immunoglobulin should be administered in all people with Category III exposure and to those with Category II exposure who are immunodeficient (WHO 2010).

Table 3 : Guidelines for post-exposure vaccination (WHO 2010)

Category	Type of exposure	Post-exposure vaccination recommendation
I	Touching or feeding animals, licks on intact skin (that is, no exposure)	No prophylaxis is required.
II	Nibbling of uncovered skin, minor scratches or abrasions without bleeding	Immediate vaccination is recommended, post-exposure prophylaxis may be discontinued if the suspect animal is proved by appropriate laboratory examination to be free of rabies or, in the case of domestic dogs, cats or ferrets, the animal remains healthy throughout a 10-day observation period starting from the date of the bite.
III	Single or multiple transdermal bites or scratches, contamination of mucous membrane with saliva from licks, licks on broken skin, exposures to bats	Immediate vaccination and administration of rabies immunoglobulin are recommended, post-exposure prophylaxis may be discontinued if the suspect animal is proved by appropriate laboratory examination to be free of rabies or, in the case of domestic dogs, cats or ferrets, the animal remains healthy throughout a 10-day observation period starting from the date of the bite.

10.4.1 Intramuscular administration of cell culture vaccine for post-exposure prophylaxis

The post-exposure vaccination involves injecting cell culture vaccine intramuscularly into the deltoid muscle (or anterolateral thigh in children aged <2 years) of patients with Category II and III exposures according to a recommended dosage schedule. The dose of the intramuscular vaccine is 1 ml or 0.5 ml (depending on the type of vaccine) while the recommended regimen consists of either a 5-dose or a 4-dose schedule. The 5-dose regimen prescribes 1 dose on day 0 followed by one dose each on days 3, 7, 14 and 28 while the 4-dose regimen prescribes 2 doses on day 0 (1 in each of the 2 deltoid or thigh sites) and subsequently 1 dose on each of days 7 and 21 (WHO 2010). In India, normally the 5-dose regimen is in practice.

The day of administration of the first dose should be taken as day 0 in cases where the vaccination could not be initiated on the day of bite itself. It would be better to use the same vaccine in all doses in a case but when it is not possible to complete full course with the same vaccine, another type of cell culture vaccine should be used to complete the post-exposure prophylaxis (WHO 2010).

10.4.2 Administration of rabies immunoglobulin (RIG)

It is common that administration of RIG in bite cases is almost ignored. As per the WHO guidelines, besides rabies vaccine, RIG must be administered in the cases of Category III exposures and in Category II exposures in immunosuppressed patients. While vaccine takes 10-14 days to produce protective antibody titre, RIG contains readymade antirabies antibodies that provide immediate passive immunity and give immediate protection. Thus, RIG covers the vulnerable initial period after exposure by causing local viricidal effect and preventing the virus from entering the nerve cells. However, these should not be used alone without proper vaccination. Two types of rabies immunoglobulins, equine RIG (ERIG) and human RIG (HRIG) are available. Human RIG is generally in short supply and available mainly in industrialized countries. Where it is not available or affordable, equine immunoglobulin or F(ab′)2 products of equine immunoglobulin should be used. Most of the new equine immunoglobulin preparations are potent, highly purified, safe and considerably less expensive than human rabies immunoglobulin. However they are of heterologous origin and carry a small risk of anaphylactic reaction. There are no scientific grounds for performing a skin test prior to administering equine immunoglobulin but the treating physician should be prepared to manage anaphylaxis which, although rare, could occur during any stage of administration (WHO 2010).

The recommended dose of ERIG and F(ab′)2 products is 40 IU/kg of bodyweight and that of HRIG is 20 IU/kg bodyweight. The RIG should be instilled carefully using 26G needle into the depth of all wounds and also infiltrated around the wounds with least traumatization. The full dose of RIG, or as much as is anatomically feasible, should be administered into and around the wound site. Any remaining RIG should be injected into the thigh region intramuscularly at a site distant from the vaccine administrative site. If the dose and the volume of RIG is too small to infiltrate in all wounds (as in case of severely bitten child), it may be diluted in physiological buffered saline to ensure more wound coverage.

10.4.3 Post-exposure prophylaxis for previously vaccinated individuals

The rabies-exposed patients who can document previous complete pre-exposure vaccination or complete post-exposure prophylaxis with a cell culture vaccine require less number of doses (only 2) of post-exposure vaccine on day 0 and day 3. The administration of RIG is also not necessary in such cases. This 1-site 2-day intradermal or intramuscular regimen also applies to people vaccinated against rabies who have demonstrated rabies-virus neutralizing antibody titres of =0.5 IU/ml (WHO 2010).

10.4.4 Pre-exposure prophylactic vaccination in human beings

Pre-exposure vaccination is recommended to the individuals of high-risk group who are at continual, frequent or increased risk of exposure to the rabies virus, either as a result of their residence or occupation. Such individuals include veterinarians, animal handlers, dogcatchers, laboratory workers, postmen, delivery personnel, pet owners, schoolchildren etc. Pre-exposure vaccination requires invariably three doses of intramuscular vaccination on days 0, 7 and 21 or 28, in the deltoid area of the arm in adults and the children (above two years). For children aged <2 years, the anterolateral area of the thigh is recommended. Rabies vaccine should not be administered in the gluteal area, as the induction of an adequate immune response may be less reliable.

Periodic booster injections are recommended as an extra precaution only for people whose occupation puts them at continual or frequent risk of exposure. Because vaccine-induced immunity persists in most cases for years, a booster would be recommended only if rabies virus neutralizing antibody titres fall to <0.5 IU/ml. Antibody monitoring of personnel at risk is preferred to the administration of routine boosters. For people who are potentially at risk of laboratory exposure to high concentrations of live rabies virus, antibody testing should be done every 6 months while those not at continual risk of exposure should have serological monitoring every 2 years (WHO 2010).

10.5 Promote cost-effective intradermal administration of vaccine

The total cost of an average post-exposure prophylaxis course typically ranges between US$ 40-49 in Africa and Asia as shown in studies, but costs could be much higher in certain settings. These estimates include the cost of biologicals and of their administration (materials for injection such as syringes, needles, swabs *etc.* and staff salaries), and patient's expenses towards transport to and from medical facilities and loss of income (Blueprint for Rabies Prevention and Control 2010). Thus, the full course of post-exposure rabies vaccination by the intramuscular route is quite expensive for the people in the developing countries, thereby, limiting the administration of cell-culture vaccines in many areas where canine rabies is widespread.

Intradermal administration of these vaccines offers an equally safe and immunogenic alternative that requires less amount of vaccine, resulting in considerably reduced cost of a full course of post-exposure prophylaxis. WHO has approved intradermal vaccination but only modern vaccines that meet the WHO requirements regarding safety, potency and efficacy for this application may be used for intradermal vaccination.

Intradermal rabies vaccination has been in use for several years in Thailand, Sri Lanka and Philippines. Intradermal vaccination regimen has been successfully introduced in India too. The Drugs Controller General of India (DCGI) has approved several modern vaccines currently available in India for intradermal use. The 2-site regimen prescribes injection of 0.1 ml at 2 sites (deltoid and thigh) on days 0, 3, 7 and 28. This regimen may be used for people with Category II and III exposures in countries where the intradermal route has been endorsed by national health authorities (Phanuphak *et al.* 1987, Briggs *et al.* 2000, Quiambao *et al.* 2005, WHO 2010).

The complete vaccination course thus takes only 1-2 vials reducing the cost by 60-80%. To lead to significant savings, it is essential that enough individuals are available for vaccination to utilize an opened vial within 6-8 hours and the vaccine is not wasted. The reconstituted vaccine should be stored at 2-8°C and the unused vaccine must be discarded at the end of 6-8 hours. It will be helpful if the vaccine vials specially pre-packaged for intradermal use are made available. Further, sufficient and adequately trained staff should be available to ensure correct storage and reconstitution of the vaccine and proper intradermal injection.

10.6 Prevent dog rabies through dog vaccination

Vaccination of dogs and elimination of rabies in dogs constitute the mainstay of any rabies control programme. Dog vaccination and stray dog populations control are more efficient and cost-effective than post-bite treatment in humans. According to OIE (2009), the cost of a post-bite treatment in humans is about twenty to one hundred times more than the vaccination of a dog. It has been estimated that with only 10% of the financial resources used worldwide to treat people after a dog bite, Veterinary Services would be able to eradicate rabies in animals and thus stop almost all human cases.

A national strategy on canine vaccination should be developed. Many industrialized countries have either eliminated or are close to elimination of human rabies through vaccination of domestic dogs and the implementation of other control measures. Mass vaccination of dogs and widespread immunization of humans following exposure have significantly reduced the number of human deaths from rabies in Asian countries such as Thailand.

Organisation of mass dog vaccination programmes using cell culture vaccines with annual or more frequent vaccination should rank high on the agenda of developing countries (Fig. 7). The cost of such programmes many times may present hurdles in their full implementation. For example, the estimated annual expenditure for rabies prevention in the United States is over US$ 300 million, most of which is spent on dog vaccinations. An annual turnover of approximately 25% in the dog population necessitates revaccination of millions of animals each year, and reintroduction of rabies through transport of infected animals from outside a controlled area is always a possibility should control programmes lapse. Reservoirs of wildlife rabies are also potential sources of rabies infection for dogs (CDC 2011b).

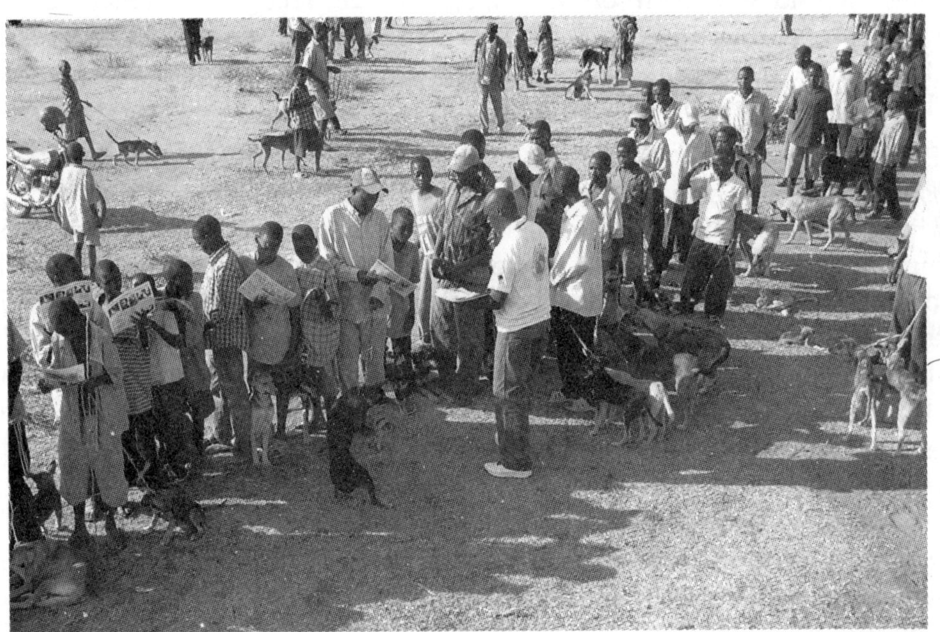

Fig. 7 : Dog rabies vaccination campaign in Tanzania (Photo courtesy: World Rabies Day Team)

The cost of dog vaccination campaigns following a central-point vaccination strategy (which is the most cost-effective strategy) typically ranges between US$ 1.19 and 4.27 per dog vaccinated in a range of rural and urban settings. This includes consumable costs (vaccine, syringes, needles, certificates, registers, collars, stationery), delivery (staff costs, transport), storage (fridges, cool boxes), and societal costs (days of work lost). The house-to-house vaccination campaigns tend to be more expensive and vary widely between different communities, but may be necessary in some situations to reach sufficient vaccination coverage. The cost can be reduced through involvement of volunteers in the vaccination campaigns, careful consideration of logistics and transport costs and by holding well-planned synchronized campaigns (Blueprint for Rabies Prevention and Control 2010).

Modern veterinary vaccines are highly immunogenic inactivated cell culture vaccines for immunization of dogs via the parenteral route. These are now widely available and are affordable to the dog owners in the developing countries. For mass canine vaccination, the use of inactivated rabies vaccine is recommended over the modified live-virus vaccine. Inactivated vaccines can be managed more easily in the field conditions because these are less sensitive to changes in temperature. Further, these do not cause any risk to the vaccinator due to accidental self-inoculation. Combined vaccines including rabies vaccine and vaccines against other diseases are also available.

To be effective, the vaccination of dogs should be done in a planned organized way. At least 75% of the dog population in each community should be vaccinated within a month. In areas where the dog population turnover is rapid, it may be necessary to carry out a mass vaccination campaign each year. However, if the effective immune period of the vaccine is longer and the system for identifying vaccinated dogs can be trusted to last more than one year, the advantage of vaccinating only the dogs entering the population after the last campaign should be considered, with revaccination of dogs vaccinated during the last campaign at intervals of about 2 years (WHO 2011).

Large dog population in India makes the task exceptionally challenging. It is, therefore, essential to chalk out programmes for dog population management besides innovating cost effective animal vaccine delivery systems in the country.

10.7 Develop and promote oral rabies vaccine for stray dogs

Administration of vaccination by the parenteral route to dogs is a major obstacle for dog rabies control. The task of covering the desirable level of dog vaccination, therefore, becomes difficult, particularly in the countries with large population of dogs that are unsupervised and have unrestricted movements. Oral vaccination with safe and effective vaccines in baits may help in mass vaccination of animals facilitating wider coverage.

Though live oral rabies vaccines have been successfully used for many years to control wildlife rabies in Europe and the USA, these vaccines are not considered safe for use in stray and ownerless dogs in India. The close association between humans and dogs increases the likelihood of direct exposure of humans to vaccine baits during oral vaccination programmes. Therefore, apart from the availability of a safe and effective oral vaccine for dogs, it is essential to investigate the potential role of oral vaccination of dogs in the country in view of the safety guidelines (WHO 2007). As oral vaccination involves administration of vaccine in baits, the safety aspects of the vaccine baits released into the environment would require utmost attention. Further, field trial for the oral vaccination of dogs would be required before the country contemplates the use of oral vaccination of dogs.

The requirements for an oral rabies vaccine include the following (rabies-vaccination.com 2011).

- *Safety*- Oral rabies vaccines intended for dogs should be safe. The close association between humans and dogs increases the likelihood of direct exposure of humans to vaccine baits during oral vaccination programmes. For the vaccination of stray or ownerless dogs, baits could be presented manually in areas where the dogs tend to congregate to eat and/or sleep e.g. garbage disposal sites. After a certain time period, uneaten baits would be removed for safety.
- *Efficacy* - The vaccine must be effective when taken in orally.
- *Palatability* - The bait used must be readily acceptable by the target species.
- *Effective distribution* - The vaccine baits must be effectively distributed to ensure that a sufficient proportion of the population is vaccinated to make the campaign effective.
- *Measurability* - A system should be in place to allow the measurement of vaccine uptake in target populations.

The development of recombinant DNA technology has initiated a new era in rabies control. Recombinant vaccines cannot exhibit residual pathogenicity caused by rabies because they contain only single non-virulent gene products. The majority of the safety requirements for modified live-virus vaccines are also applicable to recombinant vaccines (WHO 2011).

10.8 Manage dog population

Reduction of unsupervised stray dog population is utmost important in the countries where canine rabies is prevalent. Indiscriminate mass culling of dogs and dog destruction alone is not effective in rabies control. There is no evidence that removal of dogs alone has ever had a significant impact on dog population densities or the spread of rabies. In addition, dog removal may be unacceptable to local communities. However, the targeted and humane removal of unvaccinated, ownerless dogs may be effective when used as a supplementary measure to mass vaccination (WHO 2011).

Three recognized practical methods of dog population management include: (i) movement restriction, (ii) habitat control, and (iii) reproduction control. Attempts to control dog populations through culling, without alteration of habitat and resource availability, have generally been unsuccessful. Since the 1960s, Animal Birth Control (ABC) programmes coupled with rabies vaccination have been advocated as a method to control dog populations and ultimately human rabies in Asia. The rationale is to reduce the dog population turnover as well as the number of dogs susceptible to rabies and influence the male dog behaviour such as dispersal and fighting, which otherwise facilitate the spread of rabies (WHO 2005).

Dog reproduction control involves catching, neutering and releasing the dogs in their original habitats. The cost of surgical sterilization varies significantly with country, mainly due to differences in staff and drugs costs, and also depending on the number of animals being sterilised. In a range of medium to high-throughput systems based in developing world locations, the cost per surgical sterilisation has been found to range from US$ 3 to 15 for the medicines and consumables, at an average of US$ 7.50. The full costs (including veterinarians and veterinary support staff, clinic running costs, all medicines and consumables) ranged from US$ 10 to 52, with an average of US$ 30 per sterilisation. Unwanted reproduction of dogs can be controlled using chemical contraception or sterilisation or immunocontraception and efforts are being made to produce and license safe and effective contraceptives and sterilants (Blueprint for Rabies Prevention and Control 2010).

The Animal Welfare Board of India (AWBI) is promoting the implementation of Animal Birth Control (ABC) and Anti-Rabies (AR) Programme in major cities of India. Over 1 lakh stray dogs are sterilized and vaccinated against rabies every year under the Animal Birth Control (2001) Dog Rules. The ABC Programme is currently being implemented in over 60 cities all over India, including Delhi, Jaipur, Chennai, Mumbai, Bangalore, Hyderabad, Kolkata, Jodhpur and Kalimpoong. In Tamil Nadu and Goa, the ABC-AR Programme has been successfully implemented for the entire state since 2007. This has led to Tamil Nadu state pioneering a new concept of a Participatory Model of the ABC Programme in 50 Municipalities and 5 Municipal Corporations, with 50% cost sharing by local bodies on participatory basis. Similarly, Delhi too has adopted the Participatory Model of the ABC Programme since 2008 (AWBI 2009).

AWBI has brought out the Standard Operating Procedures (AWBI 2009) to carry out ABC projects for effective population control of street/stray dogs with a uniform and standard code of professional practice, efficiently, diligently and humanely. These also provide the guidelines for humane euthanasia of incurably sick, mortally wounded or rabid dogs as per the ABC Rules.

Euthanasia may also be carried out on dogs suffering from a severe or life threatening injury or illness that has no cure, dogs severely injured in an accident, and dogs found to be extremely aggressive and bad tempered, prone to biting people and with a history of having bitten people.

10.9 Strengthen surveillance and diagnostic facilities

Epidemiological surveillance is quite important in establishing the estimate of rabies burden in humans and animals. Improvement in rabies surveillance and data collection systems will help in determining the most affected areas and other epidemiological features of the disease. The information is essential to plan rabies control measures and also to demonstrate the effectiveness of such programmes. Diagnostic facilities, therefore, require strengthening for quick diagnosis of the disease as well as to evaluate the efficacy of vaccines and duration of immunity of the vaccination.

10.10 Raise public awareness of rabies

People's participation is paramount for the success of any programme. However, unfortunately, the people are generally not well-informed of the risk of rabies and about the actions to be taken in the event of an animal bite. The Asian Rabies Expert Bureau (AREB) conducted multi-country survey in Bangladesh, China, India, Indonesia, Pakistan, the Philippines, Sri Lanka, and Thailand. Two major issues were identified where active information of the population could make a difference: the necessity to apply appropriate wound care and to consult the nearest rabies prevention centre as soon as possible (Dodet *et al.* 2008).

Educational campaigns assume the greatest importance in the developing countries like India, where a large chunk of population is illiterate or semiliterate. There is need to promote responsible dog ownership at the community level. Pet owners should be responsible for keeping the movements of their dogs restricted and supervised and should follow the rules of pet animal registration and vaccination guidelines. The people should be pursued to provide full cooperation to the agencies involved in dog population management and rabies control by desisting from feeding stray animals, avoiding garbage disposal in open and participating in the vaccination campaigns. They also need to be educated about the wound care practices and the importance of seeking medical help immediately instead of wasting time in home remedies after an animal bite (Fig. 8 & 9). Delays in starting or failure to complete correct prophylaxis may result in death, particularly following bites in highly innervated regions, such as the head, neck or hands, or following multiple wounds (Wilde 2007).

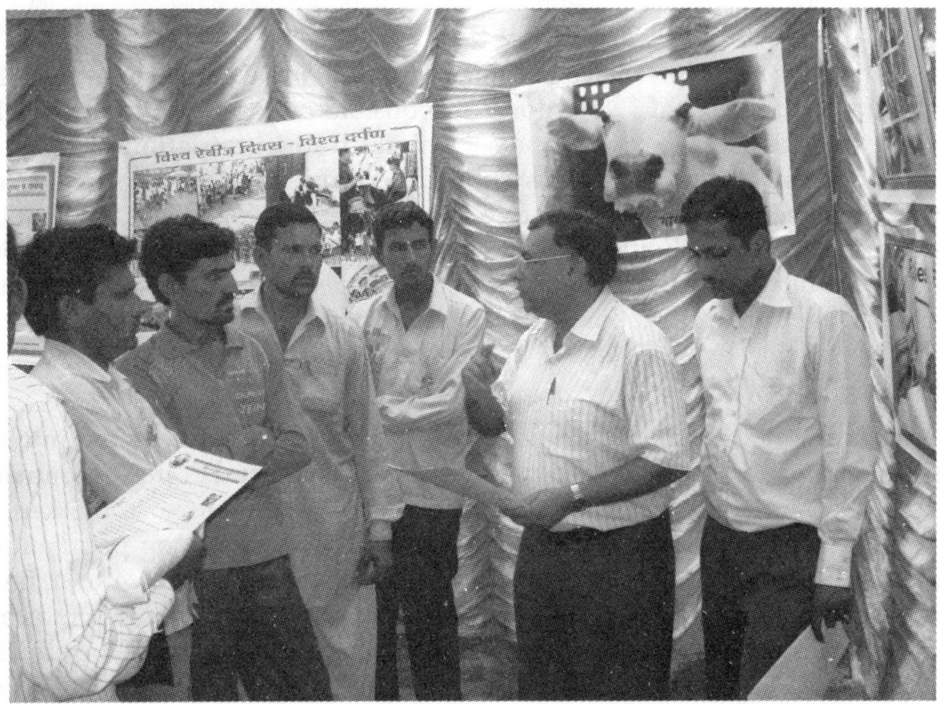

Fig. 8 : The author interacting with rural people regarding rabies prevention

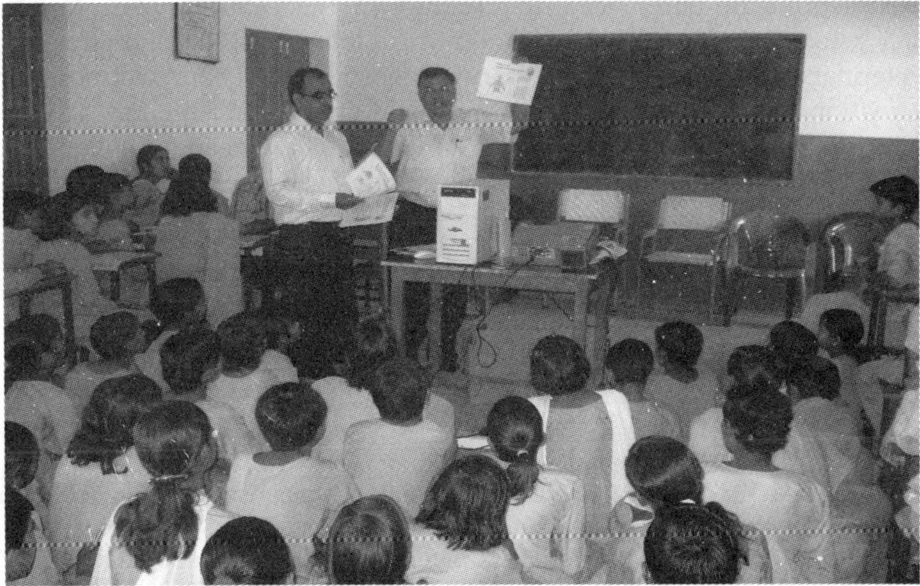

Fig. 9 : The author imparting education to schoolchildren on rabies prevention

10.11 Enforce legislative measures

Legislative measures such as tie-up orders, individual animal identification and registry are necessary to enforce responsible pet ownership among the people. Border checks, control of pet animal trade, restriction on animal movements and other measures should be implemented to prevent the introduction of rabies into rabies-free areas (Blueprint for Rabies Prevention and Control 2010). It should be made mandatory to notify the cases of rabies and animal bites. This will facilitate the surveillance of the disease, estimation of disease burden and chalking out disease control strategies.

11. Conclusion

Rabies is not, in the natural sense, a disease of humans as the human infection is incidental to the reservoir of disease in wild and domestic animals. Prevention and control of rabies in animal source, therefore, is the key to success in combating rabies. The control of excessive stray dog populations along with vaccination of animals remains the method of choice to control and eradicate rabies. The OIE advises against trying to control and eradicate rabies by killing potentially infected animals, as a sole method for ethical, ecological and economical reasons. Moreover, the cost of a post-bite treatment in humans is much higher than the vaccination of dogs making the control of rabies infection in dogs more appropriate, particularly in the developing countries. Consequently, it is the prime responsibility of the veterinarians to break the transmission pathway between the animal source of the disease and susceptible humans. According to the OIE, the Veterinary Services are a buffer between the animal source and human infections, so good governance of veterinary services, better laboratory diagnostic capacity and well structured vaccination campaigns in domestic and wild animals are the key actions to be taken. Raising public awareness of rabies and of the need for collaboration with other professions, particularly the public health sector, should also be emphasized.

The factors such as the prohibitive cost of rabies control programme and insufficient coordination among different sectors should not be allowed to let the deadly rabies prevail. Comprehensive national programmes should be launched with full might to eliminate rabies.

References

1. Agarwal AK, Mishra A (2009). Demographic characteristics of animal bite cases attending the anti rabies clinic of G. R. Medical College Hospital, Gwalior (Madhya Pradesh). Souvenir, 11th National Conference of the Association for Prevention and Control of Rabies in India (APCRI), Thiruvananthapuram, July 4-5, 2009, p. 28.

2. APCRI (2004). Assessing burden of rabies in India, WHO sponsored national multi-centric rabies survey 2003, Final report. Association for Prevention and Control of Rabies in India. www.apcri.org.

3. APCRI (2006). Rabies prophylaxis guidelines. Association for Prevention and Control of Rabies in India, http://rabies.org.in/rabies/wp-content/uploads/2009/11/APCRI-Guidelines-for-Rabies-Prophylaxis.pdf.

4. AWBI (2009). Standard operating procedures for sterilization of stray dogs under the animal birth control programme. Animal Welfare Board of India, Chennai.

5. Belotto A, Leanes LF, Schneider MC, Tamayo H, Correa E (2005). Overview of rabies in the Americas. Virus Res 111:5-12.

6. Blueprint for Rabies Prevention and Control (2010). www.rabiesblueprint.com. Accessed 15 March 2011.

7. Briggs DJ, Banzhoff A, Nicolay U *et al.* (2000). Antibody response of patients after postexposure rabies vaccination with small intradermal doses of purified chick embryo cell vaccine or purified Vero cell rabies vaccine. Bull WHO 78:693-698.

8. CDC (2011a). Rabies in the U.S. Centers for Disease Control and Prevention, Atlanta, USA. http://www.cdc.gov/rabies/location/index.htm. Accessed 1 May 2011.

9. CDC (2011b). Rabies around the world. Centers for Disease Control and Prevention, Atlanta, USA. www.cdc.gov. Accessed 12 May 2011

10. CFSPH (2009). Rabies. The Center for Food Security and Public Health, Iowa State University, Iowa. http://www.cfsph.iastate.edu/Factsheets/pdfs/rabies.pdf. Accessed 15 March 2011.

11. Clifton M (2010). How not to fight a rabies epidemic: a history in Bali. Asian Biomedicine 4:663-670.

12. Dodet B, Goswami A, Gunasekera A, de Guzman F, Jamali S, Montalban C, Purba W, Quiambao B, Salahuddin N, Sampath G, Tang Q, Tantawichien T, Wimalaratne O, Ziauddin A (2008). Rabies awareness in eight Asian countries. Vaccine 26:6344-6348.

13. Garg SR (2009). Rabies awareness among literate people in India. Souvenir, National Symposium and VIII Annual Conference of Indian Association of Veterinary Public Health Specialists, Gangtok, November 6-7, 2009, p. 34.

14. Global Alliance for Rabies Control (2011). Rabies reduced by first round of vaccinations on Bali. Rabid Bytes, Issue 22, April 2011, p. 3. www.rabiescontrol.net

15. Ichhpujani RL, Mala C, Veena M, Singh J, Bhardwaj M, Bhattacharya D, Pattanaik SK, Balakrishnan N, Reddy AK, Samnpath G, Gandhi N, Nagar SS, Shiv L (2008). Epidemiology of animal bites and rabies cases in India. A multicentric study. J Commun Dis 40(1):27-36.

16. Knobel DL, Cleaveland S, Coleman PG *et al.* (2005). Re-evaluating the burden of rabies in Africa and Asia. Bull WHO 83:360-368.

17. Lucas CH, Pino FV, Baer G, Morales PK, Cedillo VG, Blanco MA, Avila MH (2008). Rabies control in Mexico. Dev Biol (Basel) 131:167-175.

18. Mittal V (2009). Burning issues in rabies control in India. Souvenir, 11th National Conference of the Association for Prevention and Control of Rabies in India (APCRI), Thiruvananthapuram, July 4-5, 2009, p. 7-9.

19. OIE (2009). Eliminating rabies in dogs is the optimal control method for preventing spread of the disease. Press Release, World Organisation for Animal Health, Paris, 13 March 2009. http://www.oie.int. Accessed 12 May 2011.

20. OIE (2011a). World Organisation for Animal Health, HANDISTATUS II. Accessed 15 March 2011.

21. OIE (2011b). World Organisation for Animal Health, World Animal Health Information Database (WAHID) Interface. Accessed 15 March 2011.

22. Phanuphak P, Khawplod P, Sirivichayakul S, Siriprasomsub W, Ubol S, Thaweepathomwat M. (1987). Humoral and cell-mediated immune responses to various economical regimens of purified Vero cell rabies vaccine. Asian Pacific J Allergy Immunology 5:33-37.

23. Pratap AK, Behera TR, Malini DS, Satapathy DM, Tripathy RM (2009). Clinical profile of children attending ARC, MKCG Medical College, Behrampur. Souvenir, 11th National Conference of the Association for Prevention and Control of Rabies in India (APCRI), Thiruvananthapuram, July 4-5, 2009, p. 30.

24. Quiambao BP, Dimaano EM, Ambas C, Davis R, Banzhoff A, Malerczyk C (2005). Reducing the cost of post-exposure rabies prophylaxis: Efficacy of 0.1 ml PCEC rabies vaccine administered intradermally using the Thai Red Cross post-exposure regimen in patients severely exposed to laboratory-confirmed rabid animals. Vaccine 23:1709-1714.

25. rabies-vaccination.com (2011). Requirements for an oral rabies vaccine. Intervet India, Pune. http://www.rabies-vaccination.com. Access 13 May 2011.

26. Reece JF, Chawla SK (2006). Control of rabies in Jaipur, India by the sterilisation and vaccination of neighbourhood dogs. Vet Record 159:379-383.

27. Schneider MC, Belotto A, Adé MP, Leanes LF, Correa E, Tamayo H, Medina G, Rodrigues MJ (2005). Epidemiologic situation of human rabies in Latin America in 2004. Epidemiological Bulletin / PAHO 26 (1):2-4.

28. Singh MP, Goyal K, Majumdar M, Ratho RK (2011). Prevalence of rabies antibodies in street and household dogs in Chandigarh, India. Trop Anim Health Prod 43:111-114.

29. Sudarshan MK, Madhusudana SN, Mahendra BJ *et al.* (2007). Assessing the burden of human rabies in India: Results of a national multi-center epidemiological survey. Int J Infect Dis 11: 29-35.

30. Sudarshan MK, Mahendra BJ, Madhusudana SN, Ashwath Narayana DH, Rahman A, Rao NS, X-Meslin F, Lobo D, Ravikumar K, Gangaboraiah (2006). An

epidemiological study of animal bites in India: Results of a WHO sponsored national multi-centric rabies survey. J Commun Dis 38(1):32-39.

31. Vinay M, Mahendra BJ (2009). Effectiveness of 'awareness sessions' for enhancing knowledge regarding rabies among college students. Souvenir, 11th National Conference of the Association for Prevention and Control of Rabies in India (APCRI), Thiruvananthapuram, July 4-5, 2009, p. 35.

32. WHO (2001). Strategies for the control and elimination of rabies in Asia. Report of a WHO Interregional Consultation Geneva, Switzerland, 17-21 July 2001. World Health Organization, Department of Communicable Disease Surveillance and Response, WHO/CDS/CSR/EPH/2002.8.

33. WHO (2005). Expert Consultation on Rabies: First report. Geneva, World Health Organization, WHO Technical Report Series, No. 931; http://whqlibdoc.who.int/trs/WHO_TRS_931_eng.pdf.

34. WHO (2007). Oral vaccination of dogs against rabies. Rabies guidance for research on oral rabies vaccines and field application of oral vaccination of dogs against rabies. World Health Organization, Geneva.

35. WHO (2008). Rabies in the South-East Asia Region. World Health Organization, New Delhi.

36. WHO (2010). Rabies vaccines: WHO position paper. Weekly Epidemiological Record No. 32, 6 August 2010, 85:309-320.

37. WHO (2011). Rabies. World Health Organization. www.who.int. Accessed 13 May 2011.

38. Wilde H (2007). Failures of rabies post-exposure prophylaxis. Vaccine 25: 7605-7609.

❑❑❑

Chapter 14

Brucellosis : The Future Course of Action

D. K. SINGH
Division of Veterinary Public Health, Indian Veterinary Research Institute, Izatnagar-243122

Contents

1. Introduction

Brucellosis, a direct anthropozoonosis of worldwide distribution, is caused by a Gram-negative facultative intracellular bacterium capable of growth and multiplication inside both phagocytic as well as non-phagocytic cells (Celli *et al.* 2005). The disease has probably accompanied the human civilization for over 2,000 years (Capasso 2002, Boral *et al.* 2009). Though controlled in many developed countries, brucellosis remains endemic in many parts of the world particularly in Mediterranean countries, Latin America, the Middle East, Spain, parts of Africa and western Asia. In the year 1861, J. A. Marston, an Assistant Surgeon, first described brucellosis in Malta as Mediterranean gastric remittent fever (Marston 1863). Sir David Bruce isolated the bacterium from the spleen of a British soldier died due to Malta fever (Bruce 1887) and named it *Micrococcus melitensis*. Later, it was renamed *Brucella melitensis* in his honour. However, the zoonotic link of *Brucella* was recognized by Zammit (1905) who isolated ıt from milk of healthy goats. In India, the presence of brucellosis was first established early in the 20th century and since then has been reported from almost all parts of the country.

2. The Bacteria

The members of the genus *Brucella* are small, Gram-negative, facultative intracellular coccobacilli belonging to α-2 subdivision of the *Proteobacteria*, alongside *Ochrobactrum, Rhizobium, Rhodobacter, Agrobacterium, Bartonella* and *Rickettsia* (Moreno *et al.* 1990). The genus consists of six species based on the host preference and phenotypic differences (Osterman and Moriyan 2006) namely, *B. abortus* (cattle), *B. melitensis* (sheep and goat), *B. suis* (pigs), *B. ovis* (rams), *B. canis* (dogs) and *B. neotomae* (wood rats). Of late, three new species named *B. microti* (voles), *B. pinnipediae* (doplhins) and *B. cetaceae* (seal) have been identified (Ewalt *et al.* 1994, Ross *et al.* 1996, Scholz *et al.* 2008), of which *B. pinnipediae* and *B. cetaceae* are reported to be zoonotic (Brew *et al.* 1999, Sohn *et al.* 2003, McDonald *et al.* 2006). Additional new or seemingly novel species have also been described more recently (De *et al.* 2008, Scholz *et al.* 2008) indicating an ever expanding *Brucella* epidemiology. All *Brucella* species seem to have arisen from a common ancestor to which *B. suis* biotype 3 shares similarity (Moreno *et al.* 2002). Based on DNA hybridization studies, Verger *et al.* (1985) proposed *Brucella* to be monospecific genus with *B. melitensis* as the nomen species with all other as its biovar. However, on the basis of host specificity, phenotypic characteristics, varying virulence, and available genotyping data (Chain *et al.* 2005, Halling *et al.* 2005) the classic taxonomic scheme for the six *Brucella* species and 17 existing biovars was ultimately reapproved in 2003 (Osterman and Moriyon 2006).

Brucellae are fairly hardy and the organisms have been recovered from foetal and manure samples that remained in a cool environment for longer than two months. However, exposure to sunlight kills the organism within a few hours (Waring 2005) and the organism is susceptible to many common disinfectants (Anonymous 2007).

3. Disease Occurrence and Transmission

Animal brucellosis is endemic worldwide with bovine brucellosis, caused by *B. abortus*, as the most widespread in animals (Corbel 1997). However, in many countries where *B. abortus* infection in bovines was eradicated, *B. melitensis* infection in these species has emerged as a new challenge (Banai 2002). In animals, brucellosis infection is responsible for huge economic losses through reduced productivity, abortions and weak offspring. It also results in the loss of much needed animal protein for human consumption.

Human brucellosis is mainly caused by *B. melitensis, B. abortus, B. suis* and *B. canis* with *B. melitensis* as the principal cause of human brucellosis worldwide accounting for upto 90% of all cases, *B. melitensis* type 1 predominating in India (Mantur *et al.* 2006) and Spain (Colmenero *et al.* 1996), type 2 in northwestern Greece and type 3 in Turkey (Bodur *et al.* 2003). Although *B. ovis* is widespread in sheep, it has not been identified in humans. An estimated 5,00,000 human infections occur annually worldwide with great variation in the incidence in the endemic areas ranging from <1/100,000 population in UK, USA and Australia to >20-30/100,000 in southern European countries such as Greece and Spain, and upto >70/100,000 in Middle East countries like Kuwait and Saudi Arabia (Cutler *et al.* 2005).

Consumption of unpasteurized milk and their products especially soft cheese, yoghurts and ice-cream (Eckman 1975), undercooked traditional delicacies such as liver and spleen are mainly responsible for human brucellosis (Malik 1997). Camel milk is considered to be the most important source of infection in Middle East countries and Mongolia. Rarely, human-to-human transmission takes place through tissue transplantation or sexual contact (Mantur *et al.* 1996) but it is epidemiologically insignificant. The disease can also be caused by contact with vaginal discharge, urine, faeces and blood of infected animals through broken skin and mucous membrane of conjunctiva and through inhalation. The disease is an occupational hazard for livestock owners, abattoir workers, dairy workers, shepherds, farmers, veterinarians and laboratory workers. Brucellosis is one of the most common laboratory acquired infections (Noviello *et al.* 2004, Fugier *et al.* 2007). With the increase in global tourism, brucellosis is emerging as a common travel associated imported disease in the developed world (Memish and Balkhy 2004).

Among cattle and buffaloes, ingestion or inhalation of organisms that are present in foetal fluids or other birth products is the predominant route of natural infection. The herds are typically exposed following the introduction of an infected animal that subsequently aborts or gives birth to an infected foetus contaminating the pasture or water body. However, the transmission of infection through natural services is not important epidemiologically in these species. In contrast, in dogs and sheep, transmission of rough strains of *Brucella* may be more common via the venereal route. Among dogs, the urine of males and vaginal secretions of females are the main sources of infection via the venereal, oral, nasal, or conjunctival routes (Wanke 2004, Hollett 2006).

4. Global Scenario

Brucellosis is major health problem in Mediterranean, Middle East, Latin America, Africa, parts of Mexico, and parts of Asia including India (Refai 2002, Grovel 2008). Syria has the highest annual incidence worldwide (OIE 2005a). The rate of human infection is high in Peru, Kuwait and Saudi Arabia in comparison with sub-Saharan Africa, where the rate is relatively low (McGill 2003).

Only 17 countries claim to be free of brucellosis (Cutler *et al.* 2005). Though it has been eradicated from almost all of Europe, reports still indicate the presence of human brucellosis in Greece, Spain and Turkey. Brucellosis-free status has been granted by the European Union (EU) to Sweden, Denmark, Finland, Germany, the UK (excluding Northern Ireland), Austria, Netherlands, Belgium, and Luxembourg (European Commission 2003). Norway and Switzerland are also considered brucellosis-free countries. France is an example where brucellosis has been successfully eradicated (Anonymous 2005). An increase in the annual number of reported cases in Turkey has been observed, exceeding 15,000 cases in 2004 (OIE 2005a) whereas the situation in Iran showed improvement during this period (OIE 2005b). Iraq has high endemicity with the annual incidence of 278.4 cases per million of population (OIE 2005a). Brucellosis has shown an increasing trend of incidence in Pakistan particularly in large dairy herds (Jamal *et al.* 2003). Brucellosis is re-emerging in Israel, Kuwait, Saudi Arabia, Brazil and Columbia with an increasing incidence of *B. melitensis* or *B. suis* biovar 1 infection in cattle (Corbel 1997). It has re-emerged in Oman and Malta (Amato Gauci 1995). Serological evidence of brucellosis has been reported in poultry (Choudhary and Narayan 1984, Junaidu *et al.* 2006).

While the occurrence of bovine brucellosis has been reported by 93 countries, the concept of host restriction of different *Brucella* species is gradually eluding with the evidence that *B. suis* biovar 1 has become established in cattle in Brazil and Columbia, thus, becoming a more important reservoir than pigs (Lopez-Merino 1989). *B. suis* has the widest host range, with established host-pathogen relationships in reindeer (Tessaro and Forbes 1986) and hares (Vitovec *et al.* 1976) in addition to swine.

B. melitensis infection in cattle is emerging as impending threat in some southern European countries, Israel, Kuwait and Saudi Arabia (McGill 2003). It particularly poses problem as *B. abortus* vaccines does not effectively protect against *B. melitensis* infection and *B. melitensis* Rev.1 vaccine has not been fully evaluated for use in cattle.

5. Indian Perspective

The true incidence of human brucellosis in India is elusive. It has been estimated that the true incidence may be 25 times higher than the reported incidence. Mantur *et al.* (2004) showed a seroprevalence of 1.6% by SAT and isolated *B. melitensis* in 43 of the 93 children during a period of 13 years majority of whom were shepherds habitual of consuming fresh goat milk. They also reported brucellosis in 495 among 26948 adults (1.8%) in Bijapur during a period of 16 years from 1988 to 2004 and isolated *B. melitensis* from 191 cases (Mantur *et al.* 2006). Mathur (1964) reported 8.5% seroprevalence of brucellosis among dairy personnel in contact with infected animals and isolated *Brucella* from 7 cases while Randhawa *et al.* (1974) detected antibodies in 4.2% of abortion cases. In Gujarat, 8.5% prevalence of *Brucella* agglutinins was recorded in human cases (Panjarathinam and Jhala 1986). In Haryana, 34% prevalence of human brucellosis was recorded among veterinarians, attendants and compounders in contact with animals (Chauhan 1999) indicating an occupational association. Thakur and Thapliyal (2002) too observed the disease prevalence in 4.97% persons exposed to animals with a markedly higher prevalence (17.39%) among field veterinarians. Hemashettar and Patil (1991) found 8.2% veterinary workers with *Brucella* specific antibodies. High seroprevalence rate was also noted in specific risk groups such as abattoir workers (Barbuddhe *et al.* 2000, Chadda *et al.* 2004). Kumar *et al.* (1997), too, observed high prevalence (25%) among abattoir personnel in Delhi. Handa *et al.* (1998) diagnosed 4 (3.3%) cases of acute brucellosis in 121 patients with fever of unknown origin (FUO). Similarly, Sen *et al.* (2002) detected 28 (6.8%) seropositive cases in a group of 414 patients with FUO, while Kadri *et al.* (2000) reported 28 (0.8%) seropositive cases in 3,532 patients with FUO.

Mudaliar *et al.* (2003) showed the presence of *Brucella* antibodies in 5.33% of the animal handlers of which 4.51% were dairy farm workers and 14.63 % were veterinary doctors. Rana *et al.* (1985) showed a seropositivity of 27.7% among veterinarians in Delhi. Agasthya *et al.* (2007) reported brucellosis in occupationally exposed individuals with high prevalence of 41.23% in veterinary inspectors, 30.92% in veterinary assistants, 12.37% in veterinary officers, 6.18% in veterinary supervisors, 6.18% in group-D workers, 2.06% in shepherds and 1.03% in butchers. Bedi *et al.* (2007) also reported brucellosis in animal handlers in Punjab.

In India, the evidence of brucellosis based on serosurvey has been reported in all domestic animals besides poultry and wild animals (Table 1). The prevalence of brucellosis in animals reportedly varies from as low as 0.13% (Chatterjee *et al.* 1986) to as high as 44% (Zaki *et al.* 1975). In general, incidence of brucellosis is reportedly higher in cattle than in buffaloes (Maansi 1999, Prithviraj 2010). In a serological survey of brucellosis in cattle and buffalo in 23 states of India, Isloor *et al.* (1998a) demonstrated an overall prevalence of antibodies in 1.9% of cattle and 1.8% of buffaloes in 23 states. They also showed a seropositivity of 4.1% in cattle in 47 organised farms in contrast to 0.7% seropositivity in cattle owned by individual farmers in Karnataka.

Table 1 : Prevalence of brucellosis in man and animals in India

Animal species	Seropositivity	Isolation of *Brucella*
Cattle	+	+
Buffalo	+	+
Sheep	+	+
Goat	+	+
Swine	+	+
Equine	+	+
Camel	+	-
Dog	+	+
Poultry	+	-
Wild animals	+	-
Man	+	+

The samples predominantly from large herds with a history of abortion and infertility showed a highly variable seroprevalence ranging from 6.6% in Madhya Pradesh (Mehra *et al.* 2000) to 60% in Assam (Chakraborty *et al.* 2000). Mehra *et al.* (2000) reported 6.5% prevalence in cattle from organized farms compared to 5.1% prevalence in the unorganized sector. National Survey of Bovine Brucellosis (1994-2001) showed national average of brucellosis as 5% in cattle and 3% in buffaloes (Renukaradhya *et al.* 2002). In a similar national survey of sheep and goat brucellosis, Isloor *et al.* (1998b) reported 7.9% cumulative incidence in sheep and 2.2% in goats. In another study, Singh (2008) reported 7.41%, 8.58% and 8.85% seroprevalence of brucellosis in cattle, goat and sheep, respectively.

Serological evidence of *B. ovis* infection in 6 out of 102 rams was reported in Himachal Pradesh (Katoch *et al.* 1996). The seroprevalence of brucellosis in pigs has been recorded as 3.2% in Madhya Pradesh (Soni and Pathak 1969), 11.3% in Tamil Nadu (Kumar and Rao 1980) and 6.3% in Karnataka (Krishnappa *et al.* 1981). In another study, it was estimated as 9.5% in 756 pigs slaughtered in Karnataka (Thoppil 2000). Brucellosis has also been reported in dairy farms in Goa region (Barbuddhe *et al.* 2004). Similarly, Aulakh *et al.* (2008) reported a high prevalence of bovine brucellosis in Punjab. Serological evidence of brucellosis has also been demonstrated in Andaman and Nicobar Islands (Jai-Sunder *et al.* 2005). More recently, the seroprevalence of brucellosis in sheep and goats in 7 states of India has been estimated at 7.58, 11.08, 11.88 and 15.77 per cent on testing by RBPT, STAT, CFT and I-ELISA, respectively (Singh 2009). Brucellosis has also been reported in mithuns (Rajkhowa *et al.* 2005) and yaks (Bandyopadhyay *et al.* 2009).

B. abortus biotypes I and III have been isolated from cattle (Chatterjee *et al.* 1995) besides biotype IV (Batra *et al.* 1989). Though biotype I predominates in cattle in organized farms, biotype III has been usually reported to infect the cattle reared by the village population (Anonymous 1986). Occasionally, *B. melitensis* biotype I has also been isolated from cattle (Hemashettar *et al.* 1987). *B. melitensis* biotypes I, II and III have been isolated from sheep and goats (Sharma *et al.* 1995) besides *B. abortus* biotype I (Panjarathinum and Gulrajani 1974). Of the 3 biotypes of *B. melitensis*, biotype I has been shown to predominate in the sheep and goat population (Sen and Sharma 1972). *B. canis* has been isolated from dogs in Chennai (Pillai *et al.* 1991) while isolation of *B. suis* biotype II from a sow has been reported from Tamil Nadu (Kumar and Rao 1980). Subsequently, isolation of *B. suis* biotype II from an aborted foetus of goat was reported (Reddy and Rao 1984) while *B. suis* biotype I was isolated from dog (Pillai *et al.* 1990). The only report of *B. abortus* and *B. melitensis* isolation from horses is that of Polding (Polding 1947). Isolation of *B. ovis* has not been reported in India. The biotypes of *Brucella* isolated from man and animals in India are shown in Table 2.

6. Bioterrorism Potential

B. abortus, *B. melitensis*, and *B. suis* have been identified as Category B bioterrorism agents (Rotz *et al.* 2002) and as select agents by the US Government (CDC 2005). Also, *B. suis* was one of the earliest agents investigated and developed as a bioweapon in the United States in the 1950s (Christopher *et al.* 2005). In 1954, *Brucella* species became the first agent weaponised by the US offensive biological weapons programme (Sarinas and Chitkara 2003). The propensity of *Brucella* for airborne transmission and ability to induce chronic debilitating disease in man requiring prolonged treatment with a combination of antibiotics, absence of any pathognomonic clinical presentation defying early and rapid diagnosis are some of the important characteristics that make it a potential bioweapon (Pappas *et al.* 2006).

Table 2 : Biotypes of *Brucella* isolated from man and animals in India

Species	Biotypes	Animal
B. abortus	1,3,4,6	Cattle
	1,3	Buffalo
	1	Sheep
	1	Goat
	1,3	Man
	#	Equine
B. melitensis	1	Cattle
	1,2,3	Sheep
	1,2,3	Goat
	1,2,3	Man
	#	Equine
B. suis	2	Goat
	2	Pig
	1	Dog
B. canis	--	Dog

Biotype not known

7. Economic Impact

The impact of brucellosis in cattle and buffalo on the national economy of India has been estimated to the tune of Rs. 240 million every year (Schwabe 1984). This amounts to more than half per cent of the total value of all meat and milk products produced in the country. The annual loss due to human brucellosis has been put at 30 million man days. Kunen (1994) estimated that brucellosis costs India at least Rs. 350 million annually in terms of loss of food animals and man days. Earlier to this, the economic loss due to brucellosis among bovines was estimated at Rs. 311.47 million (Mathur and Sharma 1974).

8. Prevention and Control Strategies

Brucellosis being a direct zoonosis with no human-to-human transmission, decline in human brucellosis cases is always expected consequent upon the control programmes instituted against animal brucellosis. Indeed, with the fact that there is no human vaccine available for brucellosis, control and eradication programme for animal brucellosis remains a challenge.

Control of animal brucellosis is dependent on two main principles: (a) elimination of infected animals from the herd, and (b) prevention of exposure of animals to infection. Control and eradication of brucellosis in animals may be achieved by test and slaughter of infected animals with or without mass vaccination with approved vaccine depending on the situation with respect to the incidence and prevalence of the disease. In test and slaughter policy, detection of truly infected animals assumes paramount importance and requires a quick, cheap and reasonably sensitive screening test supported with an efficacious confirmatory test. In cattle, Rose Bengal plate agglutination test (RBPT) is recommended as screening test with positive sera tested with complement fixation test (CFT) for confirmation (Fig. 1). The milk ring test (MRT) could be used for identifying infected dairy herd with good results followed by sero-testing individual animals. However, this cannot be used on dry animals and its efficacy is doubtful in sheep and goats. Mass immunization should be the desired strategy in case of high prevalence of disease. For cattle, *B. abortus* S-19, a live attenuated vaccine, given at the age of 3 to 6 months (in certain cases upto 8 months) is recommended. In spite of certain drawbacks, it has been used with satisfactory results. When used routinely to attain coverage of ≥ 80% of population, herd immunity develops with gradual decline in the incidence. If eradication is the target, vaccination should be stopped once the incidence falls below 0.2% and the infected animals must be eliminated. In February 1996, the USDA approved the use of *B. abortus* strain RB51 (RB51) as the official calfhood vaccine for protection against brucellosis (http://www.aphis.usda.gov:80/vs/nahps/Brucellosis/rb51.html). The *B. abortus* RB51 strain lacks S-LPS and has much lower pathogenicity in vaccinates. It is considered only mildly abortifacient and presumed to have much lower pathogenicity in humans in response to accidental exposure. In addition, the *B. abortus* RB51 vaccine has a substantial advantage in brucellosis control programmes because it does not elicit an antibody response against S-LPS and does not, therefore, interfere with results of serologic testing.

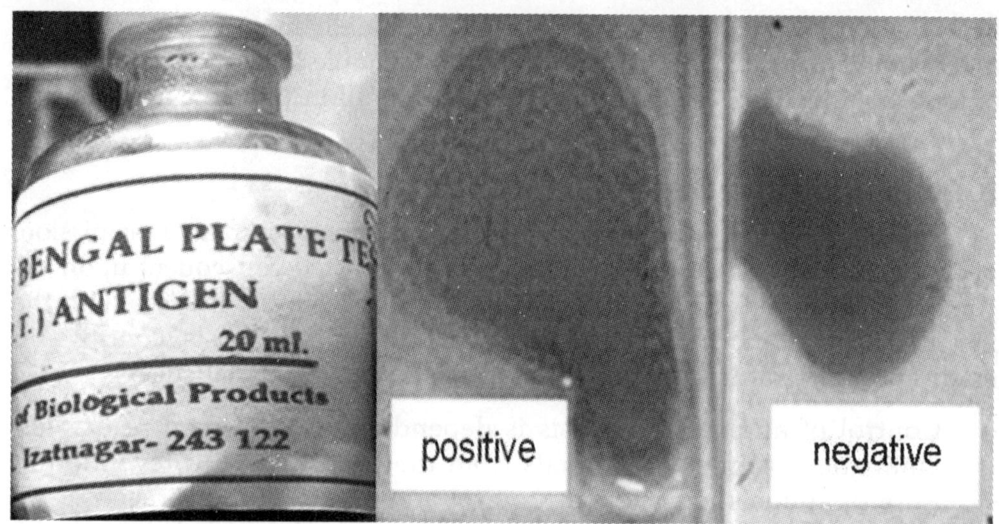

Fig. 1 : Rose Bengal plate agglutination test

The epidemiology and planning for prevention and control of brucellosis in sheep and goats are similar to that of cattle with minor adjustments. A live attenuated *Brucella* vaccine *B. melitensis* Rev-1 is highly effective and is widely used to vaccinate small ruminants in parts of the world where *B. melitensis* is enzootic. Immunization of young recently weaned rams (weaner rams) with the *B. melitensis* Rev-1 vaccine is also recommended for control of *B. ovis* in some countries (Waring 2005). Like the strain 19 vaccine, this vaccine, too, causes abortions in pregnant animals and short-term shedding of the Rev-1 strain in milk (Banai 2002) leading to human infections with *B. melitensis* Rev-1 as reported in Israel and the Middle East (Refai 2002, Banai 2002, Bardenstein *et al.* 2002). The probability of success in the flocks where contact with other flocks is frequent remains poor. In sheep and goats, allergic test, along with RBPT, could be used to identify infected herd followed by sero-testing of individual animals.

Control of brucellosis in swine poses particular difficulty because there is neither a satisfactory test to identify infected individual animal nor a satisfactory vaccine. It is, therefore, advisable to slaughter the herd. No effective vaccine against *B. canis* has been identified to date.

Control and eradication of brucellosis in domestic animals, especially bovine brucellosis in India poses particular problem as the cow slaughter is not permitted. Under such situation, it appears prudent to aim control rather than eradication of disease. For this, continued long term vaccination programme with movement control between endemic to non-endemic zone should be instituted so as to achieve vaccination of ≥ 80 per cent animal population to develop herd immunity. Such continued mass vaccination with movement control is expected to bring down the incidence of brucellosis to a level where it may cease to be a cause of worry for animal population. Once the disease is brought under control in animals, the incidence of brucellosis in human population is liable to decline.

9. Future Perspective

Brucellosis has always been a challenge to the scientific fraternity. The disease has eluded control and eradication in many parts of the world and has been re-emerging (Seleem *et al.* 2009). Much progress has been made since the identification of brucellosis. A battery of diagnostic tests and vaccines, both live-attenuated and killed, are available. The necessary technical knowhow for control and eradication programmes under different sociocultural and epidemiological situations is available. However, a lot needs to be done. The available vaccines are far from ideal. Vaccine for all species is not available. Prompt reporting of human brucellosis to health authorities is extremely important as there is no vaccine for use in humans. In the areas where brucellosis is enzootic, good animal husbandry practices are critical to prevent transmission both among animals and between animals and humans. In the management of groups of domestic animals, provision of separate birthing areas, and implementation of good management practices are important to minimize opportunities for transmission should an infected animal be introduced. Cheeses and other foods made from unpasteurized dairy products from countries where brucellosis is enzootic should be avoided, and meat should not be consumed from animals that appear to be sick at the time of slaughter.

The diagnostic tests, too, are fraught with problems and present many difficulties. It is difficult to differentiate between *Brucella* infection and *Yersinia enterocolitica* O:9 infection; and vaccinated and infected animals. All antigens are not well characterized. The pathogenicity of brucellosis is not clearly elucidated. The mechanism of intracellular survival and elimination of brucellae are yet to be explained. Clearly, until the pathogenicity of the *Brucella* infection is elucidated and the antigens characterized with respect to their virulence properties and immune capability, it would probably not be possible to develop a foolproof diagnostic test or an ideal vaccine. Now that the complete sequence of the *Brucella* genome is available, the days are probably not far off when these shortcomings would be overcome.

References

1. Agasthya AS, Isloor S, Prabhudas K (2007). Brucellosis in high risk group individuals. Indian J Med Microbiol 25:28-31.

2. Amato Gauci AJ (1995). The return of brucellosis. Maltese Med J 7:7-8.

3. Anonymous (1986). Joint FAO/WHO expert committee on brucellosis. VI Report. WHO TRS No. 740, World Health Organization, Geneva.

4. Anonymous (2005). Brucellose. http://www.invs.sante.fr/surveillance/brucellose/default.htm. Accessed 24 December 2005.

5. Anonymous (2007). Brucellosis. CFSPH, Iowa State University, Iowa.

6. Aulakh HK, Patil PK, Sharma S *et al.* (2008). A study on the epidemiology of bovine brucellosis in Punjab (India) using milk-ELISA. Acta Vet Brno 77:393-399.

7. Banai M (2002). Control of small ruminant brucellosis by use of *Brucella melitensis* Rev. 1 vaccine: laboratory aspects and field observations. Vet Microbiol 90:497-519.

8. Bandyopadhyay S, Sasmal D, Dutta TK *et al.* (2009). Seroprevalence of brucellosis in yaks (*Poephagus grunniens*) in India and evaluation of protective immunity to S19 vaccine. Trop Anim Hlth Prod 41:587-592.

9. Barbuddhe SB, Chakurkar EB, Bale MA *et al.* (2004). Prevalence of brucellosis in organized dairy farms in Goa region. Indian J Anim Sci 74: 1030-1031.

10. Barbuddhe SB, Kumar P, Malik SV *et al.* (2000). Seropositivity for intracellular bacterial infections among abattoir associated personnels. J Com Dis 32:295-299

11. Bardenstein S, Mandelboim M, Ficht TA *et al.* (2002). Identification of the *Brucella melitensis* vaccine strain Rev.1 in animals and humans in Israel by PCR analysis of the *Pst*I site polymorphism of its omp2 gene. J Clin Microbiol 40:1475–1480.

12. Batra HV, Chand P, Ganju L, Mukherjee R *et al.* (1989). Dot-enzyme linked immunosorbent assay for the detection of antibodies in bovine brucellosis. Res Vet Sci 46:143-146

13. Bedi JS, Sharma JK, Gill JPS *et al.* (2007). Seroepidemiological survey of *Brucella* agglutinins in animal handlers in Punjab, India. Indian J Anim Sci 77:1283-1285.

14. Bodur H, Balaban N, Aksaray S *et al.* (2003). Biotypes and antimicrobial susceptibilities of *Brucella* isolates. Scand J Infect Dis 35:337-338.

15. Boral R, Singh M and Singh DK (2009). Status and strategies for control of brucellosis-A review. Indian J Anim Sci 79: 1191-1199.

16. Bruce D (1887). Note on the discovery of a microorganism in Malta fever. *Practitioner* 39:161-170.

17. Brew SD, Perret LL, Stack JA *et al.* (1999). Human exposure to *Brucella* recovered from a sea mammal. Vet Rec 144:483.

18. Capasso L (2002). Bacteria in two millennia old cheese, and related epizoonoses in Roman populations. J Infect 45:122-127.

19. CDC (2005). Office of Inspector General, Department of Health and Human Services. Possession, use, and transfer of select agents and toxins. Final rule. Fed Register 70:13293–13325.

20. Celli J, Salcedo SP, Grovel JP (2005). N *Brucella* coopts the small GTPase Sar1 for intrcellular replication. PNAS 102:1673-1678.

21. Chadda VS, Soni PK, Gupta A *et al.* (2004). Incidence of brucellosis in arthritis and chronic low back pain in high risk group. J Assoc Phy India 52:338.

22. Chain PSG, Comerci DJ, Tolmasky ME *et al.* (2005). Whole-genome analyses of speciation events in pathogenic Brucellae. Infect Immun 73:8353-8361.

23. Chakraborty M, Patgiri GP, Barman NN (2000). Application of delayed-type hypersensitivity test (DTH) for the diagnosis of bovine brucellosis. Indian Vet J 77:849-851.

24. Chatterjee A, De BN, Mondol P *et al.* (1986). Studies on seroprevalence of bovine brucellosis in rural areas of West Bengal. Indian Vet J 63:95-100.

25. Chatterjee A, Mondol P, De BN *et al.* (1995). Cultural isolation of *Brucella* in relation to serum agglutinin level. Indian Vet J 72:211-215.

26. Chauhan RS (1999). Brucellosis in India and its impact on export of buffalo meat. J Anim Prod 31:316-317.

27. Choudhary SP, Narayan KG (1984). Prevalence of *Brucella* agglutinin in poultry flocks. Indian J Anim Sci 54:289-290.

28. Christopher GW, Agan MB, Cieslak TJ *et al.* (2005). History of US military contributions to the study of bacterial zoonoses. Military Med 170:39-48.

29. Colmenero JD, Reguera JM, Martos F *et al.* (1996). Complications associated with *Brucella melitensis* infection: A study of 530 cases. Medicine 75:195-211.

30. Corbel MJ (1997). Brucellosis: an overview. Emerg Infect Dis 3: 213-221.

31. Cutler SJ, Whatmore AM, Commander NJ (2005). Brucellosis-new aspects of an old disease. J Appl Microbiol 98:1270-1281.

32. De BK, Stauffer L, Koylass MS *et al.* (2008). Novel *Brucella* strain (BO1) associated with a prosthetic breast implant infection. J Clin Microbiol 46:43-49.

33. Eckman MR (1975). Brucellosis linked to Mexican cheese. JAMA 232:636-637.

34. European Commission (2003). Report on trends and sources of zoonotic agents in the European Union and Norway. European Commission.

35. Ewalt DR, Payeur JB, Martin BM *et al.* (1994). Characteristics of a *Brucella* species from a bottlenose dolphin (*Tursiops truncates*). J Vet Diagn Invest 6: 448-452.

36. Fugier E, Pappas G, Grovel JP (2007). Virulence factors in brucellosis: implications for aetiopathogenesis and treatment. Expert Rev Mol Med 9:1-10.

37. Gorvel JP (2008). *Brucella*: a Mr "Hide" converted into Dr Jekyll. Microbes Infect 10:1010-1013.

38. Halling SM, Peterson-Burch BD, Bricker BJ *et al.* (2005). Completion of the genome sequence of *Brucella abortus* and comparison of the highly similar genomes of *Brucella melitensis* and *Brucella suis*. J Bacteriol 187:2715-2726.

39. Handa R, Singh S, Singh N *et al.* (1998). Brucellosis in North India: results of a prospective study. J Com Dis 30:85-87.

40. Hemashettar BM, Patil CS (1991). Brucellosis among practicing veterinarians. Indian J Med Microbiol 9:45-47

41. Hemashettar BM, Patil CS, Jaikumar K *et al.* (1987). Isolation of *Brucella melitensis* biotype I from a cow and two of its attendants. Indian Vet J 64:822-825.

42. Hollett RB (2006). Canine brucellosis: outbreaks and compliance. Theriogenol 66:575-587.

43. Isloor S, Renukaradhya GJ, Rajasekhar M (1998a). A serological survey of bovine brucellosis in India. Rev Sci Tech Off Int Epiz 17:781-785.

44. Isloor S, Renukaradhya GJ, Rajasekhar M (1998b). Brucellosis research. In: Annual report (1997–1998) of AICRP on Animal Disease Monitoring and Surveillance (ADMAS), Bangalore, India, 13-18.

45. Jamal SM, Afzal M and Ahmed S (2003). The immune response of guinea pigs and buffalo calves to the locally prepared *Brucella abortus* strain 19 vaccine. Rev Sci Tech Off Int Epiz 22:893-897.

46. Jai-Sunder, Rai RB, Kundu A *et al.* (2005). Incidence and prevalence of livestock diseases of Andaman and Nicobar Islands. Indian J Anim Sci 75:1041-1043.

47. Junaidu AU, Ahmed F, Ambursa MA *et al.* (2006). Brucellosis in local chickens in North Western Nigeria. Int J Poultry Sci 5: 547-549.

48. Kadri SM, Rukhsana A, Laharwal MA *et al.* (2000). Seroprevalence of brucellosis in Kashmir (India) among patients with pyrexia of unknown origin. J Indian Med Assoc 98:170-171.

49. Katoch RC, Joshi VB, Sharma M (1996). Seroprevalence of *Brucella ovis, Brucella melitensis* and *Chlamydia psittaci* in rams. Indian J Anim Sci 66:1130-1131.

50. Krishnappa G, Zaki S, Keshavamurthy BSK (1981). Serological evidence of swine brucellosis in and around Bangalore. Mysore J Agri Sci 15:77-80.

51. Kumar P, Singh DK, Barbuddhe SB (1997). Seroprevalence of brucellosis among abattoir personnel of Delhi. J Com Dis 29: 131-138.

52. Kumar R, Rao CVN (1980). Porcine brucellosis in Tamil Nadu. Indian Vet J 57:1-4.

53. Kunen AV (1994). Brucellosis In: Infectious Diseases, Diagnosis and Management in Clinical Practice. CBS Publishers, New Delhi. 448-449.

54. Lopez-Merino A (1989). Brucellosis in Latin America. In: Young J and Corbel MJ (Eds.). Brucellosis: Clinical and Laboratory Aspects, CRC Press Inc: Boca Raton. 151-161.

55. Maansi (1999). Seroepidemiology of brucellosis in animals and man in tarai region. MVSc Thesis, GBPUAT, Pantnagar.

56. Malik GM (1997). A clinical study of brucellosis in adults in the Asir region of southern Saudi Arabia. Am J Trop Med Hyg 56:375-377.

57. Mantur BG, Akki AS, Mangalgi SS *et al.* (2004). Childhood brucellosis - a microbiological, epidemiological and clinical study. J Trop Pediatr 50:153-157.

58. Mantur BG, Biradar MS, Bidri RC (2006). Protean clinical manifestations and diagnostic challenges of human brucellosis in adults: 16 years' experience in an endemic area. J Med Microbiol 55:897-903.

59. Mantur BG, Mangalgi SS, Mulimani B (1996). *Brucella melitensis:* A sexually transmissible agent? Lancet 347:1763.

60. Marston JA (1863). Report on fever (Malta). Great Britain Army Med Dept Rep. 3:486-521.

61. Mathur AC, Sharma GL (1974). Studies on the estimates of the economic losses caused by brucellosis among bovines and its control in India. Indian J Anim Sci 44:654-661.

62. Mathur TN (1964). *Brucella* strains isolated from cows, buffaloes, goats, sheep and human beings at Karnal: Their significance with regard to the epidemiology of brucellosis. Indian J Med Res 52:1231-1240.

63. McDonald WL, Jamaludin R, Mackereth G *et al.* (2006). Characterisation of a *Brucella* sp. strain as a marine mammal type despite isolation from a patient with spinal osteomyelitis in New Zealand. J Clin Microbiol 44:4363-4370.

64. McGill PE (2003). Geographically specific infections and arthritis, including rheumatic syndromes associated with certain fungi and parasites, *Brucella* species and *Mycobacterium leprae.* Best Practice Res Clin Rheumatol 17:289-307.

65. Mehra KN, Dhanesar NS, Chaturvedi VK (2000). Seroprevalence of brucellosis in bovines in Madhya Pradesh. Indian Vet J 77: 571-573.

66. Memish ZA, Balkhy HH (2004). Brucellosis and International Travel. J Travel Med 11: 49-55.

67. Moreno E, Cloeckaert A, Moriyon I (2002). *Brucella* evolution and taxonomy. Vet Microbiol 90:209-227.

68. Moreno E, Stackebrandt E, Dorsch M *et al.* (1990). *Brucella abortus* 16S rRNA and lipid A reveal a phylogenetic relationship with members of the alpha-2 subdivision of the class *Proteobacteria.* J Bacteriol 172: 3569-3576.

69. Mudaliar S, Bhore A, Pandit D (2003). Detection of antibodies to *Brucella abortus* in animal handlers. Indian J Med Sci 57:181-186.

70. Noviello S, Gallo R, Kelly M *et al.* (2004). Laboratory-acquired brucellosis. Emerg Infect Dis 10: 1848-1850.

71. OIE (World Organisation for Animal Health) (2005a). Handistatus II: zoonoses (human cases): global cases of brucellosis in 2004. http://www.oie.int/hs2/gi_zoon_masld.asp?c_cont=6&c_mald=172&annee=2004 Accessed 13 December 2005.

72. OIE (World Organisation for Animal Health) (2005b). Handistatus II: zoonoses (human cases): global cases of brucellosis in 2003. http://www.oie.int/hs2/gi_zoon_mald.asp?c_cont=6&c_mald=172&annee=2003 Accessed 13 December 2005.

73. Osterman B, Moriyon I (2006). International Committee on Systematics of Prokaryotes: Subcommittee on the taxonomy of *Brucella*. Int J Syst Evol Microbiol 56:1173-1175.

74. Panjarathinam R, Jhala CI (1986). Brucellosis in Gujrat state. J Pathol Microbiol 29:53-60.

75. Panjarathinum R, Gulrajani TS (1974). Studies on brucellosis. II. Isolation of *Brucella* organism in milk of cows, sheep and goats. Indian J Anim Hlth 13:29-35.

76. Pappas G, Panagopoulou P, Christou L *et al.* (2006). *Brucella* as a biological weapon. Cell Mol Life Sci 63:2229-2236.

77. Pillai MT, Nendunchelliyan S, Raghvan N (1990). Brucellosis in a dog caused by *B. suis* biovar I in Madras. Cherion 19:97-98.

78. Pillai MT, Nendunchelliyan S, Raghvan N (1991). Serological and bacteriological detection of *Brucella canis* infection of dogs in Madras. Indian Vet J 68:399-401.

79. Polding JB (1947). Brucellosis in India. Indian J Vet Sci 147-155.

80. Prithviraj (2010). Comparison of different serological tests for diagnosis of bovine brucellosis. MVSc Thesis, Indian Veterinary Research Institute, Izatnagar, India.

81. Rajkhowa S, Rahman H, Rajkhowa *et al.* (2005). Seroprevalence of brucellosis in mithuns (*Bos frontalis*) in India. Prev Vet Med 69: 145-151.

82. Rana UVS, Sehgal S, Bhardwaj AM (1985). A seroepidemiological study of brucellosis among workers of veterinary hospital and slaughter house of Delhi. Int J Zoon 12:74-79.

83. Randhawa AS, Kalra DS, Kapur MP (1974). Some seroepidemiologic observations on brucellosis in humans and animals. Indian J Med Sci 28: 133-138.

84. Reddy PRC, Rao PVRC (1984). A note on isolation of *Brucella suis* from foetus of a she-goat. Kerala J Vet Sci 15:173-174.

85. Refai M (2002). Incidence and control of brucellosis in the Near East region. Vet Microbiol 90:81-110.

86. Renukaradhya GJ, Isloor S, Rajasekhar M (2002). Epidemiology, zoonotic aspects, vaccination and control/eradication of brucellosis in India. Vet Microbiol 90: 183-195.

87. Ross HM, Jahans KL, MacMillan AP (1996). *Brucella* species infection in North Sea seal and cetacean populations. Vet Rec 138:647-648.

88. Rotz LD, Khan AS, Lillibridge SR (2002). Public health assessment of potential biological terrorism agents. Emerg Infect Dis 8:225-230.

89. Sarinas PSA, Chitkara RK (2003). Brucellosis. Seminars Resp Infect 18:168-182.

90. Scholz HC, Hubalek A, Sedlacek I (2008). *Brucella microti* sp. nov., isolated from the common vole *Microtus arvalis*. Int J Syst Evol Microbiol 58:375-382.

91. Schwabe CW (1984). Veterinary Medicine and Human Health. Waverly Press Inc. Mount Royal Guilford Avenues, Baltimore, MD 21202 US. 16-39

92. Seleem MN, Boyle SM, Sriranganathan N (2009). Brucellosis: a re-emerging zoonosis. Vet Microbiol. Doi: 10.1016/j.vetmic.2009.06.021

93. Sen GP, Sharma GL (1972). Speciation of seventy eight Indian strains of *Brucella*, an epidemiological study. Indian J Anim Sci 45:537.

94. Sen MR, Shukla BN, Goyal RK (2002). Seroprevalence of brucellosis in and around Varanasi. J Com Dis 34:226-227.

95. Sharma M, Batta MK, Asrani RK *et al.* (1995). *Brucella melitensis* abortions among organized sheep farms in north-west states in India. Indian J Anim Sci 65:874-875.

96. Singh M (2009). Comparison of ELISA with other serological tests in diagnosis of brucellosis in small ruminants. MVSc Thesis, Deemed University, IVRI, Izatnagar, India.

97. Singh RK (2008). Prevalence of brucellosis among ruminants and comparision of serological test. MVSc Thesis, Deemed University, IVRI, Izatnagar, India.

98. Sohn AH, Probert WS, Glaser CA *et al.* (2003). Human neurobrucellosis with intracerebral granuloma caused by a marine mammal *Brucella* spp. Emerg Infect Dis 9:485-488.

99. Soni JL, Pathak PN (1969). Serological investigations into porcine brucellosis. Indian Vet J 46:191-195.

100. Tessaro SV, Forbes LB (1986). *Brucella suis* biotype 4: a case of granulomatous nephritis in a barren ground caribou (*Rangifer tarandus groenlandicus* L.) with a review of the distribution of rangiferine brucellosis in Canada. J Wildlife Dis 22: 479-483.

101. Thakur SD, Thapliyal DC (2002). Seroprevalence of brucellosis in man. J Com Dis 34:106-109.

102. Thoppil ST (2000). Serodiagnosis of brucellosis in pigs and man and differentiation of cross reactions due to *Yersinia enterocolitica* O:9. MVSc thesis, University of Agricultural Sciences, Bangalore, India.

103. Verger J-M, Grimont F, Grimont PAD and Grayon M (1985). *Brucella*, a monospecific genus as shown by deoxyribonucleic acid hybridization. Int J Syst Bacteriol 35: 292-295

104. Vitovec J, Vladik P, Zahor Z *et al.* (1976). Morphological study of 70 cases of brucellosis in rabbits caused by *Brucella suis*. Vet Med (Praha) 21:359-368.

105. Wanke MM (2004). Canine brucellosis. Anim Reprod Sci 82-83:195-207.

106. Waring SC (2005). Brucellosis. In: Kahn CM and Line S (Eds.). Merck Veterinary Manual, 9th ed. Whitehouse Station, NJ: Merck. 2546.

107. Zaki S, Murty BSK, Rao S *et al.* (1975). Serological incidence of brucellosis in sheep and goats in Karnataka. Cur Res 4:196-197.

108. Zammit T (1905). A preliminary note on the examination of the blood of goats suffering from Mediterranean fever, reports of the Commission on Mediterranean fever, Part-III, Harrison and Sons, London, 1905, pp 83.

❑❑❑

Chapter 15

Strategic Control of *Peste des Petits Ruminants*

R. P. SINGH
Division of Biological Products, Indian Veterinary Research Institute, Izatnagar-243122

Contents

1. Introduction

Peste des petits ruminants (PPR) also called "goat plague" is an acute, febrile, viral disease of small ruminants. The disease is characterized by severe bronchopneumonia, mucopurulent nasal discharge, stomatitis, enteritis followed by recovery or death. It was first described by Gargadennec and Lalanne in the year 1942 in Ivory Coast as rinderpest like disease of goats and sheep. This disease was not transmissible to the in contact cattle. PPR disease is classified in the list-A of Office International des Epizooties and World Animal Health Organization. Although similar to rinderpest, due to its affinity to small ruminants it was named as "*Peste des Petits Ruminants*" i.e. pest of small ruminants, commonly called PPR. The widespread distribution of PPR has been reported in several Asian, African and Middle East countries. Based on the distribution and epidemiology, the PPR viruses can now be categorized in to four distinct lineages namely lineage 1, 2, 3 and 4. Of these, three lineages (lineage 1, 2 and 3) are prevalent in Africa and lineage 4 is common in Asia (Shaila *et al.* 1996, Dhar *et al.* 2002). Therefore, PPR is one of the major hurdles in improvement of the production potential of small ruminants in India and several other developing countries.

Of the total small ruminant population of 752 million in the PPR affected countries of the world, India has approximately 200 million small ruminants. PPR is responsible for high mortality in goats and sheep. Mortality may reach upto 50% or even more (Abu-Elzein *et al.* 1990, Joshi *et al.* 1996), thereby leading to high economic losses (Fig. 1). In India, PPR disease was first reported from Tamil Nadu in the year 1987 (Shaila *et al.* 1989) and the disease continued for 4-5 years in south Indian states, after which it became endemic in the country (Dhar *et al.* 2002, Singh *et al.* 2004c). Goats and sheep are most susceptible to PPR, however, only one outbreak has been reported in Indian buffaloes (Govindarajan *et al.* 1997).

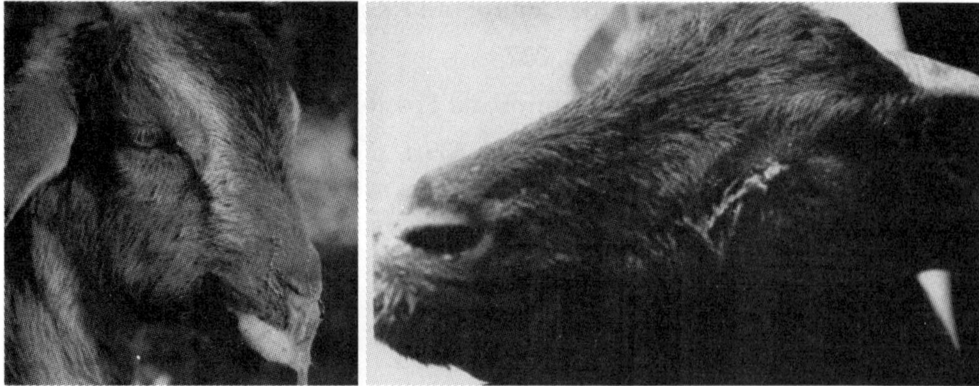

Fig. 1 : PPR infected goats with characteristic mucopurulent nasal and sticky ocular discharges

The state of the art diagnostics using monoclonal antibodies and PCR ELISA have been developed for the diagnosis of PPR in India (Singh *et al.* 2004a, 2004b, Saravanan *et al.* 2004). Simultaneously very potent and safe vaccines have also been developed using lineage 4 virus (Sreenivasa *et al.* 2000) and lineage 1 virus (Diallo *et al.* 1989). With the available tools (vaccines and diagnostics) and knowledge gained from rinderpest eradication, PPR can now be controlled and eradicated from the globe. Both the vaccines practically produce life long immunity with a single inoculation. Further, there is no serotype variation in PPR. The presence of single serotype provides a scope of use of single vaccine and single diagnostic technique irrespective of the type of disease occurrence. The technologies for mass scale vaccine production are available with the industries and leading research and development organizations for both lineage 4 (Table 1) and lineage 1 vaccine. Base line information on clinical and seroprevalence of PPR has now been generated in India and several other countries like Tanjania, Ethiopia, Saudi Arabia, Jordan, North Cameroon etc. (Table 2).The information is likely to provide actual disease status whenever disease control programme is initiated at national level. However, in order to formulate effective disease control strategy, we need to understand the nature of PPR virus and epidemiology of PPR disease in detail.

Table 1 : Manufacturers of PPR vaccines and diagnostics in India

Vaccine/diagnostics manufacturers	Address	Product details
Indian Immunological Limited	Indian Immunological limited, Rakshapur am, Gachibouwli, Hyderab ad-500032, India http://www.indimmune.com	Indian origin "PPRV Sungri 96" Lineage-4 virus
Intervet Schering - Plough Animal Health	Intervet India Pvt Limited, Intervet House 33, Pune-Nagar Road (Behind Eden garden) Pune-411014, India http://www.intervet.co.in	Indian origin "PPRV Sungri 96" Lineage-4 virus
Indian Veterinary Research Institute, Izatnagar	Division of Biological Products Indian Veterinary Research Institute, Izatnagar -243122, India http://www.ivri.nic.in	Indian origin "PPRV Sungri 96" Lineage-4 virus
Indian Veterinary Research Institute, Mukteswar	Division of Virology Indian Veterinary Research Institute, Mukteswar -263138, India http://www.ivri.nic.in	Monoclonal antibody based Competitive-ELISA kit and Sandwich-ELISA kit for PPR antibody and antigen detection

Table 2 : Seroprevalence rate of PPR as determined by competitive-ELISA

Country	Sample size	Seroprevalence rate		
		Goat	Sheep	Average
India (2004)	4407	32.4	36.3	33.0
India (2008)	3560	34.91	41.35	38.13
Tanzania	1549	49.5	39.8	44.6
Saudi Arabia	1958	55.1	36.6	45.8
Jordan	1329	49	29	39.0
North Cameroon		44	29	36.5
Ethiopia	1277	9	13	11
Ethiopia	13651	0-52.5		26.2
Turkey	892	14.9		14.9

2. The Causative Virus of PPR

The causative agent, PPR virus is a member of the genus Morbillivirus, Family Paramyxoviridae and Order Mononegavirales (Tober *et al.* 1998). Other important members of the genus morbillivirus include rinderpest virus (RPV), measles virus (MV) of humans, canine distemper virus (CDV) and phocine distemper virus (PDV). These viruses are pleomorphic particles with a lipoprotein membrane enveloping a ribonucleoprotein core, which contains RNA genome (Haffar *et al.* 1999). The genome of morbilliviruses is a single stranded-RNA, approximately 16 Kilo bases (Kb) long with negative polarity (Haas *et al.* 1995). It is divided into six transcriptional units encoding two non-structural proteins (V, C) and six structural proteins; the surface glycoproteins which include fusion (F) and haemagglutinin (H) proteins, the matrix (M) protein, the nucleoprotein (N), the phosphoprotein (P) which forms the polymerase complex in association with the large (L) protein (Diallo *et al.* 1994). A schematic diagram of a typical morbillivirus and its genome is presented (Fig. 2). The genome sequences of two strains of PPR viruses have been fully elucidated.

The surface glycoproteins, 'H' and 'F' protein, mediate virus attachment and penetration of host cells (Scheid *et al.* 1972). Antibodies to these surface proteins probably play a key role in the development of protective immunity against morbilliviruses (Norrby *et al.* 1986). The 'M' protein of paramyxoviruses forms an inner coat to the viral envelope and thus serves as a bridge between the surface viral glycoproteins and the ribo-nucleoprotein core. By virtue of its position, 'M' appears to play a central role in the formation of new virion, which are liberated from the infected cells by budding. Defects in 'M' proteins have been described which prevent the virus from completing its infectious cycle leading to a persistent non-productive virus infection. Such a phenomenon seems to be involved in some cases of persistent measles virus infection causing sub-acute sclerosing pan encephalitis (SSPE) in man and old dog encephalitis (ODE) due to CDV in persistently infected dog (Carter *et al.* 1983, Baczko *et al.* 1986, Cattaneo *et al.* 1988). No similar disease has been reported with persistence of PPR virus in infected animals. The 'N' protein is the most abundant viral protein and is the major component of nucleocapsid core. It is believed to play a major role in virus transcription and replication (Kingsbury 1990). There is a great interest in utilizing 'N' protein and the 'N' gene for the diagnosis of morbilliviruses. Monoclonal antibodies specific to 'N' protein of PPR virus have been used for detection of viral antigens (Libeau *et al.* 1990, Singh *et al.* 2004a). The 'P' gene of the morbilliviruses is expressed to give rise to three protein products. The full length mRNA is translated to give the 'P' protein. A smaller polypeptide, called 'C' protein is encoded in an alternative open reading frame (ORF). The third protein, 'V' is encoded by a mRNA that differs from primary transcript by having an additional non-templated G residue (Hass *et al.* 1995).

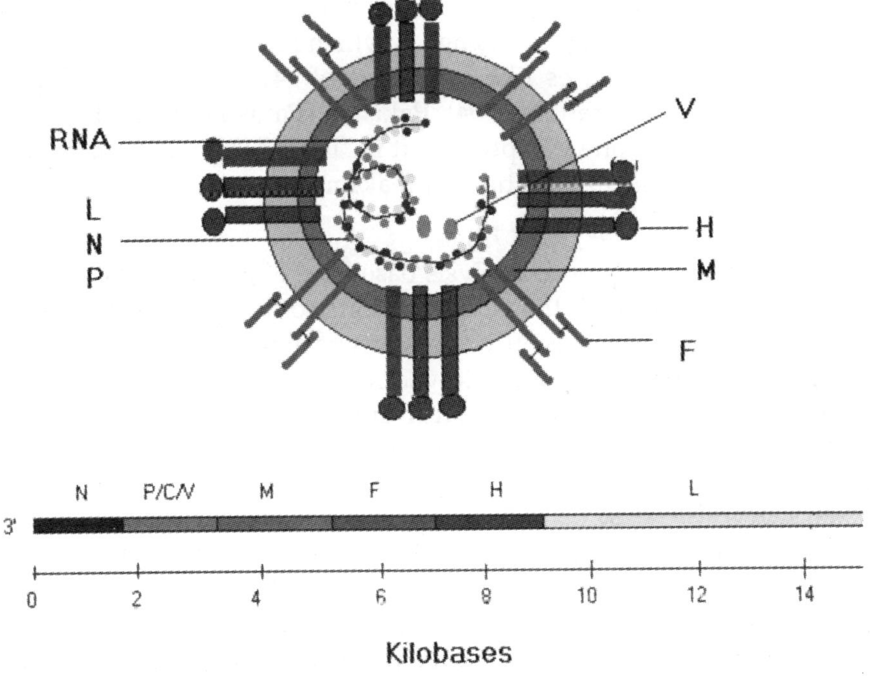

Fig. 2 : Schematic diagram of a Morbillivirus and its genome

3. Epidemiology and Geographic Distribution of PPR

The PPR virus clinically affects goats and sheep. However, outbreaks in other species like Indian buffalo (Govindarajan *et al.* 1997) and zoological collections, which include gazelles, gemsboks have also been reported (Furley *et al.* 1989). Cattle show sub clinical infection and sero-conversion, however the virus does not spread to other in-contact animals. The small ruminants between the age of four months to one year are generally more susceptible to PPR. Before Rinderpest eradication, the epidemiology of PPR was more complicated by the fact that goats and sheep are also susceptible to rinderpest virus, which is antigenically very similar to PPR virus (Forsyth and Barrett 1995). Both rinderpest and PPR have been reported to be endemic in the same geographical area of Africa, Asia and Middle East. Now a days, large-scale vaccination programmes are being established to control PPR outbreaks in several countries where vaccine is available.

Phylogenetic relationship among the PPR virus isolates from different geographical regions of the world have been determined using sequence data derived from part of the 'F' protein gene. Based on phylogeny, four distinct groups, three in Africa and two in Asia have been identified. These include Lineage 1 in West Africa, lineage 2 in Nigeria and Cameroon and lineage 3 in East Africa and lineage 4 in Asia. Based on F gene sequence there is a solitary report of lineage 3 PPR virus (India/TN/92) from southern India. There have been no further reports of lineage 3 virus from India after this. The PPR virus circulating in India belongs to lineage 4, which forms cluster with the viruses from other Asian countries like Israel (Israel 94), Bangladesh (Bangladesh 93), Nepal (Nepal 95), Iran (Iran 94), Pakistan (Pakistan 94) and Saudi Arabia (Saudi 94). However, one exception to it is "India/TN/92", which belongs to lineage 3 (Shaila *et al.* 1996). The outbreaks are more common and severe in goats than sheep.

The nucleotide sequence analysis based on 'F' gene of PPR virus isolated from India reveals that all the isolates belong to lineage 4 (Fig. 3). In spite of the genetic variation, there is only one serotype of the PPR virus. This provides the opportunity for use of a single vaccine to control PPR. Probable global distribution of the PPR virus infection is represented diagrammatically (Roeder and Obi 1999, Dhar *et al.* 2002) in Fig. 4.

3.1 Seroepidemiology

Seroepidemiology is an important indicator for judging the severity and endemic nature of any infectious disease. It provides basic input for launching any disease control programme. Several factors including vaccination campaigns, type of animal husbandry practices and geography of the place may affect the epidemiology of a contagious disease. Information on seroepidemiology/seroprevalence of PPR in different countries is available from the recent studies using state of the art diagnostic techniques (Table 2). Most of these reports indicate an overall seroprevalence of around 30-40%, showing that about a third of the animals are infected and/or recovered.

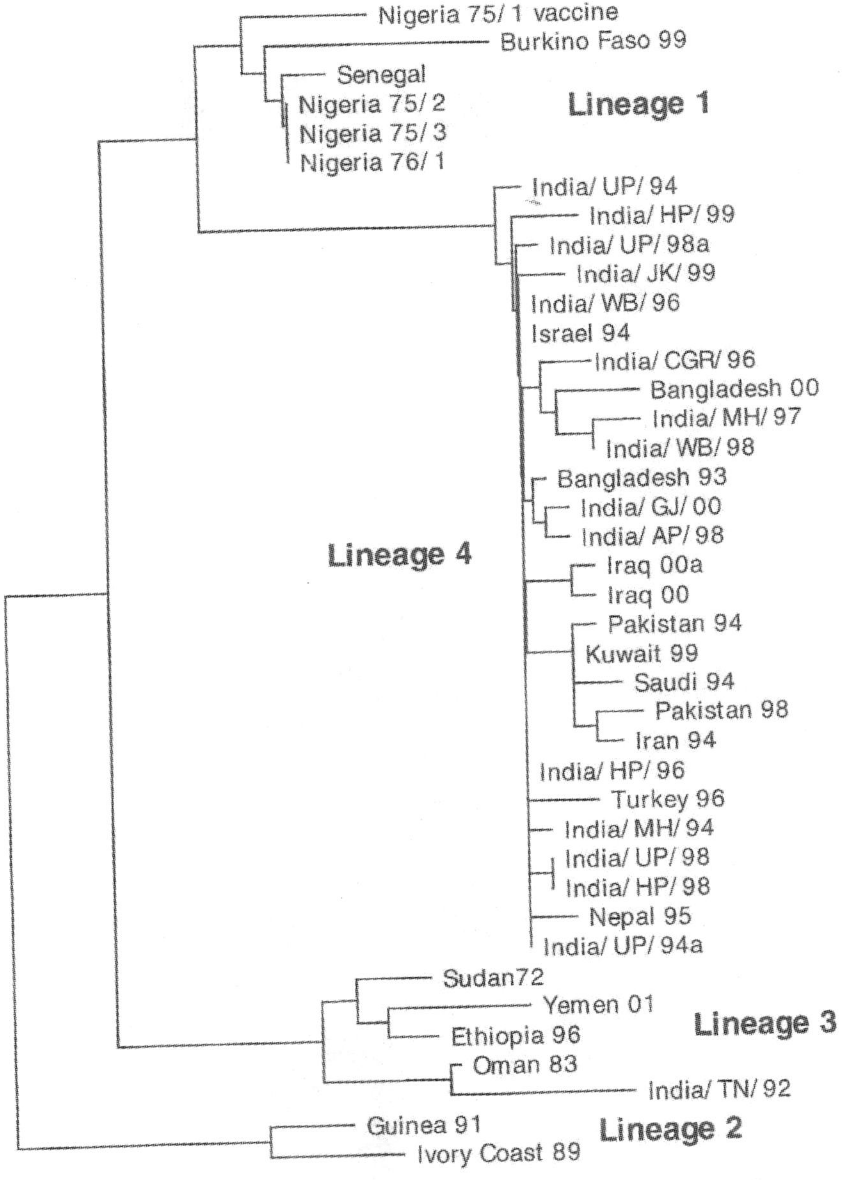

Fig. 3 : Phylogenetic tree of PPR virus isolates from different parts of the world based on part of F gene sequence analysis. All the isolates in India fall under Lineage 4 except "India/TN/92".

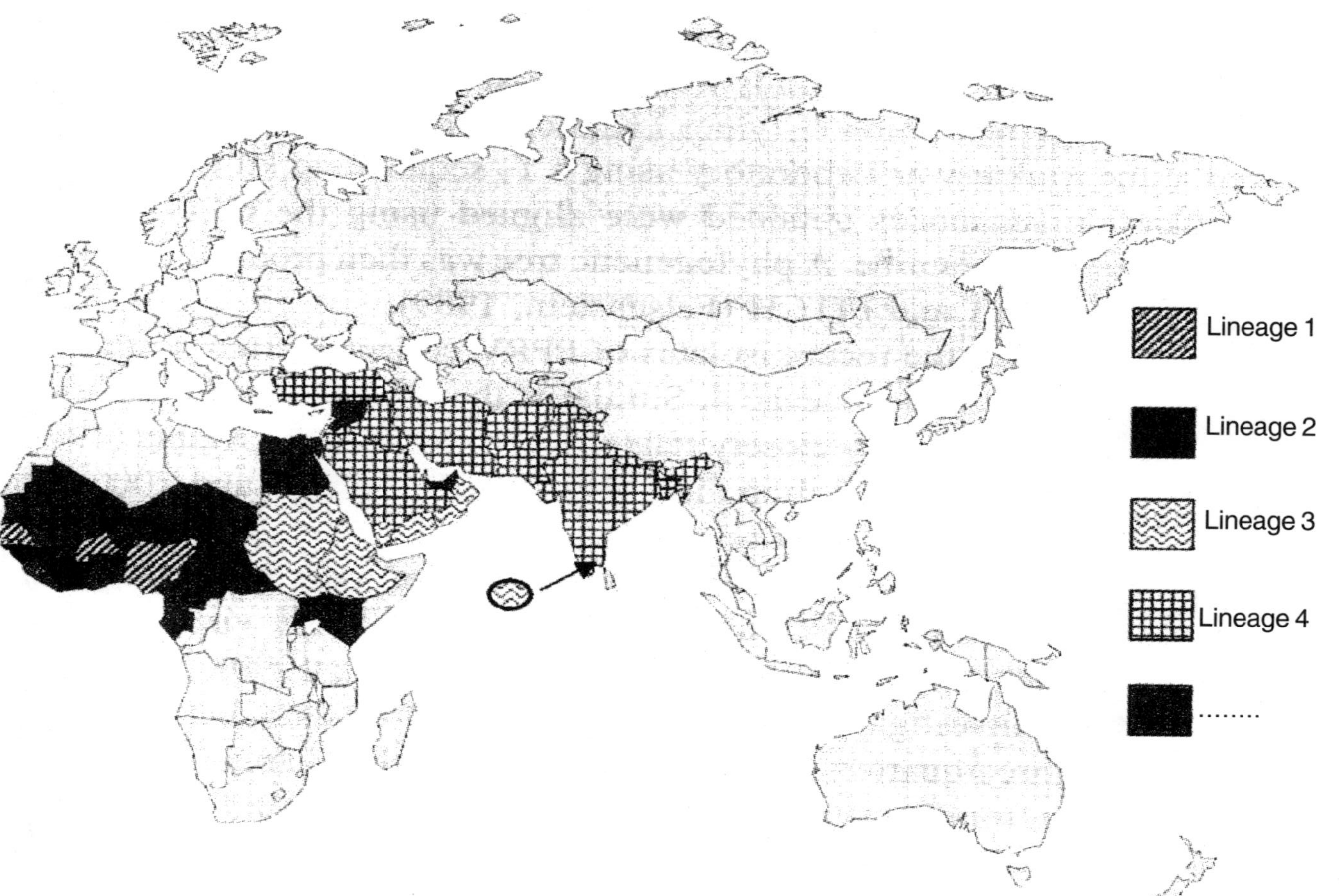

Fig. 4 : Geographical distribution of different lineages of PPR virus

3.2 Strategies for serosurveillance and seromonitoring

Serological survey and monitoring of vaccination response play crucial role in disease control programme. Random sampling method is normally adopted for these activities. Based on the available tools (vaccines and diagnostics), it is difficult to differentiate between the individual vaccinated and infected animals. However, if diagnostic tools are applied carefully in population, it may be possible to differentiate the vaccinated and infected groups.

3.3 Disease situation in India and other Asian and African countries

After the first report of PPR from Tamil Nadu in the year 1987, the disease continued in southern states. The rest of India was taken to be free from infection until 1994, when a series of outbreaks were noticed in almost all parts of the country (Dhar *et al.* 2002, Singh *et al.* 2004c). According to rough estimates, PPR causes an economic loss of Indian rupees 1,800 million (US$ 39 million) every year in the country (Bandyopadhyay 2002, Singh *et al.* 2004c). The estimate is based on the information available in the literature on PPR outbreaks without any laboratory confirmation of the disease outbreaks. The baseline data on prevalence of PPR (Singh *et al.* 2004c) indicates that a third (33% seroprevalence) of the small ruminants are seropositive for PPR virus antibodies. With the availability of baseline data, mortality and case fatality rate of the target population can now be interpolated and actual losses due to PPR in India can be calculated to a more realistic figure. This will effectively justify disease control measures and subsequent eradication programme to convince the policymakers. Government of India has a plan to launch control programme for PPR.

The disease outbreak pattern from 19 Asian and African countries, which reported regular outbreaks to Office International des Epizooties, is shown in Table 3. If we look at the pattern of the disease in India, an increasing trend in PPR outbreaks has been observed from 1996 onwards upto 2004. Number of outbreaks became significantly high after 2002, mainly due to the use of indigenous diagnostic kits which were made available for field use (Singh *et al.* 2004c). Declining pattern of PPR outbreaks was recorded after 2005 in India. This decline seems to be an aftereffect of the mass vaccination carried out from the year 2004 under SCAD (Strengthening and Control of Animal Diseases) programme of Department of Animal Husbandry Dairying and Fisheries, Ministry of Agriculture, Government of India (Fig. 5).

The trend of the disease outbreaks in Nepal, Nigeria, Oman and Iran indicates a more severe pattern up to the year 2001 and subsequently a decline, probably due to mass immunizations.

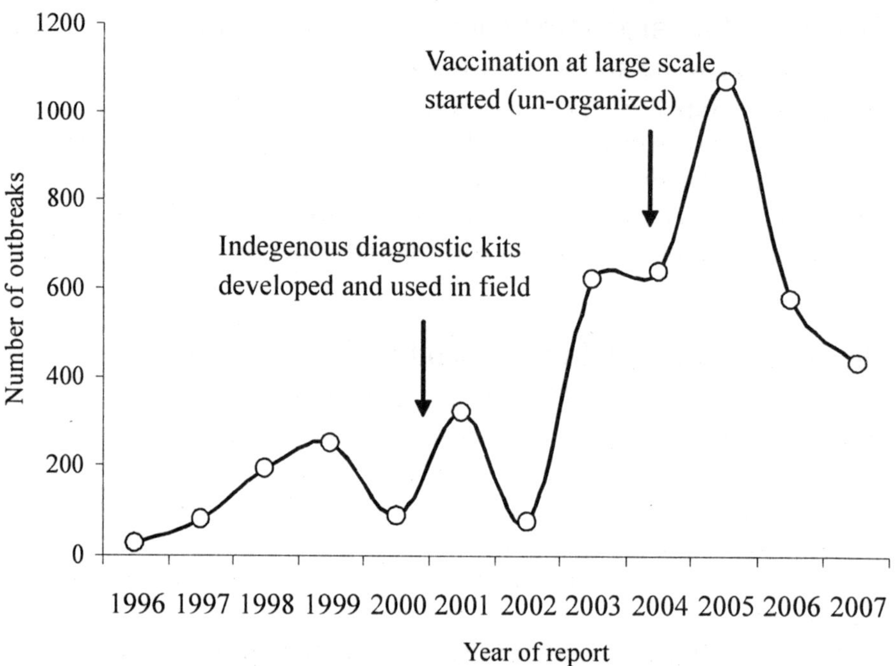

Fig. 5 : Pattern of PPR outbreaks in India. Note that number of reported outbreaks increased sharply after the introduction of PPR diagnostic kits between the years 2001/2002 till 2005. Subsequently number of outbreaks reduced significantly once mass vaccinations were introduced in the year 2004 under a government scheme.

4. Opportunities for the Control of PPR in Global Scenario

We have very good opportunities for control and eradication of PPR in line with Global Rinderpest Eradication Programme (GREP). To achieve this goal, two very potent PPR vaccines are available with the world community, one each using lineage 1 and lineage 4 viruses. The vaccine against lineage 1 uses a Nigerian isolate named "Nigeria 75/1" and the vaccine against lineage 4 uses an Indian isolate named "PPRV/Sungri 96". Both these vaccines are available for mass vaccination campaigns through industries and the government organizations located in different countries across the Asian and African countries (Diallo *et al.* 2004, Singh 2011). Similarly, two monoclonal antibody based diagnostic kits are available one each from the world reference laboratory of PPR, CIRAD-EMVT in France (Libeau *et al.* 1994, 1995) and Indian Veterinary Research Institute (Singh *et al.* 2004a, Singh *et al.* 2004b). These diagnostics have a proven track record for clinical surveillance and serological surveillance, a key inbuilt mechanism for control of these diseases. With the available immunoprophylactics, diagnostics and knowledge of PPR and rich experience on Global Rinderpest Eradication Programme, we can achieve the goal of PPR free country. The availability of biologicals without any constraint will be an added advantage to initiate the control programme. The countries (at least one in the African subcontinent and one in the Indian subcontinent) which have taken lead in research and development on PPR vaccine and diagnostics by their own resources can initiate the control programme, which may act as a model for other countries to take similar initiatives. This will open the door for eradication of PPR in global perspective. The ease in handling of goat and sheep as compared to large ruminants will further simplify the task for vaccination and serological survey of PPR. However, good logistics are required to touch the rural community and to generate high flock or herd immunity.

5. Recent Developments

Very sincere efforts have been made to develop improved vaccines, diagnostics and disease control strategies during the recent years (Diallo 2004, Singh 2011). These include the work on development of thermostable vaccine, chimeric vaccine or marker vaccines (Parida *et al.* 2007) and plant based vaccines. These efforts may lead to simplify control of PPR in future, although with variable results. Thermostable vaccines include the use of deuterium water or use of a suitable vaccine stabilizer and development of a thermostable chimera expressing protective gene of PPR. In addition to this, protective antigen of PPR have also been expressed in plants. Recent diagnostics for PPR include monoclonal antibody based ELISAs using non-infectious source of antigen/expressed proteins and chromatographic strip tests for use in the field conditions (Yadav *et al.* 2009). PCR-ELISA technique may be a good option for sensitive diagnosis of PPR outbreaks during the eradication phase of disease when the status of even a single sample is important. Several countries have been able to reduce the frequency of disease outbreaks using the vaccines and have generated very useful baseline data on the disease status during recent years (Abraham *et al.* 2005, Zahur *et al.* 2008, Raghvendra *et al.* 2008, Waret *et al.* 2008, Swai *et al.* 2009).

6. Challenges in PPR Control and Possible Remedies

Although goat is considered to be poor man's cow, policymakers in the developing countries mainly focus on cattle and buffaloes as main source of milk and meat. Being a disease of sheep and goat only, PPR fails to attract the attention of policymakers. This is likely to limit the financial support for the disease control schemes. Although very potent vaccines are available for disease control, availability of uniform quality of vaccine at the livestock owner's door is another challenging task due to thermolabile nature of the vaccine. Therefore, quality of vaccine must be ensured at two points, firstly at the stage of getting finished product from the manufacturers, and secondly, when the vaccine is being inoculated in the animals in order to ensure that vaccine has not lost its efficacy. In addition to vaccination, effective control of PPR will require quarantine and phytosanitory measures to be enforced strictly when the animal is transported from one place to another. The effective control and eradication of PPR in a country and maintenance of PPR free status in any geographical region will depend on the initiative and interest of the neighboring countries due to porous borders. Sometimes due to poor national policies and civil unrests, it may not be possible to execute the disease control programmes effectively as has been observed with rinderpest in recent past. Under these situations, control of PPR in India may not yield PPR free status if the neighboring countries like Pakistan, Afganistan, Nepal, Myanmar, Bhutan and Bangladesh do not show willingness for a similar disease control programme as all these countries have reported PPR during recent past. Another challenge would be to ensure that there is no PPR in wildlife population through a stringent surveillance mechanism. Any epidemic cycle or chance of reservoir in such population may lead to failure of control and eradication of PPR. In order to culminate the epidemic cycle from all the geographical regions simultaneously, we will have to ensure the use of uniform vaccines and diagnostics throughout the PPR control programme. Under these circumstances quality control of PPR diagnostics is of utmost significance along with the vaccines. It would be advisable to use the vaccine originating from the same lineage as the outbreaks (lineage 4 in South Asia and Lineage 1, 2, 3 in African countries), but not based on availability or convenience. Vaccination, seromonitoring and disease surveillance may require good logistic system to reach the remote areas, especially in the hilly terrains of temperate regions. In some countries, the trained staff for specific purpose is utilized in other activities due to political interference. These practices interfere with the progress and quality of vaccination and disease surveillance process.

The first and foremost step in the control of PPR virus infection in small ruminants in the developing countries should be reduction in the disease intensity by focused and organized vaccinations. This approach may reduce the direct economic losses occurring to small ruminant owners. This strategy will, thus, lead to high public acceptance of the disease control programme. Focused vaccination in high risk groups especially in the areas of high population density is important. Investigations reveal that goats are more susceptible to PPR than sheep (Singh *et al.* 2004c). Goats may, therefore, be preferred for vaccination over sheep where both populations are intermixed, however, sheep population is considered to be equally sensitive in the states like Jammu & Kashmir, Himachal Pradesh, Andhra Pradesh and Rajasthan, where the virus is circulating in the sheep population.

7. Action Plan for PPR Control

In order to develop a comprehensive strategy and the document for control of PPR, a round table conference of experts and experienced personnel needs to be organized at national level. This should be a participatory programme of all the stake holders including policymakers, R&D laboratories, vaccine manufacturers, and the departments responsible for execution of the programmes at ground level. The proceedings of the meeting should be used to develop an action plan based on the recommendations of all stake holders. In order to have uniformity in diagnosis and immunization, quality control of vaccines and diagnostic kits must be ensured from authentic sources. Accordingly national reference laboratories for this purpose must be identified. Sources of poor quality vaccines must be discouraged in vaccination programmes.

7.1 Vaccination strategy

The following strategy for control of PPR in endemic countries like India may be useful to control the disease in the shortest possible time (Singh 2011).

a) Vaccinate all small ruminants indiscriminately with good quality PPR vaccine.

b) Keep the record of vaccinated animals.

c) Vaccinate the newborn kids and lambs at around 6 months of age and keep the record.

d) Monitor the vaccine response using competitive-ELISA test or kit.

e) Evaluate vaccine failures due to improper maintenance of the cold chain and revaccinate entire population especially in winter season to minimize the problem of thermostability of vaccine. Further, explore the possibilities of all vaccination campaigns to be executed in winter season as the vaccine produces lifelong immunity. Vaccination teams will also be comfortable during winter season.

f) Explore the possibility of intermediary host if any involved in the epidemic cycle e.g. wild animals or other domesticated animals. PPR has been reported in buffaloes and gazelles, gemsboks etc. (Furley *et al.* 1987, Govindrajan *et al.* 1997).

g) Also explore the possibilities of so called thermostable vaccines for mass vaccination campaigns using either

i. Thermostable clones of virus

ii. Deuterium/Heavy water as stabilizer

iii. Magnesium sulphate as a component for vaccine stabilizer

The vaccination strategy for reducing the initial disease burden has to be designed very intelligently keeping the sociocultural and socioeconomic factors in mind for a specific area. Sero-surveillance using the competitive-ELISA should not be made an integral part of disease control strategies initially; rather vaccination should be carried out blindly using the available manpower, although a proportion of vaccine used in the pre-exposed animals will be waste. Quality of vaccine and proper vaccination are of utmost significance. Keeping records of vaccination will help to avoid repeated vaccinations, as vaccine produces life long immunity.

7.2 Intensive vaccination

Experiences of vaccination teams and farmers during the first stage of control programme (reduction in disease intensity) should form the basic input for launching intensive vaccinations for greater degree of success of disease control programme. Success in the first stage in the form of reduced "number of outbreaks" and reduced "number of deaths", which add directly to the economy of the livestock farmers, will be the main motivating factor, because PPR alone accounts for a significant proportion of mortality/deaths in goat and sheep population. With the success in reduction of disease intensity and limited control of PPR in endemic zones, mass vaccination campaigns should be launched. India is now self sufficient in quality PPR vaccine production and equipped with modern diagnostics.

7.3 PPR outbreak control

Containment of contagious disease requires a lot of commonsense depending upon the disease situations. Once we experience a PPR outbreak, first and the foremost action should be to segregate the infected population from the healthy stock following all possible phytosanitory measures as per the national regulations. This may include disinfection of the premises, treatment of the diseased animals, and stamping out policies, as the case may be. Some countries like India do not prefer stamping out policies due to socio-religious reasons and public sentiments. Most often vaccination is carried out during the phase of outbreak so as to save the animals which are not infected. These practices sometimes result in spread of the infection due to use of common needles and syringes. Under these situations ring vaccination is the ideal approach for containment of infection. It involves carrying out ring vaccination around the periphery of the outbreak and not in between the outbreak to contain the disease. Expansion of the ring to develop wider zone of immunity is advisable for effective control measures.

Table 3 : Pattern of PPR virus outbreaks during the years 1996 to 2004 in different countries which reported PPR to Office International des Epizooties (OIE).

Country	1996	1997	1998	1999	2000	2001	2002	2003	2004
India	26	81	193	248	86	319	76	623	639
Iran	0	0	0	125	93	240	164	201	71
Israel	0	0	2	2	7	10	0	4	1
Jordan	0	0	3	11	5	0	0	0	0
Nepal	8	13	18	76	344	1035	366	293	12
Oman	0	117	137	116	169	233	81	169	97
Yemen	0	0	0	0	0	32	182	133	36
Benin	18	38	6	65	93	104	51	107	65
Cameroon	3	4	3	7	1	2	2	3	7
Côte d'Ivoire	4	7	7	1	2	2	0	0	1
Eritrea	0	0	9	1	2	3	2	2	3
Ethiopia	12	22	24	1	1	2	5	17	21
Ghana	191	93	73	38	60	76	27	22	33
Guinea	62	46	55	49	64	187	215	165	171
Mali	0	0	1	4	2	1	2	1	1
Niger	9	9	11	1	0	3	3	146	0
Nigeria	0	68	23	94	88	463	139	37	39
Senegal	8	14	17	12	22	9	21	14	6
Togo	0	71	0	0	13	0	205	172	161

Note : declining trend of PPR after 2001 in several countries, probably due to mass immunizations

8. Conclusion

With the available immunoprophylactics in the form of most potent vaccines, diagnostics for mass scale application and knowledge on PPR, world community can achieve the goal of PPR control and eradication. Ease in handling of goat and sheep as compared to large ruminants further simplifies the task of vaccination and serological survey of PPR. Several countries have initiated mass vaccination campaigns, although not in a well organized form with variable success. This needs to be strengthened by systematic approaches of vaccination and sero-monitoring in order to reduce the frequency of outbreaks. The presence of epidemic cycles in animals other than goat and sheep needs to be investigated in order to have effective disease control strategy.

During the last two decades, world scientific community has developed capabilities in the form of potent vaccines, diagnostic kits and base line information on the disease situation in several countries of Asia, Africa and

Middle Eastern regions. These strengths can help us to fight against PPR which disturbs the economy of the poorest of the poor in the society. This is the appropriate time to act for control of PPR globally. The disease control programmes should be one of the important components under poverty alleviation programmes being run by different developing countries. PPR free world can be achieved step by step by reduction in the disease endemicity and intensity by focused vaccinations in high risk population of goat and sheep first, followed by intensive vaccinations. Mass vaccination campaigns should be launched to cover almost entire ovine and caprine population and thereby achieving high flock immunity (70-80%) in order to block the epidemic cycle. With the available tools, national eradication programme on PPR in India may be a successful preposition in line with National Rinderpest Eradication Programme (NPRE). In order to be successful, we need to keep in mind the sociocultural and socioeconomic aspects of goat and sheep owners. We need to be vigilant about the endemic nature of PPR in neighboring countries too. With the coordinated and concerted efforts of all stake holders in combination with the political will and administrative support, the goal of PPR free India is achievable.

References

1. Abraham G, Sintayehu A, Libeau G, Albina E, Roger F, Laekemariam Y, Abayneh D, Awoke KM (2005). Antibody seroprevalences against peste des petits ruminants (PPR) virus in camels, cattle, goats and sheep in Ethiopia. Prev Vet Med 70:51-57.

2. Abu-Elzein EME, Hassanien MM, Al-Afaleq AI, Abd-Elhadi MA, Housawi FMI (1990). Isolation of peste des petits ruminants from goats in Saudi Arabia. Vet Rec 127: 309-310.

3. Baczko K, Liebert VG, Billeter M, Cattaneo R, Budka H, TerMeulen V (1986). Expression of defective measles virus genes in brain tissues of patients with subacute sclerosing panacephalitis. J Virol 59: 472-478.

4. Bandyopadhyay SK (2002). The economic appraisal of a PPR Control Programme in India. XIV annual conference of Indian Virological Society and national seminar on management of viral diseases with emphasis on global trade and WTO regime, January 18-20, 2002, IVRI, Hebbal, Bangalore.

5. Carter MJ, Willcocks MM, TerMeulen V (1983). Defective translation of measles virus protein in a subacute sclerosing panacephalitis. Nature 305:153-155.

6. Cattaneo R, Schmid A, Billeter MA, Sheppared RD, Udem SA (1988). Multiple viral mutations rather than host factors cause defective measles virus gene expression in a subacute sclerosing panacephalitis cell line. J Virol 62:1388-1397.

7. Dhar P, Sreenivasa BP, Barrett T, Corteyn M, Singh RP, Bandyopadhyay SK (2002). Recent epidemiology of peste des petits ruminants virus (PPRV). Veterinary Microbiology 88:153-159.

8. Diallo A (2004). Vaccination for the control of Peste des Petits Ruminants. In: Schudel A, Lombard M (eds) Control of Infectious Animal Diseases by Vaccination. Karger, Basel.

9. Diallo A, Barrett T, Barbron M, Meyer G, Lefevre PC (1994). Cloning of the nucleocapsid protein gene of peste des petits ruminants virus: relationship to other morbilliviruses. J Gen Virol 75:233-237.

10. Diallo A, Taylor WP, Lefevre PC, Provost A (1989). Attenuation d'une souche de la virus de peste des petits ruminants: candidat pour un vaccin homologue vivant. Rev Elev Med Vet Pays Trop 42:311-319.

11. Forsyth M and Barrett T (1995). Detection and differentiation of rinderpest and peste des petits ruminants viruses in diagnostic and experimental samples by polymerase chain reaction using P and F gene-specific primers. Virus Research 39:151-163.

12. Furley CW, Taylor WP, Obi TU (1987) .An outbreak of peste des petits ruminants in a zoological collection. Vet Rec 121:443-447.

13. Gargadennec L, Lalanne A (1942). La peste des petits ruminants. Bulletin des Services Zootechniques et des Epizooties de l'Afrique Occidentale Francaise 5: 16-21.

14. Govindarajan R, Koteeswaran A, Venugopalan AT, Shyam G, Shaouna S, Shaila MS, Ramachandran S (1997). Isolation of pestes des petits ruminants virus from an outbreak in Indian buffalo (*Bubalus bubalis*). Vet Rec 141:573-574.

15. Haas L, Baron MD, Liess B, Barrett T (1995). Editing of morbillivirus P gene transcripts in infected animals. Vet Microbiol 44:299-306.

16. Haffar A, Libeau G, Moussa A, Cecile M, Diallo A (1999). The martix protein gene sequence analysis reveals close relationship between peste des petits ruminants virus (PPRV) and dolphin morbillivirus. Virus Research 64:69-75.

17. Joshi VB, Nagal, KB, Sharma M, Katoch RC, Batta M, Sharma AK, Sharma M (1996). Peste des petits ruminants (PPR) among Gaddi sheep and goats in Himachal Pradesh. Indian J Anim Sci 66:1126-1127.

18. Libeau G, Diallo A, Colas F, Guerre L (1994). Rapid differential diagnosis of rinderpest and peste des petits ruminants using an immunocapture ELISA. Vet Rec 134:300-304.

19. Libeau G, Lefevre PC (1990). Comparison of rinderpest and peste des petits ruminants viruses using anti-nucleoprotein monoclonal antibodies. Vet Microbiol 25:1-15.

20. Libeau G, Prehaud C, Lancelot R, Colas F, Guerre L, Bishop DH, Diallo A (1995). Development of a competitive ELISA for detecting antibodies to the peste des petits ruminants virus using a recombinant nucleoprotein. Res Vet Sci 58:50-55.

21. Norrby E, Utter G, Orvell C and Appel MJG (1986). Protection against canine distemper virus in dogs after immunization with isolated fusion protein. J Virol 58:536-541.

22. Office International des Epizooties. Multiannual animal disease status. http://www.oie.int/hs2/sit_pays_mald_pl.asp?c_pays=88&c_mald=6. Accessed 8 July 2008.

23. Office International des Epizooties. World animal health situation http://www.oie.int/wahis/public.php?page=country_personnel.

24. Parida S, Mahapatra M, Sai Kumar, Das SC, Baron MD, Anderson J, Barrett T (2007). Rescue of a chimeric rinderpest virus with the nucleocapsid protein derived from peste-des-petits-ruminants virus: use as a marker vaccine. J Gen Virol 88:2019-2027.

25. Raghavendra AG, Gajendragad MR, Sengupta PP, Patil SS, Tiwari CB, Balumahendiran M, Sankri V, Prabhudas K (2008). Seroepidemiology of peste des petits ruminants in sheep and goats of southern peninsular India. Rev Sci Tech 27:861-867.

26. Roeder PL, Obi TU (1999). Recognising peste des petits ruminants. A field manual. FAO, Rome.

27. Saravanan P, Singh RP, Balamurgan V, Dhar P, Sreenivasa BP, Muthuchelvan D, Sen A, Aleyay AG, Singh RK, Bandyopadhyay SK (2004). Development of a N gene-based PCR-ELISA for Detection of Peste-des-Petits-Ruminants virus in clinical samples. Acta Virologica 48:249-255.

28. Scheid A, Caliguiri LA, Compans RW, Choppin PW (1972). Isolation of paramyxovirus glycoproteins. Association of both haemagglutinating and neuraminidase activities with the larger SV5 glycoprotein. Virology 50:640-652.

29. Shaila MS, Purushothaman V, Bhavasar D, Venugopal K, Venkatesan RA (1989). Peste des petits ruminants in India. Vet Rec 125:602.

30. Shaila MS, Shamaki D, Forsyth MA, Diallo A, Goatley L, Kitching RP, Barrett T (1996). Geogrphic distribution of peste des petits ruminants viruses. Virus Research 43:149-153.

31. Singh RP (2011). Control strategies for *Peste des petits ruminants* in small ruminants of India. Rev sci tech Off int Epiz (In Press).

32. Singh RP, Sreenivasa BP, Dhar P, Bandyopadhyay SK (2004a). A sandwich ELISA for the diagnosis of *peste des petits ruminants* (PPR) infection in small ruminants using anti-nucleocapsid protein monoclonal antibody. Archives of Virology 149(11):2155-2170.

33. Singh RP, Sreenivasa BP, Dhar P, Shah LC, Bandyopadhyay SK (2004b). Development of monoclonal antibody based competitive-ELISA for detection and titration of antibodies to *peste des petits ruminants* virus. Vet Microbiol 98:3-15.

34. Singh RP, Saravanan P, Sreenivasa BP, Singh RK, Bandyopadhyay SK (2004c). Prevalence and distribution of *peste des petits* ruminants (PPR) virus infection in small ruminants of India. Rev sci tech Off int Epiz 23(3):807-819.

35. Sreenivasa BP, Dhar P, Singh RP, Bandyopadhyay SK (2000). Evaluation of an indigenously developed homologous live attenuated cell culture vaccine against *peste des petits ruminants* infection of small ruminants. In: Proceedings of the XX annual conference of Indian Association of Veterinary Microbiologists, Immunologists and Specialists in Infectious Diseases and national symposium on trends in vaccinology for animal diseases, Pantnagar, India, 84 pp.

36. Swai ES, Kapaga A, Kivaria F, Tinuga D, Joshua G, Sanka P (2009). Prevalence and distribution of Peste des petits ruminants virus antibodies in various districts of Tanzania. Vet Res Commun (In Press).

37. Tober C, Seufert M, Schneider H, Billeter MA, Johnston IC, Niewiesk S, Ter Meulen V, Schneider-Schaulie S (1998). Expression of measless virus V protein is associated with pathogenicity and control of viral RNA synthesis. J Virol 72:8124-8132.

38. Waret-Szkuta A, Roger F, Chavernac D, Yigezu L, Libeau G, Pfeiffer DU, Guitián J. Peste des petits ruminants (PPR) in Ethiopia (2008). Analysis of a national serological survey. BMC Vet Res 12:4:34.

39. Yadav V, Balamurugan V, Bhanuprakash V, Sen A, Bhanot V, Venkatesan G, Riyesh T, Singh RK (2009). Expression of Peste des petits ruminants virus nucleocapsid protein in prokaryotic system and its potential use as a diagnostic antigen or immunogen. J Virol Methods 162:56-63.

40. Zahur AB, Irshad H, Hussain M, Ullah A, Jahangir M, Khan MQ, Farooq MS (2008). The epidemiology of peste des petits ruminants in Pakistan. Rev Sci Tech 27: 877-884.

□□□

Chapter 16

Bluetongue Control : Indian Perspective

GAYA PRASAD[1] AND MINAKSHI[2]
[1]Indian Council of Agricultural Research, New Delhi-110001
[2]Department of Animal Biotechnology, College of Veterinary Sciences, Lala Lajpat Rai University of Veterinary & Animal Sciences, Hisar-125004

Contents

1. Introduction

Historically, bluetongue (BT) can be traced back to 1876 when it was for the first time noticed in South Africa in sheep imported from Europe. As there was no earlier record of such a disease in native breeds of sheep in South Africa, it was recognized as a new disease and named bluetongue due to cyanotic (bluish color) tongue in the affected exotic sheep. Since then BT has spread to other parts of the world through the movement of the virus-infected animals and insect vectors or due to importation of live vaccines. It is now one of the most important ruminant diseases affecting susceptible domestic and wild ruminants in tropical, semi-tropical and temperate regions of the world. Sheep is the most susceptible ruminant species for clinical BT, though there may be variation in susceptibility amongst different breeds of sheep.

The host range of bluetongue virus (BTV) is quite diverse including sheep, cattle, buffalo, goats, camel, mithun and several species of wild ruminants. In addition, BTV has also been recognized as a potential pathogen of carnivores. Serologic evidence of BTV infection has been demonstrated in several species of African wild carnivores including lions. This clearly demonstrates that the host range of BTV appears to be much larger than previously believed. Owing to its global economic importance, the World Organisation for Animal Health (OIE) has classified BT as notifiable disease, due to which mandatory restrictions are imposed on the movement of ruminants, their germplasm, embryos and other animal products from BT-endemic countries to BT-free countries. Recent outbreaks of BT in European countries have indicated the possible impact of climate change on the spread of vector and BTV to the regions where BT was not reported earlier.

Huge antigenic and genetic diversity of BTV, diverse domestic and wild ruminant host range and involvement of insect vectors in transmission of infection make its control a complicated task. Any strategy that aims at controlling BT in any geographic region should effectively address the multiplicity of virus serotypes, host and the vector. Apart from the selection of relatively resistant breeds and improving husbandry practices to minimize the exposure of animals to the competent vectors, such strategies should include vaccination of susceptible animals and effective management of *Culicoides* vector. Traditionally vaccination of animals has been the best way to minimize economic loss to the livestock industry taking into consideration the environmental concerns involved in using chemicals for vector control.

In India, BT is endemic and causes significant economic loss to the livestock sector every year. Owing to its economic importance, the Indian Council of Agricultural Research started an All India Network Programme on BT with 11 centres located in different regions of the country to understand the diversity of virus serotypes and the vector prevalent on regional basis and accordingly develop vaccine and diagnostics for its control.

2. Indian Scenario

India is a geographically vast country having diverse geo-climatic zones. The country has huge population of domestic and wild ruminants, which are susceptible to BTV infection. Over the past six decades, several exotic breeds of sheep and cattle have been introduced in the country for improvement of indigenous stock through crossbreeding (Prasad 2000). The number of animals susceptible to BTV infection is far greater now than in the early 1960s, when the first outbreak of BT was observed in indigenous and exotic breeds of sheep in Maharashtra (Sapre 1964). Since then, the outbreaks of BT have been reported from different parts of the country wherein the evidence of prevalence of 22 out of the 25 known serotypes of BTV has been recorded (Prasad *et al.* 2009).

2.1 Seasonality and geographic distribution

India lies between 8.4° to 37.6° N and 68.7° and 97.3° E and is comprised of five distinct geographic zones including the northern mountains, northern plains, great plateau, coastal plains and Indian desert (Prasad *et al.* 2009). Though broadly the climate of India has been classified into tropical, subtropical and temperate, predominantly it is tropical monsoon type. Rain-fed areas including the costal regions of Andhra Pradesh, Karnataka, Kerala and Tamil Nadu, where land is used for cultivation of rice, experience relatively more outbreaks of BT than the drier regions of the country. Variations in temperature and rainfall occur not only from season to season, but also from place to place. Some regions have hot summers and cold winters, while others have almost the same climate throughout the year (Prasad *et al.* 2009).

BT has been reported from different parts of India including northern states (Haryana, Himachal Pradesh, Jammu and Kashmir, Punjab, Rajasthan and Uttar Pradesh) and central (Madhya Pradesh), western (Gujarat and Maharashtra) and southern areas (Andhra Pradesh, Karnataka, Kerala and Tamil Nadu). In the north-eastern region, serological evidence of prevalence of BT exists but clinical BT has not yet been reported. Most of the annual BT outbreaks in the country are recorded during or immediately after monsoon season. The number of adult vectors in the southern India reaches a peak during the monsoon season. Outbreaks of BT in Karnataka, Tamil Nadu and Andhra Pradesh have been associated with the periods of peak *Culicoides* activity (Sreenivasulu *et al.* 2004). Though extensive studies have not been conducted in northern India with regard to *Culicoides* vector abundance, the authors have observed that prevalence of the vector is very high during monsoon in Haryana and Punjab.

2.2 Clinical bluetongue outbreaks

Since the first clinical BT outbreak reported by Sapre (1964) in Maharashtra, the disease outbreaks have been recorded in different parts of the country which have been extensively reviewed by Prasad *et al.* (2009). Morbidity and mortality in these outbreaks ranged from 10 to 80%. Clinical BT is now reported annually in native and exotic breeds of sheep in Andhra Pradesh, Karnataka, Tamil Nadu and Maharashtra, although it has rarely been reported in native sheep breeds in the northern Indian states where BT outbreaks have mainly occurred in exotic and crossbred animals. The clinical picture of BT in native sheep in the north also appears to be slightly different from that in the south; the major difference being that swelling of lips and face is less conspicuous though the mucocutaneous borders are very sensitive to touch and bleed easily on handling. The classical signs of cyanosis of the tongue and reddening of the coronary band are uncommon in both northern and southern Indian sheep breeds (Prasad *et al.* 2009), however, the authors noticed inflammation and reddening of coronary band quite often in BT affected Rambouillet breed of sheep imported from Texas in Haryana (Fig. 1).

BT is characterized by high rise of body temperature (105-108°C), inflammation of face, oral lesions and inflammation and reddening of coronary bands of the affected exotic breeds of sheep. Severely affected sheep show arched back (Fig. 2) and is disinclined to move due to inflammation of coronary bands. In acute cases, dramatic increase in respiration rate is often observed. A nasal discharge, which is at first watery and later mucopurulent and in some cases blood stained, appears and eventually dries out to form crusts (Fig. 3). Nose gets often occluded by a grayish-brown scab composed of desquamated epithelium and inspissated serum along with excoriation of lower lip. Swelling of face, muzzle, nostrils and upper and lower lips (Fig. 4), oedema of tongue, and hyperaemia of upper and lower lips are also observed. In some cases tongue protrudes out of mouth.

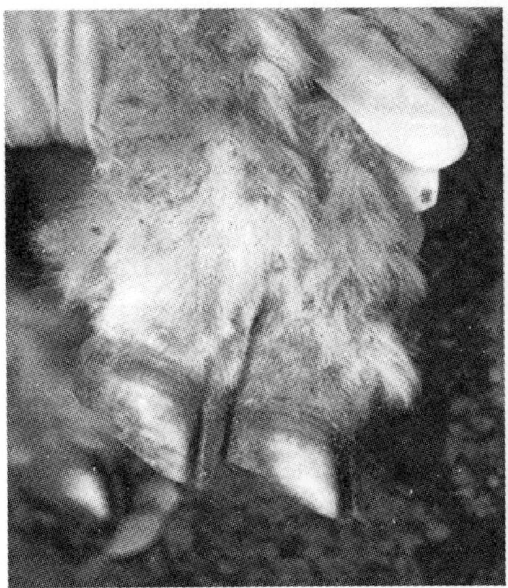

Fig. 1 : Bluetongue-affected exotic Rambouillet sheep with inflammation and reddening of coronary bands

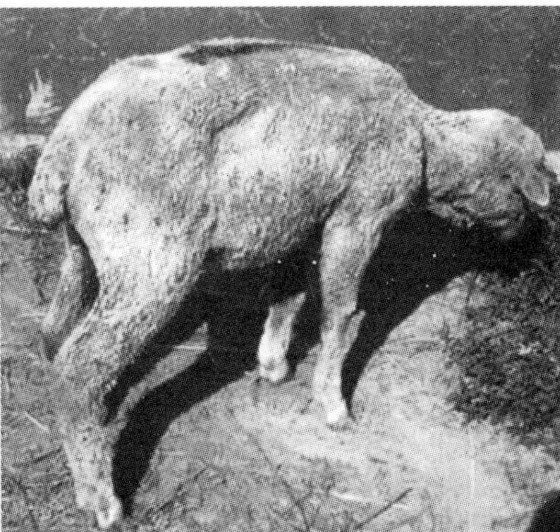

Fig. 2 : Bluetongue-affected exotic Rambouillet sheep with classical arch back

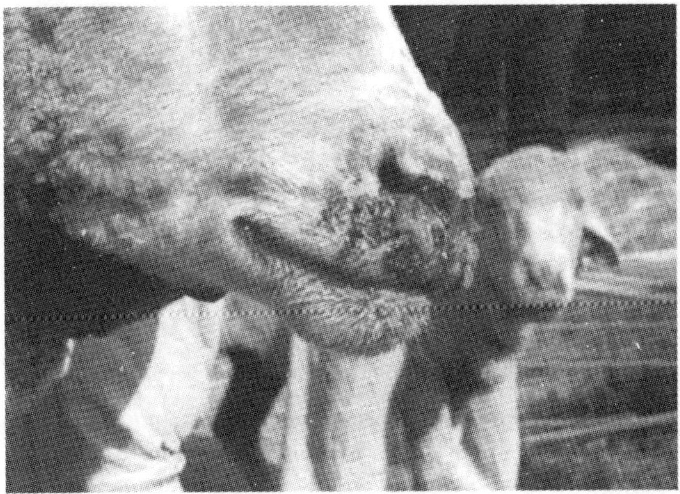

Fig. 3 : Bluetongue-affected exotic Rambouillet sheep exhibiting blood stained and dried nasal discharge in the form of crusts

Excoriation of the epithelium of gums, the inner side of the lips and cheeks, the bars of the hard palate and the dental pad occurs in later stages of infection. Careful examination of feet of the affected sheep may reveal inflammation and reddening of coronary band that may be observed more frequently in hind feet (Fig. 1). Due to inflammation of coronary band, the affected sheep shows lameness. No correlation between oral lesions and feet lesions has been observed. BT affected sheep sometimes also shows cracking of skin. BTV infection can also cause reproductive losses in the animals that have been mainly attributed to abortions, foetal malformations and stillbirths.

3. Etiologic Agent

BT is caused by the virus having 10 segmented double stranded RNA genome. It belongs to the genus *Orbivirus* in the family *Reoviridae*. Of the 25 serotypes prevalent all over the world, 22 serotypes have been reported from different states (11 each on the basis of virus isolation and neutralizing antibodies). The serotype-wise prevalence of BTV in different states of India is presented in Table 1. The largest number of BTV serotypes has been reported from Tamil Nadu, followed by Maharashtra and Gujarat. Serotype 22, 24, and newly identified serotype 25 have not been so far reported in India.

The viral genome encodes 7 structural proteins (VP1-VP7) and three nonstructural proteins (NS1, NS2, NS3, NS3a). The virus genome is surrounded by double layer proteins called outer capsid and inner capsid. The outer capsid is composed of predominantly VP2 and VP5 proteins which invoke neutralizing immune response, hence important for protection. VP2 has been identified as a major determinant of serotype specificity. Therefore, this protein has been targeted for development of recombinant vaccines. The inner capsid is composed of VP1, VP3, VP4, VP6 and VP7. VP7 protein along with nonstructural protein has been identified as group specific and is largely conserved across the serotypes. Due to this, group specific antibodies as well as nucleic acid based assays have been developed and are being used for diagnosis of BTV. Due to shared epitopes with epizootic haemorrhagic disease (EHDV), VP7 based assays are being replaced by NS1 protein/gene based diagnostics.

4. Vector

BTV is transmitted by several species of *Culicoides* midges in different geographic regions of the world. Amongst more than 40 species of *Culicoides* observed in India, *C. peregrinus*, *C. oxystoma* and *C. imicola* are reported to have potential to transmit BTV. The involvement of *Culicoides* species in the transmission of BTV in India was indicated by virus isolation from adult insects in Haryana (Jain *et al.* 1988), although the species was not identified. The presence of *C. schultzei*, *C. peregrinus* and *C. actoni* (known BTV vectors elsewhere in the world) was subsequently reported in Marathwada region of Maharashtra state (Narladakar *et al.* 1993). *Culicoides oxystoma* was also identified in the animal farms where BTV seroconversions had occurred (Bhatnagar *et al.* 1997). On this basis, it was suggested that *C. oxystoma* could be a vector for BTV in India. Moreover, *C. oxystoma* was repeatedly trapped near sentinel herds/flocks in Punjab, Haryana, Himachal Pradesh and Rajasthan, indicating a close association with sheep and cattle. There were also continuing seroconversions in these herds, further supporting the hypothesis that *C. oxystoma* (Fig. 5) is a BTV vector in India (Kakker *et al.* 1996, Bhatnagar *et al.* 1997). However, final confirmation would require virus isolation from *C. oxystoma* and experimental transmission of virus to susceptible animals.

It is now well known that environmental temperature plays important role in vector competence besides other factors. BTV development in *Culicoides* vectors is unable to occur at temperatures below 10-15°C depending on the serotype. Furthermore, there needs to be a minimum amount of time at suitable temperature (expressed as 'day degrees or hour degrees') for completion of the development cycle in *Culicoides* vector before the virus transmission can occur. This 'physiological' time is the cumulative product of virus development time multiplied by the temperature in degrees above the threshold for virus replication. Increasing environmental temperature (climate change) is also likely to extend the vector season. In addition, within the range of temperatures over which BTV development can occur, the levels of vector competence of a *Culicoides* vector population for some BTV serotypes increases linearly with temperature and so the impact of warmer temperatures may be even greater. Temperature can also affect the competence of 'non-vector' *Culicoides* species. For example, *C. nubeculosus* generally is considered to be incapable of transmitting BTV due to a mid-gut infection barrier. However, exposure of the immatures to rearing temperatures close to their upper lethal limit (33-35°C) can result in >10% of adults becoming competent to transmit BTV. It is likely that the integrity of the gut wall of some adults is damaged by the extreme rearing temperatures, thereby allowing virus particles to bypass the mid-gut barriers, enter the haemocoel and develop as in a normal vector.

Due to the presence of several diverse ecological zones with different climatic conditions in India, it is considered likely that different *Culicoides* species are involved in BTV transmission in different areas (Prasad *et al.* 2009). The rise in global temperature may have far-reaching consequences in the prevalence of competent vectors and their BTV transmission potential in India.

5. Diagnosis

BT can be easily diagnosed on the basis of typical clinical signs and symptoms such as pyrexia, swelling of muzzle, oral lesions, coronitis (Fig. 1), stiffness of limbs and in some cases oedema of head and neck (Fig. 4). However, detection of unapparent cases of BT is difficult. Such cases and the certification of animals for import and export require laboratory testing for diagnosis. Antibody based tests such as agar gel immunodiffusion test, monoclonal antibody based competitive enzyme linked immunosorbent assay (cELISA), dot immunobinding assay or dipstick-ELISA are used. Nucleic acid based assays such as reverse transcription polymerase chain reaction (RT-PCR) and real time RT-PCR (rRT-PCR) have been developed during the past few years and are now in use in several countries including India.

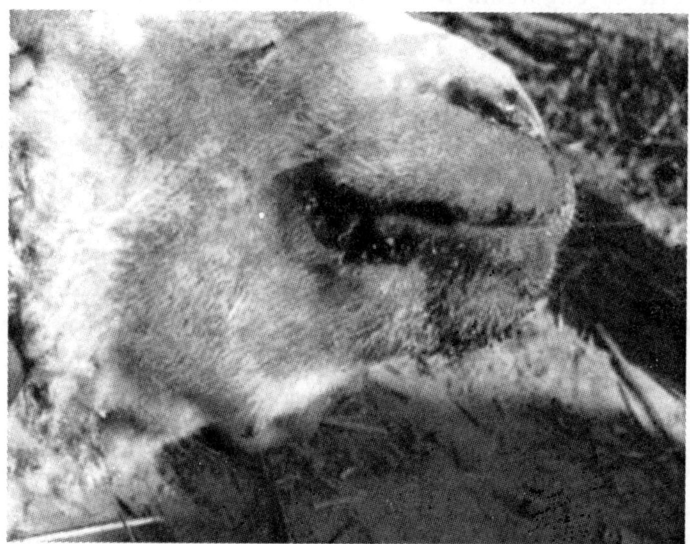

Fig. 4 : Bluetongue-affected exotic Rambouillet sheep exhibiting oedema of face

The tests for specific diagnosis of BTV infection are of generally three types viz. (i) virus isolation in susceptible chicken embryo, animal or tissue culture; (ii) tests to demonstrate the presence of viral antibodies or viral antigen; and (iii) the test to demonstrate the presence of viral nucleic acid. The conventional diagnosis usually involves isolation of virus or detection of specific antibodies in the serum of convalescent animals.

5.1 Virus isolation

Despite the explosion of new technologies for same day diagnosis of viral diseases by demonstration of virus, viral antigen or viral nucleic acid in specimens taken directly from the animal, it is still true to say that few of them achieve quite the sensitivity of virus isolation in embryonated chicken eggs (ECE) or cell culture. BTV can be isolated from blood, semen and various other tissue samples including liver, spleen, brain, lymph nodes and mucosal epithelium. The cells in fresh blood samples (with EDTA to prevent clotting) can be washed to remove humoral neutralising antibodies, thereby improving the chances of successful virus isolation. BTV isolation has been performed by inoculation of ECE effectively via an intravenous route. Sheep inoculation and cerebral inoculation of suckling mouse brains have also been used for BTV isolation. After initial isolation (e.g. by passage in ECE), the virus is usually adapted to mammalian cell lines such as BHK-21 or Vero cells, or insect cell line. Cells of insect origin, e.g. *Aedes albopictus* cells - C6-36 or *C. sonorensis* cells – KC, can also be used for primary isolation of BTV directly from biological samples including blood, tissues and insect vectors (Mertens *et al.* 2009).

Theoretically at least, a single viable virus present in a specimen can be grown in cultured cells, thus expanding it many fold to produce enough viral antigen. Virus isolation remains the gold standard and must be compared with other available methods. Initially sheep inoculation was used as the diagnostic method for BTV but subsequently the developing chicken embryo has been successfully used for isolation of the virus.

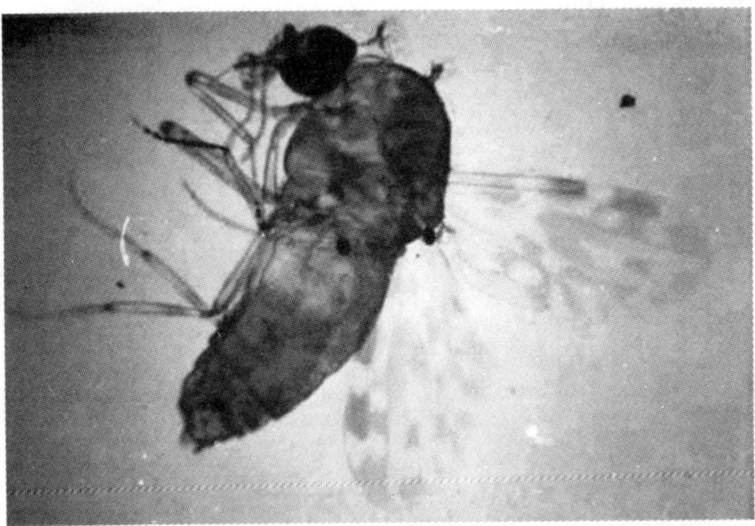

Fig. 5 : *Culicoides oxystoma* trapped from northern India

The isolation of virus from the clinical specimens is most reliable classical way of confirmatory diagnosis of BTV. There is no optimal protocol for the isolation of the virus. The chance of isolating BTV depends critically on the attention given by the attending clinician or veterinarian to the collection of the specimen. Clearly, such specimens must be taken from the right place at the right time. The right time is as soon as possible after the animal first develops clinical signs evidenced by high rise of temperature because at about this time, the virus is present in maximum number in blood circulation that subsequently declines. Inoculation of the suspected clinical material in susceptible sheep, suckling mice, ECE and a variety of vertebrate and non-vertebrate insect cell lines have been used for isolation of the virus. ECE after BTV infection shows stunting growth with oedema and haemorrhages all over the body (Fig. 6). The cell lines used for isolation of the virus include BHK-21, Vero, KC and C6-36.

5.2 Detection of virus and its antigens

Since the virus isolation is time consuming and laborious, direct detection of the virus and its antigens in clinical specimens provides a rapid means of diagnosis. The commonly employed assays include immunoperoxidase, immunofluorescence and enzyme immunoassays. Avidin-biotin immunoperoxidase procedure with more specificity has also been used to detect BTV antigens in the tissues of BTV infected calves. Electron microscopy is perhaps the most obvious method of virus detection by direct visualization of the virus itself. This has also been useful in tracking the BTV, BTV like particles and BTV antigens in infected tissue culture cells and other type of cells infected *in vivo* (Fig. 7).

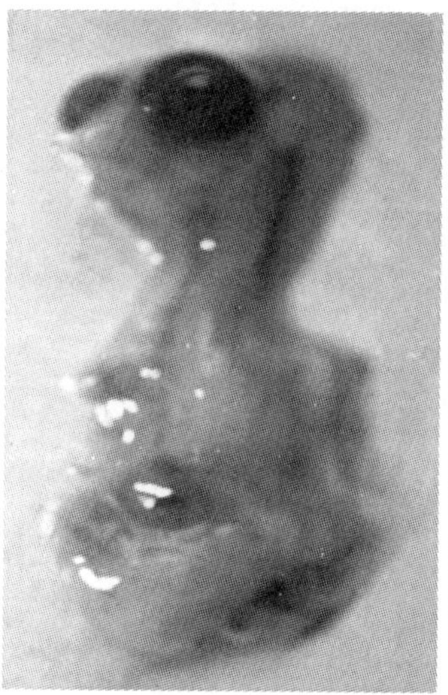

Fig. 6 : Chicken embryo inoculated with BTV positive sample, showing stunting of growth and generalized haemorrhages

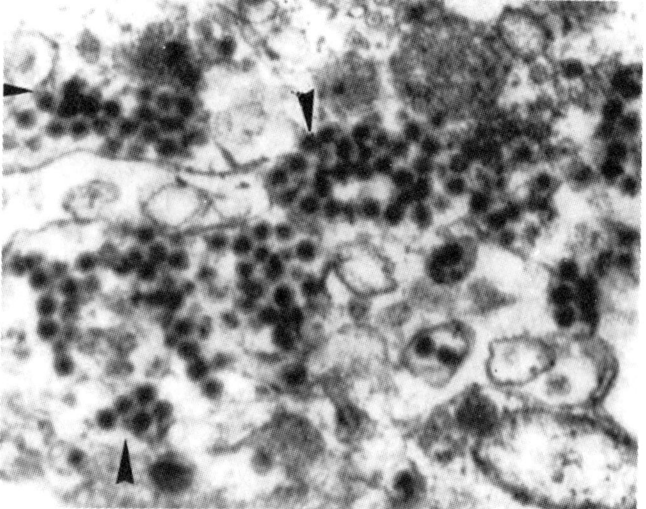

Fig. 7 : BTV-infected BHK-21 cells exhibiting several virus particles in the cell-cytoplasm by transmission electron microscopy

5.3 Detection of anti-viral antibodies

Presumptive diagnosis of BTV infection has been made by serological tests rather than by isolation and identification of virus. Serological tests have played an important role in determining the distribution of BTV infections and these are the primary methods used to certify animals for export/import. Detection of BTV antibodies is based on group reactive tests and the serotype specific neutralisation tests. A number of traditional serological methods such as agar gel immunodiffusion (AGID) test, counter current immuno-electrophoresis, complement fixation, fluorescent antibody tests etc. have been used. The serological tests used to detect BTV antibodies are of two types viz. group specific and serotype specific. Serum neutralization test (SNT) and haemagglutination inhibition test are serotype specific. Of the two, SNT is the most widely used test.

Tests devised for the detection of group specific antibodies include AGID test, complement fixation test, dot-immunobinding assay (Naresh *et al.* 1996), ELISA and c-ELISA (Naresh and Prasad 1995). All these tests are based on the detection of major inner core group specific protein VP7 that is highly conserved and reacts with antisera against all the known serotypes of BTV. The reports that AGID test failed to detect antibodies in a significant number of animals that were positive for BTV, and the problems of cross-reactivity suggested that the most likely serological test to replace AGID is ELISA. Dot-immunobinding assay has been found quite sensitive as compared to AGID and SNT in the authors' laboratory.

A rapid IgM class specific antibody assay based diagnosis of BTV can be made on the basis of a single acute phase serum by demonstrating virus specific antibody of IgM class. IgM antibodies, which appear early after infection and drop within 3 months, are usually indicative of recent infection. The most common method used is the IgM antibody capture assay, in which the viral antigen is bound on a solid phase substrate, say a microtitre well.

5.4 Nucleic acid based assays

Over the past one decade there has been an explosion of information on the BTV genome and this has enabled development of nucleic acid based diagnostic techniques that are more rapid and sensitive. These techniques rely not on the isolation and identification of a live replicating virus but on the detection of highly specific molecular subunits of the virus in infected tissues and clinical specimens. These subunits could be either gene sequences specific for BTV or certain serotypes. Obviously, direct detection of viral nucleic acid from infected cells or insect vector is more efficient diagnostic approach. For the detection of virus specific nucleic acids, RNA electrophoresis, cDNA/RNA blot hybridisation and RT-PCR have been developed using the knowledge of BTV genome and recombinant DNA technology.

The use of RT-PCR for detection of BTV eliminates detection of closely related Epizootic hemorrhagic disease virus (EHDV). RT-PCR could be used for detection of BTV in semen and embryos also. Various RT-PCR protocols have been developed targeting different genes of the virus. In the authors' laboratory, the sensitivity of the RT-PCR for detection of cell culture grown BTV was determined upto 10 infectious virus particles using NS1 gene specific primers.

Multiplex RT-PCR is based on the basic principle of RT-PCR. In this method, two or more primers pair sets specific for different target sequences are included in the same amplification reaction. Co-amplification of several target sequences is more cost-effective where multiple serotypes of a pathogen or different pathogens are possible etiological agents. In this procedure, a large number of samples can be subjected to RT-PCR in a specifically designed plate. Using the multiplex RT-PCR product detection kits, the result of the amplification can be read directly after completion of the RT-PCR. In this process, running of gel for detection is not necessary. Hence, multiplex RT-PCR appears to be very useful in processing a large number of samples at a time and can be used for detection of multiple pathogens. Multiplex RT-PCR is being used in epidemiological investigations for a variety of bacterial and viral pathogens. The availability of commercial kits for conducting multiplex RT-PCR will expand its application in future. Group specific Real Time RT-PCR has also been developed for very quick detection of BTV in clinical samples. In addition to it, serotype specific Real Time RT-PCR assays are being developed.

6. Vaccines

Owing to huge antigenic diversity, as evident from the global circulation of 25 different serotypes, developing an effective vaccine that protects against all the known serotypes has been a daunting task. International research and development efforts have lead to the formulation of conventional (attenuated and inactivated) and some recombinant technology based vaccines. An ideal BTV vaccine should have the following features:

- Protective against all serotypes of BTV present in a geographical region
- Safe for use in all susceptible animals including pregnant ones
- Free from risk of reverting back to virulence
- Permits discrimination of vaccinated from the naturally infected animals
- Economical production
- Thermostability

Merits and demerits of conventional as well as recombinant vaccines are very briefly described below.

6.1 Attenuated vaccines

Since BT was first discovered in Africa, most of the earlier efforts for development of BTV vaccines have been made in this continent. The South

African scientists have pioneered the development and production of attenuated live BTV vaccines because of their historic experience with BT through several decades. In earlier studies, the field viruses were passaged upto 80 times in ECE. However, recent work has suggested that 20-50 passages either in ECE or BHK-21 cell line is adequate to render the virus avirulent (Johnson *et al.* 1992). The attenuation process selects viruses that adapt to grow *in vitro* and have decreased ability to grow in sheep and cause clinical disease. Lower passage level viruses induce strong immune response but retain the capability to cause clinical manifestation whereas too many passages *in vitro* generate viruses that do not result in clinical disease and induce poor protective immune response (Murray and Eaton 1996).

Live attenuated vaccines are very effective in controlling clinical outbreaks of BT in endemic areas and in face of the outbreaks. Only one dose is sufficient to induce protective immune response against homologous challenge. Such attenuated BTV vaccines have been extensively used in Africa and Middle East resulting in dramatic reduction in economic losses due to BT. Presently in South Africa, sheep are vaccinated with 3 pentavalent attenuated BTV vaccines composed of 15 different serotypes at three weeks intervals. The immunized sheep are thus exposed to 15 live attenuated serotypes of BTV in a period of 6 weeks (Schultz and Grieder 1987).

The attenuated BT vaccines suffer from several drawbacks as compared to the inactivated alternatives. Firstly, attenuated strains of Australian serotypes have been shown to be teratogenic. Secondly, following vaccination and during viraemia, attenuated viruses may shed in semen of vaccinated bulls and rams. Thirdly, the attenuated virus strains could be transmitted by *Culicoides* midges as natural viruses. It is known that homologous and heterologous serotypes readily reassort and the progeny viruses may contain random combination of parentral genes (Sugiyama *et al.* 1982, de Mattos *et al.* 1991). Thus, the ability of BTV to mutate or reassort *in vitro* and *in vivo* conditions, argues against the use of live vaccines, especially in combination of multiple serotypes. The release of attenuated viruses in the environment may also lead to reversion of virulence.

The studies conducted in our laboratory using BHK-21 adapted attenuated local isolate of BTV 1 suggested that the virus produced very mild clinical signs in crossbred sheep and elicited neutralising antibodies which persisted at least 60 days (Chander *et al.* 1991). Despite wide prevalence of BT in India, no vaccine is available here and the practice of vaccination is not being followed mainly due to multiplicity of serotypes and cost of the imported attenuated vaccine. Moreover, the attenuated vaccines currently available suffer from several drawbacks described earlier.

6.2 Inactivated vaccines

Unlike attenuated virus vaccines that replicate in vaccinated animals and produce large amount of antigen *in vivo*, the only antigenic stimulus received with killed virus is derived from the vaccine itself. Because of this reason, the dose of inactivated virus has to be much higher and perhaps as higher as 100 times than the live virus vaccines. The use of adjuvant is necessary in inactivated vaccines. Viruses have been inactivated by a number of agents including beta propiolactone (BPL) and binary ethylenimine (BEI). Parker *et al.* (1975) reported that neutralizing immune response persisted for one year after immunization with BPL-inactivated virus in an oil-based adjuvant. However, they could not conduct challenge experiment. Neutralizing antibody response was not detected in the animals vaccinated with BEI inactivated virus. The inactivated BTV vaccines have been reported to have variable degree of protection ability. Stott *et al.* (1979) observed that sheep inoculated with inactivated BTV vaccine developed precipitating but not neutralising antibodies. However, when vaccinated sheep were challenged after 6 weeks of vaccination, some sheep were protected probably due to cell-mediated immunity. Recently, Krishnamohan Reddy *et al.* (2010) evaluated an inactivated vaccine containing predominant serotypes (BTV1, BTV2, BTV 10, BTV 16, BTV 23) circulating in India and showed that protective neutralizing antibody response persisted in vaccinated sheep at least for 6 months. This indigenous vaccine has been extensively evaluated in laboratory conditions and the inactivated vaccine production technology has been transferred to the Indian Immunologicals, Hyderabad and Biovet, Bangalore.

The inactivated vaccines have a number of advantages including no risk for transmission by *Culicoides* vector, transmission of the virus to the foetus and absolutely no possibility of reverting back to the virulent form. Though the inactivated vaccines do not cause clinical disease or viraemia, they suffer from other drawbacks such as repeated injections, poor immune response and side effects due to inactivating agents (Prasad *et al.* 2007). In addition, in endemic BTV areas, for example South Africa where 21 different serotypes circulate, the impact of an additional circulating attenuated virus arising from live vaccine does not substantially add to the problem.

6.3 Recombinant vaccines

Because of the inherent problems associated with the conventional attenuated and inactivated BTV vaccines, alternative methods employing molecular approaches have been explored. It is now well known that VP2 and VP5 proteins together provoke neutralizing immune response. This has raised the possibility of using recombinant immunogens as vaccine against BTV. Both of these proteins have been expressed in prokaryotic and eukaryotic expression systems. Roy *et al.* (1990) first demonstrated that the baculovirus expressed VP2 elicited immune response that protected the immunized sheep against homologous virulent virus challenge. These workers further reported that combination of VP2 and VP5 produced better neutralizing immune response that conferred protection. The purified VP2 and VP5, either produced traditionally or through recombinant DNA technology, produce protective immune response which is short lived. Thus, peptide vaccines have limited utility and are not economically attractive to manufacturers.

To develop better recombinant immunogens for immunisation against BTV, Roy (1992) developed an innovative approach to produce BTV like particles (VLPs) without the viral genome using duel baculovirus expression system. The genes corresponding to outer capsid proteins (VP2 and VP5) and major core proteins (VP3 and VP7) have been cloned in two separate baculovirus expression vectors. The simultaneous co-infection of the *Spodoptera frugiperda* cells with both the recombinant baculoviruses produced the VLPs not morphologically distinguishable from the conventionally cell culture produced authentic BTV particles. The small scale studies conducted in sheep in South Africa and Australia using the BTV-VLPs as candidate vaccine, have clearly suggested that the VLPs when used in combination with appropriate adjuvant elicit protective immune response and the vaccinated animals resist the homologous virulent virus challenge (Johnson and Roy 1996). The VLPs lack the genetic material; hence these cannot cause infection to the vaccinated animals and cannot pass it on to the foetus. Being noninfectious, there is no risk of reverting back to virulent form and transmission by the vector. Another advantage of VLPs is that a combination of different serotypes can be made in the form of cocktail, which protects against a number of serotypes prevalent in a particular geographical region. One can visualize the potential of the technology to produce vaccine chimeras representing different serotypes (Roy 1996). Another possibility of making hybrid VP2 and VP5 representing the immunogenic epitopes of different serotypes also remains workable alternative.

Using similar baculovirus expression system, BTV core like particles can also be produced in *S. frusiperda* insect cells infected with recombinant baculovirus carrying genes encoding for VP3 and VP7 group specific proteins of BTV. These two proteins, when produced in *S. frusiperda* insect cells, assemble to form BTV core like particles without the viral genome (French and Roy 1990). Preliminary studies carried out in Merino sheep in Australia using recombinant CLPs along with adjuvant have suggested that the immunized sheep partially resist the virulent virus challenge (Hosseini *et al.* 1996). Unlike VLPs, the partial protection induced by CLPs is not serotype restricted. This makes CLPs very attractive vaccine candidate because the protection is broad based possibly due to cell mediated immune response.

Keeping their broad based protection capability in view, CLPs have been proposed as potential broad-spectrum BTV vaccine. It has been suggested that in the face of outbreak of BTV infection, where serotype specific vaccines are not available or the serotype is unknown, CLPs could be used to reduce the impact of the infection (Hosseini *et al.* 1996). Since these particles are noninfectious and devoid of genetic material, these do not have the risk associated with live attenuated vaccines. More over, CLPs can be engineered to distinguish between vaccinated and BTV infected sheep by developing appropriate ELISA.

7. Prevention and Control of Bluetongue

BT has achieved global dimensions causing economic losses of alarming proportions. The major problems in its control are multiplicity of serotypes and different species of the vector involved in the transmission of BTV in different parts of the world. However, South African and the EEC countries have been able to significantly control the disease by way of vaccination and strict quarantine measures. Australia and Canada are also taking effective safety and quarantine measure to contain the disease.

Recurring outbreaks of clinical BT in sheep and production losses in other domestic ruminants have caused great economic loss in southern India. Native breeds of sheep that are particularly susceptible to clinical BT are reared mainly on a small scale; therefore, the disease is one of the major causes of economic loss to less-affluent farmers. These losses can be attributed to mortality in sheep, overall loss of productivity, weight loss and wool break (Prasad *et al.* 2009). The larger and more organized farming sector also experiences losses as the result of a ban on the export of live animals, their germplasms and other animal products. It is difficult to assess the effect of BTV infection on the overall productivity of cattle and buffalo, as they are largely asymptomatic, but previous studies in the United States have suggested that infection can result in a significant overall drop in milk yield and productivity (Tabachnick *et al.* 1996). Once established in a particular area, it is very difficult to eradicate BTV.

Interruption of the BTV transmission cycle is considered the most effective method of prevention and control of the disease. Most of the vector control approaches used in India involve systematic and repeated application of insecticide and are expensive to implement and so may be of use only in large, well-organized farms. However, most of the ruminant animals in India are kept by the less well-organized farming sector, owned by people who cannot afford these methods of vector control. This may be another contributing factor to the higher incidence of disease and losses in this sector (Prasad *et al.* 2009).

Several approaches have been used to control *Culicoides* vectors in India, including the use of chemical insecticide sprays in livestock housing and 'pour-on' insecticides applied to animals during the vector-abundant, monsoon season. The treatment of sheep in insecticide dips is an effective method for the control of ectoparasites and has been used against *Culicoides* on several of the more 'organized' sheep farms (Prasad *et al.* 2009). Farm managers have informally reported a significant decline in the incidence of BT after the use of Ektomin and Butox (as dips) during rainy season. Similarly, parentral administration of certain insecticides (e.g. Ivermectin) has been reported to reduce the abundance of ectoparasites and the incidence of BT. The authors have experienced that administration of Ivermectin to sheep greatly reduced the prevalence of BTV in an organized sheep-breeding farm near Hisar in Haryana state (Prasad *et al.* 2009).

Although synthetic chemical insecticides are very effective in destroying midges and their larvae, these also pose considerable risk to human and animal health and to the environment. Consequently, efforts are being made to develop alternative pest management strategies that are non-polluting and environment friendly. One such strategy that has attracted much interest involves the use of naturally occurring bioinsecticides such as products from Neem (*Azadirachta indica*) tree (Attri and Ravi Prasad 1980, Blackwell *et al.* 2004). The existence of 25 BTV serotypes, which largely fail to cross-protect (most of which are circulating in India), has made the goal of protective immunization against the disease particularly difficult to achieve in the region. However, a pentavalent inactivated vaccine based on Indian strains of the virus has been recently developed under the ICAR's All India Network Programme on BT and transferred to two companies for commercial production and field trials.

8. Conclusion

The prospect of climate change and unprecedented movement of people, animals and materials in highly globalized world has enhanced the possibility of transmission of vector borne diseases which were previously not reported from India. It is believed that BT in India has been imported through animals, though now difficult to prove. BT is now endemic in India and most of the states where survey has been conducted have been found positive for BTV antibodies. Climate change and importation of exotic breeds of ruminant livestock susceptible to BT may further aggravate the occurrence of BT in the country particularly in the regions where BT is currently dormant or absent. During the past over one decade, BT outbreaks have been frequently recorded in southern India while clinical outbreaks have not been reported in north Indian states. However, BTV antibodies in cattle, buffalo, sheep and goats have been reported from most of the north Indian states. For effective control of BT in India, vaccination of susceptible livestock with inactivated vaccine

Table 1 : Prevalence of different serotypes of bluetongue virus (BTV) in India

Serotype	States where demonstrated on basis of neutralizing antibodies	States where the serotype isolated
BTV 1	Haryana, Jammu and Kashmir, Rajasthan, Uttar Pradesh, Gujarat, Maharashtra, Tamil Nadu, Karnataka,	Uttar Pradesh, Haryana, Rajasthan, Maharashtra, Tamil Nadu
BTV 2	Andhra Pradesh, Haryana, , Gujarat, Maharashtra, Tamil Nadu, Karnataka	Andhra Pradesh, Tamil Nadu
BTV 3	Himachal Pradesh , Uttar Pradesh, Gujarat, Maharashtra, Tamil Nadu	Uttar Pradesh, Himachal Pradesh, Tamil Nadu
BTV 4	Haryana, Himachal Pradesh, Gujarat, Maharashtra, Tamil Nadu, Karnatak a, Andhra Pradesh	Haryana, Himachal Pradesh, Maharashtra
BTV 5	Himachal Pradesh, Gujarat , Maharashtra, Tamil Nadu	Himachal Pradesh
BTV 6	Gujarat, Maharashtra, Andhra Pradesh, Tamil Nadu	-
BTV 7	Maharashtra, Tamil Nadu	-
BTV 8	Gujarat, Haryana, Maharashtra	-
BTV 9	Himachal Pradesh, Uttar Pradesh, West Bengal, Gujarat, Maharashtra, Andhra Pradesh	Uttar Pradesh, Himachal Pradesh, Andhra Pradesh, West Bengal
BTV 10	Karnataka, Andhra Pradesh, Gujarat, Maharashtra	Andhra Pradesh, Karnataka
BTV 11	Gujarat, Tamil Nadu	-
BTV 12	Haryana, Gujarat, Maharashtra, Andhra Pradesh, Karnataka, Tamil Nadu	-
BTV 13	Gujarat, Maharashtra, Andhra Pradesh	-
BTV 14	Tamil Nadu, Andhra Pradesh	-
BTV 15	Gujarat, Tamil Nadu	-
BTV 16	Himachal, Haryana, Gujarat, Maharashtra, Tamil Nadu, Karnataka	Himachal Pradesh, Maharashtra, Tamil Nadu
BTV 17	Himachal Pradesh, Gujarat, Maharashtra, Andhra Pradesh, Karnataka, Tamil Nadu	Himachal Pradesh, Maharashtra
BTV 18	Uttar Pradesh, Madhya Pradesh, Karnataka, Maharashtra, Andhra Pradesh	Uttar Pradesh , Karnataka, Maharashtra, AP
BTV 19	Andhra Pradesh, Tamil Nadu	-
BTV 20	Gujarat, Karnataka, Tamil Nadu	-
BTV 21	Andhra Pradesh	Andhra Pradesh
BTV 23	Uttar Pradesh, Uttarakhand, Madhya Pradesh, Karnataka, Tamil Nadu	Uttar Pradesh , Uttarakhand, MP, Karnataka, Tamil Nadu

based on predominant Indian strains, continuous monitoring and surveillance of virus and the vectors and *Culicoides* control using ecofriendly agents available locally are the primary requirements. There are several researchable areas. These include understanding relative virulence of BTV serotypes/strains circulating in south and north India, species of vector responsible for transmission of BTV in different parts of the country, environmental factors contributing to outbreaks of BT, role of wildlife in BT epidemiology, maintenance of BTV in indigenous cattle and buffaloes as reservoirs, and analyzing the genetic basis for their relative resistance to clinical disease.

References

1. Attri BS, Ravi Prasad G (1980). Neem oil extract - an effective larvicide. Indian J Entomol 42:371-375.
2. Bhatnagar P, Prasad G, Kakker NK, Dasgupta SK, Rajpurohit BS, Srivastava RN (1997). A potential vector of bluetongue virus in north-western India. Indian J Anim Sci 67:486-488.
3. Blackwell A, Evans KA, Strang RH, Cole CM (2004). Toward development of neem-based repellents against the Scottish highland biting midge, *Culicoides impunctatus*. Med Vet Entomol 18:449-452.
4. Chander S, Prasad G, Jain NC (1991). Dot immunobinding assay for detection of bluetongue virus antibodies in sheep experimentally inoculated with bluetongue virus type 1. Vet Microbiol 28:289-294.
5. de Mattos CC, de Mattos CA, Osburn BI, Ianconescu M, Kaufman R (1991). Evidence of genome segment 5 reassortment in bluetongue virus field isolates. Am J Vet Res 52:1794-1798.
6. French TJ, Roy P (1990). Synthesis of bluetongue virus (BTV) core like particles by a recombinant baculovirus expressing the two major structural core proteins of BTV. J Virol 64:1530-1536.
7. Hosseini M, Dixion RJ , Kirkland PD, Roy P (1996). Studies on vaccination of sheep with bluetongue virus core-like particles produced by a recombinant baculovirus. In: St. George ST, Kegao P (ed) Proceedings of the First Southeast Asia and Pacific Regional Bluetongue Symposium, Kunming, China.
8. Jain NC, Prasad G, Gupta Y, Mahajan NK (1988). Isolation of bluetongue virus from *Culicoides* in India. Rev Sci Tech Off Int Epiz 7:375-378.
9. Johnson SJ, Polkinghorne IG, Flanagan M, Townsend WL (1992). The Australian experience: results of a bluetongue vaccination program. In: Walton TE, Osburn BI (ed) Bluetongue, African Horse Sickness and Related Orbiviruses. CRC Press, Boca Raton.
10. Johnson SJ, Roy P (1996). Bluetongue recombinant vaccines. In: St. George ST, Kegao P (ed) Proceedings of the First Southeast Asia and Pacific Regional Bluetongue Symposium, Kunming, China.

11. Kakker NK, Prasad G, Srivastava RN, Bhatnagar P (1996). Sentinel herd as tool for studying bluetongue virus infection in four northern states of India. Indian J Anim Sci 66:1254-1257.

12. Krishnamohan Reddy Y, Murali Manohar B, Pandey AB, Narsimha Redday Y, Prasad G, Chauhan RS (2010). Development and evaluation of inactivated pentavalent adjuvanted vaccine for bluetongue. Indian Vet J 87:434-436.

13. Mertens PPC, Maan S, Batten C, Darpel KE, Shaw A, Maan NS, Nomikou K, Anthony SJ, Veronosi E, Oura CAL, Carpenter S, Mellor PS (2009). Bluetongue virus diagnosis. In: Mertens PPC, Mellor PS (ed) Bluetongue. Elsevier, Amsterdam.

14. Murry PK, Eaton BT (1996). Vaccines for bluetongue. Aust Vet J 73:207-210.

15. Naresh A, Prasad G (1995). Detection of bluetongue virus antibodies by monoclonal antibody and recombinant antigen based c-ELISA. Indian J Exp Biol 33:880-882.

16. Naresh A, Roy P, Prasad G (1996). Evaluation of recombinant bluetongue virus antigens using dot immunobinding assay. Am J Vet Res 57:1556-1558.

17. Narladakar BW, Shastri UV, Shivpuje PR (1993). Studies on *Culicoides* spp (Dipetra: Ceratopogonidae) prevalent in Marathwada region (Maharashtra) and their host preference. Indian Vet J 70:116-118.

18. Parker J, Herniman KA, Gibbs EP (1975). An experimental inactivated vaccine against bluetongue. Vet Rec 96:284-287.

19. Prasad G (2000). Whither bluetongue research in India. Indian J Microbiol 40:163-175.

20. Prasad G, Minakshi, Malik Y (2007). Bluetongue. ICAR, New Delhi.

21. Prasad G, Sreenivasulu D, Singh KP, Mertens, PPC, Maan S (2009). Bluetongue on the Indian subcontinent. In: Mertens PPC, Philip Mellor (ed) Bluetongue. Elsevier, Amsterdam.

22. Roy P (1992). Genetically engineered bluetongue virus-like particles and their potential for use as vaccine in sheep. In: Pandey R, Stephan H, Prasad G (ed) Veterinary Vaccines (Progr Vaccinol Vol IV). Springer Verlag, New York.

23. Roy P (1996). Development of bluetongue virus multicomponent vaccines using a novel baculovirus system. In: St. George ST, Kegao P (ed) Proceedings of the First Southeast Asia and Pacific Regional Bluetongue Symposium, Kunming, China.

24. Roy P, Urarawa T, Van Dijk AA, Erasmus BJ (1990). Recombinant virus vaccine for bluetongue disease in sheep. J Virol 64:1998-2003.

25. Sapre SN (1964). An outbreak of bluetongue in goats and sheep. Indian Vet Rev (M&B) 15:69-71.

26. Schultz KT, Grieder FB (1987). Immunobiology of bluetongue virus Vet Immunol Immunopathol 15:115-127.

27. Sreenivasulu D, Subba Rao MV, Reddy YN, Gard GP (2004). Overview of bluetongue disease, viruses, vectors, surveillance and unique features: The Indian subcontinent and adjacent regions. Vet Ital 40:73-77.

28. Stott JL, Barber L, Osburn I, Swayer M (1979). Immunologic response of sheep to an experimental inactivated bluetongue virus vaccine. Am J Vet Med Assoc 175:611.

29. Sugiyama K, Bishop DH, Roy P (1982). Analysis of the genomes of bluetongue viruses recovered from different states of the United States and at different times. Am J Epidemiol 115:332-347.

30. Tabachnick WJ, Robertson MA, Murphy KE (1996). *Culicoides variipennis* and bluetongue disease. Ann NY Acad Sci 791:219-226.

❑❑❑

Chapter 17

Foot and Mouth Disease Control

R. SHARMA AND N. K. KAKKER
Department of Veterinary Microbiology, College of Veterinary Sciences, Lala Lajpat Rai University of Veterinary and Animal Sciences, Hisar-125004

Contents

1. Introduction

Foot and mouth disease (FMD) is a highly contagious infection of cloven footed animals. The disease is endemic and widely distributed in India and causes heavy economic losses, mainly due to loss in milk production and reduction in the working capability of animals. In addition, milk, milk products, meat and hide from the country are not accepted by the FMD-free countries, adversely affecting the export potential of the country's livestock industry. FMD is characterized by fever, lameness, and vesicular lesions on the tongue, feet, snout, and teats. However, in young animals mortality can be high, where the virus can affect the myocardium.

2. Virus Characteristics

The disease is caused by the FMD virus (FMDV), an *Aphthovirus* of the family *Picornaviridae* that includes small (20-30 nm in diameter), non-enveloped, positive stranded RNA viruses consisting of many important pathogens of human and animals. The FMDV exists in seven immunologically distinct serotypes viz. O, A, C, Asia 1 and South African Territories (SAT) -1, -2 and -3. Within these seven serotypes, more than 140 subtypes have been identified. Some of these subtypes are strongly divergent and the vaccines made against one subtype may protect against the others only after repeated vaccinations (Barteling and Vreeswijk 1991). FMDV is highly labile at temperatures above 50°C, at very low salt concentrations or when the pH drops below neutral. Its sedimentation coefficient lies between 140 and 146 S (Bachrach 1952).

The FMDV genome consists of a single strand RNA of about 8.2 kb that undergoes very high level of mutational changes (Sobrino *et al.* 1986). The viral genome encodes a unique polyprotein from which different viral polypeptides are cleaved by viral proteases (Sanz-Parra *et al.* 1999) including nine different mature non structural proteins (NSPs). Each of these NSPs, as well as some of the precursor polypeptides, are involved in functions that are relevant to the virus life cycle in infected cells (Porter 1993).

The RNA genome is enclosed within an icosahedral capsid comprising of 60 copies each of the four viral proteins; VP1, VP2, VP3 and VP4. The VP1-3 are viral surface proteins consisting of approximately 200-300 amino acid residues, while VP4 is an internal protein generally less than 100 residues in size. In fact, VP1 is the only virus protein that elicits neutralizing antibodies and protection in cattle (Meloen *et al.* 1979). It has also been established that a conserved triplet, Arg-Gly-Asp (RGD) within the FMDV loop is involved in cell attachment (Fox *et al.* 1989).

3. Epidemiology in India

In India, FMD is endemic and occurs in all parts of the country, throughout the year. Of the seven FMDV serotypes prevalent worldwide, only four serotypes i.e. O, A, C and Asia 1 were earlier reported to be circulating in India. Of these, FMDV serotype O has been the most prevalent, followed by Asia 1 and A in the northwest region of the country, while FMDV serotype C has not been detected for the last about 16 years.

The disease incidence is the highest in cattle and buffaloes followed by pigs, sheep and goat. The disease is more severe in exotic and cross-bred animals. In addition, many species of cloven hoofed wildlife such as deer, antelopes and wild pigs may become infected.

The incidence of FMD outbreaks and virus type distribution during 2009-2010 in different parts of India has been depicted in Table 1. During this period, 1005 outbreaks of the disease were recorded, about 60% of which were in the eastern states. Among 1616 samples, serotype O was prevalent in 974, serotype A in 32 and serotype Asia 1 in 37 samples while 573 specimens were untypable.

Table 1 : FMD outbreaks and distribution of virus types in India (2009-2010)[1]

S. No.	State	No. of Outbreaks	No. of Samples	Distribution of virus types		
				O	A	Asia 1
Northern Region						
1.	Haryana	2	7	2	4	-
2.	Himachal Pradesh	1	1	1	-	-
3.	Jammu	13	-	-	-	-
4.	Punjab	1	2	-	2	-
5.	Uttar Pradesh and Uttarakhand	57	104	45	11	5
Western Region						
6.	Gujarat	20	104	30	-	27
7.	Maharashtra	13	20	10	2	1
8.	Rajasthan	35	-	-	-	-
Southern Region						
9.	Andhra Pradesh	31	60	10	2	-
10.	Karnataka	187	80	50	-	-
11.	Kerala	25	165	62	6	-
12.	Tamil Nadu	0	-	-	-	-
Eastern Region						
13.	Assam	47	54	39	-	-
14.	Arunachal Pradesh	18	108	43	-	-

15.	Bihar	158	274	219	-	-
16.	Manipur	3	6	6	-	-
17.	Mizoram	1	1	1	-	-
18.	Megalaya	5	6	6	-	-
19.	Orissa	44	51	9	4	-
20.	Tripura	29	26	19	-	-
21.	West Bengal	294	501	379	1	1
22.	Sikkim	1	1	1	-	-
Central Region						
23.	Madhya Pradesh	20	45	42	-	3
	Total	1005	1616*	974	32	37

Source: Annual Report 2009-10, Project Directorate on FMD, Mukteswar, Nainital
* Of the 1616 samples, 573 clinical samples were untypable.

4. International Status of FMD

FMD occurs in most of the cattle raising regions of the world. The disease was eradicated in Australia, New Zealand and North America. Australia had its last outbreak in 1972. The first and last outbreak in Canada occurred in 1952. The United States of America has been declared FMD-free since 1929.

In Europe, the United Kingdom remained practically free from FMD since the last major outbreak of 1967-68 with the exception of isolated outbreaks in Channel Island in 1974, 1981 and recently in 2001 and 2007 that has affected the 'FMD-free status' of UK, France and Germany. In other European countries, the incidence of the disease has declined with the exception of Italy, Greece and the countries of South-eastern Europe. The western European countries eradicated the disease in the last decade but outbreaks have been recorded in 2001. FMD is endemic in many parts of South Africa, South America, Middle East and Asia and some parts of Europe.

5. Transmission

FMDV can replicate and be excreted from respiratory tract of animals. Airborne excretion of virus occurs during the acute phase of infection. The virus spreads mainly by direct contact (inhalation and ingestion), although indirect spread through fomites is important. The virus in dried blood, milk, meat and carcasses can be stable and may serve as source of infection. All secretions and excretions may be infective before the animal is clinically ill. The greatest concentration of the virus is found in vesicular fluid. Infected or carrier animal (e.g. in livestock fairs) and migratory herds are contributory factors for spread of FMDV infection.

6. Influence of Environmental Factors

The environmental factors, namely, temperature (maximum and minimum), relative humidity (morning and evening), wind speed and rainfall have some influence on the incidence of FMD outbreaks. On the basis of the incidence of FMD outbreaks in Haryana during 1996-2003, using SAS Computer Programme, a significant correlation coefficient of -0.29 was found between the number of outbreaks and maximum temperature ($P < 0.01$). Similarly, significant correlation (-0.31) was observed between number of outbreaks and minimum temperature ($P < 0.01$). The per cent relative humidity (morning) showed a significant correlation coefficient of 0.25 ($P < 0.01$) with the number of outbreaks, however, there was no significant correlation (- 0.01) between the relative humidity (evening) and the number of outbreaks. A significant correlation (-0.31) was observed between the number of outbreaks and wind velocity ($P < 0.01$). Likewise, a non-significant correlation coefficient of -0.17 was observed between the number of outbreaks and rainfall.

7. Immune Response against FMDV

7.1 Humoral immune response

The importance of neutralizing antibodies in protection against FMDV has been recognized for many years. Natural and experimental animals infected with FMDV develop a long lasting immune response that is closely related to presence of anti-FMDV antibodies. Induction of these antibodies is dependent on the structure of the viral antigenic sites (Francis *et al.* 1990). McCullough *et al.* (1986) observed that phagocytosis of FMDV is enhanced when the virus is complexed with antibodies of appropriate specificity and affinity and thus stressed the role of opsonization of the antibodies rather than neutralization.

Natural infection has been reported to induce higher titres of neutralizing antibodies and long-lasting specific antibody protection than vaçcination (Morgan and Moore 1990). Besides good correlation between the specific neutralizing antibody titre and protection against challenge in FMDV infected and vaccinated cattle, there are some reports which suggest that various immune mechanisms other than the antibody driven virus neutralization could operate *in vivo* to provide protection against FMDV.

7.2 Cell mediated immunity

In contrast to the well characterized role of humoral immune response, the role of cellular immune response in protection against FMDV challenge has not been well established. The production of neutralizing antibodies in FMDV infection requires the cooperation of B and T lymphocytes. Collen *et al.* (1989) showed that primed B cells are unable to secrete virus specific antibodies in the absence of primed T cells or cytokines from T cell culture.

The participation of Th cell mediated component of the immune response to FMDV has also been demonstrated in delayed type hypersensitivity skin reaction in guinea pigs (Knudsen *et al.* 1979) and buffaloes (Sharma *et al.* 1985). Collen and Doel (1990) demonstrated that *in vitro* recognition of FMDV antigen by peripheral blood lymphocytes is heterotypic and the serotype cross reactive response is due to T cell epitope in VP3 capsid protein. Bartels *et al.* (1994) analysed the immune response against FMDV in guinea pigs by *in vivo* and *in vitro* studies and demonstrated that the proliferating T cells were predominantly $CD4^{+}$ T cells. Stimulation of both cellular and humoral immune responses against FMDV in cattle may reduce the risk of disease and virus shedding.

8. Diagnosis

The accurate diagnosis of FMDV infection is of great importance for both control and eradication campaigns in FMD endemic areas. The control and eradication of FMD depends upon quick reporting, an accurate and swift diagnosis, followed by rapid and effective implementation of control measures. The recognition of FMD signs in cattle, buffaloes and pigs provide straightforward clinical diagnosis. However, it can often be difficult in sheep and goats as the clinical signs are mild and transient. Laboratory diagnosis is, therefore, necessary for disease confirmation. Laboratory diagnosis procedures are based on either identification of virus serotype involved or antibody response following an active phase of the disease.

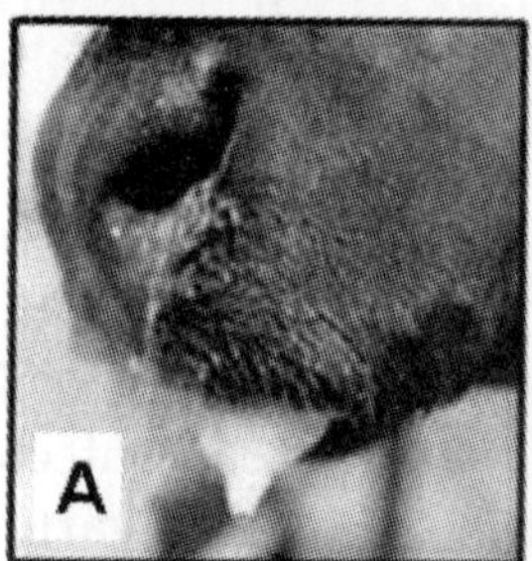

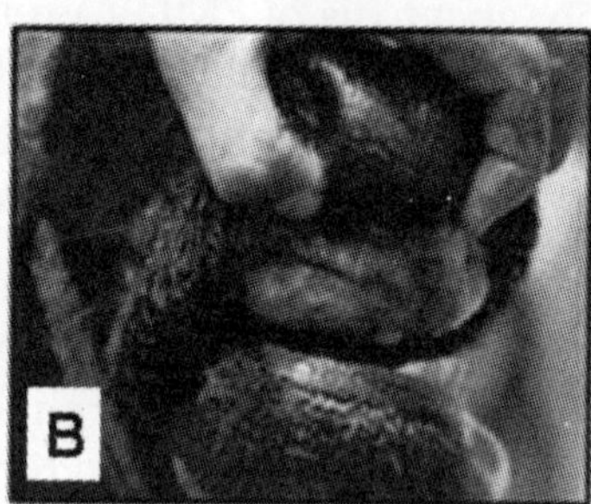

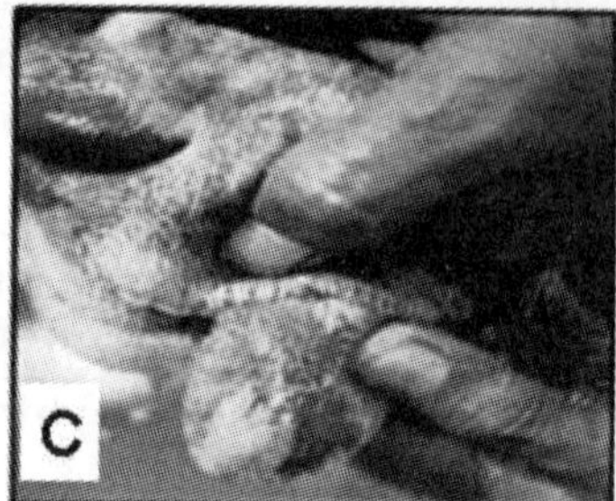

Fig. 1 : Signs of FMD: (A) salivation, (B) lesions on gums, and (C) lesions on tongue

8.1 Diagnosis through identification of virus serotype

Identification of virus serotype is done by virus isolation or by the demonstration of FMD viral antigen/nucleic acid in samples of tissue or vesicular fluid. Detection of specific antibody in serum (serotyping) can also be used for diagnosis. Serodiagnosis is enhanced by newly developed non-structural proteins (NSPs) assays that enable detection of past or current infection irrespective of vaccination status.

Although complement fixation test (CFT) has also been used to detect the FMDV antigen but enzyme linked immuno-sorbent assay (ELISA) is preferred over CFT because it is more sensitive and is not affected by anti-complementary factors. At the World Reference Laboratory on FMD, Institute for Animal Health, Pirbright, UK, the preferred procedure for the detection of FMDV antigen and identification of viral serotypes is sandwich ELISA (OIE 2004). The results can be obtained within 3-4 hours after sample is received in the laboratory; a negative sample is confirmed by inoculation of sample into sensitive cultures (BHK-21, MDBK etc.), followed by confirmation of the virus serotype by ELISA. Recently, a monoclonal antibody based rapid chromatographic strip test has also been developed for the pen-side detection of FMDV antigen.

8.2 Diagnosis of virus serotype specific antibodies through serological tests

FMDV serotype can also be diagnosed by the detection of specific antibody response. Several tests/techniques have been developed to detect the presence of FMDV serotype specific antibodies e.g. passive haemagglutination, complement fixation inhibition test, counter immunoelectrophoresis, solid phase radioimmunoassay, indirect immunofluorescence, serum neutralization, CFT, ELISA etc. Of these, ELISA is more versatile, reproducible and simple to perform and ELISA reagents have longer shelf life.

8.3 Diagnosis through nucleic acid based tests

The polymerase chain reaction (PCR) offers potential advantages over the other conventional tests. A particularly high sensitivity has been reported by RT-PCR (Alexandersen *et al.* 2000). An antigen capture RT-PCR (Suryanarayana *et al.* 1999) has also been described for serotyping of FMDV having the possibility of use in the field. Tosh *et al.* (1997) developed one tube RT-PCR that reduces assay complexity and potential errors.

A Real-time PCR capable of detecting all the seven serotypes of FMDV has been developed (Alexandersen *et al.* 2001, 2002, Zhang and Alexandersen 2003, Barnett *et al.* 2004). It has a high sensitivity (97%) and specificity for detection of FMDV genome in all seven serotypes. Viral RNA can be detected in oral and nasal samples from experimentally infected animals 24-96 hours before the onset of clinical signs (Callahan *et al.* 2002). The only disadvantage of Real-time PCR is that it is very expensive and not suited for field purpose.

In future, use of robotic extraction of RNA will increase the throughput of samples whilst reducing the timescale for the issue of laboratory diagnostic results.

8.4 Differentiating infected animals from vaccinated animals (DIVA strategy)

The conventional diagnostic tests are unable to differentiate FMDV infected and vaccinated animals. The detection of antibodies to NSPs of FMDV has been used to detect the past or present infection of any of the seven FMD virus serotypes. Further, detection of antibodies against NSP antigens could also be used for differentiation of antibodies due to vaccination/infection (Kumar 2006). When animals are vaccinated, they mount antibody response only against coat (structural) proteins of the virus. On the other hand, in infected animals antibodies also develop against NSPs (viral polymerases and proteases) of the virus because virus actually replicates inside the host cells. Detection of antibodies against NSPs is an important tool for DIVA strategy.

ELISA based assays using recombinant NSPs have been developed. Even, there are three commercially available tests to detect antibodies against NSP (3ABC) - United Biomedical, Inc., New York; Cedi-Diagnostics B.V., The Netherland; and SYANOVA Biotech AB, Sweden.

9. Control of FMD

The strategy evolved for the control of FMD varies from country to country: geographical location, economic development and the status of FMD incidence. In developed countries, the most effective way remains the slaughter of affected and in-contact susceptible animals and restriction of animal movements. In India, FMD control can not be effected either by slaughter or stamping out policy as adopted by the western countries. The control of FMD in India is a challenging task due to several factors such as i) large geographical area with different agro-climatic and socio-economic zones, ii) large array of susceptible livestock population, iii) antigenic plurality of the virus, iv) limited availability and huge cost of FMD vaccine, v) short duration of immunity, vi) unrestricted animal movement and vii) lack of legislation for compulsory reporting and vaccination.

Recently, efforts have been made to develop alternative FMD control strategy, which is directed towards creation of "disease free zone" (DFZ) in a particular geographical location depending upon the endemicity status. The DFZ may be carved out in three ecosystems based on the disease incidence in a particular zone such as epidemic zone, endemic zone and sporadic zone. The scheme consists of i) control of livestock movement into and out of the DFZ, ii) systematic mass vaccination of all the susceptible animals in the area, iii) creation of buffer zones, iv) seromonitoring of vaccination programme, v) applying emergency measures in the event of outbreak and vi) epidemiological surveillance in the DFZ for residual foci and surrounding area for FMDV circulation.

10. FMD Control Programme

In lines with the above strategy, the Government of India launched FMD Control Programme (FMD-CP) during 10th Five Year Plan (2002-2007) in three different geographical regions of the country comprising 54 districts with the total outlay of Rs. 200 crores. The region I comprises 8 districts, namely, Kanyakumari (Tamil Nadu); Quilon, Pathanamthitha, Thiruvananthapuram (Kerala) and Union Territories of Andaman and Nicobar Islands, Dadra and Nagar Haveli, Daman and Diu, and Lakshadweep. The region II is the largest comprising of 33 districts of three states Punjab (8), Haryana (8), western Uttar Pradesh (16) and Delhi as one district. The region III includes 13 districts in three states of Maharashtra (5), Gujarat (4) and Andhra Pradesh (4).

The programme envisages total funding by the government for vaccine including other supporting assistance (manpower, infrastructure and logistic support), framing of legislation to restrict animal movement and compulsory vaccination of all animals in the defined regions. Besides, pre- and post-vaccination monitoring and surveillance of vaccinated animals is being done to assess the extent of exposure of the population to FMDV.

11. FMD Control Programme in Haryana: A Success Story

The FMD Control Programme was launched in eight districts (Bhiwani, Fatehabad, Hisar, Jhajjar, Jind, Rohtak, Sirsa, Sonepat) of Haryana in January 2004. The immunization was completed in the shortest possible time in each segment and was in tune with the schedule of the supply of vaccine, storage capacity and capability to cover the area. No vaccine was stored for more than a week at the district head quarter. Efforts were made to use the entire lot of vaccine within five days of supply. Because of the mass vaccination programme by the Department of Animal Husbandry and Dairying, Haryana, the incidence of FMD outbreaks in the state during the past seven years period (2004-2011) has become considerably very low: three outbreaks in 2010, one in 2009 (Anon 2009, 2010, 2011), two in 2008, one in 2007 (Sharma and Kakker 2009), one in 2006 and three in 2005 (Kakker and Sharma 2007). In 2004, 15 outbreaks were recorded while these were 111 in 2003 (Sharma and Kakker 2005).

The Regional Research Centre on FMD, Hisar provided logistic support in the form of surveillance and seromonitoring work during the implementation of FMD-CP. The Centre successfully accomplished the work of analyzing pre- and post-vaccination serum samples upto the tenth phase of FMD vaccination in Haryana by Liquid Phase Blocking ELISA. The results of these studies revealed that animals in Haryana state developed >80% herd immunity against the prevalent FMDV serotypes after vaccination under FMD-CP. The data provided logistic support to the FMD-CP that mass FMD vaccinations after ten rounds of vaccination in the eight FMD-CP districts as well as seven vaccinations in the other 13 districts funded under the Assistance to States for Control of Animal Diseases (ASCAD) programme provided sufficient protection against FMD at herd level in Haryana state despite the prevalence of the disease in the neighbouring states. With the initial success of FMD-CP in eight districts of Haryana, the Government of India has recently extended the FMD-CP in 225 districts throughout India and has included whole of Haryana (remaining 13 districts under ASCAD) under FMD-CP from 2011-12 onwards.

The Centre also analysed the serum samples periodically for anti-NSP (3A/ 3AB3) antibodies for monitoring the FMD carrier status in the vaccinated subjects under National FMD serosurveillance. The percentages of animals found positive for anti-NSP antibodies during pre- 1st vaccination (before start of FMD-CP) and pre- 4th vaccination (after two years of FMD-CP) were 31.94% and 18.4%, respectively, which further lowered to 12.12% during pre- 8th vaccination (after four years of FMD-CP). A significant ($P<0.01$) reduction in anti-NSP antibody profile in Haryana was reported four years after the launch of FMD-CP. This further supports the fact that the incidence of FMD virus circulation in the state has significantly reduced due to vaccination.

12. Conclusion

The data on the epidemiology, FMD-CP and National serosurveillance in Haryana state can serve as a model for FMD control in the country. With the Regional Research Centre, Hisar supporting the other network units too in the northwest zone i.e. Punjab, Jammu and Kashmir, Himachal Pradesh, Delhi and Rajasthan, the reduced incidence of the disease in these states supports the candidacy of the northwest states for "Zonal freedom from FMD". It is envisaged that the success of FMD-CP will pave the way for launching a National FMD Eradication Programme in the country.

References

1. Alexandersen S, Forsyth MA, Reid SM, Belsham GJ (2000). Development of reverse transcription-PCR (oligonucleotide probing) enzyme-linked immunosorbent assays for diagnosis and preliminary typing of foot-and-mouth disease: a new system using simple and aqueous-phase hybridization. J Clin Microbiol 38:4604-4613.

2. Alexandersen S, Oleksiewicz MB, Donaldson AI (2001). The early pathogenesis of foot-and-mouth disease in pigs infected by contact: a quantitative time-course study using TaqMan RT-PCR. J Gen Virol 82:747-755.

3. Alexandersen S, Zhang Z, Donaldson AI (2002). Aspects of the persistence of foot-and-mouth disease virus in animals - the carrier problem. Microbes Infect 4: 1099-1110.

4. Anon (2009). Annual Report, 2008-09 Regional Research Centre on Foot and Mouth Disease, Eds Sharma R, Kakker NK, Department of Veterinary Microbiology, CCS Haryana Agricultural University, Hisar, Haryana, India.

5. Anon (2010). Annual Report, 2009-10 Regional Research Centre on Foot and Mouth Disease, Eds Sharma R, Kakker NK, Department of Veterinary Microbiology, CCS Haryana Agricultural University, Hisar, Haryana, India.

6. Anon (2011). Annual Report, 2010-11 Regional Research Centre on Foot and Mouth Disease, Eds Sharma R, Kakker NK, Department of Veterinary Microbiology, CCS Haryana Agricultural University, Hisar, Haryana, India.

7. Bachrach HL (1952). The determination of the sedimentation constant of a homogeneous component having the characteristics of the foot-and-mouth disease virus. Am J Vet Res 13:13-16

8. Barnett PV, Keel P, Reid S, Armstrong RM, Statham RJ, Voyce C, Aggarwal N, Cox SJ (2004). Evidence that high potency foot-and-mouth disease vaccine inhibits local virus replication and prevents the "carrier" state in sheep. Vaccine 22:1221-1232.

9. Barteling SJ, Vreeswijk J (1991). Developments in foot-and-mouth disease vaccines. Vaccine 9:75-88.

10. Bartels T, Schafer H, Liebermann H, Burger R, Beyer J (1994). T-lymphocyte responses in guinea pigs vaccinated with foot-and-mouth disease virus. Vet Immunol Immunopathol 40:213-223.

11. Callahan JD, Brown F, Osorio FA, Sur JH, Kramer E, Long GW, Lubroth J, Ellis SJ, Shoulars KS, Gaffney KL, Rock DL, Nelson WM (2002). Use of a portable real-time reverse transcriptase-polymerase chain reaction assay for rapid detection of foot-and-mouth disease virus. J Am Vet Med Assoc 220:1636-1642.

12. Collen T, Doel TR (1990). Heterotypic recognition of foot-and-mouth disease virus by cattle lymphocytes. J Gen Virol 71:309-315.

13. Collen T, Pullen L, Doel TR (1989). T cell-dependent induction of antibody against foot-and-mouth disease virus in a mouse model. J Gen Virol 70:395-403.

14. Fox G, Parry NR, Bernett PV, McGinn B, Rowlands DJ, Brown F (1989). The cell attachment site on foot-and-mouth disease virus includes the sequence RGD (arginine-glycine-aspartic acid). J Gen Virol 70:625-637.

15. Francis MJ, Hastings GZ, Clarke BE, Brown AL, Beddell CR, Rowlands DJ, Brown F (1990). Neutralizing antibodies to all seven serotypes of foot-and-mouth disease virus elicited by synthetic peptides. Immunology 69:171-176.

16. Kakker NK, Sharma R (2007). Foot-and-mouth disease outbreaks after the launch of FMD-Control Programme in Haryana. Haryana Veterinarian 46:65-68.

17. Knudsen RC, Groocock CM, Anderson AA (1979). Immunity to foot-and-mouth disease virus in guinea pigs: clinical and immune responses. Infec Immun 24: 787-792.

18. Kumar N (2006). Molecular and immunological studies on persistence of FMD virus. PhD Thesis. CCS Haryana Agricultural University, Hisar, Haryana, India.

19. McCullough KC, Crowther JR, Butcher RN, Carpenter WC, Brocchi E, Capucci L, De Simone F (1986). Immune protection against foot-and-mouth disease virus studied using virus-neutralizing and non-neutralising concentrations of monoclonal antibodies. Immunology 58:421-428.

20. Meloen RH, Rowlands DJ, Brown F (1979). Comparison of the antibodies elicited by the individual structural polypeptides of foot-and-mouth disease and polio viruses. J Gen Virol 45:761-763.

21. Morgan DO, Moore DM (1990). Protection of cattle and swine against foot-and-mouth disease using biosynthetic peptide vaccines. Am J Vet Res 51:40-45.

22. OIE (2004). Manual of standards for diagnostic tests and vaccines. Fifth ed. World Organisation for Animal Health (OIE), Rue de Prony, 75017 Paris, France.

23. Porter AG (1993). Picornavirus nonstructural proteins: emerging roles in virus replication and inhibition of host cell functions. J Virol 67:6917-6921.

24. Sanz Parra A, Jimenez-Clavero MA, Gracia-Briones MM, Blanco E, Sobrino F, Ley V (1999). Recombinant viruses expressing the foot-and-mouth disease virus capsid precursor polypeptide (P1) induce cellular but not humoral antiviral immunity and partial protection in pigs. Virology 259:129-134.

25. Sharma R, Kakker NK (2005). Scenario of foot-and-mouth disease outbreaks in Haryana during the years 2003 and 2004. Haryana Veterinarian 44:47-51.

26. Sharma R, Kakker NK (2009). Incidence of foot-and-mouth disease outbreaks in Haryana during the years 2007 and 2008. Haryana Veterinarian 48:97-99.

27. Sharma R, Prasad S, Ahuja KL, Rahman MM, Kumar A (1985). Cell mediated immune response following foot-and-mouth disease vaccination in buffalo calves. Acta Virologica 29:509-513.

28. Sobrino F, Palma EL, Beck E, Davila M, de la Torre JC, Negro P, Villanueva N, Ortin J, Domingo E (1986). Fixation of mutations in the viral genome during an outbreak of foot-and-mouth disease: heterogeneity and rate variations. Gene 50:149-159.

29. Suryanarayana V, Madanamohan B, Bist P, Natarajan C, Tratschin JD (1999). Serotyping of foot-and-mouth disease virus by antigen capture reverse transcriptase/polymerase chain reaction. J Virol Methods 80:45-52.

30. Tosh C, Hemadri D, Sanyal A, Pattnaik B, Venkataramanan R (1997). One-tube and one-buffer system of RT-PCR amplification of 1D gene of foot-and-mouth disease virus field isolates. Acta Virologia 41:153-155.

31. Zhang Z, Alexandersen S (2003). Detection of carrier cattle and sheep persistently infected with foot-and-mouth disease virus by a rapid real-time RT-PCR assay. J Virol Methods 111:95-100.

□□□

Chapter 18

Action Plan for Control of Haemorrhagic Septicaemia and Pasteurellosis

A. A. KUMAR[1] AND S. B. SHIVACHANDRA[2]

[1]Former Principal Scientist, Indian Veterinary Research Institute, Izatnagar-243122

[2]Clinical Bacteriology Laboratory, Indian Veterinary Research Institute, Mukteshwar-263138

Contents

1. Introduction

Haemorrhagic septicaemia (HS), an acute, fatal and septicaemic disease of cattle and buffaloes caused by Gram-negative bacterium *Pasteurella multocida,* has been recorded in almost all parts of the world. The different serotypes of *P. multocida* are associated with a variety of diseases or syndromes, generally termed as 'pasteurellosis', in a wide range of domestic as well as wild animals and birds. In many instances, *P. multocida* plays a secondary role in the pathogenesis of the disease or acts in combination with other bacterial, viral or parasitic infections. HS, which is a primary pasteurellosis with 100% mortality in infected animals, is endemic in most of Asian and African countries. Although, the disease has been suspected clinically in other countries, it was not confirmed by serology. HS has never been reported from UK, Australia, Japan, New Zealand, Denmark, France and some other European countries. Most Asian countries including India rank HS as one of the most economically important bacterial disease. The OIE classifies the HS, with a number of other bacterial and parasitic diseases, as a List B disease. Asia has 423 million cattle and 145 million buffaloes comprising 33% and 95%, respectively, of the world's population. The distribution and frequency of disease occurrence has been attributed to climatic conditions, husbandry practices and types of animals reared.

India is a major country in Asia as well as in the world with the highest domestic animal population which comprises of cattle (185 million), buffaloes (98 million), sheep and goat (181 million), poultry (425 billion) and pigs (13 million). Cattle and buffaloes, which account for the largest in the world, are reared mainly for use as draught animals as well as milk production in the region. It is estimated that during the years 1936 to 1944, there were an average of 700 reported outbreaks of HS and 40,000 deaths per year. The average mortality per year ranged from 30,000 to 60,000 until 1960s, however, the death rate started to decline to approximately 4000 per year from 1970s, presumably due to improved control measures in the region (FAO 2005). It has been reported that during the past four decades HS has accounted for 46-55% of all bovine deaths. Following the successful control or eradication of rinderpest and continued low mortality with foot and mouth disease (FMD), HS emerged as a disease of considerable economic importance in India. The present cumulative HS profile and eco-pathozone in different states of India is depicted in Fig. 1.

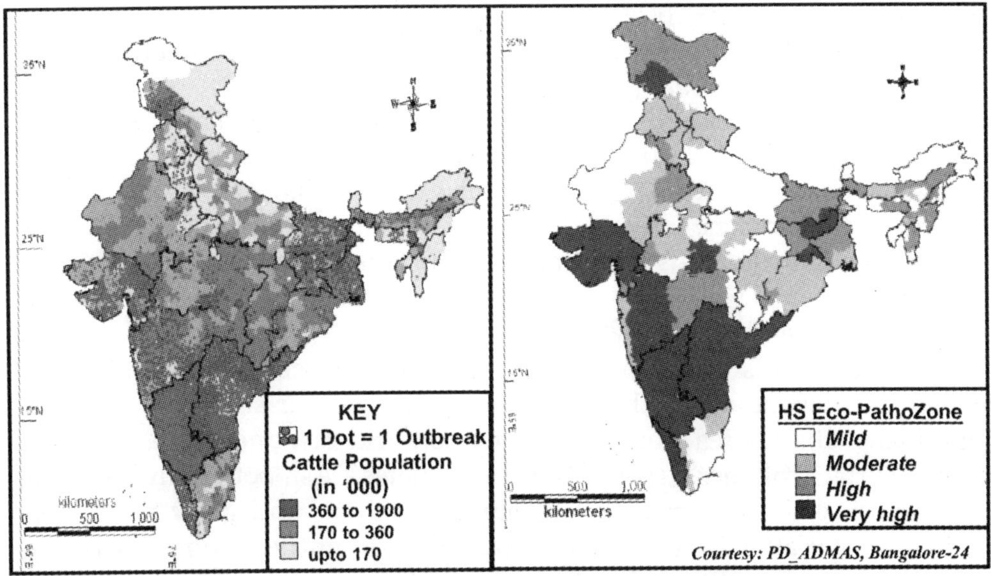

Fig. 1 : Cumulative disease prevalence profile of Haemorrhagic septicaemia (HS) from 1987 to 2007 in India (Courtesy: Director, PD_ADMAS, Bangalore)

2. Background

2.1 Etiological agent *Pasteurella*

2.1.1 History

The history of *Pasteurella* organism dates back to 1782, when it was first studied by Chabert in France. In 1836, Mailet, first used the term 'fowl cholera' for an outbreak of disease in fowl, however, the causative bacterium was first described in 1878-79 by Revolta and Revolee. About the same time, Bollinger from Germany described a disease in cattle and buffaloes. In 1885, Kitts isolated the causative organism. A septicaemic disease in rabbits was described by Gaffky in 1881 and a similar disease in swine by Loeffler in 1886. Later, in 1887, Oreste and Armani from Italy proposed the name *'Bacillus septicaemiae'*. In 1887, Trevisan proposed the name *'Pasteurella'* in recognition of pioneering work done in early 1880s by Louis Pasteur on the etiology of fowl cholera.

2.1.2 Nomenclature

Initially, the bacterium was named according to the host species in which it caused the disease. The isolates from cattle were named 'Boviseptica', those from pigs as 'suiseptica'; and from poultry as 'aviseptica'. Subsequently, there were several changes in the name until in 1939 Rosenbach and Merchant proposed the name *'Pasteurella multocida'* (L. adj. *multus* - many; L. adj. suf. *cidus* - kill; *multocida* - many killing, referring to pathogenicity for many species of animals). It is further divided into three subspecies; *P. multocida* subsp. *multocida, P. multocida* subsp. *septica* (*septica* - poisoning, infecting) and *P. multocida* subsp. *gallicida* (*gallina* - hen; *cida* - kill; *gallicida* - hen killing, referring to pathogenicity for poultry). At present, the organism *P. multocida* belongs to the family *Pasteurellaceae*, which includes a large group of Gram-negative bacteria with three genera namely *Pasteurella, Actinobacillus* and *Haemophilus* that are facultatively anerobic, fermentative and known to cause diseases in mammals, birds and reptiles (Christensen and Bisgaard 1997).

2.1.3 Morphological characteristics

Pasteurella cells are non-motile, small and coccoid to rod shaped, pleomorphic depending on the growth stage, they occur singly, in pairs, or short chains. Gram's reaction is negative, non acid fast and non-endospore forming. Surface colonies on sheep blood agar plates are smooth round, grayish or yellowish, glistening translucent, non-haemolytic, and grow nearly 1-2 mm in diameter after 24 h of incubation at 37°C. In nutrient broth, there is a slight clouding after 18 h of incubation at 37°C, however, a good growth is achieved in brain heart infusion (BHI) broth. There is no growth on MacConkey's agar. The fresh cultures, blood smears, exudates and infected animal tissues show bipolar staining of organism with Leishman or Methylene blue or Giemsa stain.

2.1.4 Biochemical characteristics

Members of the genus are mesophilic, chemo-organotrophic with both oxidative and fermentative types of metabolism. Molecular oxygen is used as a terminal electron acceptor but can be replaced by nitrate and fumerate. Oxidase, alkaline phospatase and catalase positive, most species are V-factor (b-nicotinamide adenine dinucleotide) and X-factor (protohemin or proto porphyrin IX) independent, although V-factor requiring species and strains do occur. Members of the genus are always positive for fermentation of D-glucose, D-galactose, D-fructose, D-mannose, and sucrose; acid is produced from L-sorbose, L-rhamnose, m-inositol, or adonitol. No hydrolysis of starch, salicin or aesculin occurs. Arginine dihydrolase, lysine decarboxylase, liquefaction of gelatin and urease test are negative. The genome of *Pasteurella* contains 37.7 to 45.9 mol% G+C, with molecular weight ranging from $1.4x10^9$ to $1.9x10^9$ (Mutters *et al.* 1985). The phenotypic variability among the strains of *P. multocida* of bovine, avian, caprine, leporine and ovine origin has been well documented by many workers (Ekundayo *et al.* 2008).

2.1.5 Serotypes classification

Numerous attempts have been made in the past to classify *P. multocida* and to correlate these with a specific disease manifestation (Carter 1955). In

1947, Roberts started an immunological typing system based on passive protection of mice by antiserum and four types (I, II, III & IV) were recognized. Later, in 1954, Hudson added one more type V. In 1961, Namioka and Murata recognized 11 serotypes (1-11) based on tube agglutination test. Currently, the most acceptable and widely used serotype designation system is a combination of Carter capsular typing and Heddleston somatic typing, which recognizes five capsular serogroups (A, B, D, E and F) based on the indirect haemagglutination assay (IHA) and sixteen (1-16) somatic serotypes based on agar gel precipitation test (Carter 1967, Heddleston *et al.* 1972).

The causative agent for HS has been named in different classifications as Robert type-I, Heddleston type 2, Carter type B and Namioka & Carter type 6:B and 6:E. The Asian serotype for HS is designated as B:2 and the African serotype E:2 by the Carter-Heddleston system which corresponds to 6:B and 6:E of Namioka-Carter system.

2.1.6 Virulence Factors (VFs)

P. multocida has several mechanisms or components to evade the host defensive immune systems, which are generally cumulatively termed as virulence factors (Harper *et al.* 2006).

2.1.6.1 Capsule

The capsule structure has a significant role in the determination of the serogroup type of *P. multocida,* namely A, B, D, E and F. Polysaccharides constitute the major part of the capsule and in some cases may be associated with lipoproteins. The capsular serotypes A, D and F are composed of hyaluronan, heparosan and unsulphated chondroitin, respectively. The genes required for the synthesis and transport of these capsular types are encoded within a single region on the chromosome. The gene expression gives rise to capsular variability of strains. It has been found that the capsular strains are more virulent than their acapsular variants. The capsule of an organism is known to play a significant role in resistance to phagocytosis. Removal of hyaluronic acid from capsule increases adhesiveness of the organism to the animal cell surfaces as well as its susceptibility to phagocytosis. The production of capsular material of *P. multocida* is affected by sub-minimal inhibitory concentration of antibiotics (Boyce *et al.* 2000).

2.1.6.2 Fimbriae and adhesin

Fimbriae, which are known to play a role in surface adhesion, have been found in *P. multocida* strains that are able to adhere to mucosal epithelium. The presence of fimbriae on *P. multocida* isolated from rabbit pharyngeal cells, pigs tonsilar and nasal cells, and calves nasal and tracheal cells has been identified by electron microscopic studies. Type IV fimbriae (pili) have been isolated and characterized from serotypes A, B and D and are often associated with attachment to host surfaces (Ruffolo *et al.* 1997). The subunit gene, *ptfA*, has been isolated and sequenced from number of strains. The predicted protein sequences show significant variation between strains. The treatment of the organism with pronase, heat, acidity or homogenisation, has confirmed the involvement of the fimbriae and/or the capsular material in the attachment process as the anti-fimbrial antibodies specifically inhibit the adherence capabilities of the organism, which has been found to vary among different serotypes.

2.1.6.3 Outer membrane proteins (OMPs)

Complex OMP profile of more than 15-20 protein bands is demonstrated in *P. multocida* isolated from HS. Although, the correlation between the electrophoretic pattern and serotypic properties of isolates are established, there is no single protein band which could be identified as unique to all strains that caused haemorrhagic septicaemia. The common OMP bands with molecular weights, 27kDa, 34kDa and 36kDa have been identified in all isolates regardless of serotype. Earlier studies indicated proteins of 37kDa and 39kDa as protective antigens. Some of the proteins identified in OMP are OmpH, OmpA, Oma87, Pm1069 and iron related proteins, Tbp (transferin binding protein), HgbA (haemoglobin-binding protein) (Hatfaludi *et al.* 2010).

Iron is an essential element which is required by *P. multocida* organism to grow and survive by using several mechanisms to uptake iron from host under varied conditions. Comparison of *P. multocida* grown in iron rich, iron depleted media or *in vivo* has demonstrated that many high molecular weight OMPs are regulated by iron levels and called iron regulated OMPs (IROMPs). It is considered that IROMPs play a significant role cross protective immunity (Srivastava 1998). Serum from vaccinated animals has been reported to contain antibodies reacting only with few OMP bands. A very recent study based on bioinformatics analysis of *P. multocida* genome predicted 129 proteins as secreted and located in the outer membrane, or lipoproteins (Al-Hasani *et al.* 2007).

2.1.6.4 Lipopolysaccharide (LPS) - endotoxins

LPS is a major virulence factor and plays a critical role in the pathogenesis of diseases such as haemorrhagic septicaemia in buffaloes. It is considered to be a protective antigen as it is known to stimulate humoral immunity. Examination of *P. multocida* strains from different animals has confirmed that LPS from *P. multocida* is slightly similar or shorter than that of *Enterobacteriacae*. It is reported that LPS with low molecular weight is responsible for the 1-16 somatic serotypes. Intravenous inoculation of LPS from serotype B:2 strains is reported to reproduce clinical signs of HS in buffaloes. Antibody reacting with the LPS of different strains is known to provide protection against the infection. Clinical isolates of *P. multocida* from cattle exhibited serum resistance. LPS is found to stimulate the release of many interleukins, TNF-α and other tumour inhibition factors from bovine alveolar macrophages due to mitogenic action of the endotoxins.

2.1.6.5 Exotoxins

P. multocida toxins (PMT), in particular those of capsular serotype D, produce a factor designated as 'dermonecrotic toxin' (DNT). Purified DNT is a protein of estimated molecular weight ranging from 112kDa to 160kDa and can be recovered from sonic and culture fluids. Dermonecrotizing activity is considered one of the toxic actions, which include cytotoxicity for embryonic bovine lung cells, lethality, mucoid diarrhoea or splenic atrophy in mice, turbinate bone atrophy in a range of animals including pigs, rats, rabbits and goats, and vascular endothelial damage in the liver of pigs and rats. The toxin is also reported to be mitogenic, lethal and to cause inhibition of bone cell differentiation as well as osteoblast activity, stimulation of osteoclast activity and inhibition of adoptive immunity development (Foged 1992). Other than serotype-D, the serotype-B has also been reported as potentially active toxin producing serotype. DNT has been associated with atrophic rhinitis in pigs due to the toxic action on turbinate nasal bones. Other hosts such as poultry, calves, cats, dogs, and rabbits are also susceptible to the toxins.

2.1.6.6 Multocidin or siderophores

Iron is an essential element for *P. multocida* growth. The organism, grown in iron deprivation conditions, is able to secrete a growth enhancing factor that functions as a siderophore (multocidin). Siderophores selectively bind ferric iron and are involved in receptor-specific iron transport into the bacterial cell. Several types of siderophores are synthesized by *P. multocida*. The organism is also capable of obtaining iron for growth by a non-siderophore mediated mechanism. Such acquisition is associated with the production of a number of high molecular weight, iron-regulated OMP including an 82kDa receptor protein for transferrin-bound iron (TbpA). This capacity is observed in bovine strains but not in avian strains, and is restricted to acquisition from bovine transferrin.

2.1.6.7 Extracellular enzymes

Several lipase enzymes produced by many strains of *P. multocida* isolated from different animal are considered potential virulence factors. Hyaluronidase is another enzyme produced by *P. multocida*. Its production appears to be limited to type B virulent strains (B:2) isolated from haemorrhagic septicaemia cases, whereas neuraminidase activity is detected in most serogroups isolated from different species. Hyaluronidase activity test can be used to presumptive diagnosis of B:2 strains causing HS. High neuraminidase production is correlated to higher virulence of strains. Sialidases produced from several *P. multocida* strains are known to involve in scavenging sialic acid from host and increase the virulence of bacteria by blocking the effectiveness of the host defences such as mucin. Avian strains are reported to be lacking extracellular enzymatic activity. Yet many genes have been identified for secreting extracellular enzymes from different species that expressed high virulence potentials (Carter and Chengappa 1980).

2.1.6.8 Plasmids

Plasmids have been recovered from *P. multocida* strains isolated from various animal species. These plasmids are known to confer antibiotic resistance (R-factor) as well as encoding many toxins. Avian strains contain plasmids correlated to complement resistance. Plasmid profile is considered as virulence marker of *P. multocida* as well as an essential epidemiological tool for identifying different strains from the same phenotype. *P. multocida* can be easily transformed with plasmids by electroporation process.

2.1.7 Pathogenicity to laboratory animals

The most strains of *P. multocida* are highly virulent to mice as well as rabbits by experimental inoculation. The minimum lethal dose (LD_{50}) is between 1 and 10 viable organisms. Guinea pigs are also susceptible to infection to a less extent. The serotype B:2 strains are not known to cause infection in birds. Comparative virulence studies have indicated chicken strain of *P. multocida* to be the most virulent to mice followed by duck and bovine strains. Strain differences are generally noticed in terms of lesion severity and time leading to death within 24 h post-inoculation.

2.1.8 Antibiotic sensitivity pattern

Antibiotic resistance in *Pasteurella* is increasing with the emergence of R-plasmids which have been reported to be as both conjugative and non conjugative (Hirsh *et al.* 1981). The conjugative R-plasmids are commonly responsible for inter-species and inter-genic spread of multiple drug resistance and transfer of such plasmids among the pathogenic strains may give rise to epidemic spread of infection. Most of *P. multocida* isolates are found to be resistant to sulpha drugs with varied sensitivity to chloramphenicol, gentamycin, tetracycline, kanamycin, penicillin-G, streptomycin, sulphonamides and trimethoprim as assessed by agar dilution technique and determination of the susceptibility of transconjugants and transformants by disc diffusion assay. Coexistence and the spread of small plasmids are used by *P. multocida* to become multi-resistant (SanMilan *et al.* 2009).

2.2 *Pasteurella* associated diseases

Several serotypes of *P. multocida* are associated with different disease manifestations in cattle, buffaloes, sheep and goat, rabbit, poultry and wild animals as well as human beings.

2.2.1 Haemorrhagic septicaemia (HS)

It is a highly fatal, acute septicaemic disease of great economic importance occurring mainly in buffaloes and cattle, caused by two specific serotypes of *P. multocida* designated B:2 (Asian Serotype) and E:2 (African Serotype). It is prevalent mostly in the regions where husbandry practices are poor (Benkirane and De-Alwis 2002). Incidence and distribution of HS varies greatly from a few cases to large number of reports depending on the geographical area and agro-climatic conditions prevailing in various regions of the country. The presumptive epidemiological cycle of HS is depicted in the Fig. 2.

The disease occurs in acute, sub acute and chronic forms. The clinical case of HS is characterized by initial phase of temperature elevation (often unnoticed), a phase of respiratory involvement, and a terminal phase of septicaemia and recumbence leading to death. The incubation period is usually 1-3 days, and the course of the disease may range from sudden death, with no observable clinical signs, to a protracted course extending upto 5 days.

The acute form is manifested by sudden onset and death within 24 hours. The animals show a high rise in body temperature (41-42°C), pulse is thin, rapid and shallow respiration with cyanosis of visible mucus membranes. Restlessness, mild colic pain, muscular tremors, lacrymation, nasal discharge and diarrhoea are also observed. In sub-acute form, known as subcutaneous edematous form, animal survives for 2-3 days with oedematous swelling of throat and brisket region and bronchopneumonia. In chronic form, course of infection is longer with signs of short, rapid painful respiration coupled with mucopurulent or blood stained nasal discharge.

At post mortem examination, the first obvious lesion is subcutaneous oedema, particularly in the mandibular and brisket region. Other lesions include petechial to echymotic haemorrhages, congestion and/or consolidation of lungs, fibrinous pneumonia, pleurisy and pericarditis.

Buffaloes are generally believed to be more susceptible to HS than cattle, and in this species, the disease course is shorter. In endemic areas, most deaths are confined to older calves and young adults. In non endemic areas, massive epizootics may occur. Case fatality approaches to 100% if treatment is not carried at early stage. The presence of naturally acquired immunity is observed among buffaloes. It has been opined that HS morbidity and mortality pattern, in endemic and non-endemic areas in a given population, is largely dependent on the proportion of naturally acquired immune to non-immune animals (Bain 1954).

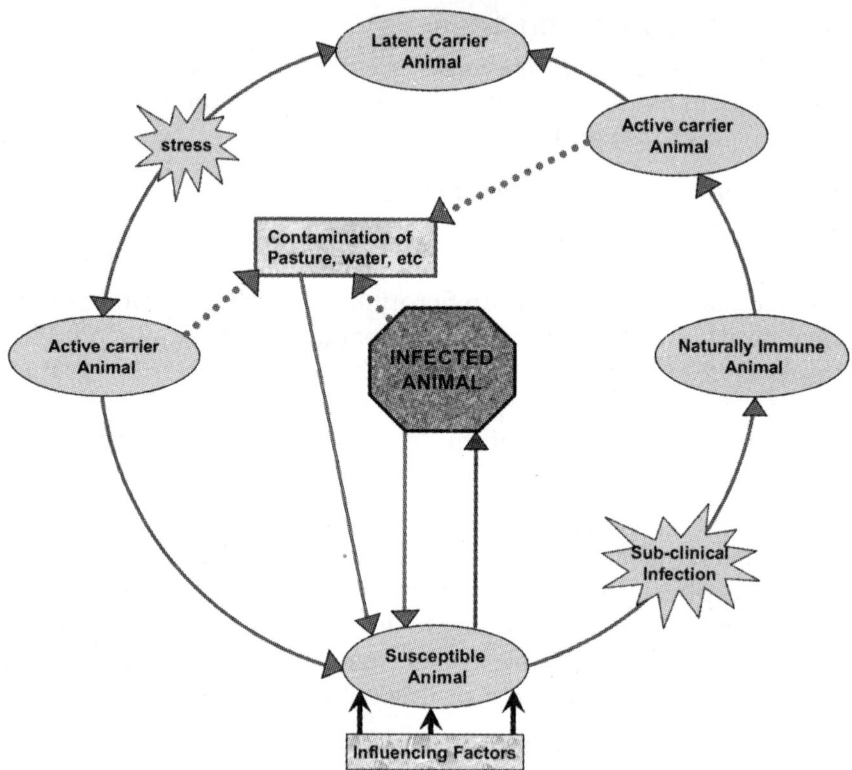

Fig. 2 : Presumptive epidemiological cycle of haemorrhagic septicaemia (HS)

The presence of HS-causing pasteurellae in small proportion in the naso-pharynx of apparently normal healthy cattle and buffaloes and recent exposure to outbreaks of HS has been documented for a long time. Further investigations in the experimentally exposed buffaloes and induced carrier animals, which remained clinically normal, have shown the persistence of pasteurellae in the crypts of tonsils for several months despite treatment with antibiotics, before they appeared actively in the nasopharynx and are shed intermittently in the nasal secretions. The factors, responsible for influencing the latent carriers to become active, are still an enigma.

2.2.2 Fowl cholera in birds

Fowl cholera may result from infection with several strains of *P. multocida*. However, serotype A strains are regarded as the primary cause of Fowl cholera, the most severe form of the disease. The strains, belonging to serogroups D and F have also been isolated from diseased birds, but with low incidence compared with serogroup-A. Serotypes A:1, A:3 and A:4 appear to be prevalent in most of the countries. Moreover, these strains are reported to vary in virulence.

Clinically, fowl cholera is often classified into two forms, acute and chronic, despite the fact that field outbreaks often present clinical signs and lesions that are intermediate between these two forms. In the classic acute form, death may be the only indication of the disease, however, a few hours before death, the birds can reveal signs such as fever, anorexia, ruffled feathers, mouth discharge, diarrhoea, and increased respiratory rate. In the chronic form, signs of localized infection appear viz. swelling of sinuses, wattles and leg and/or wing joints (Christensen and Bisgaard 2000).

2.2.3 Pasteurellosis in pigs

Atrophic rhinitis and pneumonia are two well defined disease manifestations caused by *P. multocida* in pigs. It is known to cause septicaemia and death in young pigs. However, it is more commonly associated with pneumonia in pigs of two to six months age, usually secondary to other infections (Ross 2006). *P. multocida* serotype A and D are mostly associated with the pneumonic condition. Occasional outbreaks of acute septicaemia in swine due to *P. multocida* serotype B have been reported. It has been well documented that some strains of *P. multocida* serotype D and serotype A are also toxigenic, and release exotoxins (PMT also known as dermonecrotic toxin) following the rapid proliferation causing atrophic rhinitis, which is characterized by the atrophy of the nasal turbinates resulting in shortening or twisting of snout accompanied by sneezing and epistaxis. It is rarely known to cause death but significantly reduces the growth rate of the infected pig (Hungerford 1989).

2.2.4 Pasteurellosis in rabbits

It is also known as 'snuffles', a very contagious respiratory disease that commonly affects domestic rabbits. Different strains of *P. multocida* are involved in causing the upper respiratory signs in rabbits. Some strains are commonly found in the nasal tract of rabbits, but may not cause infection unless the animal is stressed or has suppressed immune system. Serogroups A and D are frequently isolated but serogroup A:1,2 is predominant. Susceptibility of individual rabbits varies greatly, though all age groups are susceptible. The disease is known to cause acute pneumonia, septicaemia, otitis media, encephalitis abscesses and pyometra.

2.2.5 Pasteurellosis in sheep, goat and wild animals

Septicaemic and pneumonic menifestations are observed among sheep, goat and wild animals. Climatic changes and stressful management practices such as transport, dipping and shearing may precipitate the disease outbreaks in sheep and goat.

Apart from domestic animals, occasional or sporadic outbreaks of the disease have been recorded among different wild animals like deer, yaks, horses, minks, elephants, bison, snow leopards, lions, tigers, camels and monkeys. The types of infections recorded are highly variable ranging from septicaemia to respiratory infections. Clinical signs of pneumonic and septicaemic forms are observed and the severity of infection varies depending on the serotype involved and species affected. At necropsy, serofibrinous peritonitis, fibrinous pleurisy with areas of pneumonia, congestion, oedema, and widespread haemorrhages are seen. Moreover, latent infection is known to occur in wild as well as many domestic animals.

2.2.6 Zoonotic P. multocida *infection*

In recent years, the number of human cases infected with *P. multocida* has been reported to be on the rise due to increased intimacy with domestic/ pet animals (Shivachandra *et al.* 2003b). *P. multocida* is a common component of the normal oral flora in majority of dogs and cats, but particularly in cats. Most human soft tissue or wound infections ensue subsequently to traumatic introduction of *P. multocida* through the skin, secondary to dog or cat bites or scratch. In a non-bite/non-scratch scenario, human infections are known to occur due to contact with oral secretions of dogs/cats, or licking. Some of the complications reported in humans with chronic illness, or immuno-compromised persons are cellulites, osteomyelitis, septic arthritis, subcutaneous abscesses, epiglottitis, pharyngitis, sinusitis, pneumonia, peritonitis and conjunctivitis.

2.3 Diagnosis

The sudden death seen with peracute and acute HS must be differentiated from that due to lightening, snakebites, blackleg, RP and anthrax by both conventional and molecular approaches.

For diagnosis, specimens collected from infected live animals are blood samples and nasal secretions, whereas from dead animals, heart blood, liver, spleen, lung and bone marrow of long bones may be collected. The diagnosis is usually done by:

a) Clinical diagnosis

It is based on the characteristic signs, gross pathological lesions, herd history, morbidity and mortality pattern, species susceptibility, age group affected.

b) Laboratory confirmation

- Blood smear examination by staining with Gram's, Leishman's or methylene blue stain

- Isolation by culture or mice inoculation, identification by colony morphology, pathogenicity test, biotyping and antibiogram

c) Immunological methods of identification

- Rapid slide agglutination test
- Indirect haemagglutination test (IHA)
- Agar gel immunodiffusion test (AGID)
- Counterimmunoelectrophoresis

Serological tests are for detecting antibodies but are not normally used for diagnosis. However, IHA test with high titres from 1/160 upto 1/1280 or higher among in-contact animals surviving in the affected herds, are indicative of recent exposure to HS. Other serological tests like passive haemagglutinations, AGID and ELISA have been used with varying degrees of success in attempts to predict level of immunity. The ease of obtaining definite diagnosis through isolation and identification of organisms precludes the need for serodiagnosis. Non-serological methods such as acriflavine flocculation test and hyaluronidase tests could can be employed. However, all these conventional methods of diagnosis with potential problems limit their application in clinical diagnosis of HS and pasteurellosis (Dziva *et al.* 2008).

d) Molecular diagnostic approaches

Recently, polymerase chain reaction (PCR) assays for the specific identification of *P. multocida* and HS causing serotypes have been developed, which can be applied directly to the bacterial colony, bacterial culture lysate and mixed bacterial culture for rapid and specific identification within 3-4 hours. PCR assays have also been employed directly on clinical samples to augment rapid disease diagnosis (Lee *et al.* 2000, Choi and Chae 2001). Nucleic acid based typing tools like, REA, REP-PCR, ERIC-PCR, ribotyping, PFGE, RAPD-PCR and AFLP etc. can be effectively employed for routine genotypic differentiation of *P. multocida* isolates (Shivachandra *et al.* 2003a).

2.4 Treatment

Treatment is of little use once visible signs have appeared. However, treatment is effective in the early stages. The only practical procedure is to check the rectal temperature of all in-contact animals after the first case has been reported, and to start antibiotic therapy immediately. Effective antibiotics should be selected for the treatment after conducting antibiotic sensitivity test for the isolate from a particular outbreak.

Although, a serum therapy using 60-100ml of hyperimmune serum has been suggested in treating animals at varying periods from 6 hours before to 18 hours after infection but is found to be less significant in treatment.

2.5 Prophylaxis

Vaccination of susceptible animals in endemic areas is the only practical approach in the prophylaxis of pasteurellosis. A variety of vaccines with different formulations and combinations are available (Verma and Jaiswal 1998), and some of them are as follows:

a) *Plain bacterins*: prepared either from broth/agar culture, immunity is not more than 6 weeks, occasionally given in the face of outbreaks.

b) *Alum precipitated vaccine*: immunity over five months, but immunity can be enhanced with adjuvants.

c) *Oil adjuvant vaccine*: immunity for one year, commonly used in majority of areas.

d) *Multiple emulsion vaccine* (MEV): immunity lasts for 1 year approximately.

e) *Attenuated/Chemically altered/Live vaccines*: prepared by either prolonged *in vitro* cultivation or chemically/genetically altered mutant vaccines, known to provide immunity for more than one year.

However, these vaccines have few shortcomings and the consequent difficulties in mass vaccination programmes.

3. Past Achievements

Since the pioneering work of Pasteur, several notable milestone achievements in the realm of organism's characteristics, virulence, pathogenicity, disease diagnosis and development of vaccines have been reported by many workers.

3.1 Complete genome analysis

Knowing the complete sequence of *P. multocida* genome provides much information about the unique biology of the organism. In the recent past, a physical and genetic map of an Australian serotype A:1 fowl cholera isolate (PBA100) was generated by using restriction enzymes. This study found the chromosome to be a 2.35 Mb single circular molecule with no extra chromosomal elements. The genetic organization of *P. multocida* A:1 strain appeared to have many features common to other bacterial species. A putative location for the origin of replication was suggested and various genes involved in transcription were also located in the surrounding regions. Several genes involved in virulence and immunity in *P. multocida* and other bacterial pathogens were localized onto the physical map, such as Type 4 fimbrial gene *ptfA*, capsule biosynthesis genes, genes involved in iron acquisition (transferrin binding protein, *tbpA*), the *skp* gene and those encoding outer membrane porin *ompH* and the *oma*87 OMP. The rRNA genes of *P. multocida* were found to exist as five operons with the gene order *rrs-rrl-rrf* similar to that of many other eubacteria. The *rrn* operons were arranged in two groups being transcribed divergently away from the *oriC* region. Comparison of rare restriction sites and marker genes between genomic maps of different species or strains provides one measure of genetic variation at the molecular level. Avian strains of *P. multocida* in particular have been found to exhibit considerable genomic diversity. Genomic diversity may have arisen through recombination events such as insertions, deletions, inversions and duplications or may be due to the large number of separate serotypes being grouped together in the species (Hunt *et al.* 2000).

More recently, complete genome sequence of *P. multocida* A:1 (*Pm*70) has been reported by the Advance Genetic Analysis Center at the University of Minnesota (http://www.cbc.umn.edu/Researchproject/AGAC/Pm/index.html). The generation of genetic maps of other *P. multocida* strains and serotypes to compare the organization may help to determine if these restriction polymorphisms relate to a distinct association between the genome architecture and properties such as virulence, host specificity and other metabolic or pathogenic phenotypic aspects (May *et al.* 2001).

3.2 Advances in molecular analysis

With the advent of PCR technology and genomic and proteomic tools, the applied research has taken a new dimension with fortified ability to better understand and accurately diagnose the diseases affecting humans as well as animals. The key advances in applicability and suitability of molecular tools with respect to *P. multocida* are mentioned here under.

3.2.1 Molecular identification or diagnosis

DNA based molecular techniques are emerging as an attractive option with high specificity and rapidness when compared to the complexities associated with the conventional identification and serotyping methods (Blackall and Miflin 2000). Polymerase chain reaction (PCR) technology has been particularly useful in this regard with the use of primer sequences designed to facilitate identification at any level of specificity i.e. strain, species, genus or all members of domain. The list of primer sequences used in different PCR assays is given in Table 1.

3.2.1.1 *Pasteurella multocida*-specific PCR (PM-PCR) assay

Townsend *et al.* (1998) were able to develop a PCR for *P. multocida* based on a DNA sequence obtained by a fortuitous finding of KMT1 clone, during the work directed at looking for difference between HS and non-HS isolates of *P. multocida*. This PCR termed as KMT-PCR showed a positive signal (amplicon size ~460bp) with field isolates of *P. multocida* (representing capsule types A, B, D and F) and the type strains for the three *P. multocida* subspecies

(Fig. 3). KMT-PCR has been shown to give a positive reaction with reference strain for *P. canis* biovar 2.

3.2.1.2 Haemorrhagic serogroup B specific PCR (HSB-PCR) assay

Two independently isolated gene sequences unique to HS-causing serogroup B *P. multocida* (Brickell *et al.* 1998, Townsend *et al.* 1998) have been utilized in the development of serogroup B-specific PCR assays. The HSB-PCR developed by Townsend *et al.* (1998) remains specific for HS-causing serogroup B cultures with the predominant somatic antigen being either serotype 2 or 5 specifically identified by the amplification of ~620 bp fragment by the KTSP61 and KTT72 primers (Fig. 4).

3.2.1.3 Multiplex capsular PCR typing system

The capsular typing system based on PCR has been developed by Townsend *et al.* (2001) following identification, sequence determination and analysis of the capsular biosynthetic loci of each capsular serogroups (A, B, D, E and F). The targeted gene, amplicon size and primers used in this assay are listed in Table 1 and Fig. 5. The multiplex capsular PCR assay is highly specific and its results, with the exception of those for some serogroup F strains, correlate well with conventional serotyping results. This assay represents a rapid and reproducible alternative to the serological and non-serological methods currently used for classification of *P. multocida* capsular types.

3.2.1.4 *Pasteurella multocida* serogroup-A specific PCR assay

Recently, another primer set (Table 1), designed by Gautam *et al.* (2004) in development of PCR assay for detecting *P. multocida* serogroup A isolates, was identified within genes *hya*C-*hya*D of region 2 capsule biosynthetic locus of *P. multocida* A:1. This PCR assay is known to produce an amplified product of ~564 bp with high specificity and sensitivity, and can be employed for rapid identification of bacterial colony and bacterial culture lysate.

3.2.1.5 *Pasteurella multocida* virulence typing system

Recently, a new valuable PCR-based method was introduced to determine the epidemiological correlation between *P. multocida* infection and existence of virulence genes including *tbp*A, *pfh*A, *tox*A and *hgb*B (Ewers *et al.* 2006).

3.2.2 Molecular characterization

It encompasses a large range of methods with variable specificity and discriminating power most of which have been used to differentiate the phenotypically similar *P. multocida* isolates from various animal or avian species (Shivachandra *et al.* 2003a).

Table 1 : List of primers used in specific identification of *P. multocida* isolates from pasteurellosis

Sl. No.	Specific PCR	Primer Name	Primer sequence	Target gene	Amplicon size	Reference
1	*Pasteurella multocida*	KMT1 SP6	5'-GCTGTAAACGAACTCGCCAC -3'	KMT1 clone	~460 bp	Townsend *et al.* (1998)
		KMT1 T7	5'-ATCCGCTATTTACCCAGTGG -3'			
2	*Pasteurella multocida* HS serogroup -B (B :2, B :5, B :2,5)	KTS P61	5'-ATCCGCTAACACACTCTC -3'	6b (KTSP61 - KTT72) clone	~620 bp	
		KTT72	5'-AGGCTCGTTGGATTATGAAG -3'			
3	*Pasteurella multocida* Capsular serogroup - A	CAPA-FWD	5'-TGCCAAAATCGCAGTCAG -3'	*hya*D	~1044 bp	Townsend *et al.* (2001)
		CAPA-REV	5'- TTGCCATCA TTGTCAGTG -3'			
4	*Pasteurella multocida* Capsular serogroup - B	CAPB-FWD	5'-CATTTATCCAAGCTCCACC -3'	*bcb*D	~760 bp	
		CAPB-REV	5'-GCCCGAGAGTTTCAATCC -3'			
5	*Pasteurella multocida* Capsular serogroup - D	CAPD-FWD	5'-TTACAAAAGAAAGACTAGGAGCCC -3'	*dcb*F	~657 bp	
		CAPD-REV	5'-CATCTACCCACTCAACCATATCAG -3'			
6	*Pasteurella multocida* Capsular serogroup - E	CAPE-FWD	5'-TCCGCAGAAAATTATTGACTC -3'	*ecb*J	~ 511 bp	
		CAPE-REV	5'-GCTTGCTGCTTGCTTGATTTTTGTC -3'			
7	*Pasteurella multocida* Capsular serogroup - F	CAPF-FWD	5'-AATCGGAGAACGCAGAAATCAG -3'	*fcb*D	~851 bp	
		CAPF-REV	5'-TTCCGCCGTCAATTACTCTG -3'			
8	*Pasteurella multocida* Capsular serogroup - A	RGPMA5	5'-AATGTTTGCGATAGTCCGTTAGA -3'	*hya*C-*hya*D	~564 bp	Gautam *et al.* (2004)
		RGPMA6	5'-ATTTGGCGCCATATCACAGTC -3'			

3.2.2.1 Restriction endonuclease analysis (REA)

REA uses restriction endonuclease (RE) enzymes derived from bacterial cell, which are capable of cutting double stranded chromosomal DNA wherever specific recognition sequence of the enzyme occurs, producing a set of DNA segments representing a fingerprint of the respective genome. REA is the method currently being used to characterize and differentiate the isolates of the same serotype and to determine the sources of infection in different outbreaks of HS and pasteurellosis. This technique has been shown to be highly sensitive and reproducible in a variety of bacteria. A major advantage of REA is that it involves examining the genotype of the organism which is more stable than the phenotype.

Typically, REA of *P. multocida* strains has been performed using enzyme either six- or four base cutter enzymes. REA using different enzymes viz. *Pst*I, *Eco*RI, *Sma*I; *Bgl*II, *Xho*I *Hha*I, *Hind*III and *Hpa*II have been successfully applied to differentiate the isolates of *P. multocida* indicating good typeability of the technique with some exceptions (Rimler 2000).

3.2.2.2 Pulsed field gel electrophoresis (PFGE)

PFGE of whole chromosomal DNA is a specialized form of REA, often considered a 'gold standard' of molecular typing methods. It uses the rare cutter RE enzymes to digest the bacterial DNA and is subjected to electrophoresis in which the polarity of the current is changed at predetermined intervals. The resultant digest contains few fragments (5-20) of 10 to 800 kb in size, larger than REA fragments. The PFGE patterns enable to create a reference database for the organisms to compare with any new strain. Although, the technique has been proven to be highly discriminating the *P. multocida* isolates (Gunawardana *et al.* 2000, Jablonska and Opacka 2007), its applicability in routine diagnostic laboratories is limited due to requirement of high quality DNA and expensive electrophoresis apparatus.

3.2.2.3 Southern blot-restriction fragment length polymorphism (RFLP) method

It is mainly based on REA coupled with hybridization. The restriction fragments from the bacterial DNA digest are transferred from agarose gel to nylon membrane by southern blotting. The membrane bound DNA is hybridized to one or more labeled probes homologous to the gene to be examined. RFLP refers to the polymorphic nature of the location of RE sites within a defined genetic region. Ribotyping is a variation of southern blot-RFLP in which the probes are derived either from ribosomal RNA (5s RNA, 16s RNA and 23s RNA) itself or the genes that code for rRNA (*rrf, rrs* and *rrl*). It has been applied successfully for typing of *P. multocida* strains.

3.2.2.4 PCR amplifications based on repetitive regions (REP-PCR and ERIC-PCR)

Consensus oligonucleotides matching highly conserved extragenic or intergenic repetitive sequences are being used as primers to amplify DNA between successive repetitive elements in different Gram-negative enterobacterial strains to assess genotypic distinctions directly. Two such techniques are Repetitive Extragenic Palindromic (REP)-PCR and Enterobacterial Repetitive Intergenic Consensus (ERIC)-PCR, which target the REP and ERIC elements of bacterial genome respectively.

The REP elements are potential regulatory sequences of 33 to 40 base pair repeats within untranslated regions of operons, counted as 500 to 1000 copies (1% of the genome) and are widely present in enteric bacteria (Olive and Bean 1999). ERIC elements, known as intergenic repeat units (IRUs), are located in extragenic regions with 126 bp large, highly conserved central inverted repeats (Hulton *et al.* 1991). The ERIC consensus sequence does not appear to be related to REP consensus sequence and both the sequences are present in most bacterial strains including in the genome of *P. multocida*. REP- and ERIC-PCR are known to generate multiple amplified bands depending on the distribution/location of the REP elements across the genome. REP-PCR and ERIC-PCR techniques have proved to be a valuable tools for rapid epidemiological analysis and differentiation of outbreak related isolates of *P. multocida* (Versalovic *et al.* 1991, Townsend *et al.* 1997). As PCR-based tests do not require high quality DNA preparation (must for REA, ribotyping and PFGE), the REP/ERIC-PCR can be performed directly on colonies without any need for extensive DNA extraction and, thus, highlights the time advantage over other DNA-based typing methods (Gunawardana *et al.* 2000).

3.2.2.5 Randomly amplified polymorphic DNA (RAPD)-PCR

RAPD analysis uses oligonucleotide primers that amplify certain sections of the genome by PCR to produce identifiable banding patterns, which are useful in strain differentiation. The procedure has been widely used in a variety of bacteria. RAPD-PCR assay for *P. multocida* has been developed to provide a fast and resource efficient method of classifying individual field isolates with high specificity. Many workers have reported the use of RAPD-PCR assay for *P. multocida* to provide a fast and resource efficient method of classifying and differentiation of individual isolates with high specificity (Dziva *et al.* 2001). Evidence suggests that it is a useful tool for strain differentiation and the availability of commercial kits makes it easy to apply in molecular typing of avian *P. multocida* isolates.

3.2.2.6 Amplified fragment length polymorphism (AFLP)

A novel PCR-based DNA fingerprinting technique, AFLP was developed by Vos *et al.* (1995). This technique is based on the selective amplification of the genomic restriction fragments and combines a high resolution with a high degree of reproducibility, sensitivity and good discriminatory power. The variation by AFLP analysis is based on the mutations in restriction sites or length variation of restriction fragments. The AFLP technique is robust and reliable because stringent reaction conditions are used for primer annealing. AFLP technique can be used to generate fingerprint from DNA of any origin and from any complexity without prior sequence knowledge for identification, epidemiology and taxonomy (Savelkoul *et al.* 1999).

3.2.2.7 Gene sequencing and multi locus sequence typing (MLST)

The differences in the particular gene loci have been used to differentiate the strains but it is expensive and requires identification of species specific loci. However, multiplex capability of high density DNA array can be useful in future.

MLST with high reproducibility and discriminatory power seems to be a viable option as it targets housekeeping loci and the sequence data is portable between laboratories and can permit in establishing a global database (Spratt 1999).

3.3 Advances in vaccine development

A new generation of different vaccines formulations has been developed in the recent times with varying degree of success to control pasteurellosis. These include the conventional ones and those developed by molecular approaches and emerging technologies designed for production of efficient vaccines. Some of these approaches are mentioned here under.

3.3.1 Conventional Approaches in Development of Vaccines

Since the beginning of vaccination for control of diseases, traditional vaccines are proven to be impeccable with a few exceptions and still continue to dominate in the era of the new age vaccines. However, there is a need to rejuvenate them in the present scenario.

3.3.1.1 Killed vaccines

The first approach in making the HS vaccine consists of killing *P. multocida* organisms using formalin which still retains the antigens responsible for inducing the host's immune response. Several killed vaccines have been developed in the past with different kinds of adjuvants. The commonly used vaccines include bacterin, alum precipitated, aluminium hydroxide gel, oil adjuvant vaccines (OAV) and multiple emulsion vaccines. These vaccines vary in their duration of immunity. The OAV and multiple emulsion HS vaccines have been reported to impart immunity for upto 12 months. More recently, an experimental saponified HS vaccine has also been developed which gives good protection in cattle and buffaloes upto 12 months post-vaccination. The difficulties in injecting the OAV due to its high viscosity, formation of abscess at the site of injection and post-vaccination reactions have often been reported. However, vaccination with killed vaccines is generally practised in the areas where the disease is endemic and it has reduced the incidence of disease, but due to short duration of immunity, outbreaks still occur. Moreover, immunity is generally serotype specific. Bacterins are inexpensive to produce but give very limited protection against heterologus serotypes. Further, the protective potency of different batches of vaccines is unpredictable since there is no satisfactory quality control test available for ascertaining their protective potency. There is a need to standardize the methods for suitable vaccines development and monitoring their efficacy, safety and duration of immunity.

3.3.1.2 Attenuated live vaccines

This approach of making vaccines involves methods to attenuate or weaken live *P. multocida* microorganisms by ageing, passage in unnatural hosts, chemical or antibiotics treatment, or altering the growth conditions. Vaccines made in this way are often the most successful vaccines, because they multiply in the body thereby eliciting effective immune response. However, these live attenuated vaccines also carry the risk because they can mutate back to the virulent form at any time. Such mutation would result in induction of the disease rather than protection against it, however, immunity is of longer duration. A deer strain aerosol vaccine (B:3,4) developed in Myanmar, is the sole live vaccine which has been used with success (Myint and Carter 1989). At present, there is no live vaccine for control of HS in India.

3.3.1.3 Acellular vaccines

These vaccines use only the antigenic part of *P. multocida,* for example, the capsule, the fimbriae, lipopolysaccharide (LPS), outer membrane proteins (OMPs) or part of the cell wall proteins. Numerous attempts undertaken in the past to identify the most-potent immunogen of *P. multocida* have yielded conflicting results particularly with regards to the protective role of LPS and capsule (Confer 1993). Further, no encouraging results were obtained from repeated attempts to develop conjugate vaccines by using components like ribosomes or carrier proteins in association with several polysaccharides of *P. multocida*. However, immunization trials with OMPs from *in vivo* grown and iron restricted medium are found to elicit the production of antibodies which give protection against different serotypes. Neither killed nor acellular vaccines generally induce durable immune responses and may therefore require a booster dose after every few months to ensure their continued effectiveness. These are considered to be safe for use in animals as they do not cause disease.

3.3.1.4 Adjuvants in vaccines

Adjuvants, known to enhance immune response against specific antigens, play an important role in the efficacy of some HS vaccines where the antigens become more and more purified especially in case of recombinant proteins or synthetic peptides which are safer but less immunogenic. In the past, many adjuvants namely, vegetable like saponin or glucan extract; bacterial components like monophosphoryl lipid-A, trehalose dymicolate, LPS and their derivative; chemicals like aluminium hydroxide gel, surfactants and emulsions have been used for development of HS vaccines. A new generation of adjuvants comprising mainly cytokines like γ-IFN or GM-CSF, and micro/nano-particles is under trial (Aucouturier *et al.* 2001).

3.3.2 Molecular approaches in development of vaccines

Some of the new biotechnological and genetic engineering techniques in vaccine development have resulted in purified subunits, synthetic peptides, chemical conjugation of polysaccharides with recombinant proteins, use of recombinant bacteria or defined mutants and bacterial ghosts as vaccines (Adler *et al.* 1999).

3.3.2.1 Subunit vaccines

Molecular cloning and expression of particular gene has resulted in generation of number of recombinant proteins from *P. multocida,* which represent only the parts of an organism yet stimulate a strong immune response. To create a subunit vaccine, researchers in the past identified and isolated the gene or genes which code for appropriate subunits from the genome of the infectious agent. For example, Type 4 fimbriae (*ptfA*), outer membrane protein-87 (Omp87), fragments of exotoxin (PMT), porin (OmpH), liporptein E (PIpE), filamentous haemagglutinin (fhaB2), adhesin (OmpA) and transferrin binding protein (TbpA) have been considered as a candidate antigens (Wu *et al.* 2007, Seo *et al.* 2009, Tatum *et al.* 2009). The purified recombinant proteins used as subunit vaccines are known to be safe for immuno-compromised animals because they cannot cause disease. However, no recombinant single antigen has been shown to stimulate protection against HS.

3.3.2.2 Synthetic peptides

Recently, some workers have reported development of synthetic peptides designed according to the amino acid sequences of predicted loop structures to mimic the epitopes of *P. multocida*. For example, synthetic porin (OmpH) peptides have been shown to provide a limited protection against *P. multocida*. However, development of synthetic peptides was hampered due to their less immunogenicity and requirement of effective adjuvants. Despite its major lacunae, there is a hope to gather much useful information for further construction of multi-epitope cross-protective HS vaccines.

3.3.2.3 Genetically engineered defined mutant vaccines

In recent years, genetic technologies have emerged as powerful tools to identify targets for the development of defined live-attenuated vaccines. Among these technologies, *in vivo* expression technology (IVET), substractive hybridization and signature-tagged mutagenesis (STM) have resulted in identification of innumerable number of genes responsible for virulence and pathogenesis of *P. multocida*. A number of attenuated mutants containing transposon insertions in genes encoding biosynthetic enzymes, virulence factors, regulatory components and unknown function are currently being evaluated at laboratory level. For example, acapsular *cexA* mutant of *P. multocida* B:2 generated by inactivation of *bcbH* gene, predicted to be involved in polysaccharide biosynthesis was found to elecit protective immunity against wild type challenge. Another report suggests the use of stable, non-reverting *aroA* mutants as live vaccines (Ataei *et al.* 2009). Nevertheless, the efficacy of various attenuated mutants warrants further laboratory investigations before releasing them for field use against HS.

3.3.2.4 Bacterial ghosts

Bacterial ghosts from a variety of bacteria are currently being used as non-living candidate vaccines. These intact bacterial envelope structures, devoid of cytoplasmic contents, are generated by controlled expression of cloned PhiX174 gene *E* in Gram-negative bacteria and protein E-mediated lysis. A study has reported generation of *P. multocida* ghosts and found 100% protection against homologus challenge in laboratory model (Marchart *et al.* 2003).

4. Current Indian Perspective

4.1 Diseases and epidemiology

HS is an endemic major bacterial disease causing a loss of worth more than 22 crore rupees per year in India through reduced milk production, draught power and death of cattle and buffaloes. Fowl cholera is also a major disease affecting wide range of avian species viz. chicken, duck, turkey, quails and geese, thereby posing a threat to avian biodiversity with large genetic resources in India. Pasteurellosis has also been reported in sheep, pig, rabbit, goat, poultry as well as various wild species viz. tiger, snow leopard etc. The disease prevalence and distribution in different regions of India are depicted in the Fig. 1. On the basis of distribution, endemic nature and utmost economic importance of HS and other related diseases, India has been included under the Category A (FAO-WHO-OIE 1994).

4.1.1 Conventional approaches

Currently, the conventional methods of identification and characterization of field isolates of *P. multocida* in India is being carried out as per the international standards (OIE 2008). A large number of *P. multocida* organisms (>500 isolates) have been isolated in the recent past from various outbreaks of pasteurellosis occurring in different agro-climatic geographical regions (Kumar *et al.* 1996, 2004a, Shivachandra *et al.* 2006c). Considerable variation has been observed among serotypes with respect to host predilection, pathogenicity, and biochemical, cultural and antigenic specificity. We as well as others in the past recorded a noticeable variation in the distribution and occurrence of *P. multocida* infections in different agro-climatic regions of country involving different animal and avian species. As evident from our previous analysis, the outbreaks of the diseases occur throughout the year irrespective of the season (Kumar and Shivachandra 2002). This is in contrast to the known perception that the disease is mostly precipitated during the monsoon or post monsoon period. The incidences of disease outbreaks in India are known to vary considerably in different states and also in each state from year to year (Khera 1979).

4.1.1.1 Prevalent serotypes

Numerous attempts have been made in the past to classify *P. multocida* on the basis of capsular and somatic types and correlate these with a specific disease manifestation. The prevalent serotypes of *P. multocida* isolated from different species of animals and birds are presented in Table 2. Typically, *P. multocida* serotype B:2 is involved in cases of HS among cattle and buffaloes (Singh *et al.* 1996). However, the investigations of field isolates have revealed the presence of other serotypes such as A:1,3, A:3, A:4, F:3, and F:3,4, especially serotype A:1 as next predominant to type B:2 (Kumar *et al.* 1996, 2004a). The clinical signs as observed by field veterinarians in many of these animals (serotype A:1 infected), did not suggest typical HS.

The prevalence of serotypes A:1 and A:3 in sheep, and A:1 has been recorded in goats. Previous reports on pasteurellosis in these animals and associated *P. multocida* serotypes from various countries including India are scarce. *P. multocida* types A and D have occasionally been associated with infectious pneumonia /pasteurellosis in small ruminants. Limited literature reveals that a number of *P. multocida* strains viz. A:1, A:3, A:3,4, A:3,4,12, A:12, B:2, D:3, F:1, F:4,12 have been isolated from sheep and goats (Dhanda and Sen 1972, Dwivedi *et al.* 1990).

Fowl cholera in avian species viz. chickens, duck, turkey, quail, geese, pigeons and cage birds has been reported to be caused by various capsular and somatic types of *P. multocida* (Chawak *et al.* 2000, Shivachandra *et al.* 2006c). To quote a few, serotypes A:1, A:1,3, D:1, D:3 and F:3 have been observed among Indian poultry, with majority of isolates belonging to serotypes A:1, and A:3 and A:4. Occasional outbreaks of acute septicaemic swine pasteurellosis die to serotype B have been reported from time to time (Kumar and Parai 1984). The prevalence of serotype B:2 in pigs may become a source of infection in cattle and buffaloes where composite farming is practised. Snuffles, although a common and widespread infection in rabbit farms, a very few samples analyzed in the past indicate the presence of A:1 and A:3 among infected rabbits. It may be due to less flourishing rabbit farming in the country.

Despite relatively little information about pasteurellosis among Indian wild animals, the presence of *P. multocida* organisms in different wild species viz. lion, tiger, spotted deer, hippopotamus and leopard have been reported (Pavri and Apte 1967, Arora and Kumar 1988, Chaudhari *et al.* 1992, Prabhakar *et al.* 1998). However, the association of these serotypes with disease conditions has to be ascertained following detailed investigation with respect to disease inducing ability of serotypes in wild species.

4.1.1.2 Biotyping studies

A variety of biochemical reactions have proven to be useful in characterization and epidemiological studies of *P. multocida* infections. Since the DNA hybridization studies of Mutters *et al.* (1985), there have been many studies on the biochemical characterization of isolates of *P. multocida* finding three subspecies (Fegan *et al.* 1995). The authors also have earlier carried out the biovars classification and identification of Indian isolates of *P. multocida* and found majority of isolates belonging to *P. multocida* subsp. *multocida*, followed by small numbers of *P. multocida* subsp. *septica* and *P. multocida* subsp. *gallicida* (Shivachandra *et al.* 2006d). The vast differences in the fermentation reactions of carbohydrates might be due to the geographical variation of the isolates and the use of chemotherapeutic agents coupled with host and environmental factors influencing the enzyme profiles of microbes.

4.1.1.3 Antibiogram studies

In the last two decades, shift in antibiotic sensitivity spectrum of pasteurellae is well evident. A number of studies on field isolates of *P. multocida* in India have reported variation in the pattern of sensitivity to different antibacterials. The variation in the sensitivity pattern of *P. multocida* may result in high morbidity and mortality. Studies have indicated the rise in multiple drug resistant strains of *P. multocida*. The differences in the antibiogram may be due to extensive and indiscriminate use of antimicrobials for treatment of bacterial infections, which might lead to selection of resistant strains.

Our earlier studies also indicated that sulphadiazine, the drug of choice in the field, may not work against control of HS and pasteurellosis in India (Biswas *et al.* 2004, Shivachandra *et al.* 2004a). A high trend of resistance in pasteurellae was also observed for a conventional sulpha drug. Moreover, many commonly used antibiotics like amikacin, carbenicillin, erythromycin and penicillin may not be effective in near future because of the development of gradual resistance to these antimicrobial drugs. The injudicious use of the antibiotics is leading to the severe problem of antibiotic resistance, the gene for which is plasmid-borne. This also reflects the fact that Indian strains may have plasmids encoding for drug resistance. Although, there are reports of varied antibiotic sensitivity pattern of isolates from a particular region or outbreak, a comprehensive pattern among different hosts and regions still needs to be studied.

4.1.1.4 Pathogenecity studies

Most studies on the pathogenesis of pasteurellosis have used mice as the host animal for capsular type A or B of *P. multocida*. Very small doses of *P. multocida* organisms are known to proliferate and kill the mice inoculated intraperitoneally within 24 h. Similar results have been observed by many workers who reported nearly 85% of Indian field isolates to cause death of mice in 24 h following intraperitoneal inoculation, whereas the remaining isolates took more than 24 h. The pathogenicity of an organism in mice depends upon the virulence characteristics of the organism and genetic makeup of the host and variation in pathogenicity of the isolates. Pathogenicity studies of *P. multocida* in chicken having indicated 90% mortality within 48-72 h, whereas other isolates have been found to be pathogenic between 72-96 h. Recent literature and many reviews reveal no better understanding of the mechanisms of pathogenesis, nor of the determinants of virulence of this organism.

Our study on the pathogenicity of *P. multocida* serotype B:2 and D:1 isolates from the cases of pneumonic pasteurellosis in crossbred pigs showed development of acute septicaemia characterized by high rise of temperature (105-106° F), anorexia, rapid and distressed respiration and death within 4 days (Dey *et al.* 2002). More intense lesions were seen on post mortem examination in the animals which were inoculated with serotype D:1. The pathogenicity of *P. multocida* in embryonated chicken eggs has also been reported by chorio-allontoic membrane inoculation (Shivachandra *et al.* 2005b).

4.1.2 Molecular approaches

In India, molecular assays and typing tools have been introduced in parallel to the existing conventional methods of identification and characterization of *P. multocida* isolates. It has been more than a decade since the inclusion of PCR assays for primary screening of Indian isolates of *P. multocida* for rapid and specific diagnosis of HS and pasteurellosis.

4.1.2.1 Identification of *P. multocida* strains by PCR assays

A number of workers have extensively used PM-PCR, HSB-PCR and multiplex capsular typing systems for rapid identification and capsular serotyping of more than 500 field isolates originated from different animal and avian species (Shivashankar *et al.* 2001, Dutta *et al.* 2001, Gautam *et al.* 2004, Shivachandra *et al.* 2006c). The results of PM-PCR conducted either in single reaction (Fig. 3) or in multiplex PCR reaction using HSB-PCR assay (Fig. 4), have shown to produce an amplicon size of ~460bp (PM specific) and ~620bp (HSB specific), which correlated well with the results of conventional identification and capsular serotyping. Similarly, the results of serogroup-A specific PCR and multiplex capsular typing system employed on large number of field isolates revealed the correct identification of conventional capsular serogroups (Fig. 5). Moreover, PCR assay is able to identify the acapsular isolates of *P. multocida* which could not be typed based on conventional methods of classification. PCR assays did not cross react with any other bacteria and fungi tested in previous studies revealing high specificity as well as high sensitivity which was observed even with 10 ng of DNA used in the reaction mixture. Moreover, the PCR assay could be directly employed on bacterial colony, bacterial culture lysate or mixed culture lysate without the extraction of purified genomic DNA.

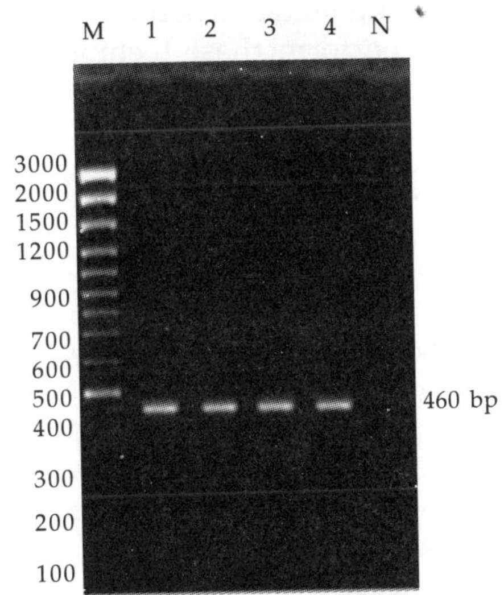

Fig. 3 : Identification of pasteurellosis field isolates by *Pasteurella multocida* specific PCR assay

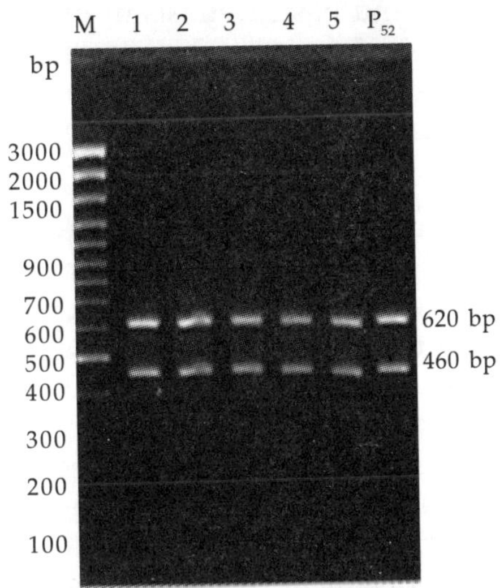

Fig. 4 : Identification of pasteurellosis field isolates by *P. multocida* specific PCR and HSB specific PCR assay

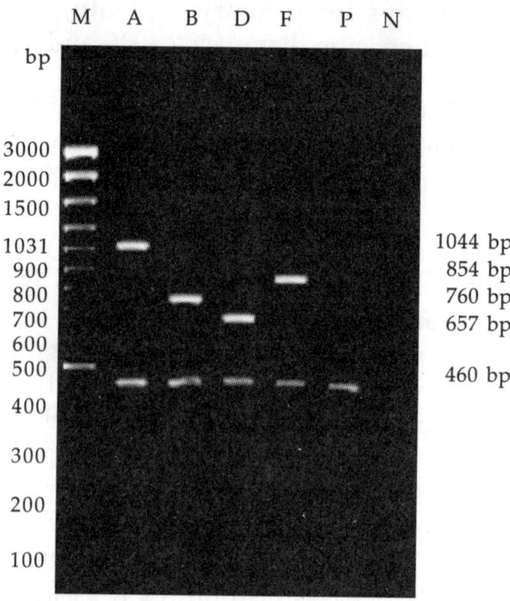

Fig. 5 : Identification and capsular serotyping of pasteurellosis field isolates by Multiplex Capsular PCR assay

In our experience, PCR assays is rapid, specific and highly sensitive for identification and capsular serotyping of *P. multocida* isolates irrespective of the host and geographical region of isolation. The simplicity and versatility of PCR assay would enable the technique to be used on routine basis for diagnosis of HS and pasteurellosis in India compared to conventional serotyping. The PCR equipment and experience required to perform these techniques is becoming readily available in most laboratories in the country, providing a marked advantage over the current methods of identification.

The presumptive diagnosis of peracute and acute form of HS and pasteurellosis is generally based on the occurrence of typical signs and lesions and / or on the microscopic demonstration of bacteria showing bipolar staining in smears of tissues such as blood, liver or spleen. The complexities associated with the conventional diagnostic methods have given up ways for the DNA based methods (Lee *et al.* 2000). Previously, we described the use of PM-PCR and *P. multocida* serogroup A specific PCR assay for diagnosis of HS and fowl cholera by evaluating its direct applicability on the homogenized lysates of tissue samples viz. spleen, lung, liver, heart, and bone morrow, collected from experimentally infected chicken without enrichment of tissues in BHI broth or involvement of DNA extraction from tissues (Shivachandra *et al.* 2004b). PCR can be successfully applied for detection of *P. multocida* serogroup A in the experimentally infected chick embryo using PM specific and serogroup A specific primers. There has been no failure in amplification from embryonic materials such as allontoic, amniotic fluids, homogenized embryo and its membranes (Shivachandra *et al.* 2006b).

Compared with *P. multocida* cultivation, PCR assays are less laborious and results are available within six hours, thereby dramatically reducing the time for diagnosis from a few days to a few hours. However, the sensitivity of the assay may be variable for different tissues. Even a low number of organisms can be detected especially in bone marrow of long bones. The storage studies of morbid materials following detection by PCR has also indicated the possibilities of detecting the organism upto 3 days at 37°C, 40 days at 4°C and even upto 100 days at -20°C especially from bone marrow without *in vitro* cultivation. PCR based detection directly from tissues is of greater advantage in early diagnosis of the disease manifestations.

4.1.2.2 Molecular typing of *P. multocida* isolates

A large number of *P. multocida* isolates originated from different outbreaks of HS and pasteurellosis in the country have been analyzed by many workers by employing various typing techniques viz. REA, ribotyping, REP-PCR, ERIC-PCR, RAPD-PCR and AFLP for their discriminative ability (Dutta *et al.* 2004a, Saxena *et al.* 2005). The banding profiles of Indian *P. multocida* isolates under different molecular typing methods are depicted in Fig. 6 and Fig. 7. REA

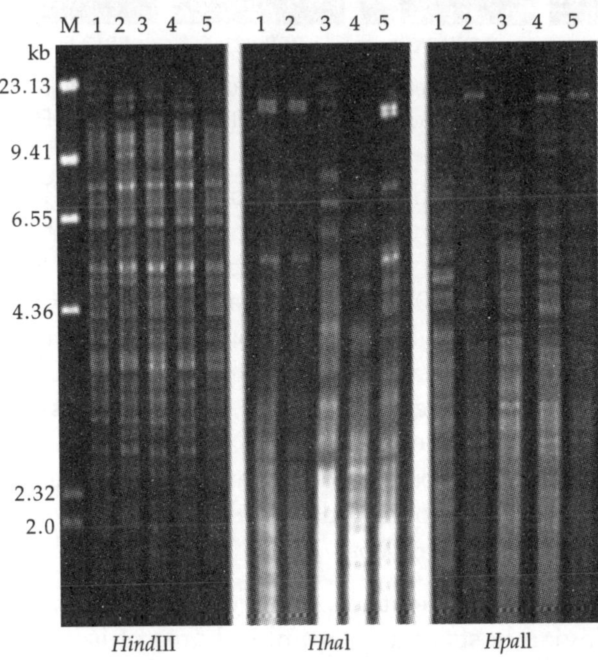

Fig. 6 : Molecular characterization of *P. multocida* isolates by REA using *Hind*III, *Hha*I and *Hpa*II

using several enzymes such *Hind*III digestion of avian *P. multocida* genome resulted in fragments of large numbers with not so clear distinctions between the succeeding fragments upon electrophoresis. Digestion of *P. multocida* genome using *Hpa*II resulted in a good number of larger clear and distinct bands that could be appreciated very easily by an unaided eye. We have noted the high reproducibility and easy to read banding pattern generated by *Hpa*II as compared to other two restriction enzymes. REA analysis using *Hpa*II is a very simple discriminative method and can enable accurate typing of avian *P. multocida* isolates as a complement to classical capsular and somatic typing (Gautam *et al.* 2006).

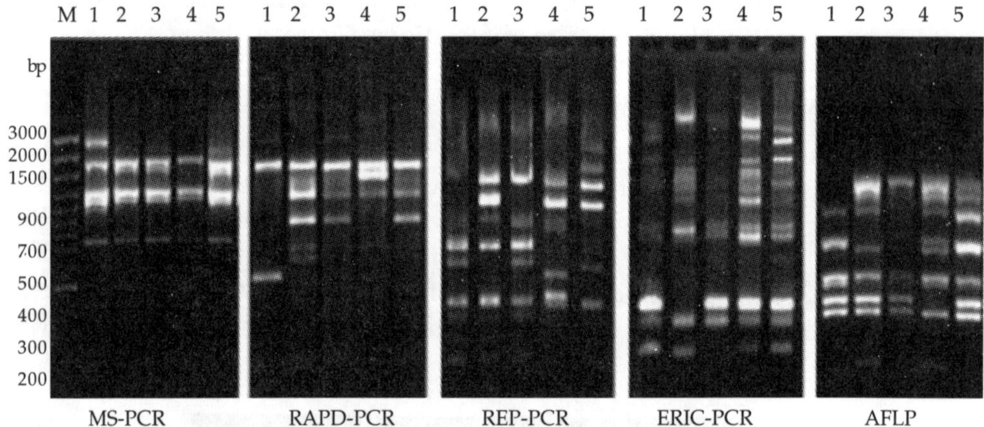

Fig. 7 : Banding profiles of *P. multocida* isolates following molecular characterization by Microsatellite (MS)-RAPD, single primer-RAPD, REP-PCR, ERIC-PCR and AFLP typing

PCR based fingerprinting techniques like REP-PCR, ERIC-PCR, and RAPD-PCR have been employed on the same and different sets of *P. multocida* isolates for characterization studies (Dutta *et al.* 2004b, Saxena *et al.* 2006, Shivachandra *et al.* 2007, 2008). REP-PCR and ERIC-PCR typing techniques appear to be rapid with good discriminatory power and could be employed for routine typing of isolates. Although, RAPD-PCR is also equally discriminative tool to type the isolates, it requires standardization of methodology. Single enzyme AFLP, a novel typing tool with combination of REA and PCR, is found to be a discriminatory method but time consuming that could be employed for occasional or high stringency characterization of isolates (Shivachandra *et al.* 2006a).

On comparison and correlation of phenotypic and genotypic profiles with that of animal/avian hosts and geographical area of isolation, no correlation could be drawn among them as there was sharing of same clusters by different isolates under various typing techniques. Moreover, our studies as well as others in the past have documented the existence of maximum genotypic differences among *P. multocida* isolates especially among the isolates originated from fowl cholera outbreaks. Involvement of multiple strains of *P. multocida* in HS outbreaks (Biswas *et al.* 2004), fowl cholera outbreaks (Shivachandra *et al.* 2005a) as well as outbreaks of pasteurellosis in pigs (Kalorey *et al.* 2008) could also be investigated by employing PCR based typing tools to detect and differentiate between isolates which phenotypically appear similar by conventional methods.

4.1.2.3 Candidate gene amplification and sequence analysis

One vaccine strategy that has been adopted in several other bacterial species in the *Pasteurellaceae,* is to target the surface proteins involved in acquisition of iron in the host as vaccine antigens. One of our earlier studies involving analysis of gene encoding transferrin binding protein (TbpA) from *P. multocida* serogroup B:2 revealed high antigenic index of matured TbpA (89.16 kDa) as well as greater sequence similarity with that of serogroup A:1, which could be used as a candidate antigen in development of vaccines against HS (Shivachandra *et al.* 2005c). Cloned and purified proteins have been tested for their efficacy as protective antigens. In particular, the OMPs and IROMPs have been a focus for development of subunit vaccines. The sequence analysis of Type 4 fimbrial gene (*ptfA*) from *P. multocida* serotype B:2 (strain P_{52}) indicated 78.4% similarity with that of serogroup A:1 (Joseph *et al.* 2007). Comparative gene sequence analysis of 16S rRNA gene from the isolates of *P. multocida* serotype B:2 belonging to buffalo, cattle, pig, sheep and goat indicated close relationships of HS causing *P. multocida* serotype B:2 isolates of buffalo and cattle with that of other uncommon hosts (Dey *et al.* 2008). Differences in surface proteins are a direct reflection of the nucleotide sequence differences in the gene encoding them. Comparative gene analysis of various virulent factors would reveal their role in terms of host specificity, predilection site and pathogenesis.

4.2 Antibacterial treatment

Antibacterial chemotherapy is still being used extensively for treating clinical cases of HS and pasteurellosis in India with varying success depending mainly on the kind of drug used. However, therapy has been compromised due to emergence of multi-drug resistant strains as a result of wholesale use of antibiotics either as a supplement in feed, both for prophylaxis and growth promotion or subtherapeutic use in the feed and metaphylactic antibiotic therapy. The strains of *P. multocida* vary in susceptibility to chemotherapeutic agents and resistance to treatment may develop especially during prolonged use of these agents. The conventional antibiotics had shown more resistance which is posing problems in treating the animals and birds suffering from pasteurellosis.

In India, so far there is scanty literature pertaining to the drug resistance against pasteurellosis as the disease is treated with oxytetracycline, co-trimexazole and with a combination of penicillin and streptomycin or with sulphaquinoxazoline which have proved to be effective. According to earlier reports, most of the strains are resistant to sulpha drug, the drug of choice in pasteurellosis. However, the sensitivity to other therapeutic agents was in the order: amoxicillin (90.9% ampicillin (72.7%), chloramphenicol (45.4%), norfloxacin (27.2%), kanamycin (18.15%) and gentamicin (18.1%). The strains were also comparatively resistant to oxytetracycline and sulfamethoxazole + trimethoprim.

In view of these facts, it is necessary to have a check on the indiscriminate use of antibiotics in treatment of pasteurellosis. Moreover, this warrants the need for pre-testing of antibiotic sensitivity against pasteurellae so as to find out an effective antimicrobial agent to be used by veterinarian/specialists for therapeutic purpose.

4.3 Current vaccines

HS vaccines in India are prepared using *P. multocida* serogroup B:2 (strain P_{52}). Indian Veterinary Research Institute (IVRI) has been involved since long in development and production of HS hyperimmune serum as well as various formulations of HS vaccines such as polyvalent HS vaccine, low volume saponified monovalent HS vaccine and Bivalent HS (B:2, D:1) vaccine combined with FMD vaccine (Kumar and Shivachandra 2004). However, HS oil adjuvant vaccine and multiple oil adjuvant HS vaccine are currently available for vaccination of animals. Most of the veterinary biological laboratories in different states are involved in production of alum precipitated HS vaccine, which has been prepared from highly antigenic B:2 (strain P_{52}) inactivated by formaldehyde solution and precipitated by addition of alum. This vaccine, given at the dose of 5 ml s/c in cattle and buffaloes and 2-5ml s/c in sheep and goat is known to provide immunity lasting for only 6 months and requires additional annual booster dose. Toxoids prepared from purified toxin are also effective against the systemic effect of the toxin in turbinate atrophy of pigs. More recently, a biofilm based vaccine against *P. multocida* serotype A, a causative agent of pasteurellosis in sheep and goat has been developed.

The investigations on isolation and serotyping of *P. multocida* from the cases of HS have revealed the presence of other serotypes (A:1) as well. Moreover, it has been observed in the field that despite proper vaccination, HS does occur among cattle and buffaloes. This could be due to lack of cross protection conferred by the vaccines against other serotypes. In view of the present scenario, there is an imminent need to revamp existing vaccination strategy against HS.

5. Scenario in the Developed Nations

Although, HS has been recorded in most countries of the world, especially in the less developed and developing countries, the developed nations seem to be less affected with the disease. HS has been reported in the Middle East and southern Europe. In the United States, the disease was reported among bison in national parks in 1912, 1922 and 1965-67. Outbreaks were also reported among dairy cattle and beef calves in US and Canada. However, apart from sporadic outbreaks, the disease is not endemic in North America. Most of the oceanic countries such as Australia, New Zealand and others like Japan and Western Europe have not yet reported the disease (De Alwis 1999). However, fowl cholera, a fatal disease of birds, is widely reported from almost all developed countries of the world causing huge economic losses. The sporadic cases of pasteurellosis in sheep and goats as well as in pigs have been recorded in all intensive farms of developed countries. Isolated cases of HS have also been reported from the central and south American states, and from southern and Eastern European countries. It is presumed that HS may occur in developed countries with high water buffalo population and where conditions are similar to that of tropical Asia.

6. Comparative Analysis

Compared to *P. multocida* infections in Asia, *P. haemolytica* infections are known to be prevalent more among livestock in the developed countries. The disease conditions like shipping fever, transit fever, enzootic pneumonia and bovine respiratory disease (BRD) complex have been reported (Dabo *et al.* 2007). In US, it is believed that the losses to beef and dairy industries from this disease complex are greater than the losses due to all other diseases put together. The disease complex is associated with multiple factors with involvement of more than one species and serotype of pasteurellae. The organisms, which reside normally in the healthy host, are known to play a secondary role to other infections due to either bacteria or viruses or stress. Following the stress and other incriminating factors, pasteurellae are known to undergo rapid proliferation resulting in a disease complex with high severity and fatality.

Pasteurellosis in sheep and goat in temperate countries is mainly due to *P.haemolytica* causing pneumonia in all ages of sheep and septicaemia in lambs. Pasteurellosis in pigs is known to involve *Bordetella bronchiseptica,* a normal inhabitant of upper respiratory tract (URT). Since most of the disease conditions are multi-factorial, the use of vaccine to control the infections has limited value. Unlike in India, where most of the conditions are attributed to *P. multocida* as primary cause of HS and pasteurellosis in animals, it is a challenging task in developed countries to design and develop an effective vaccine for control of manifestation. The only remedy has been the use of supportive chemotherapy and implementation of good husbandry practices that avoids stress as well as incriminating environmental factors prevalent in the intensive farms.

Comparative analysis of worldwide distribution indicates the occurrence of the pathogen and disease in highly varied agroclimatic geographical regions ranging form temperate to tropical environment with different livestock densities involving different breeds and age groups. The region based husbandry practices are known to influence the disease outbreaks.

7. Challenges and Constraints

The lingering problem of HS and pasteurellosis has several challenges which are self intrigued by the natural as well as anthropogenic factors. Although, challenges could be overcome by the advances in scientific research, the constraints appear to perplex the progress made in alleviating the disease prevalence.

7.1 Challenges

It is commonly believed that the reported number of HS outbreaks and affected cases represent only a fraction of the actual number in India. The available reports indicating the number of outbreaks, morbidity and mortality statistics of HS from different parts of the country are hardly complete. With the existing sources of information, it would be a great challenge to assess the actual prevalence and distribution of HS to estimate the realistic economic losses in different regions. It also causes difficulty in studying the epidemiological characteristics with a view to formulating and implementing effective methods of control and prevention.

It would appear that the extent of rainfall and its geographic and temporal distribution are important factors influencing the incidence and change from enzootic to epizootic occurrence of HS. The annual fluctuations in the incidence are difficult to interpret. It has been postulated that the first outbreaks of HS occur with the first rains and the maximum spread of HS is associated with monthly rainfall of 60-270 mm and a total rainfall from 340 to 700 mm in the first two months (Khera 1979). Other factors known to influence the occurrence and spread of HS include the mean air temperature, relative humidity, parasitic infections, carrier rate of *P. multocida* and herd immunity level etc. It is always a great challenge to predict the unpredictable environmental factors that kick off the disease outbreaks.

Despite the unraveling of complete genome sequence of *P. multocida*, the pathogen still continues to be enigmatic with vague information about the genes involved in virulence factors, pathogenicity, host adaptability, predilection sites, carrier state and cross protective antigens or immunogens which would provide complete protection against heterologus challenge strain. The elusive determinants of protective immunity pose a greater challenge to the scientific community.

Moreover, the occurrences of HS and pasteurellosis outbreaks despite vaccination generate a new set of questions which remain unanswered because neither the precise mechanism of immunity nor the specific bacterial antigens involved in immunity to HS have been clearly identified so far. It is also clear that due to the genotypic differences among strains of the same serotype, conventional serotyping, which is widely used in India, in many cases does not provide sufficiently detailed information to determine the epizootiology of infections.

The overall occurrence of the cases of HS has, however, shown a declining trend in India. Perhaps, a more consistent and rapid decline could have been brought about if the production of more effective vaccines with a good adjuvant (like saponin- under trial), biofilm based vaccines or live mutant strains, was stepped up and if these were to completely replace the broth culture bacterins and the oil adjuvant vaccines which are self intrigued by complexities of administration and duration of immunity.

7.2 Constraints

There are multiple hurdles with varied restrictions, either natural or man made, that pose continuous threat to effective implementation of HS control and possibly eradication measures. Some of them are as follows:

a) Lack of public awareness about the diseases and good animal husbandry practices
b) Lack of strong legislation for animal movement and mandatory disease reporting
c) Illegal trafficking of livestock and their products across the international borders
d) Injudicious and indiscriminate use of antibacterial agents
e) Drastically variable stress and incriminating factors prevalent in an endemic area
f) Lack of research data on protective determinants/immunogens of *P. multocida*
g) Lack of single efficient, affordable vaccine for mass application

8. Remedies

The panacea for pasteurellosis lies in the concerted efforts and multidisciplinary approaches involving farmers, veterinarians, scientists, policy makers and administrative personnel aiming to control or eradicate HS from an endemic area. Some of the key remedies are as follow:

- Application of emerging methods of typing tools for rapid identification and differentiation of field isolates from animal/avian hosts for epidemiological studies to track the origin
- Selection of sensitive or a relatively new broad spectrum antibiotic based on antibiogram for use in the treatment of HS and pasteurellosis caused by resistant strains
- Design and development of an ideal vaccine that is easy to prepare in bulk, free from side effects and provides longer duration of immunity from a single injection of a small volume
- Mass awareness extension programmes to educate farmers
- Mass vaccination programmes to strengthen herd immunity
- Strict enforcement of legislation on animal movement/quarantine/ disposal of contaminants
- Improved or advanced husbandry practices that lessen stress and incriminating factors

9. Developmental Guidelines

The control and/or eradication of HS from India is a long term pragmatic plan, which requires a proper blue print with timely scheduled milestones to be accomplished. Some of the key aspects, which need the attention of policy makers, are envisaged as follows:

- Establishment of National Repository on *P. multocida* isolates and maintenance of regional data base on prevalent serotypes especially in endemic areas
- Establishment of conventional serotyping facility within the country as per the international standards (OIE 2008)
- Strengthening the disease outbreak investigation process by streamlining the process of samples collection, transport of materials in time, and rapid process at laboratory level
- Funding the research activities for better understanding of the intricacies of epidemiology, pathogenesis, pathogen and host interaction, cross

species transmission, virulence factors, emergence of antibiotic resistance pattern and human interventions in the disease process

- Inclusion of commonly prevalent or most circulating indigenous or local strains of *P. multocida* in formulation of vaccines
- Identification of potential or candidate strains of *P. multocida* for inclusion in either monovalent, bivalent or multivalent vaccines for HS alone or in combination with other bacterial (black quarter) or viral (FMD) diseases that affect a particular host
- Selection of compatible and effective adjuvant for incorporation in different vaccine formulations
- Establishment of international collaboration with developing as well as developed countries where the disease is prevalent, for exchange of research information and to evolve a strategic control or eradication methods
- Development of PCR assays for rapid identification of somatic serotypes of *P. multocida* as well as presence of virulent factors
- Development of improved diagnostics, mass applicable cost effective vaccines and drugs to treat the infected animals or population at risk
- Identification of major protective antigens in different serotypes especially serotype B:2 and assessing their role in development of protective immunity
- Selection of an effective, stable, safe, easily injectable and cost effective adjuvant which enhances the specific immune response and protection against HS even by administering a vaccine with a reduced dose or antigenic concentration
- Identification of either naturally attenuated strain or more efficient means of attenuating the existing vaccine strain with least affordable procedure so as to produce a rationally attenuated *P. multocida* mutant for use as live attenuated vaccine

There is an imminent call for thorough investigation and reporting of each and every outbreak of HS from remote areas of the states to fill up the lacunae in the present data, because the reporting of HS is quite inadequate to launch an effective strategy to control the disease.

10. Action Plans and Strategies for India

HS and pasteurellosis with an enormous potential for severe losses in the livestock sector, calls for an imminent action oriented policy that is prophylactic vaccination in most parts of the country especially in the endemic areas. By giving a protection at the times of the greatest risk, it is possible to reduce the incidence of HS. Regarding vaccination schedule, various schedules have been adopted in different regions of the country ranging from annual prophylactic vaccination and vaccination in the face of an outbreak, to vaccination just before the HS season. Since the disease has a seasonal distribution in most parts of the country, vaccination just before the HS season seems to be the appropriate schedule.

Apart from an action oriented vaccination programme, the following steps need to be considered while designing strategic measures to control HS:

- Development of an efficient system of disease reporting starting from local, district, state and each regional station leading to Central Pasteurella Referral Laboratory
- Strengthening of National disease surveillance unit such as PD_ADMAS with the co-operation and collaboration of the state animal husbandry departments, state agricultural universities and central government agencies to have constant vigil in the country
- Enhanced infrastructure development at regional diagnostic laboratories with equipments like PCR machine, electrophoresis and gel doc system etc and recruitment of experts in the area or training of the existing personnel in the advanced diagnostic/characterization techniques
- Conducting authentic surveys on disease incidence and distribution in the defined population with the support of standard laboratory procedures
- Identification of prevalent serotypes in various hosts in different states and molecular characterization of field isolates by DNA based typing tools for a detailed epidemiological investigation of an outbreak and to trace its source of infection
- Provision of adequate facilities to field veterinary officers, institutes and diagnostic laboratories at district level by way of providing early forecast/ public warning and necessary requirements during different seasons under varied agroclimatic conditions
- Adoption of improved husbandry practices, hygienic measures, isolation and strict implementation of quarantine measures coupled with proper disposal of contaminated or infected materials in order to reduce the incidence and spread of the disease
- Implementing extension programmes for effective communication to the masses on the success of prophylactic vaccination and commitment to better health status of livestock

Table 2 : Prevalent serotypes of *P. multocida* isolated from pasteurellosis outbreaks in India in recent times

Host	Serotype
Cattle	A:1; A:3; A:4; A:1,3; B:2; F:3; F:3,4; F:4,12
Buffalo	A:1; A:3; B:2
Sheep	A:1; A:3; A:3,4; B:2; D:3; F:1; F:4,12
Goat	A:1; A:3
Pig	B:2
Chicken	A:1; A:3; A:1,3; A:4; D:1
Duck	A:1; A:3; F:3
Quail	A:1
Turkey	A:1
Rabbit	A:1; A:3
Deer	A:1
Leopard	A:1
Lion	A:3;4; B:2
Tiger	A:3.4, B:l

Above all, geographical area with agro-climatic variations and tradition of inhabitants and their culture with respect to livestock distribution has to be considered before making any strategic approach.

11. Conclusion

Insufficient data on incidence, occurrence and distribution of HS and pasteurellosis coupled with inefficient prophylactic and control measures make an insidious impact on the livestock sector, particularly in the developing countries like India, drastically affecting the growing economies that solely depend on agriculture, livestock and allied sector with an overall contribution of 28-32% to the nation's GDP.

The need of the hour is to focus on the key thrust areas such as strengthening the national disease monitoring and surveillance system, networking of well equipped remote/regional laboratories with easy accessibility to endemic areas, supporting the region/species based applied research, effective implementation of national mass prophylactic vaccination programme, training of veterinarians about recent advances in rapid disease diagnosis/treatment/control measures as per the international standards (OIE 2008) and mass awareness programmes by multi-pronged extension activities at rural level. Moreover, the farmers engaged in animal husbandry practices should adhere to the basic rules of hygienic measures coupled with advanced management practices and continuous monitoring of the general health status of animals or herds on routine basis. It would ultimately help in control as well as eradication of HS/pasteurellosis in a region.

In the era of new generation vaccines, improved conventional approaches coupled with robust growth of molecular biological techniques are likely to generate a wide range of vaccines against HS with an enormous applicability in the health scenario of livestock. The new approaches have greater strategic potential in vaccine development with a plenty of advantages over conventional vaccines. However, these new technology vistas warrant thorough investigations in relation to compatibility of different combinations/ formulations of vaccines and their safety in vaccinated animals. With the current frontier areas of research on evolving effective HS vaccine, 'New age HS vaccine' would certainly turn out to be an everlasting panacea for the pestering problem of pasteurellosis among the livestock.

References

1. Adler B, Bulach D, Chung J *et al.* (1999). Candidate vaccine antigens and genes in *Pasteurella multocida.* J Biotechnol 73:83-90.
2. Al-Hasani K, Boyce J, McCarl VP *et al.* (2007). Identification of novel immunogens in *Pasteurella multocida.* Microbiol Cell Factories 6:3 doi:10.1186/1475-2859-6-3.
3. Arora BM, Kumar PN (1988). Pasteurellosis in panther tigris. Ind J Comp Microbiol Immunol Infect Dis 9:215-216.
4. Ataei S, Burchmore R, Christopher Hodgson J *et al.* (2009). Identification of immunogenic proteins associated with protection against haemorrhagic septicaemia after vaccination of calves with a live-attenuated *aro*A derivative of *P. multocida* B:2. Res Vet Sci 87(2):207-210.
5. Aucouturier J, Dupuis L, Ganne V (2001). Adjuvants designed for veterinary and human vaccines. Vaccine 19:2666-2672.
6. Bain RVS (1954). Vaccination against haemorrhagic septicaemia of bovines. Nature 173:584.
7. Benkirane A, De Alwis MCL (2002). Haemorrhagic septicaemia, its significance, prevention and control in Asia. Vet Med Czech 47(8):234-240.
8. Biswas A, Shivachandra SB, Saxena MK *et al.* (2004). Molecular variability among strains of *Pasteurella multocida* isolated from an outbreak of haemorrhagic septicaemia in India. Vet Res Commun 28(4):287-298.
9. Blackall PJ, Miflin JK (2000). Identification and typing of *Pasteurella multocida*: a review. Avian Path 29:271-287.
10. Boyce JD, Chung JY, Adler B. (2000). *Pasteurella multocida* capsule: Composition, function and genetics. J Biotec 83:153-160.

11. Brickell SK, Thomas LM, Long KA *et al.* (1998). Development of a PCR test based on a gene region associated with the pathogenicity of *Pasteurella multocida* serotype B:2, the causal agent of haemorrhagic septicaemia in Asia. Vet Microbiol 59: 295-307.

12. Carter GR (1955). Studies on *Pasteurella multocida*: A haemagglutination test for the identification of serological types. Am J Vet Res 16: 481-484.

13. Carter GR (1967). Pasteurellosis: *Pasteurella multocida* and *P. hemolytica*. Adv Vet Sci Comp Med 11:321.

14. Carter GR, Chengappa MM (1981). Recommendation for a standard system of designating serotype of *Pasteurella multocida*. Am Assoc Vet Lab Diag pp. 37-42.

15. Chaudhuri S, Mukherjee SK, Chatterjee A *et al.* (1992). Isolation of *P. multocida* F:3,4 from a still born Leopard. Vet Rec 130:36.

16. Chawak MM, Verma KC, Kataria JM *et al.* (2000). Characterization of indigenous isolates of avian *Pasteurella multocida*. Ind J Comp Microbiol Immunol Infect Dis 21:111-114.

17. Choi C, Chae C (2001). Enhanced detection of toxigenic *Pasteurella multocida* directly from nasal swabs using nested polymerase chain reaction. Vet J 162: 255-258.

18. Christensen JP, Bisgaard M (1997) .Avian pasteurellosis: taxonomy of the organisms involved and aspects of pathogenesis. Avian Pathol 26: 461-83.

19. Christensen JP, Bisgaard M (2000). Fowl cholera: a review. Rev Sci Tech 19(2): 626-637.

20. Confer AW (1993). Immunogens of Pasteurella. Vet Microbiol 37:353-368.

21. Dabo SM, Taylor JD, Confer AW (2007). *Pasteurella multocida* and bovine respiratory disease. Anim Health Res Rev 8(2):129-150.

22. De Alwis MCL (1999). Haemorrhagic septicaemia. ACIAR Monograph No. 57.

23. Dey S, Biswas A, Kumar AA *et al.* (2002). An experimental study on the pathogenicity of *Pasteurella multocida* of Pig origin. Ind J Comp Microbiol Immunol Infect Dis 73:36-37.

24. Dey S, Singh VP, Kumar AA *et al.* (2007). Comparative sequence analysis of 16S rRNA gene of *Pasteurella multocida* serogroup B isolates from different animal species. Res Vet Sci 83(1):1-4.

25. Dhanda MR, Sen GP (1972). Haemorrhagic septicaemia and allied conditions in sheep, goats, pigs and poultry. Indian Council of Agricultural Research, New Delhi.

26. Dutta TK, Gautam R, Singh VP *et al.* (2004a). Molecular detection and characterization of Indian Isolates of *Pasteurella multocida* serogroup A. Ind J Ani Sci 74:244-247.

27. Dutta TK, Gautam R, Singh VP *et al.* (2004b). Molecular characterization of Indian isolates of *Pasteurella multocida* serotype B:2 using REA, RAPD-PCR and ribotyping. Ind J Ani Sci 74:572-576.

28. Dutta TK, Singh VP, Kumar AA (2001). Rapid and specific diagnosis of haemorrhagic septicaemia by using PCR assay. Ind J Anim Hlth 40:101-107.

29. Dwivedi PN, Sharma AK, Punj V (1990). Serotyping of *Pasteurella multocida* from sheep and goats. Ind J Comp Microbiol Immunol Infect Dis 11: 48-49.

30. Dziva F, Christensen H, Olsen JE *et al.* (2001). Random amplification of polymorphic DNA and phenotypic typing of Zimbabwean isolates of *Pasteurella multocida.* Vet Microbiol 82:361-372.

31. Dziva F, Muhairwa AP, Bisgaard M *et al.* (2008). Diagnostic and typing options for investigating diseases associated with *Pasteurella multocida.* Vet Microbiol April 1; 128(1-2):1-22.

32. Ekundayo SO, Odugbo MO, Olabode AO *et al.* (2008). Phenotypic variability among strains of *P. multocida* isolated from avian, bovine, caprine, leporine and ovine origin. African J Biotechnol 7(9):1347-1350.

33. Ewers C, Lübke-Becker A, Bethe A *et al.* (2006). Virulence genotype of *Pasteurella multocida* strains isolated from different hosts with various disease status. Vet Microbiol. 31; 114(3-4):304-317.

34. FAO (2005). Production Yearbook 2005, Statistics Division, FAO.

35. FAO-WHO-OIE (1994). Animal Health Yearbook, 1994.

36. Fegan N, Blackall PJ, Pahoff JL (1995). Phenotypic characterization of *Pasteurella multocida* isolates from Australian poultry. Vet Microbiol 47:281-286.

37. Foged NT (1992). *Pasteurella multocida* toxin: the characterization of the toxin and its significance in the diagnosis and prevention of progressive atrophic rhinitis in pigs. Acta Pathol Microbiol Immunol Scand 100 (25):1-56.

38. Gautam R, Dutta TK, Kumar AA *et al.* (2006). Molecular typing of Indian Isolates of *Pasteurella multocida* Serogroup-A from different animal species. Ind J Anim Sci 76(11):867-872.

39. Gautam R, Kumar AA, Singh VP *et al.* (2004). Specific identification of *Pasteurella multocida* serogroup-A isolates by PCR assay. Res Vet Sci 76(3):179-185.

40. Gunawardana GA, Townsend KM, Frost AJ (2000). Molecular characterization of avian *Pasteurella multocida* isolates from Australia and Vietnam by REP-PCR and PFGE. Vet Microbiol 72: 97-109.

41. Harper M, Boyce JD, Adler B (2006). *Pasteurella multocida* pathogenesis: 125 years after Pasteur. FEMS Microbiol Lett 265:1-10.

42. Hatfaludi T, Al-Hasani K, Boyce JD *et al.* (2010). Outer membrane proteins of *Pasteurella multocida.* Vet Microbiol 29:1-17.

43. Heddleston KL, Gallagher JE, Rebers PA (1972). Fowl cholera: Gel diffusion precipitation test for serotyping *Pasteurella multocida* from avian species. Avian Dis 16:925-936.

44. Hirsh DC, Martin LD, Rhodes, KR (1981). Conjugal transfer of R-plasmid in *Pasteurella multocida*. Antimicrobiol Agents Chemother 20:415-417.

45. Hulton CSJ, Higgins CF, Sharp PM (1991). ERIC sequences: a novel family of repetitive elements in the genomes of *Eschereichia coli, Salmonella typhimurium* and other enterobacteria. Mol Micobiol 5:825-834.

46. Hungerford TG (1989). In: Diseases of livestock, 9th ed, McGraw-Hill Book Company, New Delhi, p 829.

47. Hunt ML, Adler B, Townsend KM (2000). The molecular biology of *Pasteurella multocida*. Vet Microbiol 72:3-25.

48. Jablonska AK, Opacka BB (2007). Analysis of *Pasteurella multocida* strains isolated from cattle with haemorrhagic septicaemia by the use of PFGE. Bull Vet Inst Pulawy 51:515-517.

49. Joseph S, Kumar AA, Shivachandra SB *et al.* (2007). Cloning and Characterization of Type 4 Fimbrial Gene *(ptfA)* of *Pasteurella multocida* Serogroup B:2 (Strain P_{52}). Vet Res Commun 31(4):397-404.

50. Kalorey DR, Yuvaraj S, Vanjari SS *et al.* (2008). PCR analysis of *Pasteurella multocida* isolates from an outbreak of pasteurellosis in Indian pigs. Comp Immunol Microbiol Infect Dis 31(6):459-65.

51. Khera SS (1979). The incidence and distribution of epizootic diseases in India: Haemorrhagic septicaemia. Bull Office Intern Epizooties 91:331-347.

52. Kumar AA, Harbola PC, Rimler RB *et al.* (1996). Studies on *Pasteurella multocida* isolates of animal and avian origin from India. Ind J Comp Microbiol Immunol Infect Dis 17:120-124.

53. Kumar AA, Parai TP (1984). Swine pasteurellosis and its treatment. Ind J Vet Med 4:63-64.

54. Kumar AA, Shivachandra SB (2002). Hemorrhagic septicaemia in Eastern and North-Eastern region and strategies towards its control. National symposium on Prospects of animal resources in eastern and North-Eastern region of India, 25 Dec 2002, Kolkata, India.

55. Kumar AA, Shivachandra SB (2004). Frontier areas of research on haemorrhagic septicaemia vaccines. In Proc. of annual conference of IAVR, 24-26 Feb, IVRI, Izatnagar, India.

56. Kumar AA, Shivachandra SB, Biswas A *et al.* (2004). Prevalent serotypes of *Pasteurella multocida* isolated from different animal and avian species in India. Vet Res Commun 28(8):657-667.

57. Lee CW, Wilkie IW, Townsend KM *et al.* (2000). The demonstration of *Pasteurella multocida* in the alimentary tract of chickens after experimental infection. Vet Microbiol 72:47-55.

58. Marchart J, Dropmann G, Lechleitner S *et al.* (2003). *Pasteurella multocida* and *Pasteurella haemolytica*-ghosts: new vaccine candidates. Vaccine 8; 21(25-26): 3988-3997.

59. May BJ, Zhang Q, Li LL *et al.* (2001). Complete genomic sequence of *Pasteurella multocida*, Pm70. PNAS 98(6):3460-3465.

60. Mutters R, Ihm P, Pohl S *et al.* (1985). Reclassification of the genus *Pasteurella* Trevisan 1887 on the basis of deoxyribonucleic acid homology, with proposals for the new species *Pasteurella dagmatis, Pasteurella canis, Pasteurella stomatis, Pasteurella anatis* and *Pasteurella langaa.* Int J Syst Bacteriol 35:309-322.

61. Myint A, Carter GR (1989). Prevention of haemorrhagic septicaemia in cattle and buffaloes with a live vaccine. Vet Rec 124:508-509.

62. OIE (2008). Haemorrhagic septicaemia, Chapter 2.4.12. Terrestrial manual 739-750.

63. Olive DM, Bean P (1999). Principles and applications of methods for DNA based typing of microbial organisms: a mini review. J Clin Microbiol 37(6):1661-1669.

64. Pavri KM, Apte VH (1967). Isolation of *Pasteurella multocida* from a fatal disease of horses and donkeys in India. Vet Rec 80:437.

65. Prabhakar TG, David BP, Chandramohan A *et al.* (1998). Pasteurellosis in hippopotamus in captivity. Ind J Anim Sci 68(4):348-349.

66. Rimler RB (2000). Restriction endonuclease analysis using *Hha*I and *Hpa*II to discriminate among serogroup B *Pasteurella multocida* associated with haemorrhagic septicaemia. J Med Microbiol 49:81-87.

67. Ross RF (2006). *Pasteurella multocida* and its role in porcine pneumonia. Anim Health Res Rev 7(1-2):13-29.

68. Ruffalo GC, Carmel G, Tennet JM *et al.* (1997). Identification, purification and characterization of type 4 fimbriae of *Pasteurella multocida.* Infect Immun 65: 339-343.

69. SanMillan A, Escudero JA, Gutierrez B *et al.* (2009). Multiresistance in *Pasteurella multocida* is mediated by coexistence of small plasmids. Antimicrob Agents Chemother 53(8):3399-3404.

70. Savelkoul PH, Aarts HJ, Haas J *et al.* (1999). Amplified fragment length polymorphism analysis : the state of an art. J Clin Microbiol 37:3083-3091.

71. Saxena MK, Kumar AA, Chaudhuri, P *et al.* (2005). Ribotyping of Indian isolates of *Pasteurella multocida* based on 16S and 23S rRNA genes. Vet Res Commun 29(6): 527-535.

72. Saxena MK, Singh VP, Kumar AA *et al.* (2006). REP-PCR analysis of *Pasteurella multocida* isolates from wild and domestic animals in India. Vet Res Commun 30(8):851-861.

73. Seo J, Pyo H, Lee S *et al.* (2009). Expression of 4 truncated fragments of *Pasteurella multocida* toxin and their immunogenicity. Can J Vet Res 73(3):184-189.

74. Shivachandra SB, Kumar AA, Srivastava SK *et al.* (2003a). Nucleic acid based typing techniques: emerging tools for epidemiological studies. Livestock International 7(2):20-23.

75. Shivachandra SB, Biswas A, Kumar AA (2003b). *Pasteurella multocida*: a pathogen of zoonotic importance. The Veterinarian 27(8):9-10.

76. Shivachandra SB, Kumar AA, Biswas A *et al.* (2004a). Antibiotic sensitivity patterns among Indian strains of Avian *Pasteurella multocida*. Trop Anim Health Prod 36(8):743-750.

77. Shivachandra SB, Kumar AA, Gautam R *et al.* (2004b). PCR assay for rapid detection of *Pasteurella multocida* serogroup-A in morbid tissue materials from experimentally induced Fowl cholera in chicks. Vet J 168(3):349-352.

78. Shivachandra SB, Kumar AA, Chaudhuri P (2007). Differentiation of Avian *Pasteurella multocida* strains by Single primer PCR. Vet Res Commun 31(8):941-949.

79. Shivachandra SB, Kumar AA, Chaudhuri P (2008). Molecular characterization of avian strains of *Pasteurella multocida* serogroup-A based on amplification of repetitive regions by PCR. Comp Immun Microbiol Infect Dis 31(1):47-62.

80. Shivachandra SB, Kumar AA, Gautam R *et al.* (2005a). Detection of multiple strains of *Pasteurella multocida* in Fowl cholera outbreaks by PCR- based typing. Avian Path 34(6):456-462.

81. Shivachandra SB, Kumar AA, Singh SD *et al.* (2005b). Pathogenecity of *Pasteurella multocida* A:1 in experimentally infected chickens and chicken embryos. Ind J Anim Sci 75:411-414.

82. Shivachandra SB, Kumar AA, Amaranath J *et al.* (2005c). Cloning and characterization of *tbpA* gene encoding Transferrin binding protein (TbpA) from *Pasteurella multocida* B:2 (strain P52). Vet Res Commun 29(6):537-542.

83. Shivachandra SB, Kumar AA, Gautam R *et al.* (2006a). Characterization of Avian strains of *Pasteurella multocida* by Restriction Endonuclease and Amplified Fragment Length Polymorphism. Res Vet Sci 81(1):8-18.

84. Shivachandra SB, Kumar AA, Gautam R *et al.* (2006b). Detection of *Pasteurella multocida* in experimentally infected embryonated chicken eggs by PCR assay. Ind J Exp Bio 44(4):321-324.

85. Shivachandra SB, Kumar AA, Gautam R et al (2006c) Identification of Avian Strains of *Pasteurella multocida* in India by Conventional and PCR Assays. Vet J 172:561-564.

86. Shivachandra SB, Kumar AA, Saxena MK *et al.* (2006d). Biochemical Characterization of Avian Strains of *Pasteurella multocida* in India. Ind J Anim Sci 76(6):429-432.

87. Shivshankara N, Saxena MK, Singh VP (2001). Rapid diagnosis of haemorrhagic septicaemia by PCR assay. Ind Vet J 78:101-103.

88. Singh VP, Kumar AA, Srivastava SK *et al.* (1996). Significance of HS in Asia-India: International workshop on diagnosis and control of HS. Bali Indonesia May 28-30, 1996.

89. Spratt BG (1999). Multilocus sequence typing: molecular typing of bacterial pathogens in an era of rapid DNA sequencing and the internet. Curr Opi Microbiol 2:312-316.

90. Srivastava SK (1998). Immunogenicity of *Pasteurella multocida* grown in iron restricted medium. J Appl Anim Res 136:137-144.

91. Tatum FM, Tabatabai LB, Briggs RE (2009). Protection against fowl cholera conferred by vaccination with recombinant *Pasteurella multocida* filamentous hemagglutinin peptides. Avian Dis 53(2):169-174.

92. Townsend KM, Boyce JD, Chung JY *et al.* (2001). Genetic organisation of *Pasteurella multocida* cap loci and development of a multiplex capsular PCR typing system. J Clin Microbiol 39(3):924-929.

93. Townsend KM, Dawkins HJS, Papadimitriou JM (1997). REP-PCR analysis of *Pasteurella multocida* isolates that cause haemorrhagic septicaemia. Res Vet Sci 63:151-155.

94. Townsend KM, Frost AJ, Lee CW *et al.* (1998). Development of PCR assays for species and type specific identification of *Pasteurella multocida* isolates. J Clin Microbiol 36:1096-1100.

95. Verma R, Jaiswal TN (1998). Haemorrhagic septicaemia vaccines. Vaccine 16: 1184-1190.

96. Vos PR, Heger M, Blecker M *et al.* (1995). AFLP: a new technique for DNA fingerprinting. Nucleic Acids Res 23:4407-4414.

97. Wu JR, Shien JH, Shieh HK *et al.* (2007). Protective immunity conferred by recombinant *Pasteurella multocida* lipoprotein E (PlpE). Vaccine 25(21):4140-4148.

□□□

Chapter 19

Strategies for Mastitis Control

ANSHU SHARMA AND RAJESH CHHABRA
College Central Laboratory, College of Veterinary Sciences, Lala Lajpat Rai University of Veterinary and Animal Sciences, Hisar-125004

Contents

1. Introduction

Mastitis is a disease complex with multiple causes, varying degrees of clinical intensity, and variations in duration and residual effects. The inflammation of mammary gland parenchyma is characterized by physical and chemical, usually associated with bacteriological changes in milk and pathological alterations of glandular tissue (Radostits *et al.* 2000). It is a worldwide problem responsible for heavy economic loss to dairy industry. In India, Dhanda and Sethi (1962) published first detailed report regarding annual losses due to mastitis in the country which were estimated at Rs. 5.9 crores. In later years, the losses increased many folds due to rise in the high-yielding bovine population following the launch of Operation Flood programme and implementation of crossbreeding programme. This is evident from the report of Dua (2001), who estimated the annual loss due to mastitis in cows and buffaloes in India at Rs. 6053.21 crores, of which a sum of Rs. 4365.32 crores was attributed to subclinical mastitis. Later, Wadhwa *et al.* (2003) reported that subclinical mastitis accounted for 76.55 per cent of the total losses due to mastitis in India. Besides the financial implications, mastitis has public health consequences as well. The extensive and indiscriminate use of antimicrobials in the treatment and control of mastitis can lead to the occurrence of undesirable drug residues in milk, emergence of drug-resistant bacteria and loss of milk during the withholding period after administration of drugs for treatment of mastitis.

Mastitis, both in clinical form and in subclinical form, is a major disease affecting milk production. While clinical mastitis is generally an individual animal's problem manifested by gross abnormalities in milk and mammary gland, subclinical mastitis is often a herd problem. The latter is far more important as it may remain unnoticed most of the time because of no apparent gross changes in the milk and udder. Subclinical mastitis is 15-40 times more prevalent than clinical mastitis. It causes drastic reduction in milk yield and can be converted into clinical form at any time. Surveys of the prevalence of mastitis in most countries, irrespective of the cause, show a comparable figure of 50 per cent among dairy cows and a quarter-wise infection rate of 25 per cent (Radostits *et al.* 2000). Studies conducted in different regions of India indicate that the prevalence of subclinical mastitis on farms could range from 19 to 78 per cent (Tuteja *et al.* 1993). The findings of some prevalence studies carried out in different regions of India from the year 2000 to 2009 have been summarized in Table 1.

Table 1 : Prevalence of mastitis in different regions of India

State	Species	Prevalence (per cent)		References
		Clinical mastitis	Subclinical mastitis	
Uttarakhand	Cow	NR	76.01	Nauriyal and Pachauri (2003)
	Buffalo	NR	33.33	Nauriyal and Pachauri (2003)
Madhya Pradesh	Cow	NR	66.67	Ashish *et al.* (2000)
	Buffalo	84.31	NR	Das and Joseph (2005)
Rajasthan	Cow	60.25	NR	Chahar *et al.* (2005)
Haryana	Cow	NR	36.69	Sharma *et al.* (2006)
	Buffalo	18.74	32.90	Sharma and Sindhu (2007)
Maharashtra	Buffalo	NR	31.03	Chavan *et al.* (2007)
Tamil Nadu	Buffalo	22.12	77.87	Rani *et al.* (2008)
	Buffalo	NR	44.47	Palanivel *et al.* (2008)
Gujarat	Buffalo	NR	39.56	Gowardhan *et al.* (2008)
Uttar Pradesh	Cow	15.18	42.93	De and Mukherjee (2009)
Jammu and Kashmir	Cow	10.93	42.18	Sharma *et al.* (2009)
Jharkhand	Cow	72.63	NR	Ranjan *et al.* (2011)

NR - Not reported

2. Etiological Agents' Status

Staphylococcus aureus and streptococci are the most frequently isolated bacteria from the mastitic milk samples of cows and buffaloes in different parts of the country (Chavan *et al.* 2007, Behera *et al.* 2008, Palanivel *et al.* 2008, Roychoudhary and Dutta 2009) while *Streptococcus uberis* and enterococci have been isolated less frequently in comparison to the developed nations. The milk samples from organized farms and clinical cases brought to our laboratory for examination showed that 49.34 per cent samples were culturally positive. From the data, staphylococci and streptococci emerge as the predominant organisms associated with clinical and subclinical mastitis, followed by *E. coli, Corynebacterium pyogenes, Klebsiella* sp., *Pseudomonas aeruginosa,* enterococci, *Bacillus* sp. and yeast. Coagulase-positive staphylococci were the main organism accounting for more than 50 per cent of the staphylococcal infections in earlier studies. Coagulase-negative staphylococci were earlier regarded as saprophytic and relatively nonpathogenic organisms but notably these have been the most prevalent organisms in mastitis cases for the last 15 years. Among streptococci, *S. agalactiae* and *S. dysgalactiae* are the most frequently encountered organisms followed by the other species of streptococci in India.

3. Strategies for Mastitis Control

Several strategies have been tried to control mastitis. In the USA in late 1930s, efforts were made to eradicate the infection caused by *S. agalactiae*, which was the most prevalent pathogen at that time, first by hygiene coupled with segregations and culling and later much more successfully by treating cows with penicillin. The treatment immediately reduced the losses in milk yield due to infection and stimulated research on practical methods of control of the disease. Due to the involvement of several other organisms in causation of mastitis, it was clear by 1955 that antibiotic therapy was not the panacea that initially it appeared to be. It was an essential component of control but alone it was not sufficient. This encouraged the scientists and dairy farmers to develop a new scheme to control infections other than *S. agalactiae*. Ultimately, dry animal therapy and post-milking teat dipping were introduced as an essential part of control programme.

A practical approach for mastitis control that can be used by all farmers and dairymen involves preventing new cases of mastitis and eliminating the existing ones. This can be achieved by the following strategic actions.

3.1 Immediate treatment of cases of clinical mastitis

On the basis of severity of symptoms ranging from few flakes to clots in milk, fever and different systemic dysfunctions, clinical mastitis is categorized as acute, subacute, per acute and chronic. To maximize the chances of curing, it is imperative that each case should be treated immediately at 12 or 24 h intervals for 3-5 days or more depending upon the etiology and severity of case. In case of subacute and chronic cases, to avoid undesirable drug residues in milk, emergence of antibiotic resistant bacteria and prolonged withholding period, it is important to identify the etiological agent and to determine its *in vitro* antimicrobial sensitivity for an effective treatment. However, in per acute and acute cases, where delay in treatment may have bad consequences, animal should be treated with broad spectrum antibiotics along with supportive therapy.

Teat ends should be thoroughly disinfected with 70 per cent alcohol or any suitable disinfectant before administering intramammary preparations in clinical cases during lactation as well as at drying off. It kills the bacteria normally present on the teat skin which are often highly resistant to common antibiotics. The method of administration of intramammary infusion influences the outcome of the treatment. If proper teat sanitation and precautions are not observed, the method of infusion of intramammary drug may cause new infections. Partial insertion of the syringe tip is a feasible method of administering intramammary infusion. When teat ends are disinfected prior to infusion, most of the bacteria are probably killed, but some remain lodged in the cracks and crevices around the teat orifices. When therapy is administered by full insertion of the syringe cannula, these bacteria may be pushed upward into the teat and may cause a more severe form of clinical mastitis than the one for which treatment was intended.

The route of drug administration is an important factor affecting the outcome of treatment. The studies conducted abroad and in our laboratory indicate that combination therapy by both the routes is more effective as compared to intramammary or systemic route alone. The studies reveal that on treatment with antimicrobials, bacteriological cure rates vary from 0 to 80 per cent with evidence of a significant loss of activity of the major classes of antibiotics used for the treatment of mastitis. The reasons for low cure rate and failure of treatment include delayed treatment, under dosing of drugs, presence of deep-seated pockets of infection in the udder, poor selection of drugs and resistance of bacteria to drugs.

3.2 Culling

Generally, a chronically affected animal not responding to treatment should be culled. It is a highly effective way of eliminating existing infection and preventing transfer of infection to other animals. It also saves time and money spent in treating and rearing the non-responder animals.

3.3 Post-milking teat dipping

Dipping teats in a solution of suitable disinfectant after completion of the milking process has been found to be the most effective single hygienic practice for preventing mastitis. Effective teat dips include the preparations of 0.1-1% iodophores, 4% sodium hypochlorite, 0.6% sodium dicholro-s-triazenetrione, 0.2-0.5% quaternary ammonium compounds and 0.5% chlorhexidine. Post-milking teat dipping controls the bacteria residing on teat skin and prevents new intramammary infections occurring between two milking. It also helps in repairing minor damages to teat skin. The practice is known to be quite effective against staphylococci, *S. agalactiae* and *S. dysgalactiae*. However, the infections due to *E. coli* and *S. uberis* are not adequately controlled by post-milking teat dipping. Such cases require additional attention to the cleanliness as discussed later in this chapter.

3.4 Dry animal therapy

It is well established that majority of infections occur during dry period because flushing of bacteria through milking is discontinued and the accumulation of milk increases the intramammary pressure which causes dilatation of teat canal and enhancement of bacterial penetration. Upto 40 per cent of new infections establish during first two weeks of dry period. Adoption of dry period therapy eliminates 50-60 per cent of the existing infections. Other advantages of this therapy are: cure rate is higher than during lactation, development of new infection during dry period is reduced, damaged milk producing tissue may be regenerated during calving, clinical mastitis at calving is reduced and the milk on calving is not contaminated with antibiotic residues.

Dry animal therapy has become an important component of mastitis control programme in bovines in developed countries. Two methods, namely, selective dry animal and Blitz dry animal therapy are used. For selective dry animal therapy, infected animals are identified by bacteriological examination and treated with antibiotic in long acting base. However, involvement of labour and money in laboratory diagnosis of infected quarters is the major disadvantage here. Secondly, some of the quarters that get infected after the testing procedure are left untreated and may act as subsequent source of infection for other quarters. Therefore, Blitz therapy involving treatment of all quarters of all animals at drying off is more advantageous because all quarters are treated simultaneously and laboratory testing to select infected quarters is not necessary, thus, saving time, money and labour.

In India, due to lack of awareness and unavailability of specially formulated antibiotics, the dry animal therapy is yet not in practice on large scale. As a result, there is generally high incidence of clinical mastitis at the time calving. Although the practice was started in early eighties, very limited information is available on dry animal therapy in the country. Bansal *et al.* (1994) observed that a combined regimen of post-milking teat dipping (iodophore, 0.5% available iodine) and complete dry animal therapy (cepravin dry cow, cephalonium in long acting base) could reduce the incidence of subclinical mastitis by 54.27 per cent animal wise and 65.72 per cent quarter wise at the end of 11 months trial in a cow herd. The level of *S. aureus* and coagulase-negative staphylococci infections reduced from 14.58 per cent to 3.33 per cent. In another cow herd, the reduction in infection was 40.71 per cent animal wise and 71 per cent quarter wise with a combined treatment of post-milking teat dipping (chlorhexidine 0.5%) and selective dry period therapy (cepravin dry cow). In this trial, the incidence of *S. aureus* reduced from 17.19 per cent to 4.17 per cent and from 9.37 per cent to 4.17 per cent, respectively. Malhotra *et al.* (1980) conducted a field trial on dry cow therapy using neomycin sulphate. Ninety quarters of 23 cows were infused with 'Bite' containing neomycin sulphate (500 mg), hydrocortisone acetate (20 mg), hydrocortisone sodium succinate (12.5 mg) and chlorbutanol (500 mg) at the time of drying-off. The formulation cleared 92 per cent of the infection due to *S. aureus* and *S. epidermidis* while it was 100 per cent effective against infections due to streptococci, micrococci and corynebacteria.

Malhotra *et al.* (1981) assessed the efficacy of 'Orbenin' (benzathine cloxacillin 500 mg) in dry cow therapy. Thirty-eight quarters of 10 cows were infused. The formulation cleared 83.3 per cent infection due to *S. aureus* and *S. epidermidis* and 100 per cent due to micrococci, *S. agalactiae, S. dysgalactiae* and *Corynebacterium* spp. which were found at the time of drying off. Misra *et al.* (1984) infused benzathine cloxacillin (500 mg in long acting base) into the quarters of 47 cows at the time of drying off. Of these, 78.7 per cent cows were found bacteriologically negative at the time of calving and no fresh infection was reported in these animals.

The efficacy of combination of neomycin sulphate and benzathine salt of penicillin, and benzathine cloxacillin alone against *S. aureus* has been reported as 83.8 per cent and 85.2 per cent, respectively. Spontaneous cure rate for *S. aureus* among controls was 38.80 per cent (Pankey *et al.* 1982). Their efficacy against *S. agalactiae* was more than 90 and the spontaneous cure rate was 28.6 per cent.

The trials conducted by our laboratory at organized farms revealed that the use of orbenin in dry cow therapy could clear 82 per cent udder infections while in the untreated control animals, there was an overall 31.25 per cent increase in the udder infections due to different pathogens at calving. Therefore, antibiotic therapy of all the quarters of all the cows with a specially formulated high persistence antibiotics combined with teat dipping is recommendable at the time of drying off in the country. It may, however be added that it is a poor practice to commence treatment on large scale until measures are taken to prevent further spread of the disease. Chemotherapy without an effective hygiene programme for mastitis control will be just a waste of time and money.

3.5 Proper management practices

Management practices at the dairy farms bear great significance in mastitis prevention and control. Some major practices for maintaining good udder health are listed below.

3.5.1 Housing and stall management

In confinement housing system, it is important to provide adequate space, bedding and lighting to ensure cleanliness and comfort. The stall size and floor should be such that animals can move easily without getting teat injury because injuries facilitate teat infection. The stall floor should not be slippery.

Livestock farmers should be advised not to keep animals on concrete/ cemented floors. The floors should be cleaned regularly. Overcrowding of the animals must be avoided to prevent transmission of infectious agents. The animal house should be free from flies.

3.5.2 Milking time hygiene

Milking time hygienic measures help in preventing exposure of the animal's teats to pathogenic organisms and in preventing transmission of pathogen from one teat to another of the same animal as well as from animal to animal. Hence, maximum efforts should be focused on controlling these pathogens.

Contagious bacteria (e.g. *S. aureus, Corynebacterium bovis, S. agalactiae* and coagulase-negative staphylococci) cause most of the infections. These infections usually spread from animal to animal during the milking process via milker's hands, udder cleaning cloth and teat cups in case of machine milking. The practice of wearing smooth rubber gloves and disinfecting gloved hands by dipping in an appropriate disinfectant before handling each animal reduces manual transfer of pathogens. Milking a dirty wet teat may lead to mastitis in the animal. Cleaning and sanitization of teats and udder is important in minimizing contamination at the time of milking. Teat orifices take half to one hour time in attaining full closure position, so maximum infections occur during this period. It can be avoided by keeping the animal in standing position during this period.

Some transmission of infection occurs during the intervals between milking. The possible sources of infection include contaminated bedding, licking of teats and udder and contact of teats with rear legs, tail switch and flies. Pathogens most commonly transmitted during inter milking period are *S. uberis* and coliforms.

3.5.3 Nutritional aspect

Diet plays an important role in improving the disease fighting ability of an animal. Vitamin E and selenium are extremely important components, which act synergistically as antioxidant and stimulate the neutrophils that in turn increase the phagocytic cell function. Plants grown on selenium deficient soil do not provide adequate dietary selenium. Fresh green forages are the major sources of vitamin E, however, vitamin E decreases in the stored forages, and is destroyed in silages. Deficiency of Vitamin E and selenium is sequel as well as predisposing factor for mastitis. Supplementation of these micronutrients in diet prevents new intramammary infection and decreases the severity of the existing infection. Silica, whose role is similar to selenium, has a marked effect on free radicals, lipid peroxidation and macrophage activity. The silica contents in diet may be increased by giving high silica feed ingredients like cereal grains.

3.5.4 Control of mastitis in heifers

Traditionally, mammary glands of heifers are considered as uninfected and their mammary secretions are not examined until the first milking or during the first episode of clinical mastitis following calving. Studies conducted abroad and in India, however, indicate the prevalence of mastitis in pregnant heifers which may lead to decreased milk production in future. *S. aureus* and coagulase-negative staphylococci followed by different species of *Streptococcus* have been encountered as main organisms in heifer mastitis. These infections are of great concern because of heavy economic losses due to the expected production losses. Control of heifer mastitis should, therefore, also be considered in mastitis management practices. This could be achieved by avoiding suckling among calves, segregating pregnant heifers, controlling flies, and rational antibiotic treatment prior to breeding or during pregnancy.

3.5.5 Vaccination

Vaccination has been used to produce antibodies which aid the host specific resistance against mastitis by acting as opsonins facilitating ingestion of organisms by mammary gland phagocytes, by neutralizing toxins and adherence factors of bacteria. Since *S. aureus* responds poorly to antibiotic therapy, several vaccines against this organism have been studied extensively (Nickerson 1991). Progress has also been made with vaccines against coliform mastitis. One is heat killed *E. coli* J-5 mutant vaccine tested at the University of California, Davis. A proprietary version of this vaccine is now being manufactured and sold by Poultry Health Laboratory, Davis, CA (Nickerson 1991). From the available literature, it appears that in near future vaccination against *E. coli* and *S. aureus* mastitis may become an important component of mastitis control programme. In the future, various vaccines that provide additional protection will likely be a part of the overall management programme against mastitis.

3.5.6 Genetic selection

Animal breeders gained success in achieving high milk production by adopting intensive selection for this trait, but it cannot be denied that high yielders are more susceptible to mastitis. Therefore, a realistic approach involving genetic selection based on genes both for mastitis resistance and high milk yield should be developed. However, for maximum expression of these selected genetic traits in animals, it is the duty of each dairy farmer to provide appropriate management and environment.

3.5.7 Management of cases of mastitis-metritis complex

There are chances of contracting mastitis in majority of metritis cases as the uterine discharge is likely to soil the udder causing infection.

3.5.8 Other control measures

(a) *Cytokines*: Cytokines are potent modulator of inflammation and immune function and have been identified as mediators of host response to bovine mastitis. Potential clinical application of recombinant cytokines for the control of experimental *S. aureus* and coliform mastitis is now well established.

Granulocyte/macrophage colony stimulating factor has been shown to increase local non-specific immune response of bovine mammary gland by its bactericidal and chemotactic activity.

Both *in vitro* and *in vivo* studies indicate that recombinant bovine IL-2 may enhance mammary gland immunity by recruitment of phagocytes and plasma cells that produce immunoglobulin, activation of polymorphonuclear leucocyte superoxide production and phagocytosis (Daley *et al.* 1991), enhanced mononuclear cell mitogenesis (Torre *et al.* 1992) and increased lymphocyte cytotoxic and bactericidal activity.

Sordillo *et al.* (1991) have described role of INFã in enhancing leucocytic activity and minimizing deleterious effect of endotoxins in coliform mastitis.

(b) *Antimicrobial proteins*: Newly recognized proteins which are collectively known as antimicrobial proteins play important role towards control of mastitis. Creactive proteins, haptoglobulin, caeruloplasmin and amyloid A transmission can be produced within an hour after microbial invasion and have a role in the inactivation of microorganisms. Some of the antimicrobial proteins such as lysostaphin and detensins produced in the microorganisms and leucocytes are active against both Gram-negative and Gram-positive bacteria.

(c) *Stress factors*: Any kind of physical (e.g. calving), physiological (e.g. high milk yield) or mental stress (e.g. early weaning or abortion or death of calve) makes the animal susceptible to mammary gland infections. Proper management at the time of calving, abortions, and weaning may reduce mastitis to a certain extent.

(d) *Intramammary device*: Introduction of abraded polyethylene intramammary device into the bovine lactiferous sinuses has been shown to raise somatic cell count of foremilk and stripping in quarters containing the device. New infection rates have been shown to be lower in the intramammary device quarter than in the control quarters. The possible side effects and long term effects on milk production, milk composition and resistance against various mastitis pathogens remain to be determined.

4. Future Strategies to Control Mastitis

Continuous work on different aspects of mastitis is required, particularly on control and preventive measures, in order to reduce the losses resulting from the disease in the country. It will be worthwhile to consider the following points:

1. There is need to have well staffed and well equipped mastitis research laboratory in each region or state. Specialist services are necessary for the effective operation of mastitis control schemes to act as focal point, to investigate problems and to provide link between the field and research findings. The activities in mastitis control should be coordinated through an organization such as National Mastitis Council.

2. As the knowledge of epidemiological patterns of the disease is fundamental to development of adequate control measures, the work in this direction is needed. To improve mastitis control, the main types of intramammary infections and the major factors that are more likely to cause such infections in a dairy herd should be considered first.

3. Standardization of sampling and diagnostic methods to detect infection is essential.

4. Dairy farmers are likely to be averse to implement mastitis control measures because of the inconspicuous nature of the disease. Our aim should be to diffuse information effectively and motivate the dairy farmers to adopt control measures.

5. The dairy farmers have very few ways of determining the state of health of the udders in the herds. It is, therefore, necessary to examine herd's bulk milk regularly to determine the state of udder health.

5. Conclusion

The current mastitis control programme based on hygienic milking practices, pre- and post-milking teat dipping, and dry animal therapy now have been widely used for over 25 years in the USA, UK and other developed countries. It has been demonstrated that application of control measures based on post-milking teat disinfection and drying off therapy supported by other sound management practices would reduce the level of infection by 50 per cent in one year and by over 70 per cent in three years.

Unfortunately, no such systematic programme exists to control mastitis in India. A variety of microorganisms are responsible for the disease but over 80 per cent of mastitis cases in India are caused by coagulase-negative staphylococci, *S. aureus, S. agalactiae and S. dysgalactiae.* Therefore, maximum efforts should be focused on controlling these pathogens. There is an urgent need to develop simple and comprehensive control strategies which should be economical, practical and adaptable to a wide range of management conditions with the purpose to minimize the devastating losses associated with mastitis.

References

1. Ashish T, Sisodia RS, Sharma RK, Tiwari A (2000). Incidence of subclinical mastitis in cows of Malwa region of MP. Indian J Dairy Sci 53(4):328-331.

2. Bansal BK, Singh KB, Randhawa SS, Joshi DV, Nauriyal DC (1994). Evaluation of post milking tat dipping and dry period therapy programme for mastitis controlling in cows. Indian J Dairy Sci 47:734-737.

3. Behera S, Swain RK, Samantaray DP, Dash SK (2008). Early diagnosis and milk quality assessment of subclinical mastitis by somatic cell counts and its correlation with pathogenic bacteria in crossbred Jersy cows. J Pure Appl Microbiol 2(2):607-613.

4. Chahar A, Gahlot AK, Tanwar RK (2005). Prevalence of subclinical mastitis in cattle in Bikaner city. Vet Practitioner 6 (1):84-87.

5. Chavan VV, Digraskar SU, Dhonde SN, Hase PB (2007). Observation on bubaline subclinical mastitis in and around Parbhani. Indian J Field Veterinarians 3(1):50.

6. Daley MJ, Coyle PA, Williams TJ, Furda G, Dougherty R, Hayes PW (1991). *Staphylococcus aureus* mastitis: Pathogenesis and treatment with bovine interleukin-1 beta and interleukin-2. J Dairy Sci 74(12):4413-4424.

7. Das PK, Joseph E (2005). Identification and antibiogram of microbes associated with buffalo mastitis in Jabalpur, Madhya Pradesh. India. Buffalo Bulletin 24(1): 3-9.

8. De UK, Mukherjee R (2009). Prevalence of mastitis in cross bred cows. Indian vet J 86 (8):858-859.

9. Dhanda MR, Sethi MS (1962). Investigation of mastitis in India, ICAR Res, Series No. 35, Indian Council of Agricultural Research, New Delhi, India.

10. Dua K (2001). Studies on incidence, etiology and estimated economic losses due to mastitis in Punjab and India -An update. Indian Dairyman 53(10):41-48.

11. Gowardhan AP, Chavan KD, Mote MG (2008). Studies on prevalence of subclincal mastitis in private buffalo farms. Indian vet J 85:687-688.

12. Malhotra BP, Kapur MP, Bali MK (1980). A field trial on dry-cow therapy using neomycin sulphate in mastitis control. Indian vet J 57:676-680.

13. Malhotra BP, Kapur MP, Bhutani JL (1981). Mastitis control with benzathine cloxacillin in dry-cows. Indian J Dairy Sci 34:104-106.

14. Misra SK, Singh KB, Randhawa SS (1984). Preliminary studies on control of mastitis with dry-therapy. Indian J Vet Med 4:54-56.

15. Nauriyal DS, Pachauri SP (2003). Incidence of subclinical intra mammary infection in cows and buffaloes. Indian J Vet Medicine 27:363-365.

16. Nickerson SC (1991). Production of quality milk and control of mastitis in Mexico. Proc. V Annual International Conference on Bovine Milk, Mexico City, Mexico. p 75-96.

17. Pankey JW, Barker RM, Twomey A, Duirs G (1982). A note on effectiveness of dry-cow therapy in New Zealand dairy herds. NZ Vet J 40:50-52.

18. Palanivel KM, Suresh RV, Jayakumar R, Ganesan PI, Dhanapalan P (2008). Retrospective study of subclinical mastitis in buffaloes. Indian J Vet Med 28(1): 34-36.

19. Radostits DM, Gay GC, Blood DC, Hinchcliff KW (2000). Veterinary Medicine (9th Edn.), WB Saunders.

20. Rani N Lakshami, Srinivas Manda, Suresh K, Sreenu Makkena (2008). An epidemiological study of mastitis in buffaloes. Indian vet J 85(12):1350-1351.

21. Ranjan R, Gupta MK, Singh KK (2011). Study of bovine mastitis in different climatic conditions in Jharkhand, India. Veterinary World 4(5):205-208.

22. Roychoudhary P, Dutta TK (2009). Prevalence and antibiotic sensitivity pattern of bacteria from bovine mastitis in Mizoram. Indian J Animal Sci 79(5):483-484.

23. Sharma A, Dhingra P, Pander BL, Kumar R (2006). Bovine subclinical mastitis: Prevalence and treatment with homeopathic medicine. Intl J Cow Sci 2:40-44.

24. Sharma A, Sindhu N (2007). Occurrence of clinical and subclinical mastitis in buffaloes in the State of Haryana (India). Ital J Ani Sci 6(suppl.):965-967.

25. Sharma N, Pandey V, Upadhyay SR (2009). Recent trends in diagnosis of bovine mastitis in field condition. Indian Dairyman 61(4):21-27.

26. Sordillo LM, Peel J, Babiuk LA (1991). Potential role of cytokines in determinng the outcome of acute coliform mastitis. In: Proc. 30th Annu Mtg Natl Mastitis Counc, Inc, Reno, NV, p 50.

27. Torre PM, Konur PK, Oliver SP (1992). Proliferative response of mammary gland mononuclear cells to recombinant bovine interleukin-2. Vet Immunol Immunopathol 32 (3-4):351-358.

28. Tuteja FC, Kapur MP, Sharma A, Vinayaka AK (1993). Studies on bovine subclinical mastitis: Prevalence and microflora. Indian vet J 70:787-791.

29. Wadhwa D, Wadhwa DR, Sharma KS (2003). Nutritional status and mastitis in dairy cows. Round Table Conference on Mastitis, IAAVR, 4:53-64.

□□□

Chapter 20

Poultry Disease Control Strategies

F. R. SHERIFF
Department of Poultry Science, Madras Veterinary College, Chennai-600007

Contents

1. Introduction

Poultry production is one of the fastest growing sectors of Indian agriculture. While egg production is increasing at a rate of 6-8 per cent per annum, broiler production is increasing at 12-15 per cent. India at present is the third largest producer of eggs (only next to China and USA) and fifth largest producer of poultry meat (next to USA, China, Brazil and Mexico) in the world. Andhra Pradesh, Tamilnadu, Punjab, Maharashtra and West Bengal are the major egg producing states, 60 per cent of the total eggs were produced by these five states in the year 1997-98 which has increased to 70 per cent in 2004-05 and during 2005-06. Broilers are the major source of poultry meat in the country. About 140 million broilers are produced every month. Tamilnadu, Andhra Pradesh, West Bengal, Maharashtra, Karnataka and Punjab are the major broiler producing states. The per capita consumption of poultry meat has increased from 126 g in 1961 to 1730 g in 2005. Per capita consumption is about 4 kg in southern states and almost three fold more than that of the national average.

There were about 60,000 broiler farms in the early nineties practicing intensive system of production. Fifty per cent of these farms were small with bird strength varying from few hundreds to 5000 and 40 per cent were medium farms with bird strength varying from 5000-20000. The rest 10 per cent were large or very large farms with bird strength ranging from 20000 to 1 lakh and more. About 70 per cent of the layer farms were small or medium with bird strength varying from 3000-10000 and 10000-50000 per farm, respectively. Only 10 per cent were large farms with bird strength ranging from 50000 to 4 lakh. Due to increase in feed prices and labour cost small farmers could not compete with large farmers. As a result most of the small layer farmers have either closed their operations or have become broiler farmers many of whom prefer to be contract growers.

Not only the number of farms raising broilers has increased but also there has been significant increase in the sizes. Broilers are raised at 10 to 20 thousand on a weekly cycle as a result of which the total capacity has increased manifolds. Production practices have also improved considerably. In very large farms automatic feeding and watering systems and environmental control houses are used to optimize growth rate and to improve the feed conversion ratio (FCR). Improvement has also been made in health control measures, feeding regimes and management system. As a result of which there has been significant improvement in broiler weight and FCR. The body weight, which was achieved at 8 weeks of age during the year 1980s, is now realized in 35 to 40 days of age. FCR has improved from 2.5 to less than 2.0 due to good management and feeding practices.

At this stage it is necessary to have good knowledge of the prevailing diseases that affect the high meat and egg producing chicken to implement strategies for prevention and control of such diseases.

2. Common Poultry Diseases

Several kinds of pathogens, such as bacteria, viruses, protozoa, endoparasites and ectoparasites affect the poultry. Major bacterial diseases include *E. coli* infection, Infectious Coryza, Chronic Respiratory Disease, Fowl Typhoid, Fowl Cholera, and Bacillary White Diarrhoea. Common viral diseases include Newcastle Disease/Ranikhet Disease, Marek's disease, Infectious Bursal Disease, Infectious Bronchitis, Fowl Pox and highly pathogenic Avian Influenza that cause serious impact on growth and economic viability of the industry. Coccidiosis is a major protozoan disease affecting poultry. The ectoparasites such as lice, mites, fleas and ticks and the endoparasites such as roundworms and tapeworms also affect the poultry health.

3. Vaccination Strategy against Viral Diseases

Despite good sanitation programme, viral diseases may affect the farm birds. Hence, vaccination against the known viral diseases is the best choice and has to be followed without fail in all the commercial and breeder farms. Rearing of birds with out vaccination should not be practiced. Viral diseases cannot be treated but can be prevented by timely vaccinations. The regular vaccination schedules for layer and broiler farms are given in Table 1 and Table 2.

Table 1 : Vaccination schedule in layer farms

Age	Vaccination
At hatch	Newcastle Disease vaccine at the hatchery
5-7 days of age	RDVF or LaSota through eye or nasal drops to prevent Ranikhet disease/ Newcastle Disease
14-21 days of age	IBD vaccine through drinking water to prevent Infectious Bursal Disease
35-42 days of age	LaSota through drinking water to prevent Ranikhet disease/ Newcastle Disease
56 days of age	RDVK through S/C route to prevent Ranikhet disease/ Newcastle Disease
16-18th week of age	R2B vaccine through S/C route to prevent Ranikhet disease/ Newcastle Disease

Before vaccination deworm all the birds reared in deep litter system is to be done. It is advisable to give anti-stress drugs along with vitamin supplements before and after vaccination.

Table 2 : Vaccination schedule in broiler farms

Age	Vaccination
At hatch	Marek's disease vaccine at the hatchery
5-7 day of age	RDVF or LaSota through eye or nasal drops to prevent Ranikhet disease/ Newcastle Disease
14-21days of age	IBD vaccine through drinking water to prevent Infectious Bursal disease
35- 42 days of age	LaSota through drinking water to prevent Ranikhet disease Newcastle disease if the marketing is going to be after 56 days

Deworm be done before vaccination. It is advisable to give anti stress drugs along with vitamin supplements. Always take the advice of the local veterinarian or the hatchery recommendation.

Major vaccines that are manufactured in the country are given in Table 3. Some imported vaccines that are available are given in Table 4.

Table 3 : Poultry vaccines manufactured by Indian companies

Manufacturer	Live vaccines
Ventri Biologicals	a) Newcastle disease vaccines (NDV) - LaSota, B1, F and R2B b) Marek's vaccines - Cell associated SB freeze dried and HVT strain c) IBD vaccines - Intermediate, Intermediate plus and Luckert strain d) IB - Mass Type H-120 e) Fowl pox vaccine f) NDV (LaSota)+IB
Hester Pharmaceuticals	a) Newcastle disease vaccines (NDV) - LaSota, B1 and R2B b) Marek's vaccines - Cell associated SB freeze dried and HVT strain c) IBD vaccines – Intermediate, Intermediate plus strain d) IB – Mass Type M-48 e) Fowl pox vaccine f) NDV (LaSota)+IB and B1+IB (M-48)
IVPM Ranipet	a) NDV-LaSota b) NDV-F c) RDVK
Biomed	NDV - LaSota, RB
Indovax	a) Newcastle disease vaccines (NDV) - LaSota, F and R2B b) Mareks vaccines – HVT vaccine c) IBD vaccines – Intermediate, Intermediate plus strain d) IB - Mass Type H-120 e) Fowl Pox Vaccine f) NDV (LaSota)+IB

Table 4 : Imported poultry vaccines

Company	Vaccines
Intervet	ND killed, IB killed, IBD killed , ND+IBD+IB killed
ABIC (Marketed by Sarabhai)	IB – Mass Type H-120, ND Killed, IBD killed ND+IBD killed, ND+IBD+IB killed
Neuva (Marketed by Stallon)	ND killed
CEVAC (Marketed by RFCL Ltd.)	ND killed
Fort Dodge	Marek's vaccines – HVT strain, ND killed, IB killed IBD killed, ND+IBD killed, ND+IBD+IB killed

4. Biosecurity Measures

Poultry farms, hatcheries and egg and meat processing plants generate deep litter manure, cage manure, hatchery waste and meat plant waste that poses major threat to the birds and also to the birds of other farms. These waste materials need careful attention for safe disposal, or these may cause serious health hazards to the flock. The poultry farming and poultry operation have expanded greatly and these can become a threat to themselves and to their neighbouring farms. Poultry farmers should take precautionary measures to eliminate as many disease causing organisms as possible from the farms. It is always better to wait a little longer period of more than 21 days before introducing new flock in the farm. The most effective form of protection against diseases, especially for poultry under modern production techniques is practicing hygienic measures.

Biosecurity literally means safety of living things. It is a programme designed to prevent the exposure of birds to disease causing organisms by reducing introduction and spread of pathogens into and between the farms. Biosecurity in a broader sense encompasses isolation, preventing the visitors into the farms, sanitation, vaccination, serological monitoring of diseases and air quality maintenance which aids in preventing the entry of the pathogens in and around the farm.

Biosecurity, vaccination and good management practices at a farm are three dimension of disease control. Poultry must be given an environment in which disease and infection is controlled to the point where vaccination and medication achieve beneficial effects.

4.1 Farm location biosecurity

1. It is best to build farm in an isolated area where no poultry farm is present. If the farms are to be located nearby, the new farms can be established at least 2 to 3 kilometer away from the existing farms.

2. In case of breeders, the farm should be away from the commercial farms and also away from the highways and the roads connecting the city which might be in use for transport of all type of poultry.
3. Sufficient and safe distance (300 ft) should be maintained between breeders, brooders, growers and layer houses and the facilities such as hatcheries and feed mills.

4.2 Farm structural biosecurity

1. Fencing of entire farm perimeter is essential.
2. Test water source for minerals, bacteria, chemical contamination and pathogen load before start of the farm and rectify.
3. Construct a concrete platform with suitable water and power supply for sanitation of incoming and out going vehicles.
4. A suitable location is to be selected for constructing a storage room for feed ingredients and bagged feed.
5. Dust free roads within the farm are to be laid for easy cleaning and to prevent spreading of microbes by vehicles and foot wear.
6. Provide facilities for safe and scientific disposal of dead birds preferably an incinerator.
7. Provide safe housing and try as much as possible to avoid entry of wild birds and rodents.
8. Feed, litter and equipment should be stored in a section separated from live bird area to prevent contamination.
9. Fire prevention and protection methods should be established.

4.3 Farm operational biosecurity

1. Action plan should be developed for day-to-day activities for the farm/ feed mill/hatchery/ and also during emergencies and to be followed without deviation.
2. Proper cleaning and disinfection of equipment and houses should be done after removal of the entire stock of flock.
3. In breeder farms, no visitor is to be allowed. As far as possible avoid visitors politely. If unavoidable, the visitors may be permitted after a shower and make them wear clean sterilized farm clothes to prevent any possible cross contamination. Only those visitors who have not visited any other farms before their arrival may be permitted.
4. In case of breeders, no vehicles or equipment should be allowed within the farm area.

5. In commercial broiler unit, a minimum interval of two weeks is recommended between the batches of fresh chick arrivals (This is called the down time). All in and all out system of farming is recommended for efficient control of disease outbreaks.
6. Use an effective integrated pest management programme to control pest and rodent through biological, chemical and mechanical means after taking due precautions. Weeds and grass around the poultry sheds should be removed to avoid rodents and pests.
7. Appropriate programme of disease diagnosis and proper vaccination schedule should be implemented.
8. Chicks should always be obtained from a reliable known source.
9. Recycled egg trays should be decontaminated at the point of entry into the farm.
10. Routine disease monitoring procedures like postmortem examination and periodic serum antibody assay to determine immune status of the flock are to be taken up periodically.
11. Regular culling of unhealthy, unproductive and diseased birds has to be done to reduce the disease organism carriers.

5. Management Factors in Disease Prevention

The following managerial tips may help to reduce the spread of disease and stress to the birds.

5.1 Isolation

Do not rear birds of different age groups in the same house. Proper layout of houses, proper and adequate ventilation, balanced feeding, provision of good quality potable water with clean feeders and drinkers, avoiding spillage of water and feed are basic essentials in disease prevention.

5.2 Litter management

Wet litter is a potential source of transmission of diseases like Coccidiosis, Coryza, Chronic Respiratory Disease, Newcastle Disease, Infectious Bronchitis and many more. Maintain litter moisture below 20 per cent always to prevent disease outbreaks in the farm. Cage rearing avoids many litter based problems in poultry farms.

5.3 Quality chicks

Ensure that chicks are received from a hatchery where adequate preventive care is taken for breeder birds to guard against mycoplasmosis, salmonellosis, Marek's disease and infectious bursal disease Only Marek's disease vaccinated chicks are to be procured. Look for signs of dehydration due to transport stress. Ensure that the received chicks are healthy and are within the normal weight range.

5.4 Proper nutrition

A well balanced feed prepared according to nutrient requirements at different ages will ensure proper health and good immune status in birds. Birds should reach normal bodyweight according to their age, breed, strain and sex by proper balanced and adequate feeding to develop good immunity.

5.5 Water quality

Poultry farmers often fail to provide good quality water for their birds. Before establishing the poultry farm the microbial and chemical quality of the water is to be tested and if found suitable, the farm can be established. Microbial contamination of water may happen at the source, for instance in ponds, rivers, open wells and the public water supply system, or during transportation and storage, as well as in the overhead tank. Do not use pond or reservoir water for the poultry as it may be highly contaminated. The microbial load shoots up during rainy seasons and during flood conditions. Faecal contamination of water will add to the presence of Coliform organisms. Mineral levels in water depend on soil conditions, and show only minor fluctuations based on the season and the water table. They lead to hardness in water and affect the taste and palatability. Deep bore well water is highly preferred for poultry farms provided it is soft and potable. The deep bore well water will always have low bacterial contamination. Before use of the potable water, test it for its suitability for the poultry farms. The desirable quality guidelines for drinking water are given in Table 5.

Table 5 : Water quality permissible levels

Parameter	Permissible level
Total hardness	60-180 mg/litre
pH	6.8-7.5
Nitrate	10 mg/litre
Nitrite	0.4 mg/litre
Total bacterial count	0/ml
Coliform count	0/ml
Calcium chloride	60 mg/litre
Sodium	50 mg/litre
Sulphate	125 mg/litre

Removal of excess dissolved minerals is not practicable and will be expensive. Hence the farmer should change to other water sources in case of excess minerals or total hardness in the water. Chlorination is the best and cheapest method to get rid of microorganisms. About eight grams of bleaching powder with about 35 per cent available chlorine should be added to 1000 liters of drinking water to maintain a chlorine level of 1 to 2 ppm at delivery. A minimum contact time of one hour should be given before providing the water to birds. Where storage facilities are not available, liquid chlorine preparations like chlorine dioxide, 5 per cent sodium hypochlorite may be used at a level of one ml per 10 liters of water. Iodophores containing 1.6 per cent available iodine are also used as water sanitizers at the same dosage level. Products containing quaternary ammonium compounds may be used as water sanitizers as per the manufacturers' specifications. By providing sanitized water to the birds, the chance of waterborne infections is reduced and the cost of medication is saved.

5.6 Dead bird disposal

The main principle involved in the prevention and control of current and emerging diseases is the scientific disposal of dead birds. When birds die, their carcasses remain as a source of infection for other birds on the farm. All carcasses should be removed from the shed as soon as possible. Mortality varies with the prevailing disease and sanitary conditions on the farm. Diseased and ill birds also discharge infectious material into the environment and act as reservoirs for disease-producing organisms. It is essential to eliminate ailing birds from the flock rather than treating them which may continue to infect the remainder of the flock. The habit of throwing dead birds on to the nearest manure pile or into an open field is dangerous and unscientific for the following reasons:

- The smell of the carcasses attracts street dogs and cats, which consume the infected carcasses and harbour the pathogenic organisms infectious to poultry. These animals are capable of carrying contaminated carcass portions to neighbouring farms thus causing spread of disease.
- Vultures, crows and other wild birds invade the carcasses and become potential carriers of the disease causing agents. These may spread infection from one farm to another.
- The carcasses lure insects and flies, which act as transmitters of infectious agents.
- The disease causing agents along with portions of viscera carried by rain water contaminate all water sources and soil.
- On decomposition, the carcasses may emit foul smell and cause air pollution.

The disposal of carcasses of birds dying from known or unknown causes should be carefully attended to. There are many methods for the efficient disposal of carcasses such as burying, pit disposal, incineration, septic tank disposal, or composting. In general, the following points should be observed while disposing the carcasses.

- Remove the dead birds from the flock as soon as possible.
- Do not deposit carcasses in or near a flowing water stream.
- Take necessary precautions to prevent spillage of infectious material from the carcasses during transportation from the farm or post-mortem room to the disposal site.
- Take sound biosecurity measures at the disposal sites to prevent disease transmission.

Moreover, with the present concern for the environment, the poultry industry needs to pursue efforts to protect the environment. Therefore, all methods that allow for environmentally safe and scientific ways of disposing of carcasses should be considered. Current methods for routine disposal of carcasses include burial, incineration, and rendering in India.

5.6.1 Burial

Burial of dead birds is a natural process that has been used for hundreds of years. On farm, burial historically has been the predominant disposal option. If this method seems to be the best option, a site should be selected in advance, based on soil type and drainage characteristics. Methods for burial are as simple as excavation of a trench, although more complex burial may include the use of a plastic liner placed under the birds, or the placement of birds in a cardboard. Burial is not a good practice but still used and its use will diminish due to concerns for groundwater quality. Despite the fact that disposal pits have been found to cause no more groundwater contamination than an individual septic tank and dug up soil pit, the decline in groundwater quality in the area of an open-bottom pit and the fact that residue remains after years of use have been cited as reasons for discontinuation of burial pits.

5.6.2 Incineration

Incineration is recognized as one of the biologically safest methods of disposal, eliminating the threat of disease. Birds died due to noninfectious diseases can be processed and the resulting residue easily disposed of without causing water contamination. Proper, acceptable cremation of carcasses is not accomplished simply by drenching carcasses with a flammable fluid and igniting them, as is done in pyre construction. Such an approach usually is incomplete, and the resulting smoke and odours may bring about environmental pollution. Other home made incinerators constructed from drums or barrels are unsatisfactory because they fail to meet temperature and air emission requirements that would support complete combustion under environmental compliance regulations for carcass incineration. Commercial units with oil or gas burners and equipped with automatic timers to ensure proper burn can be used.

5.6.3 Rendering

Rendering of dead birds involve conversion of carcasses into various by-products such as hydrolyzed whole poultry meal, fat, and water. Hydrolyzed whole poultry meal results from modern processing methods that use hydrolysis with high temperature and pressure. In this method, the whole carcasses of dead, undecomposed poultry including feathers, heads, feet, and entire carcass are utilized. In the rendering processes, after cooking and separation of fat, water, and protein materials are separated. The most often used method is grinding, mixing, pressing, decanting, centrifugation, cooking, evaporating, and drying. The resulting meal and fat obtained from hydrolyzed whole poultry can be used for preparing animal feeds. The dead birds have to be rendered before decay to get good quality end products; carcasses should be processed as soon as possible or stored appropriately to preserve them to retard decay. The cooking step in the rendering process kills most bacteria but does not eliminate endotoxins produced by some bacteria during the decay of carcass tissue. Rendering is only feasible, only if the rendering plant is located close enough for convenient pickup. The spread of pathogenic microorganisms during pickup and transportation is to be avoided.

5.7 Litter removal

After the house is emptied, the litter and droppings are to be removed as far as possible from the farm and composted. It should be disposed of as soon as possible as fertilizer or for other purposes. Composting is better, since the heat produced destroys the pathogens. It should be completely covered with mud and opened after five to six months and transported in closed containers for agricultural purpose as fertilizer, far from the Poultry farms.

5.8 Disinfection

A disinfectant is a chemical that kills disease producing organisms on contact. Disinfection is the act of destroying infectious agents. Disinfectants and disinfection procedures have been widely used for many years in the poultry industry. Natural disinfection agents, such as sunlight, heat, or just simply resting poultry houses, are considered to be of limited use. Increasing evidence of the prolonged survival time of a number of important chicken pathogens, outside the body of the birds together with an ever-increasing economic pressure for quicker restocking of units, has led to a greater dependence on chemical disinfectants. Sanitization is often done to reduce the number of bacteria present and also to prevent them from multiplying.

5.8.1 Desirable features of disinfectants

All disinfectants used in the poultry farm and hatchery should have the following features.

1. Effective germicidal property, less expensive and readily available
2. Non-toxic to man and birds, without pungent odours
3. Effective in the presence of organic materials
4. Readily soluble in water and stable when exposed to air
5. Capable of penetrating materials and crevices
6. Non-corroding and non-staining
7. Non-polluting and environmental friendly
8. Broad spectrum activity, effective under farm conditions, organic soiling, hard water and low temperatures
9. Free of residual toxicity
10. Non-transmitters of residue or odour to eggs or meat

5.8.2 Mode of action of surface disinfectants

Surface disinfectants differ in their action according to the type of organisms involved. Most of them are bactericidal but some chemically disrupt the life cycle of the bacterium. To inactivate virus, the agent must disrupt the non-nucleic acid protein coat around the nucleic acid gene material content. The content of the virus should be destroyed to make it inactive. Fungal organism is difficult to be destroyed and most fungicides only poison the fungus rather than destroy the fungal cells. There are few surface disinfectants specific for protozoa affecting poultry. Even though several chemical compounds are available, their concentration and cost make them unacceptable.

The lethal action of a disinfectant depends on the chemical composition of the disinfectant and the type of organism. No disinfectant works immediately. All require a certain amount of contact time to be effective. Disinfectants are less effective in the presence of organic matter. Organic matter interferes with the action of disinfectants by coating the disease producing organisms and preventing their contact with the disinfectant. Hence, the disinfectants are to be used after removing the debris and organic matter by mechanical means for better effectiveness.

5.8.3 Common chemicals used for disinfection

Many disinfectants are of similar composition. Directions for dilutions given by the manufacturers should be closely followed. Continuous use of certain chemicals, particularly at inadequate concentrations, may produce a population of microorganisms resistant to that chemical. A brief description of some of the commonly used disinfectants is given here.

a) Cresol and cresylic acid

Cresols and cresylic acid are liquid yellow or brown, coal tar derivatives. They are effective against Gram-positive, Gram-negative bacteria, most fungi and some viruses and work best in an acid medium. They have greater use in the poultry house than in the hatchery.

b) Phenols

These are also coal tar derivatives with a base of carbolic acid (C_6H_5OH). Synthetic related compounds also fall in this category; phenols have characteristic odour, turn milky in the presence of water and are effective germicides. Their action is rapid. Such disinfectants are effective against fungi, Gram-positive and Gram-negative bacteria but not effective against bacterial spores. Phenol in its pure form is colourless crystals, having a characteristic smell. It is usually used in water solutions with a dilution of 1:1000 but it is too expensive for general poultry house use. Another disinfectant commonly called as 'phenyl' is used as a 5% solution in water, generally for dipping of shoes and gloved hands.

c) Iodine

Iodine has long been recognized as an effective disinfectant. To overcome many of the disadvantages of the earlier products, 'iodophors' have been prepared. The term 'iodophor' refers to a combination of iodine with a solubilizing agent that slowly liberates free iodine when diluted with water. The solution will be amber (brownish-yellow) in colour. When the solution is colourless, it is no longer effective. The product can be mixed in hard water also.

Iodine compounds have a wide variety of uses. They can be applied safely to all surfaces, and are useful for disinfecting hatchery and incubator surfaces, incubator and hatchery trays, feeders, footwear, and poultry buildings. Iodophors are good disinfectants, but do not work well in the presence of organic matter. Like all other disinfectants, these compounds are most effective on clean surfaces.

Iodophors have a broad disinfecting range which includes bacteria, viruses, fungi and even coccidia and ova of parasites. Iodophor can be prepared by dissolving 100 g crystalline iodine in 450 ml heated isopropanol. Heating is continued and non-ionic detergent (450 ml) is added. Finally, cold water is slowly added to make final volume 4½ litres of iodophor. It acts best at low pH. The low pH (6.0 or below) can be obtained by adding some sulphuric or phosphoric acid.

d) Chlorine

Chlorine is an effective constituent of certain disinfectants described below.

1. Powder forms
   a. Calcium hypochlorite combined with hydrated trisodium phosphate (less active for short duration)
   b. Sodium hypochlorite combined with hydrated trisodium phosphate (very active with short disinfecting life)
2. Liquid forms
   a. Sodium hypochlorite
   b. Organic chloramines
   c. Chlorine dioxide

Chlorine compounds are good disinfectants when free chlorine is available in abundance (200-300 ppm). When elemental chlorine or hypochlorites are added to water they produce hypochlorus acid (HOCl) which produces bactericidal action.

e) Quaternary ammonium compounds

These compounds are cationic, odourless, clear, generally non-irritating, have deodourizing and detergent action and are quite effective as surface disinfectants. The most common is alkyl dimethyl benzyl ammonium chloride.

A solution of 500 ppm quaternary ammonia, 200 ppm EDTA (ethylene diamine tetra acetic acid) and sodium carbonate to adjust pH to about 8.0 (about 200 ppm) is an excellent hatchery disinfectant. It may be used on floors, walls and incubator trays. This should not be used in meat and egg processing plants. Precaution should be taken where foods are involved.

f) Formaldehyde

Formaldehyde is a gas. It is sold commercially in a 40% solution with water as formalin. Formalin is very effective, cheap and easily available. It is used with potassium permanganate for fumigation of poultry house, brooder, and hatchery. Formaldehyde is usually generated by adding formalin to potassium permanganate in an earthen pot or metal container. The reaction produces heat by the chemical reaction; hence glass containers should not be used. The container should be deep and have a volume several times that of the combined chemicals, because a lot of bubbling takes place. Not more than 1 litre of formalin should be used per container. The container is placed in the room meant for disinfection. The ratio of formalin is about twice the amount of potassium permanganate, that is, 2 ml formalin to 1 g of potassium permanganate. Potassium permanganate is poisonous and has to be handled with care. It causes eye and nose irritation and had to be protected by the user.

Application of formaldehyde for fumigation or fogging

After setting up the house, formaldehyde fumigation is done after closing all the sides so that the fumes are retained in the shed for a longer time. This method is not much in use now as it is more cumbersome. The traditional method of formaldehyde fumigation has been replaced by safer chemicals that are either applied with fogging machines, or as a fine spray. The house should remain closed after the spraying or fogging to prevent the reentry of disease organisms and to make the fumes stay in the room for more time to kill the existing organisms. No traffic is to be allowed into the shed after cleaning.

Though formaldehyde is a powerful disinfectant, it has many disadvantages. It is extremely irritating to the conjunctiva and mucous membranes, and some people are very sensitive to it. Therefore, precautions must be taken to prevent its escape into the areas where people work. Operator should wear rubber gloves when handling formalin.

Its chief advantage is that formaldehyde can be used as a gas or vapour for fumigation of hatching eggs to destroy potential harmful shell contaminants, such as *Salmonella*. It is a good disinfectant in the presence of some organic matter. Formaldehyde is also used to fumigate the interiors of incubators and hatchers and their contents. Fumigation of incubators and eggs has been an established practice in the industry. The higher the humidity and temperature, the more effective is fumigation. Fumigation should not be done in incubators with eggs inside because of the danger of injuring embryos. About 15-20 ml of pure formalin can disinfect about 100 cubic feet of a box or incubator.

Methods of generating formaldehyde gas

The methods commonly used are:

1. Potassium permanganate method
2. Paraformaldehyde method
3. Evaporation of formalin solution

Potassium permanganate method: Two parts (by volume) of formalin are mixed with approximately one part (by weight) of potassium permanganate. When the entire gas is expelled the left out powder will be brown in colour. If sufficient amount of potassium permanganate is not used, the powder will be wet in consistency. When too much of potassium permanganate is added, the residue will be purple in colour. Varying concentration of formaldehyde gas is necessary to fumigate under different conditions as mentioned below.

Normal or single strength concentration: This is obtained by mixing 40 ml of formalin with 20 g of potassium permanganate for each 2.83 m^3 (100 ft^3) of closed space. This is also called 1-X concentration.

Double strength concentration: This is achieved by mixing 80 ml of formalin with 40 g of potassium permanganate for each 2.83 m^3 (100 ft^3) of space. This is called 2-X concentration.

Other concentration: Other concentrations are 3-X and 5-X. The amount of formalin and permanganate to be used will depend on the size of the incubator or the chamber and the desired strength of the fumigation.

The capacity of the incubator is obtained by multiplying together the internal width, height and depth of the compartment to be fumigated, making no allowance for the space occupied by the eggs, the trays and all the internal fittings. The container should be made of metal and at least 50 times the volume of formalin to be used so as to prevent chemical overflowing during the reaction.

Paraformaldehyde method: Paraformaldehyde is a white powder or pellet and is more easily handled than potassium permanganate and formalin. The powder should be placed in an electric pan with the 232°C. For obtaining the normal or single strength (1-X) concentration, 10 g of paraformaldehyde is used for each 2.83 m^3 (100 ft^3) of space. The gas will be released after 20 minutes of heating. It is advisable to add a little water to the pellet before heating to raise the relative humidity between 60 and 80 per cent.

Evaporation of formalin solution: A 40 per cent solution of formalin is often used in regulated quantities for the fumigation of hatchers during the egg pipping and hatching period. Some hatchers are fitted with a special tray or cup for this purpose or the formalin may be placed in an enamel coated or earthen container on the incubator floor. The formalin is used at the rate of 60 ml per m^3 of hatcher space placed in an enamel pan 24 hours after transfer of chicks. Formaldehyde gas evaporates from formalin solution throughout the period the eggs are in the hatcher, thus reducing the microorganism population in the hatchery environment.

Temperature and humidity requirement for maximum formaldehyde disinfection: The efficiency of formaldehyde gas is increased in the presence of heat and moisture. It is impossible to get maximum results unless the temperature of the area to be fumigated is 24°C or higher and the relative humidity is 75per cent or more.

Neutralising formaldehyde gas with ammonium hydroxide: In certain cases it is necessary to stop the action of formaldehyde gas after the required period of fumigation is over. Usually this is accomplished by opening the air inlets and exhausts in the incubators or rooms but often this method is too slow. Ammonium hydroxide (NH_4OH) may be used to stop the process. A solution of 16 to 20 per cent ammonia should be used. First it is checked to see how much formalin has been used, and then the same amount of ammonium hydroxide is sprinkled on the floor of the fumigated area. In case of paraformaldehyde, 2 ml of ammonium hydroxide is used for each gram of paraformaldehyde used.

Strength of formaldehyde fumigation: Varying concentrations of formaldehyde gas are needed under different conditions and the length of the fumigation period is also variable. The gas is detrimental to living embryos and to the newly hatched chicks, so care must be exercised that the concentration of the gas and length of the fumigation period are able to kill the pathogenic organisms as possible but are not lethal to the embryos or chicks. Detailed recommendations in this regard are given in Table 6 and Table 7.

Table 6 : Strength of formaldehyde fumigation for 100 ft^3 space

	To produce formaldehyde gas (mix together)	
Strength	**Formalin (ml)**	**Potassium permanganate (g)**
Single (1-X)	40	20
Double (2-X)	80	40
Triple (3-X)	120	60
5-X	200	100

Table 7 : Formaldehyde fumigation process recommendations

Item for fumigation	Concentration of fumigant	Fumigation duration (minutes)
Hatching eggs immediately after they are laid	3-X	20
Eggs in incubator (1st day only)	2-X	20
Chicks in Hatcher	1-X	3
Incubator room	1-X, 2-X	30
Hatcher between hatches, Hatchery room, chick room, Wash Room and Chick boxes	3-X	30
Trucks	5-X	20

Special recommendations for fumigation

1. *Fumigating eggs soon after laying*: Fumigating with 3-X concentration of formaldehyde for 20 minutes will kill about 98 to 99 % of the organisms on the shells. Egg should never be fumigated between 24 and 96 hour after setting in the incubator, as it is the critical periods of incubation of breed able eggs.
2. *Fumigating chicks*: Chicks that have been hatched should not be exposed to concentrated fumigation by rapid gas release. Formaldehyde fumigation colours the down of the chicks to deep orange and is often noticeable. Chick's fumigation, therefore, should be considered on emergency measure only such as in case of omphalitis outbreaks.
3. *Fumigating between hatches*: After the chicks have been removed from the hatchers, the trays washed and sun dried, the hatchers, trays, hatcher cabin and washroom should be fumigated with formaldehyde gas.
4. *Fumigating chick trucks*: After thoroughly cleaning the truck, it may be fumigated in a specially constructed tent covering its whole body and chassis with 5-X concentration. This can be done by the owner of the truck before every trip of use.

Copper sulphate

Copper sulphate is toxic to fungi. A 0.5% solution is generally used for destroying fungi on feed, hoppers, utensils, water fountains, and surrounding areas associated if the outbreaks of fungal diseases are suspected.

Chlorinated lime (bleaching powder)

Chlorinated lime or bleaching powder, prepared by saturating slaked lime (i.e. lime treated with water) with chlorine gas, is one of the recognized disinfectants. It has corrosive effect on metals and skin, and hence caution is required after proper cleaning of floor. A 20 per cent solution is used for disinfecting floor and utensils for feed and water. However, chlorinated lime has now been largely replaced by hypochlorite. If used according to directions, hypochlorite is highly efficient. It is mainly used for egg washing and sanitizing, and for disinfecting incubators, and hatcher trays, small brooders, and water and feed containers. They can also be used on cement surfaces. All surfaces to be disinfected with hypochlorite solutions must first be thoroughly cleaned to ensure no organic matter is adhering to the floor.

Lime

Lime is commonly used as a disinfectant for litter, floor, and poultry carcasses. It is mainly used in areas that are damp and cannot be exposed to the sun, as well as for disinfection of drains and sewerages. The action of lime depends on liberation of heat and oxygen when the chemical comes in contact with water. Heat destroys bacteria and parasitic eggs and even coccidia, and keeps fungi under control. It can be applied using at least 4-7 kg/100 square feet. For disinfection of poultry manure, lime should be added at the rate of 90 kg/ton of manure. It also disinfects wall and crevices, if a solution containing 38 parts lime and 15 parts sodium chloride is used for washing the wall. As lime has a caustic action, birds should be kept away from it, until it has become thoroughly dry.

Hot water

Hot water adds to the efficiency of most disinfectants. If applied in the form of boiling water, it is effective without addition of any chemical.

Dry heat

Dry heat in the form of a flame is effective if the flame comes in contact directly with the infective agent to be killed. While using dry flame, care should be taken to prevent fire hazards.

5.9 Rodent control

Rodents should be kept out from the initial stage of farming itself, since once the farm is infested; it is difficult to get rid of them. Care should be taken to remove piles of unused equipment and empty gunny bags as they serve as breeding places for rats and mice. Removal of spilled feed daily and storage of feed in well-ventilated, rodent-proof rooms can be practised.

5.10 Insect control

Insects entry into the farms are to be prevented to maintain good sanitary environment, as insects play a significant role in transmitting disease-producing microorganisms, tape worms and other parasites. Flies irritate the birds; prevent them from taking water and feed normally, causing stress which results in reduced egg production especially where cage rearing is practiced. Some of them suck blood and permanently stay in the feathers and cause irritation. Insects also stay in the crevices and on litter and irritate the birds during night times. Insect or fly control measures include:

- Avoiding stagnation of water in and around the farm premises and provision of proper drainage facilities.
- Use of insecticide sprays or dusting with care
- Treating the birds and checking the feed and water quality to avoid watery droppings, keeping the surroundings clean by covering the area with treated soil devoid of vegetation or by growing grass lawns

- Preventing entry of country chicken and wild birds in the farm premises which are the usual carriers of parasites.

5.11 Sanitation of the building

Pathogens present in poultry house floors, ceilings, nets can transmit diseases continuously from flock to flock. The survival time of many pathogens on improperly cleaned and disinfected surfaces can run into months. Rodents (rats, mice) and insect vectors (transmitters) are often seen to transfer both viral and bacterial infections. Such a situation can be dealt with by a process generally known as 'terminal disinfection'. Apart from the selection of an effective disinfectant, the success of any 'terminal disinfection programme' depends on careful attention to every step given below.

5.11.1 Dry cleaning

Residual feed should be removed from the feeders. Portable equipments should be taken out of the house for cleaning. Litter should be completely removed from the house and transported to manure pit. After removal of the litter, dust, cob web from ceilings, water pipes, and the netting should be removed entirely.

5.11.2 Sanitization of the drinking water system

Cleaning of water storage tanks, water basins, nipples, and water pipes is essential for providing safe water for the new arrival of the chicks. The overhead tank should be drained and cleaned and whitewashed with lime. The tank should then be filled with required quantity of water, and the disinfectant added to achieve the required dilution. The solution should be allowed to flow through the water lines and drinkers to get sanitized. Then the entire water in the overhead tank should be drained and filled with fresh water, and the tanks should be covered.

5.11.3 Pre-cleaning the house and equipment

All the utensils should be thoroughly cleaned with water and sun dried for at least 6 to 8 hours. The equipments should be cleaned with a detergent sanitizer to further clean the surfaces to minimize organic matter and reduce the bacterial load. All surfaces should be sprayed with the solution at low pressure, ensuring thorough wetting. This must include coverage of pipe lines, feeders, and drinkers. After the detergent application, cleaning should be completed with high pressure water until all the areas are visibly clean.

5.11.4 Disinfection of the house and equipment

The house should be cleaned by removing the litter material. The floor and side walls are to be cleaned with running water and then allowed to dry.

The debris and adhering dirt should be scrapped thoroughly before washing the floor and walls. Detergent solution in water should be used to wash the floor, walls and nettings. Application by spraying of the selected broad-spectrum disinfectant to all surfaces and equipment in the house, strictly following the required dilution rate, application rate, and contact time is essential. Application can be with any suitable spraying equipment. The dilution at which the disinfectant is most effective against disease organisms should be used. It is advisable to always select the highest concentration necessary to eliminate the most resistant disease organisms. Effective disinfection requires surfaces to be thoroughly wet. All disinfectants must remain in contact with the disease producing organisms for the recommended contact time. In practice, at least 30 minutes contact time is generally required for effective disinfection.

It should always be kept in mind that disinfection is not a substitute for cleanliness. It is a means of destroying microorganisms but is effective only when things are relatively clean to start with.

6. Conclusion

Breeder and commercial poultry farms are likely to be affected with bacterial, viral and fungal infection if the birds are not reared under hygienic conditions. Even despite strict hygienic management conditions of rearing, there is likelihood of new emerging diseases such as Infectious Bursal Disease and Avian Influenza. The birds need to be vaccinated against known pathogens at appropriate age with well protected potent vaccines that have been kept in proper cold chain from the date of manufacture to the date of utilization to give adequate protection. Adequate quantity of nutritive feed and well-ventilated clean poultry houses constitute primary needs of poultry farming. Cleaning of the houses and utensils with clean water, sun drying and disinfection with effective disinfectants in proper dose are prerequisites for safety. Biosecurity measures should be adopted to ward off pathogens from the farms. Dead bird carcass disposal poses a problem in many farms and is often neglected which leads to spread of diseases. Use of incinerators is the safest method to dispose of the carcasses. Disposal of used litter as fertilizer for agricultural operation should be done after proper composting of the manure to avoid disease outbreaks. Sanitary procedures must start at hatchery at the time of incubation of eggs to produce healthy chicks. Many farms have been managed over decades without major disease outbreaks by following strict hygienic and biosecurity measures.

□□□

Chapter 21

Applications of Information and Communication Technology in Livestock Sector

ABDUL SAMAD[1], PRASHANT MURDESHWAR[2] AND ZOHAIB HAMEED[3]

[1]Maharashtra Animal and Fishery Sciences University, Nagpur-440006, [2]Infovet India, Thane-400605, [3]Department of Electrical and Computer Engineering, University of Alberta, Edmonton, Canada

Contents

1. Introduction

The term information and communication technology (ICT) is widely used and has assumed diverse connotations. The word 'information' is connoted by 'fact', but in the context of ICT, it is understood as 'logically jointed facts that generate knowledge in deducible and communicable form'. At times 'information' and 'data' are used interchangeably. When the information is organized logically and stored in computers, it becomes 'data'; interestingly when the same data is processed, the output (in any form) is still perceived as 'information'. When information is packaged and sent to receiver for understanding or for applying to handle a task based on the past experience, it turns into 'knowledge' which is the end of the information process. Communication is an integral part of ICT, which in simple terms means the process of transforming information from one entity to another entity. The complete cycle of communication involves three entities: sender, media and the receiver (who may not be always aware of sender's intent). The communication cycle is complete once the recipient understands the message (information or knowledge). For example, if the information about milk produced by each cow is collected and entered into computer (data), it can be processed to calculate, for example, the average milk yield per day per cow. When this information is communicated to the farmer along with the expected values (below or above of the default farm average), the farmer would know how his cows are performing. Based on this information he can take the management decisions.

The term ICT was first used in 1997 in a report submitted by Dennis Stenvensen to the Government of United Kingdom. He referred to the term as merging/convergence of audio-visual and telephone network with computer network using a single unified system of cabling, signal distribution and management. ICT is often used as an extended synonym for information technology (IT) but is usually a more general term that stresses the role of unified communications and integration of telecommunication. ICT encompasses all the technical means used to handle information and aid communication, including computer and network hardware, communication middleware as well as necessary software. India has been recognized as global leader in ICT development. The industry has grown from USD 7.8 billion to more than 64 billion in 2009. Its contribution to the national Gross Domestic Product (GDP) has grown from 1% a decade ago to more than 6%, providing direct employment to 2.3 million, mostly young, people. Unfortunately much of this progress has impacted other countries as these developments took place under export category. India's rural areas, especially the core agriculture, rural services and livestock sectors have remained untouched from this revolution (Desai 2006).

ICT is often used in specific sector context, such as, ICT in agriculture (e-agriculture), ICT in education (e-education) or ICT in livestock (e-livestock), since depending upon the sector the need for infrastructure, domain contents and communication media would vary. Many countries around the world have established organizations for ICT promotion as it has now become a core infrastructure for development. In late 1990s and early 2000s there was fear that investment in network, cabling and the progress in IT might lead to technology-divide between urban and rural, and rich and poor. These fears led to a number of community-based initiatives such as Village ICT Center which would act as knowledge access point for the rural citizens. This idea though did not pick up as it also required investment for establishment and sustenance which again depended on farmers visiting the centers (Ramkumar *et al.* 2007). ICT however is now being used for enhancing management efficiency, training and empowerment by providing information access to all stakeholders. Livestock rearing is a management activity hence use of ICT would certainly benefit the sector.

ICT can be leveraged to improve health and productivity in domestic animals accruing benefits to otherwise difficult-to-reach millions of small-hold and marginal farmers. The authors have been involved in facilitating software and hardware developments and implementing novel pilot projects in livestock sector (Swedberg 2010). The names of the software and hardware mentioned in the paper are for illustration purpose and should not be construed as authors endorsement.

2. ICT Tools and Convergence

ICT set up requires a number of tools like server, middleware, computers, camera, scanners; software such as operating systems, ERP (Enterprise resource planning) solutions, dedicated software; and communication tools like telephone, television, radio etc. Networking needs cabling or wireless technology such as Wi-Fi. There has been a perception that ICT involves huge investments in infrastructure, large skilled and trained manpower, and great funds for maintenance. Because of these constraints, its implementation in rural sector has been slow. The scenario however changed in the late 20th century as rapid progress in computer and electronics led to introduction of simple and cost-effective network technologies which proved hassle-free for operators and users. With evolution of new technologies such as 3G and 4G, and pervasive 5G, cell phones are likely to occupy central place in the ICT network around which new paradigms in communication would be witnessed. It is estimated that in the next five years, predominant population would own cell phone which will be single machine doing all the communication tasks. For example with the availability of Radio Frequency Identification (RFID)-reading enabled cell phones, farmers would be able to identify their animals and communicate data to the server (Samad *et al.* 2010). Artificial intelligence software and knowledge database would help in processing the acquired data to communicate about the putative problems of the animals and the possible solutions. For a consumer in the supermarket, cell phone would read RFID/bar code information on the animal product to instantly download the product safety information for him to decide on the purchases. In a few years time, the ICT will become highly interactive and people would largely depend on these tools. The challenge for the developing countries is to free ICT from the intricate web of cable network to offer simple solutions, functioning around one data center and cell phones in the periphery. Such a scenario will provide level playing field for the urban and rural poor.

3. ICT in Agriculture

ICT finds its application wherever information and communication is part of the business process. There is no sector which has remained untouched with its rapid development. Agriculture sector is information-dependent and if the data is properly captured, processed and communicated to the stakeholders in real time, it would benefit millions of farmers directly. ICT in agriculture (E-Agriculture) involves diverse functions such as designing and development of novel applications that can facilitate the use of ICT in rural domain. E-Agriculture is a fast emerging field poised to help farmers in raising agriculture productivity, implementing traceability concepts such as farm-to-fork and sustainable rural development through improved information along with communication and knowledge empowerment. Globally e-Agriculture is growing at much faster pace because of strict food safety laws and consumers' insistence on traceability. Industrial, services and social sectors are passing through ICT-driven transformation due to rapid progress in electronic, telecommunication, computing and remote (wireless) networking. Quick information gathering in real time, internet technologies and use of multimedia and communication devices have ensured knowledge and information availability all the time. E-Agriculture has been identified as a priority area in the World Summit on Information Society and an action plan 'Tunis Agenda for the Information Society' was published in 2005. The agenda emphasizes the leading and facilitating roles UN agencies need to play in the implementation of the Geneva Plan of Action. The Food and Agriculture Organization has been assigned the responsibility of organizing activities related to the action line under C.7 'ICT Applications on E-Agriculture' (Anonymous 2010).

The Summit has rightly noted that public private partnership should maximize the use of ICT as an instrument to improve agriculture productivity. In contrast, it is a relatively new concept in India trying to find its place in small-hold farming systems (Parikh *et al.* 2010). The scope and spectrum of the technology is still evolving. ICT applications are more crucial for sustainable development in less industrialized countries since bulk of their population is engaged in agriculture as primary vocation and majority belong to small marginal farmer category. A number of novel pilot projects involving use of ICT in agriculture sector have been implemented in India and other developing countries (Table 1), but these have remained at the pilot stage and are yet to be scaled up.

Table 1 : Some ICT-based projects in agriculture sector

Name of the project	Implementing agency
Gyandoot	Government of Madhya Pradesh
Village ICT Center	M. S. Swaminathan Research Foundation
ICT-enabled rural veterinary and extension services	Bombay Veterinary College
Jhabua Development Communication Project	Government of Madhya Pradesh
Warana Village Network	Government of Maharashtra
ISAP Kissan Call Center	Indian Society of Agri-business Professionals, New Delhi
Kissan Kerla Online Agri-video Channel	Indian Institute of Information Technology, Kerala
Smart Krushi	Orissa e-Governance Services Ltd.
E-Krishuk	Bangladesh Institute of ICT Development
mKrishi	Tata Consultancy, Mumbai
e-Chaupal	Indian Tobacco Company
Livestock Services Call Center	Chitale Dairy, Maharashtra and Infovet

4. ICT in Livestock Sector

Livestock is an integral component of agriculture. In fact, its social equity is more than agriculture since even landless people own livestock and their livelihood depends on this vocation. Thus any investment in livelihood ICT will have greater social impact compared to agriculture. Livestock sector is also important from the point of view of public health since animals can transmit diseases to humans. Hence, the control of transmissible diseases also pays dividends in terms of improved human health. Livestock farming is information-intensive since it generates huge body of information which if processed and communicated properly to the stakeholders can bring radical improvement in farming efficiency and profitability. Livestock sector in India faces numerous inherent problems like wide geographical areas under livestock production, large population of livestock, inadequate infrastructure to provide veterinary care and extension service, and small hold systems, which do not permit introduction of farm technology and farm automation easily. In contrast, the developed countries have been able to harness the power of ICT to improve farm automation (Naas 2002), health (Andonovic *et al.* 2009) and productivity of their livestock many-folds in the last two decades. It is necessary that the scientific communities and technologists in developing countries focus on the ICT applications in the livestock sector.

4.1 Information cycle in livestock farming

In livestock farming, the data is generated at the farm and after computerization may pass through a series of processes generating useful knowledge for the stakeholders. Fig. 1 depicts the ICT flow scheme for a typical livestock farm. The right hand panel describes how in case of a goat farm the

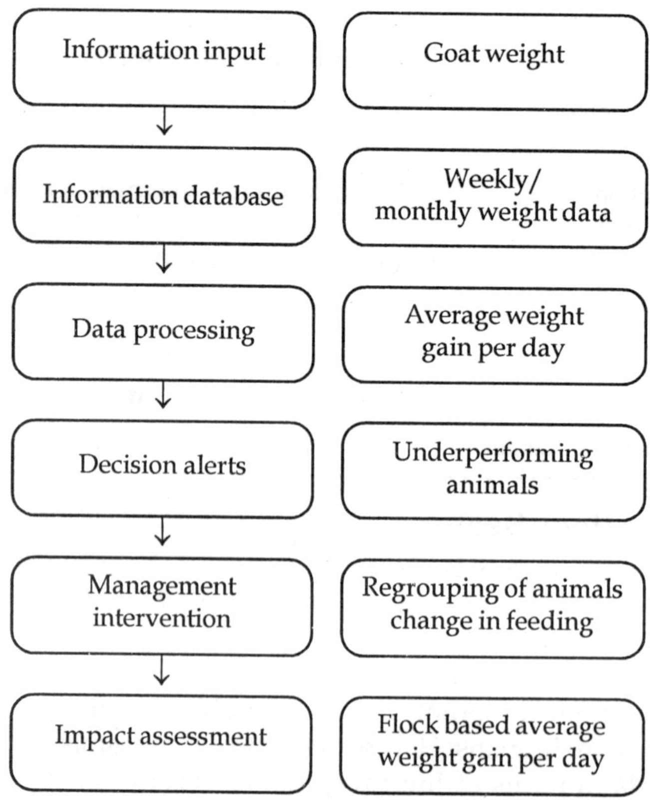

Fig. 1 : Information cycle in a model livestock operation

information will be processed and communicated to the farmer/veterinarian. Weight gains in growing goat kids is an important health and productivity determinant; hence the goat farms acquire periodic information on weight of the animals to process and calculate 'average weight gain per day per animal' and generate alert list of animals that are under-performing (compared to predefined targets), which is communicated to the farmer for management action. In case the computer has access to the knowledge database (novel feed formulations), even the solution to the problem could also be communicated to the farmer (Maru 2004). The communication cycle also helps in impact evaluation of the management intervention implemented earlier.

The diversity of information and measurable data generated in a typical livestock farm has been depicted in Fig. 2. New data is generated daily which can be merged with archival data to understand the trends in health, production and reproduction. If the farm records can be computerised and analysed periodically, it would give enormous and valuable information and insight in the farm operations. For example, in a small hold cooperative set

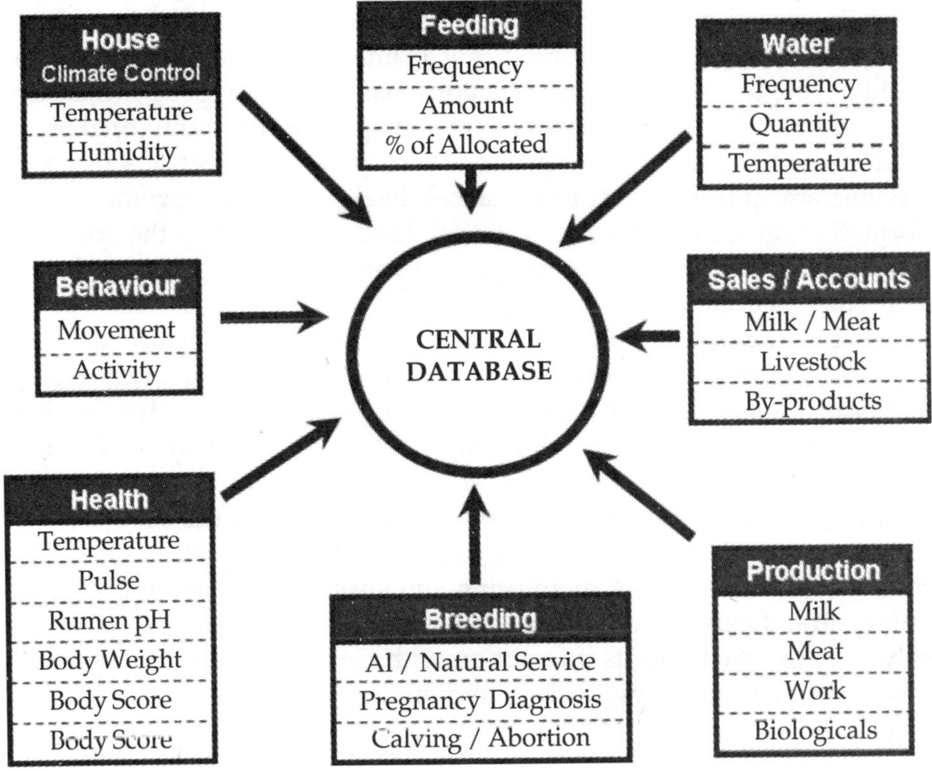

Fig. 2 : General scheme of data generated in a typical livestock farm

up, if the veterinary service provider has access to processed information on the animals in a village, especially animals due for oestrus and pregnancy check, this would improve health and husbandry services to the poor farmers. It is, therefore, evident that unless modern ICT tools are employed it would not be possible to handle and process volumes of information generated in herds/flocks of animals (Becchino *et al.* 2007). The ICT for Indian livestock sector is more critical for development since the units generating information and the end users expected to be communicated number in millions and are spread over wide, remote and at time unreachable areas. The ICT can surmount all these problems and the unreachable can be reached in a very cost effective way.

The application horizon of ICT in livestock sector is very wide. Few domain applications are discussed below to give an overview of how data network can be planned and executed.

5. ICT Application in Livestock E-Governance

Globally livestock rearing is tightly regulated by government (public) agencies as per international and national guidelines and regulations. It is an extremely crucial public function as it has enormous economic and public health implications. It is accepted that primarily the government agencies should devote to undertake core functions, namely: (a) to set up infrastructure to implement animal and product traceability programmes and (b) to organize system of collection of data on disease (especially infectious diseases of economic and public health importance), health, animal movement etc. The information can be maintained in central database owned by the government agencies, which is periodically analyzed to understand the trends and patterns and predict emerging problems in livestock. For controlling disease outbreaks, the most crucial issues include detecting the problem at an early stage, monitoring animal movements to understand the dimension of the outbreak, identifying the source of the infection and arriving at the site within the shortest possible time to reach out to all the high-risk farms of the area. To perform such functions the core requirements are: (a) system of voluntary but incentive-based registration and maintenance of database on all the premises where animals are kept (even in transit); (b) dynamic system of collection of disease occurrence data, including monitoring and surveillance data and its transfer to the central database in real time, and (c) software platform to enable spatial analysis of the data and its integration with Geographic Information System (GIS) to develop premises, disease, and epidemic maps.

Many developed countries employ elaborate ICT tools and systems to perform these functions (Henderson 1998). In North America and Europe, the concept of premises registration is now almost a decade old. Other countries like Australia, Argentina and Brazil have also launched premises registration and unique animal identification programmes more than one decade earlier. Under the guidance of the World Organization for Animal Health (OIE), many countries have created national animal health information system which enables access of animal health and disease information to global communities. Post-BSE (bovine spongiform encephalopathy) outbreak in Great Britain there has been public outcry that threatened the meat and dairy industry resulting in speeding up implementation of the project on unique animal identification and premises registration for better traceability. The developed countries have launched a collaborative programme on traceability, proactive testing for important diseases, surveillance and monitoring of important diseases by laboratory analysis and dynamic disease reporting system. The information is fed into centralized database which is interfaced with national animal health information system accessible under public domain. In Africa ICT has been employed for improving the market access to livestock farmers (Abidi 2004). With such an ICT network, these countries have been able to assess disease threats and are better prepared to mobilize resources in the event of disease outbreak. These developments have resulted in reaffirmation of public confidence in dairy and meat products. Since there is lot of international movement in livestock, it was necessary to develop guidelines to be followed across the globe for which 'International Committee on Animal Records (IntCAR)' was established in Italy. The Committee has the mandate to regulate standards of animal identification and data recording to provide unified information platform. India is also a member of this organization and the National Dairy Development Board (NDDB) is the designated national authority for this purpose. Unfortunately, NDDB did precious little to regulate such an important function, as a result, the health and breeding programmes implemented did not reap expected results and the per animal productivity of Indian livestock continues to be low.

6. Roadmap for Livestock E-Governance in India

In many developing countries, the government agencies continue to dominate and support breeding and veterinary services which are in fact 'economic activity' beyond the scope of the government. These activities should have been privatized long back. This has resulted in neglect of legitimate regulatory functions, surveillance, monitoring, testing and control of important infectious diseases, ante-mortem and postmortem checks at the slaughter points, extension services, execution of regulations and implementation of breeding policies for the state. Unlike the western countries, in India, where the state departments of animal husbandry provide diverse types of services to farmers, the ICT requirements for e-governance are much more elaborate. The use of ICT in animal health and productivity is still in very primitive stage in the country where few small pilot projects have been implemented to test the depth of water. In the year 2006, a project supported under National Agricultural Technology Programme (NATP) of the Indian Council of Agricultural Research was implemented to develop animal health information system based on weather data. This was in fact a disease forecasting programme and not a classical animal health (disease) information system. It failed to take off since the programme did not focus on improvising the disease reporting and weather forecasting system. Many state departments of animal husbandry have disease reporting system, which is neither scientific nor credible. Under the National e-Governance Plan 2006, several states attempted e-governance initiatives in the state departments of animal husbandry but these remained restricted to office automation, document traceability and internal communication system.

Department of Animal Husbandry in Maharashtra state envisioned the importance of ICT and as a first step appointed a 'Study Group' to explore the possibility of implementing information management system to support and improvise livestock operations. The Group in the leadership of the senior author of this chapter (Dr. Abdul Samad) submitted a comprehensive report to the government (available at www.mafsu.in) wherein the potential of ICT in animal health and productivity enhancement was described and an action plan was proposed. It was recommended that as a first step, the ICT initiatives of the department should be institutionalized for which establishment of a state-level authority consisting of animal science experts and IT professionals was recommended to regulate and undertake premises registration, unique animal identification and field data collection (for disease, health, breeding, production) and maintain state level animal health information system (Fig. 3). It was also envisaged that this authority would also maintain state level animal database and animal health information system.

The Government of Maharashtra accepted the proposal and notified the formation of the Maharashtra Animal Identification and Recording Authority (MAIRA; details available at http://www.mldb.in/new/mldb_maira.asp). To start with, MAIRA has been assigned three important functions: (a) voluntary premises registration in the state with special emphasis on incentives such as preference in preventive, breeding and other services, (b) encouragement and regulation of unique animal identification (UAID) in the state by assigning unique series and monitoring the distribution data, and (c) standardization and maintenance of state level animal database, especially by mandating software developers to select common database structure to ensure data interchangeability. MAIRA has developed detailed guidelines on premises registration and UAID in the state (Box 1).

Box 1 : Guidelines on premises registration & unique animal identification

Premises registration	**Unique animal identification**
Initially voluntary but should be made compulsory by legislation	Every animal to be identified with unique 15 digit number
Unique 13 digit PIN, issue PIN certificate and RFID card to farmers	The series to be obtained by the state or national authority
Village code, contact details of farmer, types of animals and type of operations	As per international standard RFID external tags to be encouraged, chip bearing tag to be applied on the left ear
Data stored with latitude and longitude data	Calf to be tagged within three weeks of birth
Premises maps for areas can be generated	Fall rate should not be more than 2%
	Insert devices should be avoided in ruminants

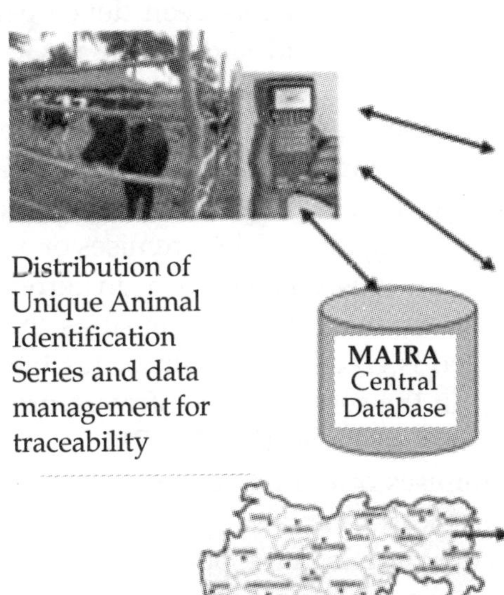

Premises registration and latitude and longitude data of the village, the farmer and contact details

The farmers' premises given 13 digit PIN number with RFID card

Farm data such as vaccination, deworming and notifiable disease incidence using RFID reader cum data recorder and GPRS data transfer

State or National Animal Health Information System for premises traceability and regional disease / health pattern.

Fig. 3 : Scheme for premises registration and animal identification for state-level animal health information system

In order to implement MAIRA programmes in the state, a custom software application *'Ahisam'* has been developed and deployed for the state by *Infovet* (www.infovet.in). The software facilitates on-line and offline premises registration using unique village code (allocated by the Election Commission of India) and the latitude and longitude information of the village provided in the database. The software integrates the premises and other data with GIS/GPS (Global Positioning System). The premises are registered as 13 digits Permanent Identification Number (PIN) and other relevant information about the premises such as type of animal/bird species reared, type of operation (*Goshala*, farm, livestock market etc.) is also collected and stored. The farmers registering their premises are issued a PIN certificate and a RFID card bearing the PIN number that can be affixed to the premises door.

The software can also be used to collect data on disease occurrence in animals, vaccination undertaken and disease testing which can be stored in the server. The most challenging part in such systems is collection of field data, transmission to data server and communication back to the stakeholders. In public-governed system, it is likely that the field staff transfer concocted data without visit to the farm if there is no proper monitoring. ICT tools can be used to develop a robust and secure system of data capture and transfer with in-built capability of monitoring. For the bovine frozen semen laboratories (BFSL) ICT network, an RFID reader cum recorder has been developed by *Senergy Intellution* (www.senergy.net.in). This handheld device is General Packet Radio Service (GPRS) enabled and has been named *'Sadat'* (Secured Animal Data Access Tool). It is simple to operate and cost effective compared to similar devices available abroad. The routine animal data such as vaccination in the premises, artificial insemination (AI) and calving can be entered in the device only when it is within the RFID reading range. The premises or animal identity is displayed and after entering, the new data can be transferred and saved in the central server using GPRS connectivity. This ensures that the information gathered and communicated is credible and timely (as the date and time of data transfer is imprinted in the server). The software program *'Ahisam'* has the facility of report integration with GIS/GPS platforms available commercially to generate premises or epidemic maps. This system helps in rapid access to the epidemic location and supplementary data to draw causal association conclusions. For example, if the point of the epidemic is a specific village, the program would generate list of all the premises of the species of animals within defined radius of the village. The names of the farmers and their contact details can also be generated for sending advisories in local language through Short Message Service (SMS) or Voice over Internet Protocol (VoiP)-based communication services. It is a unique and state-of-art ICT application suitable for developing countries for implementing animal disease control campaigns effectively. It is possible with this system to reach out to a large number of farmers who can be brought into the communication loop at a very marginal cost.

Apart from this, there is a vast network of veterinary hospitals and polyclinics where sick animals are brought for treatment in the country. It is necessary to network all the hospitals to transmit the disease data to the state server after validation by the administrator in order to develop dynamic health information system. A novel network-based software *VetChamp* has been developed *(Infovet)* to undertake this task. The unique feature of the system is that it is RFID compliant and the data can be stored in the web server. The owner of the animal can have access to the treatment history of the animal through internet or WAP (Wireless Application Protocol) and secondly, any veterinarian treating the animal can download the case paper from the web server. In addition, it has the facility of SMS messaging of appointments, vaccination and treatment reminders to owners. Implementing such a system would enhance preventive and curative compliance.

7. ICT for Breed Improvement Programmes

Modernization of livestock industry in developed countries was possible due to implementation of scientific and planned genetic improvement schemes to develop new breeds of animals. This activity has been privatized in western countries but tightly regulated by government agencies and farmers' organizations. Genetically superior bulls are officially permitted for breeding programme only after these are progeny tested, ranked and declared free from genetic and other diseases. During marketing phase too the bulls are monitored for performance by collecting health and performance data from selected daughters. The bulls' performance data is accessible to farmers, veterinarians, public officials and universities. Many breeding companies have set up transparent public domain system for farmers to access bull data online for considered selection.

The situation however is different in developing countries like India. Breed improvement efforts are mostly funded by the government or cooperative organizations. Such programmes comprise of: (a) rearing of breeding bulls for semen production, (b) distribution of semen straw, liquid nitrogen (LN_{2}) and other accessories, (c) maintenance of data of straw use and monitoring of bull fertility performance, and (d) young sire testing (progeny testing). These centers generate lot of data which if managed properly would enhance the implementation efficiency. Unlike western countries, the use of ICT in breeding programmes is still in infancy in the country. The progeny testing due to complexity of data acquisition has not been adopted by many state organizations. Few states initiated pilot efforts but failed since it was not backed by a foolproof data acquisition system employing ICT. Even the Government of India has not made marketing of progeny tested semen mandatory. The entire breeding programme is ad hoc and lacks accountability. The farmers do not have access to bull information; hence their involvement is passive. There is no designated official organization to conduct progeny testing programmes for the BFSL. Since these operations are under the control of government or cooperative, ICT for e-resource planning is the last priority area. These concerns have been raised in various fora by the scientific community but there is very little improvement in the situation. As a result, per animal productivity in Indian livestock continues to be extremely low.

Maharashtra state, however, has taken a lead recently. In line with the recommendation of the Study Group in its report, the Department of Animal Husbandry of the state decided to set up Information Management System for their BFSL. The ICT set up was designed and implemented as a turnkey project by the Bombay Veterinary College. To keep the cost low and to expedite implementation, it was decided to use the off-shelf software applications as the skeleton around which the network can be custom designed. Since *Semen^perfect^* and *Herdman* software developed by *Infovet* (www.infovet.in) were the only software developed for Indian livestock sector, it was decided to use these for building of the network. The basic concept here was that all the BFSL in the state should be networked so that data in the central server (local and web) could be stored and made accessible to administrators, AI officers, para-veterinarians and the farmers. The network is novel in many respects and specially conceived keeping the requirements of the small-hold livestock farming system in mind. It should be appreciated that implementing such systems is not difficult for a country like India which is a global leader in ICT.

8. ICT for Bovine Frozen Semen Laboratories

The general scheme of BFSL ICT network system is presented in Fig. 4. In Maharashtra, the targets set for the BFSL ICT were: (a) to create a central database of bulls and semen straw inventory for efficient and planned management, production and distribution, (b) set up online system for LN_2 and semen straw distribution within the state, (c) develop an online reporting system for AI and calving, (d) provide online access to administrators to access all BFSL data, and (e) implement field performance data collection of the daughters registered in progeny testing programmes. The unique feature of the system is that it is free from middle level hardware. The data is stored in the central server maintained by MAIRA; hence hardware related security and maintenance problems are minimized. The field officers can access the data authorized to them online using internet connectivity, similarly they can also upload monthly reports using the online reporting formats. The administrators can access data online and monitor the overall performance efficiency. The other unique feature is that the data collected in the village can be directly sent either by farmers or the veterinarians employing GPRS-enabled cell phone or 'Sadat'. It is envisaged that farmers having more than 50 animals can afford the cell phone device whereas the para-veterinarian would collect and transmit breeding data for small hold farmers.

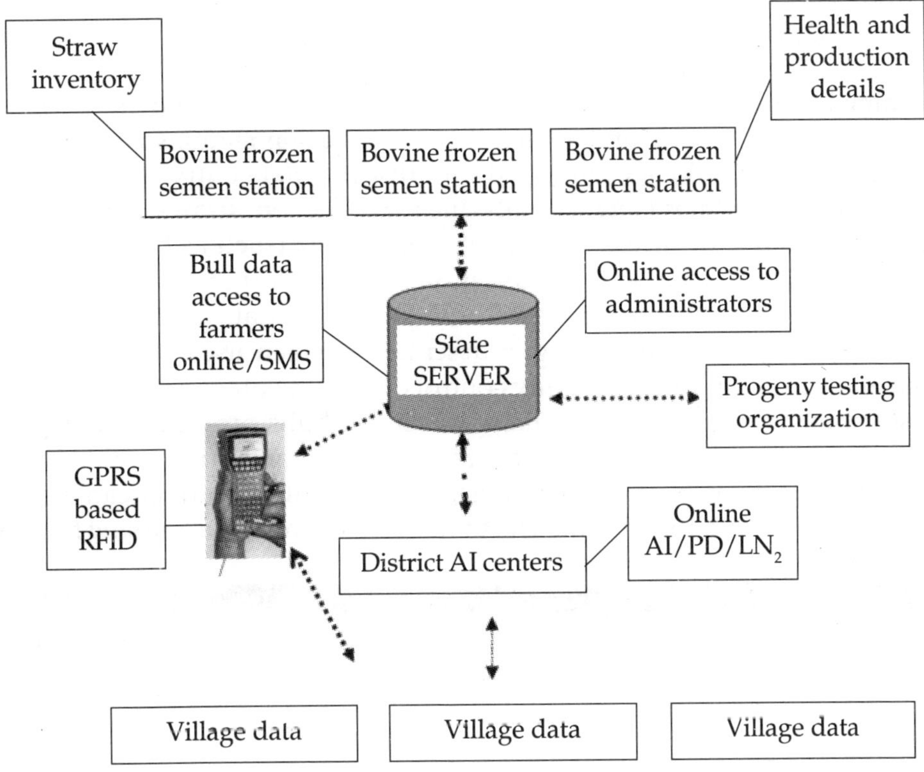

Fig. 4 : General scheme of BFSL ICT network system

For the purpose of credibility and security, it is important that the performance is recorded in digitized form at the point of generation (farm) instantly. Currently, many cell phones available in the market are GIS interactive in that when the image (data) is captured the location's longitude and latitude data is also imprinted which can be decoded using 'Flicker' platform. Using such devices it is possible to trace the place from where the data was captured and sent. The software deployed for BFSL networking has similar facilities. The second important factor to consider while implementing the breeding related ICT is that the data relevant to farmers must be accessible to them in processed form. The information management system network developed for BFSL has been provided with the facility of data access to farmers through internet or SMS or VoiP based systems. The BFSL ICT has three major modules: (a) e-management of bulls, (b) semen/LN_2 inventory management and (c) bull performance testing. The three modules are part of the ERP solution.

8.1 E-management of bulls in BFSL

In Maharashtra, the bull data management is done employing *Semen*[perfect] software *(Infovet)*. The bulls are registered with unique identification number and the lifetime health and semen production records of the bulls are maintained in individual animal files. All the operations from semen collection to quality control testing and semen/LN_2 distribution stations can be LAN (local area network)/Wi-Fi connected for error-free data entry. The program generates day schedules (such as bulls due for collection, straws due for post-thaw testing, bulls for disease testing etc.) and alerts (such as bulls with low motility, freezibility etc.). Various administrative and technical reports can be generated. There is also a facility of online entry of data pertaining to AI, pregnancy check and calving. Fig. 5 describes a screen used for storing the semen analysis, dilution and quality control data in the processing laboratory. The software is also RFID compliant and if the bulls are RFID ear tagged (which is highly recommended) and the collection arena is provided with fixed gate reader (or blue tooth reader), the bull collection data can also be captured directly into the system. The semen collection and processing formats

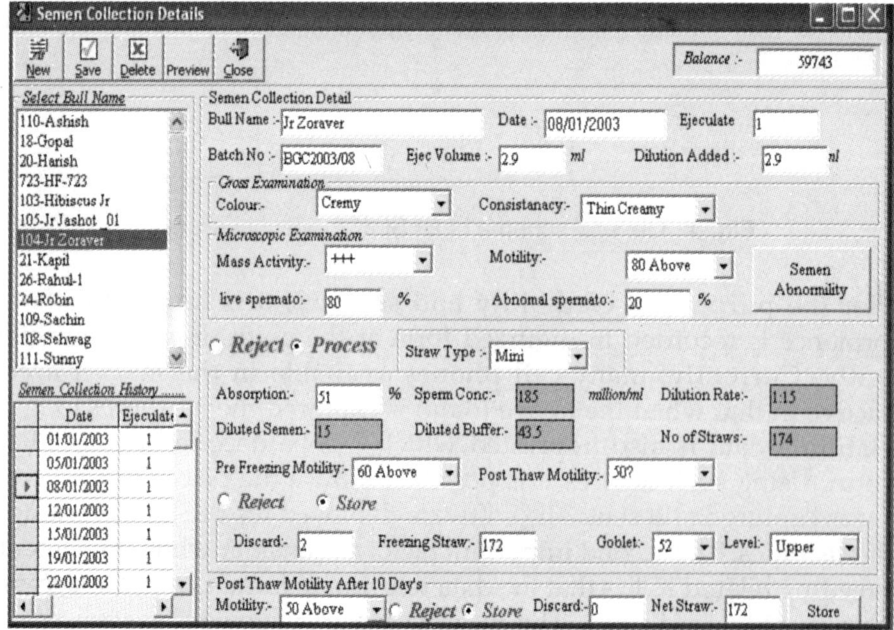

Fig. 5 : Semen processing data entry format in Semen[perfect]

are opened only after the bull is recorded in the RFID reader. This ensures that the semen processing data is real. Probably, this is the first elaborate livestock breeding ERP solution implemented in any state. A software for e-semen banking is also marketed in India by IMV, France but it is restricted only to e-networking of semen processing laboratory and has no modules for bull health, production, semen inventory and AI data management and does not support the network system.

8.2 Semen liquid nitrogen container management

In a large BFSL every year millions of semen straws are produced, stored and distributed. This is the most onerous operation because for locating desired batch of semen for distribution the operator is compelled to open the container and the goblets to verify the batch contents. This results in LN_2 loss and may also harm spermatozoa. A simple solution to the problem is the virtual container inventory. The precondition to set up this system is that all the containers used for semen storage should be unique coded and registered in the database. MAIRA has taken a decision to identify and label all the containers used in the state by allotting a unique identification code. The goblets in each container are also labeled with unique number and identified with a distinct color. The information for each container is stored in the central database. This enables the program to generate virtual container inventory. A sample virtual container is shown in Fig. 6. The small circles with different colors and numbers depict the goblets. The inventory in each goblet can be found out by taking the cursor to the goblet and clicking it. It would identify the bull name, batch number of semen and the number of straws in the goblet on the screen (at different levels). Thus without opening the container the operator can get information about the goblet contents. Many a times, the clients may demand semen of a particular bull or batch, or the operator may wish to dispose semen of earlier years. In this case, searching the container for predefined criteria becomes necessary. The software provides search facility. The search screen for container is shown in Fig. 6. The right hand panel is for entering the search criteria. For example, if the client wants semen of a particular bull, its name can be entered, whereas if the operator wants to locate semen of this bull from a particular year, he can enter the year in the appropriate box. If all the criteria are to be considered for search, the operator has to select 'Both'. The numbers on the right top panel indicate the container codes wherein particular semen straws are stored. The operator can select a container by clicking over it which would show the details of the container goblets where the selected bull's or batch of the semen straws are stored. This is a unique feature of the software which makes the work of semen distribution very convenient and prevents damage to semen due to unnecessary handling.

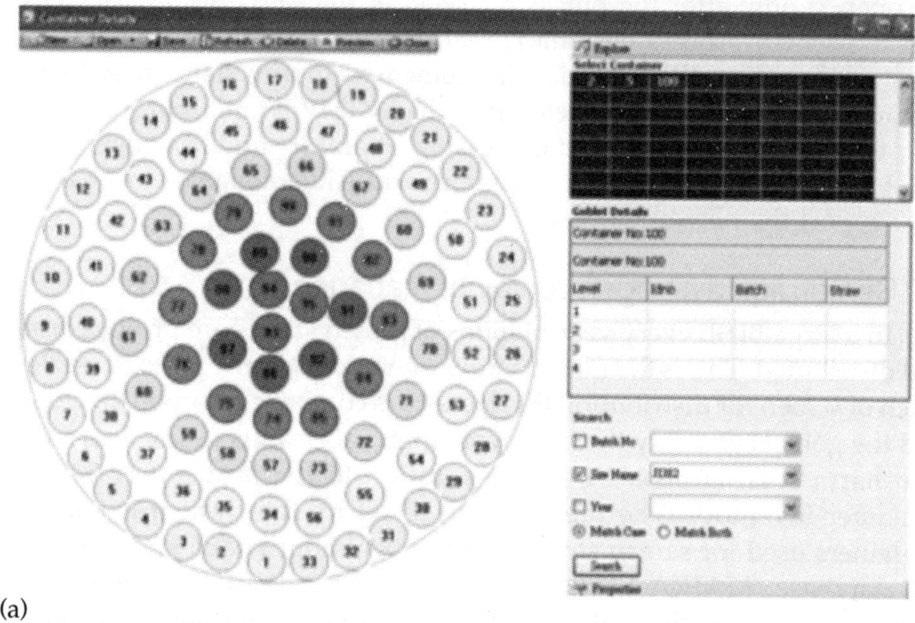

(a)

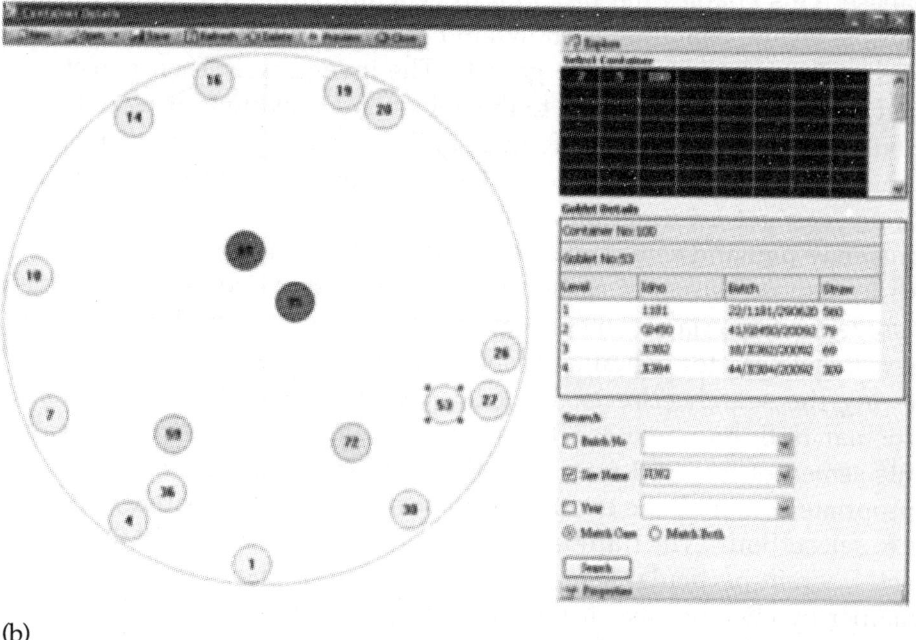

(b)

Fig. 6 : Virtual semen container inventory showing (a) Search facility for straw location (b) Post-search inventory

In order to administer and monitor semen distribution in the state beyond the districts and block levels the program provides the facility of online report submission and monitoring by the district administration officers. The administrator needs to log onto the official website (www.mldb.in) for access to web-based server. By using the authorized user name and the password, the officer can access online AI data entry form. Secondly, the officers can also access and generate species or bull-wise production and distribution reports for a desired day, month or year. Fig. 7 depicts a screen of the online report for the month of April 2010. Similarly, the administrator can also generate report to monitor distribution pattern of semen of each bull to various areas (center-wise). The program also provides facility for accessing performance and technical reports of each BFSL online.

CENTER	SELECT REPORT TYPE:	SELECT MONTH, YEAR:	
Aurangabad Nagpur ☑ Pune	Bull wise	April 2010	GO

Bull Wise Stock Reports

SEMEN JOURNAL FOR DEEP FREEZING , Pune

Bull Name	Opening Volume	Production Doses	Received From Other Institutes	Total Doses	Supplied	Wastage/ Testing	Total Disposed	Closing Balance
305	5169		9000	9000	4500		4500	9669
325								
335	3750				3000		3000	750
341	1250		6000	6000				7250
343	3415		6000	6000	3000		3000	6415
345	1500		3000	3000				4500
347	2250		3000	3000	1500		1500	3750
397	2257		4514	4514				6771
3078								

Fig. 7 : Online report for administrator providing details of bull-wise semen production and distribution in a selected month

There is also provision to deploy the information of each bull and its performance summary (official) online so that the farmer can select the bull's identity and name and get an insight about the bull. With the online data access facility the state-level administrators will be able to monitor the production efficiency of the semen banks in the state.

8.3 ICT for liquid nitrogen level alerts

Maintaining the level of LN_2 in the containers (storage, transport or the one with AI workers) is critical requirement to store semen in good quality. A variety of LN_2 containers are available in the market and each has different capacity and evaporation rate. The user has to refill the container once the level of LN_2 goes down to a critical level. In general, the AI workers know the frequency of refilling but the problem is that they have to depend on their memory, which sometimes may fail. In such cases, the stored semen quality is severely compromised and the use of such semen would adversely affect the fertility, resulting in economic losses to farmers. This problem can be solved by employing the power of ICT. Under the MAIRA all LN_2 containers are given unique identification code and a database of the evaporation rates for different types of containers is provided in Semen*perfect*. In order to generate auto-alerts for each container, the threshold level is to be defined by the administrator which would depend on the transport time for refilling. Since refilling of the LN_2 of the field AI staff is done at the block or district level, the network provides facility of online LN_2 distribution data entry. The operator at the distribution point connects to the internet and opens the online format. This updates the data on the server in real time. In case there is no internet connectivity, the server can be updated by the user by sending SMS message to a dedicated number (interfaced with the server) specifying the container code, and quantity refilled. This updates the server data. Once the level in a container reaches the predefined threshold, an alert is generated on the computer and simultaneously SMS message is also sent to the cell phone of the AI worker. With this facility the semen quality supplied at the doorstep of the farmers can be ensured, enhancing their productivity.

8.4 Progeny testing (PT) module

The availability of superior genetic bulls is the backbone of the productivity enhancement and breed improvement programmes. Since bulls do not produce milk, production capability is estimated indirectly by evaluating their daughters' health and production performance. This is an elaborate and long drawn exercise wherein first suitable dams in diverse locations (to minimize effect of environment and management) are to be identified. These dams are tagged and registered and bred by AI using semen of the young sire under testing. The newborn daughters are then registered and identified and when in milk, the milk records are collected periodically and a sample of milk is also tested in an accredited laboratory for composition (fat, protein and total solids). The data is then imported in the PT software which calculates the genetic value of the bull and a ranking is provided. The PT is a typical example of complex process of data acquisition over a long period and analysis. However this process can be simplified by employing ICT tools. The critical requirements for this task are: (a) the database platform of BFSL and field data collection of dams and daughters should be compatible for integration so that there is no need to reenter the animal's data, (b) since very few bulls based on their performance would be officially ranked and used for breeding and producing lakhs of progeny in lifetime, the credibility of the collected data is important, and (c) the data requires high security as the bulls selected would be of high value. In order to meet these critical requirements, it has been decided in Maharashtra to ear tag all the dams (preferably RFID) and to register their data in *Herdman* software. The participating farmers receive management advisories for these animals through auto generated SMS. The daughters born to these sires would be compulsorily double ear tagged; visual plastic ear tag on right ear and RFID bearing ear tag on left ear. The health and production records (of the first lactation) of these animals would be collected and stored in the central data server.

The most critical and expensive part of the program is periodic data collection from registered animals and transferring the data securely to the central server. In order to provide advisory services to the farmers, it is essential that the data is collected and updated on the server in real time. In western countries, there is an independent performance recording organization, whose job is to collect and transfer data to the computer. This makes the performance data acquisition very expensive. For a country like India, where the farms are small hold and scattered, such a proposition would be even more expensive. However, a cost effective system has been developed wherein the service providers also collect and transfer the data by using GPRS-enabled RFID reader-cum-data recorder 'Sadat' Fig. 8 describes the network scheme for PT implemented in Maharashtra.

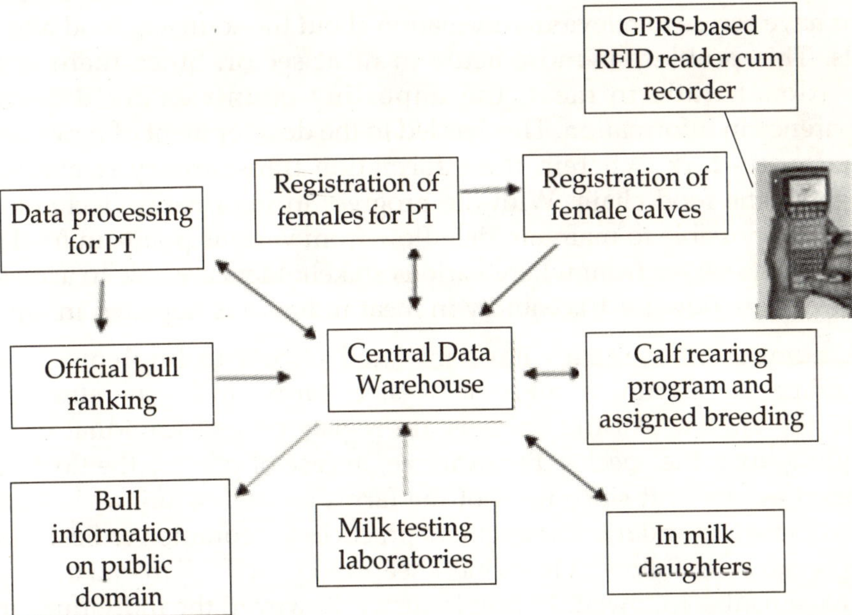

Fig. 8 : ICT network for progeny testing programme implementation in a bovine semen bank

The data can be exported to the PT software for analysis and once the sire is evaluated and officially ranked, the data would be transferred to the MAIRA database which will be accessible to the farmers through internet or cell phone. In India, the AI coverage is only 20-25% in case of cows whereas in buffaloes it is still lower. Farmers use either own or village bulls for the purpose of natural service. The Government of Maharashtra has launched a scheme of registration of the bulls used for natural service. The premises where bull is kept and the bull (with its details) are registered either online or offline. These bulls are then tested for genetic disorder, important infections like brucellosis, TB, JD etc. at the government cost at accredited laboratories and the semen is evaluated. The owner of the bull is provided with a certificate of registration and health card for the bull. The participating owners get incentive for periodic screening of the bulls for diseases. If the bull is found to carry genetic disorder or infection, the owner is encouraged not to use the bull for breeding purpose. The data of these bulls can be stored in MAIRA database and the information is made available to the farmers. A simple system of data access to farmers has been developed. The farmer is required to send a SMS message giving the identity number of the bull to a dedicated mobile phone number and in return the farmer receives details of the selected bull.

9. ICT for Traceability in Meat Industry

Globally consumers have become more concerned with the food quality especially in the context of health implications. There is demand that consumers should have access to relevant information about the source of food and other details. This problem is more acute in meat sector. Since there is lot of international trade in meat, the importing countries are demanding transparency in information. This has led to the development of new concepts like 'farm- to- fork' wherein the information transparency is maintained throughout the food chain. With the progress in information technology, it has become possible to maintain data flow from various points in food chain to central data server from where various stakeholders are able to access it. A scheme of data flow for traceability in meat industry is depicted in Fig. 9.

A number of countries have initiated efforts to implement such a programme. The starting point is the livestock farm which generates the basic data of the animal. All the animals are registered as individual or group depending upon the species. For example, in case of poultry the flock can be registered as one unit since most of the farms are following 'all in - all out' system of farming and the management practices are common to flock. Similar concepts can be so followed in swine, sheep and goat if 'all in - all out' system of management is followed. In beef industry, however, the individual animal is required to be registered. In sheep and goat now a days individual animal is registered and identified in many countries for easy management. In case individual animals are identified these should be tagged/inserted with RFID device. Dedicated handheld device that are RFID reader-cum-data recorder are supplied by the farmers' organizations in western countries. Such a handheld device is now available commercially under the name *'Sadat'* (*Senergy Intellution,* Mumbai) in India.

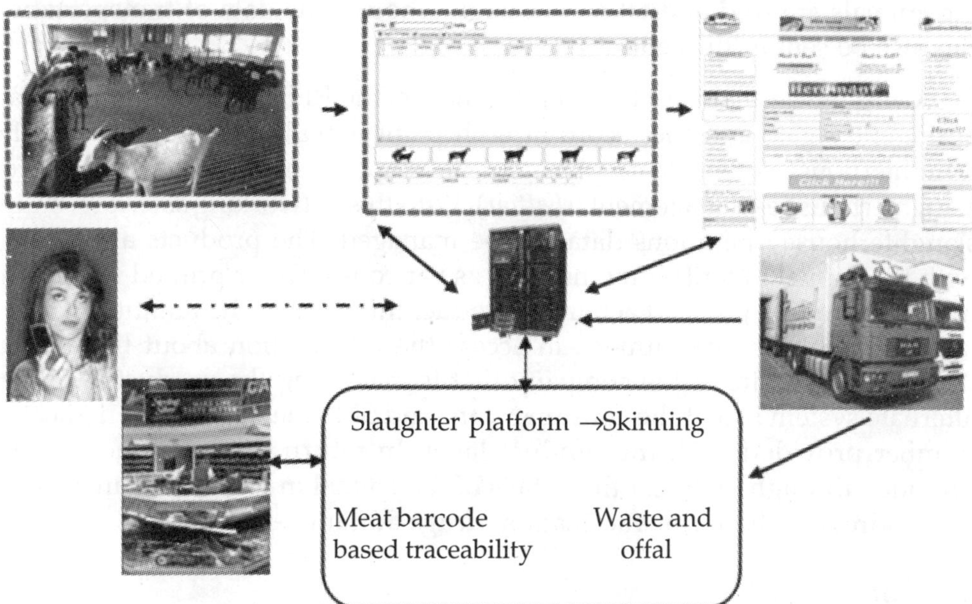

Fig. 9 : Scheme of data flow for traceability in meat sector

The data from the farm can be directly recorded in the central data server. Whenever the stock is ready for market, the farmers pass on the information to the concerned agency. Since such an agency is not available in India, the marketing is generally done either by direct contact with the butchers or through agents. In many cases the animals are taken to the nearest market and sold. This creates lot of problem for the farmers in that they have to transport the animals to the market where many a times sick animals are also brought. The facilities at the livestock markets are scanty. Once the animal is brought to the market, it is cornered by the cartel of agents. The present day livestock marketing in the country is mostly dictated by the agents who in fact make big profits at the cost of farmers. The buyers also face problems as they have to go to market and there is no other way to know what kinds of animals are available. Thus it becomes a difficult exercise if the buyer has to hop around to different locations and markets for purchase of animals. *Infovet* has attempted to address this problem by starting a web livestock market under the name *www.pashubazar.com* . The farmers through their veterinarian franchisee can upload the animals' information on the website. In case the animal is registered in *'Herdman'* or *'Flockman'* the performance records are uploaded on the site. The buyers can access the information either through WAP-enabled cell phone or internet for which they can also take help of the veterinarian franchisee. The farmers can put hold on the animals which sends SMS message to the cell phone of the selling farmer. With this facility the farmers can sell or buy livestock and related services on the website. When the animals are sold and taken to slaughterhouse, the data of transportation can also be sent to the central server.

Once the animal is in the slaughterhouse, the RFID of the animal is read at the entry gate and the record at each point is built up and stored in the slaughterhouse server. *Infovet* has also developed a networking solution for slaughterhouse e-management (*ebattoir*). With this networking software, entire slaughterhouse operations data can be managed. The products are labeled with the animal identification number as bar code or laser printed number at different product points. Each meat product thus carries the identity number of the animal. The consumer can access the information about the animal though the website of the company that is marketing the product. Another alternate system is that the consumer can send SMS message to the dedicated number provided with the product label. In return the consumer can be provided through SMS text the details of the animal in terms of source, name and address of the farm, vaccination, drugs administered etc.

10. Conclusion

Livestock farming and management is an information-intensive activity that generates large volume of data. Every animal in its lifetime generates huge physiological, production, breeding and movement data which if properly captured, stored and analyzed could be used for better planning and productivity improvement. Although in western world computerization of the livestock management data is ubiquitous, there are inherent constraints to deploy these applications in developing countries. Despite being a global leader in ICT development, India is yet to use the ICT in livestock sector. It is, therefore, necessary that appropriate software and hardware applications are developed for small-hold livestock production system considering the remoteness of the areas and unavailability of uninterrupted communication systems.

From the above description, it can be appreciated that deployment of ICT offers numerous opportunities to understand and improve livestock health and breeding programmes. The systems are very cost effective and hassle-free as the network can be managed from a single center only. The investment by the state in this core infrastructure would certainly bring about transformation of the livestock sector in the country.

References

1. Abidi A, Stuth J, Kaitho E, Ali A, Karinki G (2004). The application of emerging ICT in livestock marketing in rural areas of Eastern Africa. http://www.ictes2004-gstit.edu.et/ session%20VI_fullpapers/
2. Andonovic I, Micheie C, Gilory M, Goh HG, Kwong KH, Sasloglou K, Wu T (2009). Wireless sensor networks for cattle health monitoring. In: Daveceu D, Gomez JM (eds) ICT Innovations, Springer, UK.
3. Anonymous (2010). World Summit of the Information Society. http://www.itu.int/ wsis/c7/e-agriculture/index.html
4. Becchino W, Ciccavelli L, Kenny J (2007). Reinventing the enterprise with communication enabled applications. Nortel Technical J 5:33-42.
5. Desai AV (2006). Information and other technology developments. In: Stanley Wolpert (ed) Encyclopedia of India (vol 2), p. 269-273.
6. Henderson CW (1998). Electronic identification and records programme offers producer, consumer benefits, but poses challenges in cost and practicality. Natl Livestock Producers Assn News Release, July 12, http://www.nlpa.org/AnID.htm, May 2, 2000.
7. Maru A (2004). Potential contributions from use of new information and communication technologies (ICT) for livestock production and services in India. http://www.indiaveterinarycommunity.com/
8. Naas IA (2002). Application of mechanotronics to animal production. CIGR J Scientific Res Dev 4:1-14.
9. Parikh A, Belani K, Patel K (2010). ICT based cattle heat period, insemination and fertility management model. Fourth UKSim European Symposium on Computer Modelling and Simulation Society, Los Alamitos, CA, USA, Pisa, Italy, 218-222 http://doi.ieeecomputersociety.org/10.1109/EMS.2010.43, IEEE Computer.
10. Ramkumar S, Garfroth C, Rao SVN, Heffeman C (2007). Design and formative evaluation of an information kiosk on cattle health for landless cattle owners. J Agric Edn Extn 13:7-22.
11. Samad A, Murdeshwar P, Hameed Z (2010). High-credibility RFID-based animal data recording system suitable for small-holding rural dairy farmers. Computers and Electronics in Agriculture 73:213-218.
12. Swedberg C (2010). Chitale dairy uses RFID to improve milk yields http:// www.rfidjournal.com/article/view/7621.

□□□

Chapter 22

Bioinformatics : A Modern Tool in Livestock Health and Production

M. L. SANGWAN
Department of Animal Biotechnology, College of Veterinary Sciences, Lala Lajpat Rai University of Veterinary and Animal Sciences, Hisar-125004

Contents

1. Introduction

Bioinformatics is an integration of statistics, computer science and biology to manage and analyse biological information. It is acquisition, storage, management, accessing, and processing of molecular biological data. It is indispensable for almost every aspect of data management in molecular biology. As the amount of data grows exponentially, there is a parallel growth in the demand for tools and methods in data management, visualization, integration, analysis, modeling and predication. Bioinformatics has become an emerging field and has wide application in medicine, biotechnology, agriculture and veterinary sciences. Bioinformatics constitutes an integral component of research in genomics, proteomics, pharmacogenomics, cheminformatics, immunoinformatics, neuroinformatics, medical informatics, veterinary informatics, computation biology, and system biology. For example, molecular biology faces a great challenge in analysing the large volume of data generated by the genome sequencing projects. Bioinformatics will revolutionize molecular biology research by organizing the data in a manner that it can be easily accessed. Similarly, bioinformatics helps in revolutionizing drug development and gene therapy and to understand toxic responses and to predict toxicity. It also helps in the identification of useful genes leading to the development of new gene products, contributing greatly in genomics and proteomics research and in analyzing the patterns of gene expression.

From 1950 onwards, large amounts of sequence data of different living organisms have been stored in databases. Several computational techniques were developed to analyse several hundred sequences. The field of bioinformatics emerged in the early 1980s with the creation of the GenBank database. The advent of the Internet allowed researchers to access data in different databases freely. Due to the development of automatic DNA sequencing tools, sequence data in GenBank is growing exponentially. Establishment of the European Molecular Biology Network (EMBnet) and the United States National Center for Biotechnology Information (NCBI) were two major developments in bioinformatics.

2. Databases

Large numbers of databases are used to store and manage different types of data. Some major databases are described below.

2.1 NCBI (National Center for Biotechnology Information)

Established in 1988 as a national resource for molecular biology information, NCBI creates public databases, conducts research in computational biology, develops software tools for analyzing genome data, and disseminates biomedical information for better understanding of molecular processes affecting development, production and reproduction in animals and human health and disease (Fig. 1). The NCBI houses genome sequencing data in GenBank and an index of biomedical research articles in PubMed Central and PubMed, as well as other information relevant to biotechnology. All these databases are available online through the Entrez search engine.

2.2 GenBank (Genetic Sequence Databank)

GenBank operated by NCBI is one of the fastest growing repositories of genetic sequences. Most complete collection of annotated nucleic acid sequence data for almost every organism. Its content includes gDNA, mRNA, cDNA, ESTs, high throughput raw sequences data and sequence polymorphism. The sequences can be searched by two ways, viz., i. text based keywords similar to a PubMed search and ii. using sequences to search by sequence similarity with BLAST. EMBL (European Molecular Biology Laboratory) and DDBJ (DNA Data Bank of Japan) also contain same DNA sequence content as GenBank which are updated every 24 hour.

2.3 Online Mendelian Inheritance in Man (OMIM)

Another unique database accessible from Entrez is OMIM. It is a comprehensive, authoritative and timely knowledgebase of human genes and genetic disorders so as to support research and education in genomics and the practice of clinical genetics. Each OMIM (www.ncbi.nlm.nih.gov/omim) entry has a full-text summary of a genetically determined phenotype and/or gene and has a number of links to other databases like DNA and protein sequence, PubMed references, general and locus-specific mutation databases, and the highly detailed mapviewer, as well as patient support groups. It is an easy and straightforward portal to the burgeoning information in human genetics (Hamosh *et al.* 2002). It is excellent starting point to study genes related to a disease. Directly detailing SNPs and mutations, it allows the user to quickly link to the relevant dbSNP entry for the gene of interest (Xiong 2005).

2.4 Online Mendelian Inheritance in Animals (OMIA)

It is an online database of genes, inherited disorders and traits in more than 206 animal species. It is modeled on, and is complimentary to OMIM. It aims to provide a publicly accessible catalogue of all animal genes, excluding those in human and mouse, for which species specific resources are already available. The database contains textual information and references as well as links to relevant PubMed and Gene records at the NCBI (http://en.wikipedia.org/wiki/Online_Mendelian_Inheritance_in_Animals). It is a source of information on known diseases in animals which are related to human diseases. It provides first step on animal diseases with links to potential human homologs.

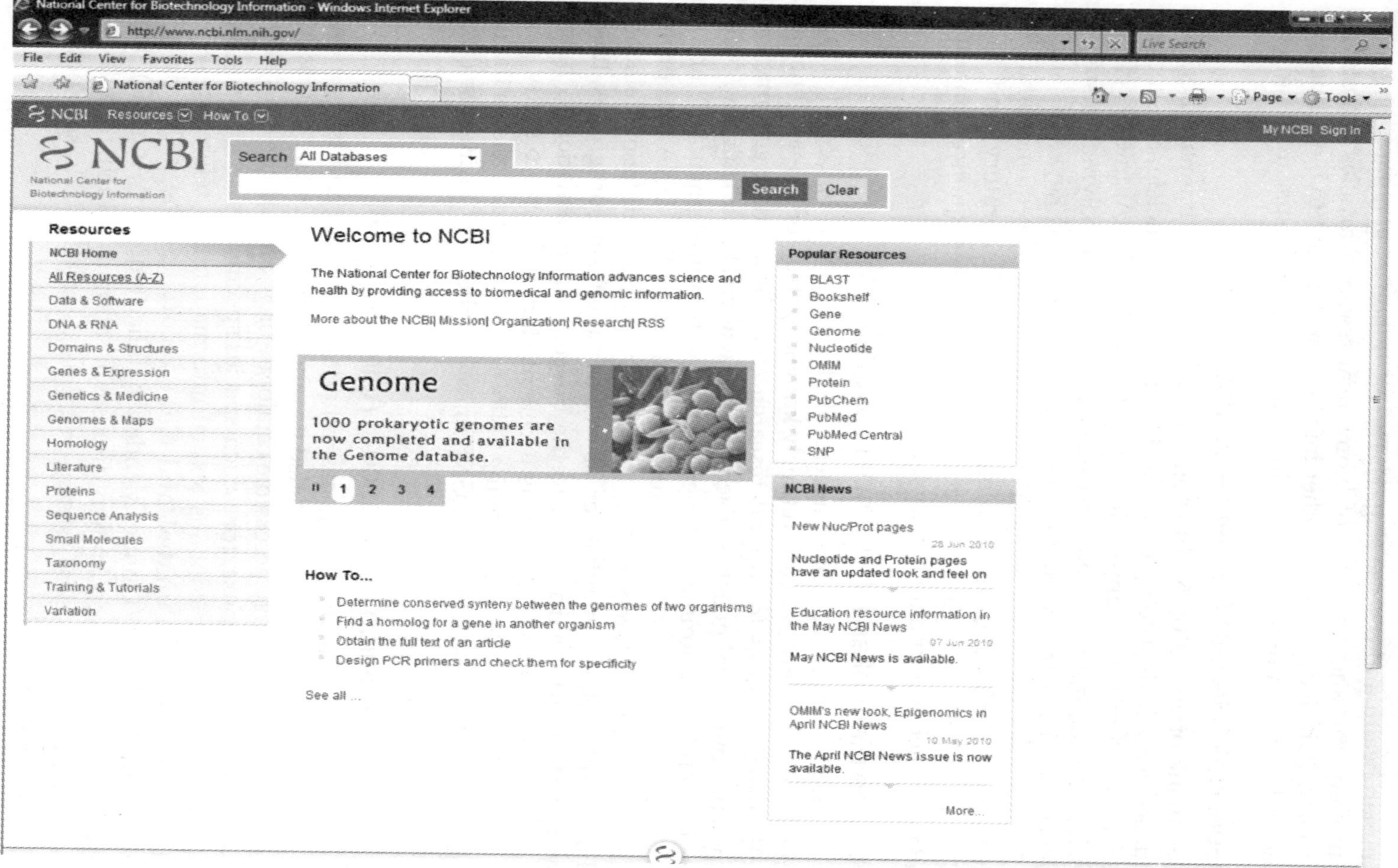

Fig. 1 : NCBI Home page (http://www.ncbi.nlm.nih.gov/)

2.5 Single nucleotide polymorphism (SNP) databases

SNPs are the common DNA sequence variations in the genome. SNP discovery programme has resulted in the submission of over 10,000,000 human SNPs to the NCBI dbSNP. SNPs are a valuable resource for investigating the genetic basis of disease, drug response and impact growth, reproduction and production. They can serve as markers for fine-scale mapping and genome-wide association studies. Genetic traits may predispose individuals to illnesses such as diabetes, hypertension, cancer, or affect disease progression. Hence their identification will play a great role in improving various traits as well as predicting health status and drug response. Bioinformatics is used to annotate genes that contain SNPs and allow researchers to retrieve data about SNPs based on gene of interest, genetic or physical map location, or expression pattern (Clifford *et al.* 2006). Genome-wide panels of SNPs have recently been used in domestic animal species to map and identify genes for many traits and to select genetically desirable livestock. However, the genetic merit of animals can still be estimated by genomic selection, which uses genome-wide SNP panels as markers. This approach is expected to double the rate of genetic improvement per year in many livestock systems (Goddard and Hayes 2009).

2.6 Immunologic databases and websites

These databases provide focused, detailed and updated information about genes relevant to the immune response. The Kabat Database of sequences of proteins of immunological interest (http://immuno.bme.nwu.edu/) contains sequences that are classified according to antigen specificity. The Immunogenetics database (IMGT) focuses on Igs, T-cell receptors, and major histocompatibility complex molecules (Kaminsky 2000).

2.7 PubMed

It is the U.S. National Library of Medicine's premiere search system for health information. Available free on the internet (http://pubmed.gov), it provides access to MEDLINE database of citations, abstracts and some full text articles on life sciences and biomedical topics. It is a biomedical literature database, which contains abstracts and full text articles from nearly 4,000 journals. PubMed provides retrieval of information based on medical subject headings (MeSH) terms.

3. Bioinformatics Tools

There exist a number of bioinformatics tools which help in extraction of meaningful information from the biological data. Some commonly used tools are mentioned below.

3.1 Entrez

It is a search and retrieval tool developed by NCBI that is capable of searching multiple NCBI databases including annotated genetic sequences information, structural information, citations abstracts, full papers and taxonomics data. The key feature of Entrez is its liability to integrate information, which comes from cross-referencing between NCBI databases based on preexisting and logical relationship between individual entries. It is highly convenient tool as users do not have to visit multiple databases. Entrez searches large number of databases listed below (Fig. 2).

- Books: online books
- Gene: gene-centered information
- Genome: whole genome sequences and mapping
- Nucleotide: sequence database (GenBank)
- OMIA: Online Mendelian Inheritance in Animals
- OMIM: Online Mendelian Inheritance in Man
- Protein: sequence database
- PubMed: biomedical literature citations and abstracts, including Medline
- SNP: single nucleotide polymorphism
- Structure: three-dimensional macromolecular structures
- Taxonomy: organisms in GenBank taxonomy

3.2 BLAST

The most commonly used programme for sequence alignment is Basic Local Alignment Search Tool (BLAST). This tool (http://www.ncbi.nlm.nih.gov/BLAST) allows researchers to identify similarities between their own nucleotide or protein sequence with those in the public databases (Fig. 3). It allows to identify whether a given sequence is new or similar to a known sequence already available in public databases. There are various forms of BLAST like BLASTn, BLASTp, BLASTx, tBLASTn, tBLASTx megaBLAST, phi-BLAST, psi-BLAST, and IgBLAST. IgBLAST is a tool developed at NCBI to facilitate analysis of immunoglobulin (Ig) sequences in GenBank.

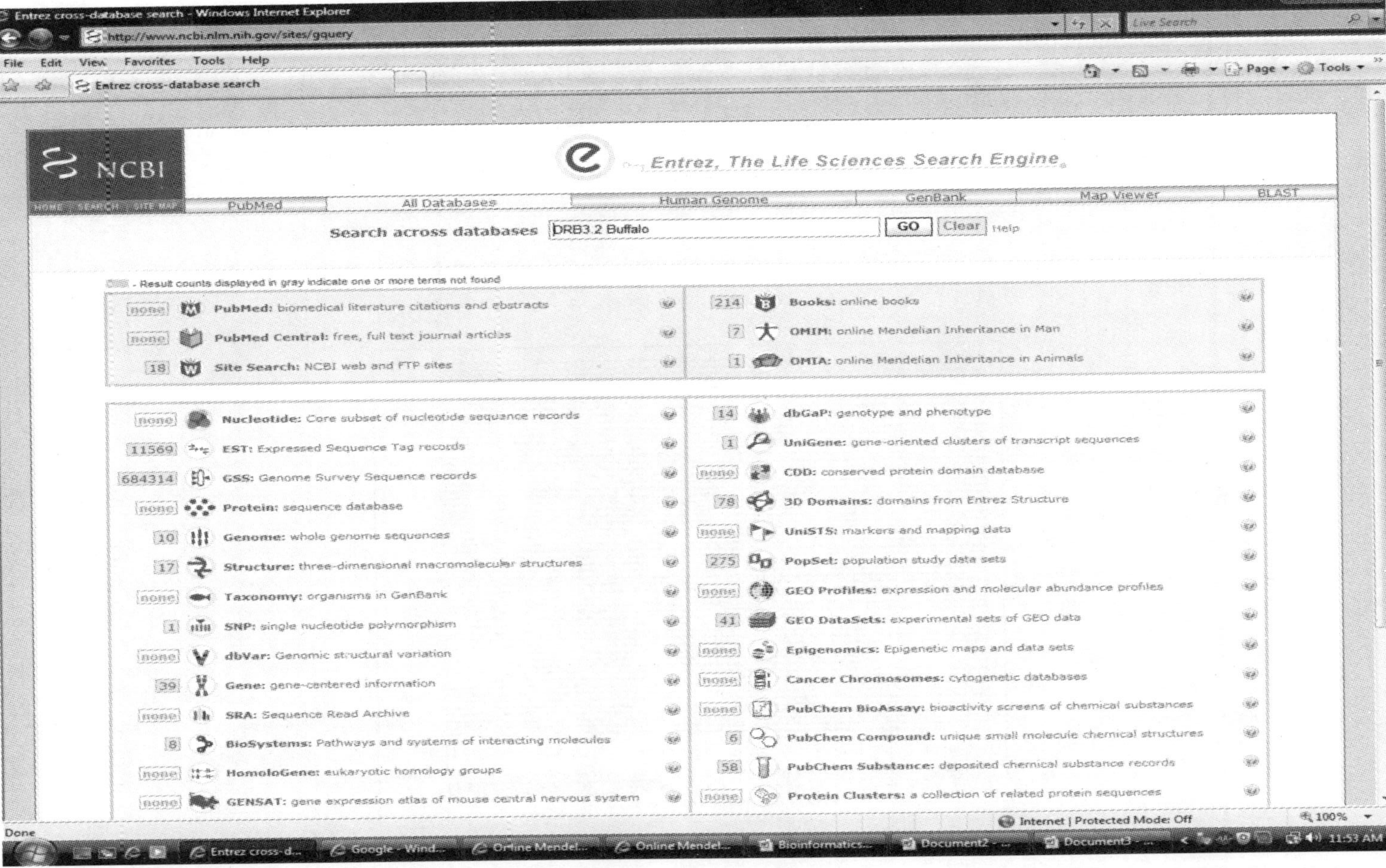

Fig. 2 : Entrez search engine (http://www.ncbi.nlm.nih.gov/sites/gquery)

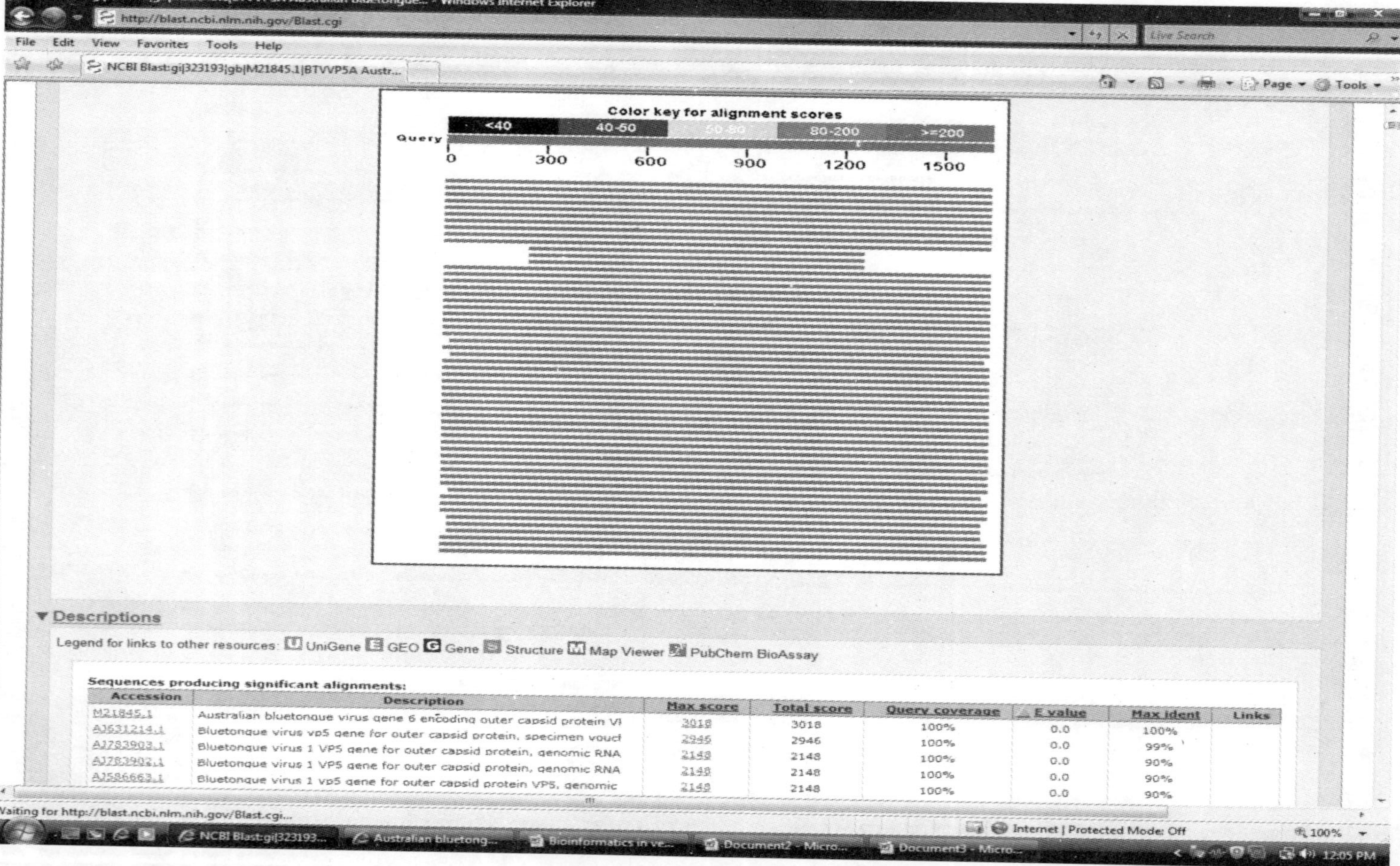

Fig. 3 : NCBI BLAST (http://blast.ncbi.nlm.nih.gov/Blast.cgi)

3.3 Genome browsers

Browsers have been developed to provide easy access to millions of sequences. Most commonly used browsers are the Entrez genome browser, UCSC genome browser and the EBI/ Ensembl browser. Entrez browser provides graphical overviews of complete genomes/chromosomes and the ability to explore regions of interest in detail. The genome browsers provide essential genomic data, such as genomic sequence, exon structure, mRNA sequence, and EST or SNP data, through simple web based text search interfaces.

3.4 Map Viewer

It is a tool that allows for visualization of an organism's complete genome, integrated maps for each chromosome, and sequence data for a genomic region of interest (www.ncbi.nlm.nih.gov/mapview/). The data are presented graphically, displaying available sequence data, cytogenetic, genetic, physical, and radiation hybrid maps (Ricketts 2009). When using Map Viewer, a researcher has the option of selecting either a "Whole-Genome View" or a "Chromosome or Map View". The Genome View displays a schematic for all of an organism's chromosomes, whereas the Map View shows one or more detailed maps for a single chromosome (Fig. 4).

3.5 Primer designing

It is the most critical parameter to obtain desired PCR product. It is a powerful and simple, real-time interface to allow rapid identification of ideal primers for PCR reactions. Primer pairs are designed for a set target region in the genome. It shows all the possible pairs of forward and reverse primers that conform to the set parameters for the specified target regions. The *in silico* screening process makes it possible to quickly narrow down the list of potential primers, and select the one that best suits the needs. Poorly designed primers can lead to little or no product. The example of primer3 is shown in Fig. 5.

3.6 NEBcutter

This programme (http://tools.neb.com/NEBcutter) accepts an input DNA sequence and produces a comprehensive report of the restriction enzymes that will cleave the sequence at specific site (Fig. 6). It produces a variety of outputs including restriction enzyme maps, theoretical digests and links into the restriction enzyme database, REBASE (http://www.neb.com/rebase). The table of recognition sites is updated daily from REBASE and it marks all sites that are affected by DNA methylation (Dam, Dcm etc.). Various options exist to choose the enzymes used for digestion, including sets of enzymes that produce compatible termini (Vincze *et al.* 2003).

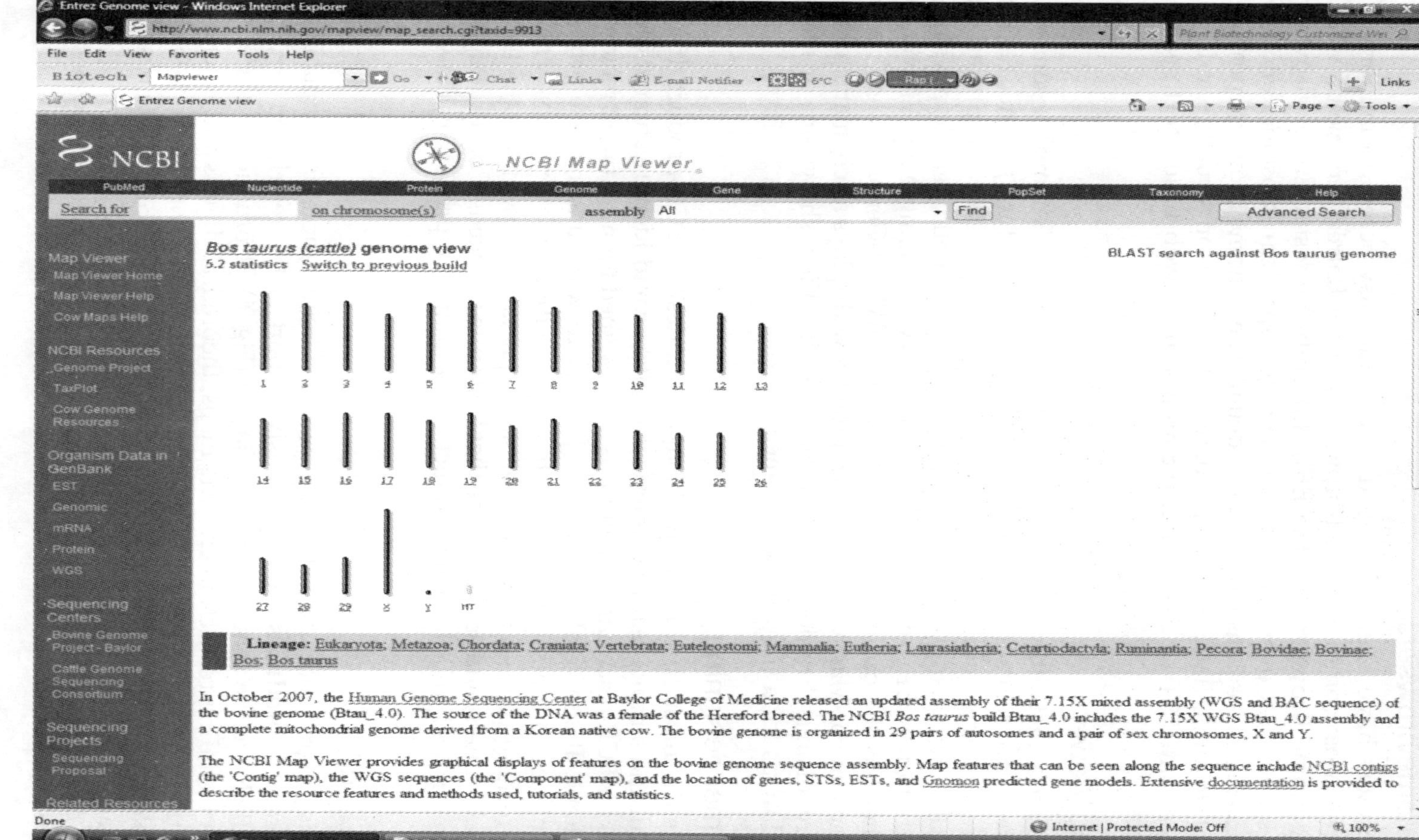

Fig. 4 : NCBI MapViewer (genome view of cattle)

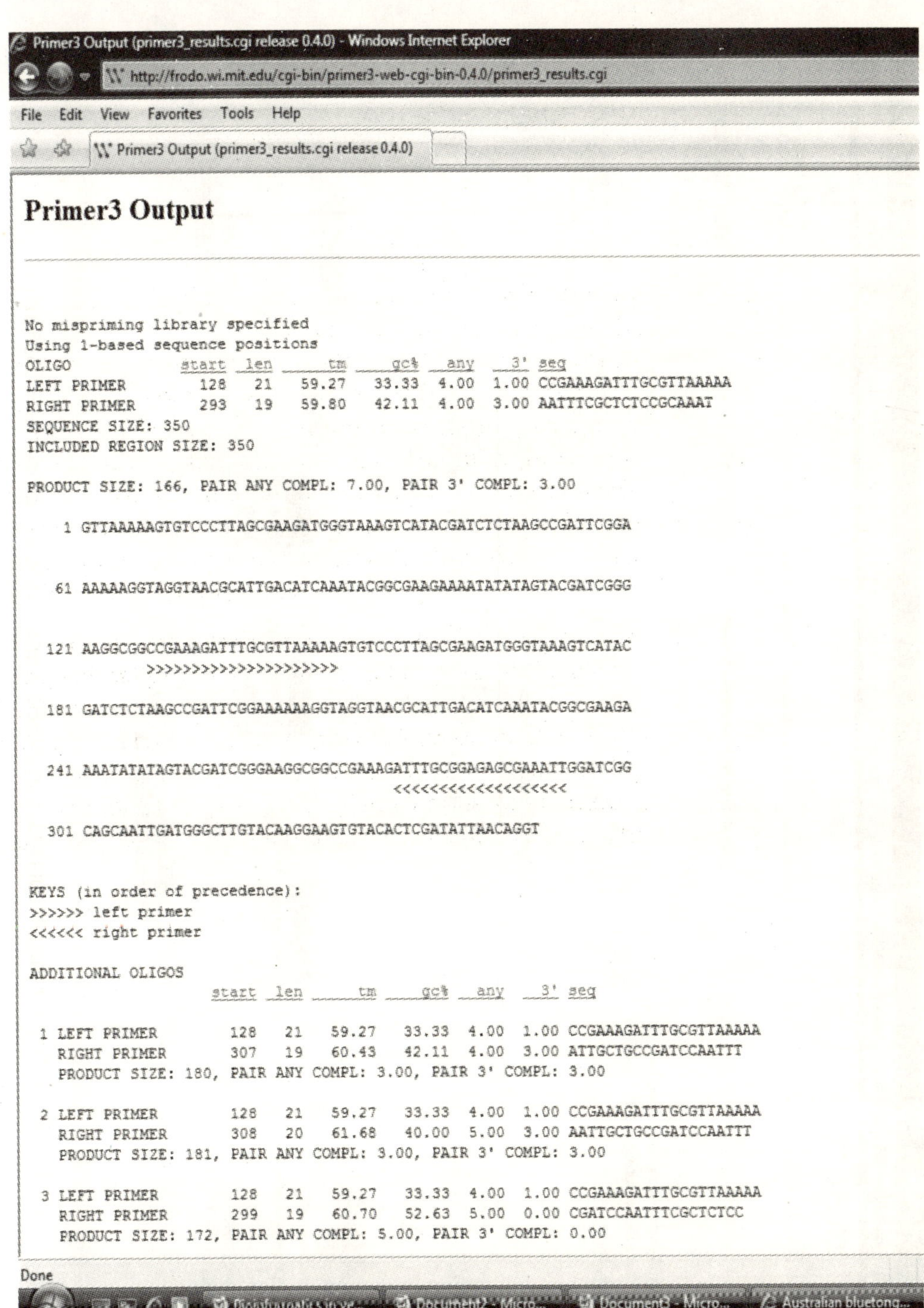

Primer3 Output

```
No mispriming library specified
Using 1-based sequence positions
OLIGO            start  len      tm     gc%   any    3' seq
LEFT PRIMER        128   21   59.27   33.33  4.00  1.00 CCGAAAGATTTGCGTTAAAAA
RIGHT PRIMER       293   19   59.80   42.11  4.00  3.00 AATTTCGCTCTCCGCAAAT
SEQUENCE SIZE: 350
INCLUDED REGION SIZE: 350

PRODUCT SIZE: 166, PAIR ANY COMPL: 7.00, PAIR 3' COMPL: 3.00

    1 GTTAAAAAGTGTCCCTTAGCGAAGATGGGTAAAGTCATACGATCTCTAAGCCGATTCGGA


   61 AAAAAGGTAGGTAACGCATTGACATCAAATACGGCGAAGAAAATATATAGTACGATCGGG


  121 AAGGCGGCCGAAAGATTTGCGTTAAAAAGTGTCCCTTAGCGAAGATGGGTAAAGTCATAC
             >>>>>>>>>>>>>>>>>>>>>

  181 GATCTCTAAGCCGATTCGGAAAAAAAGGTAGGTAACGCATTGACATCAAATACGGCGAAGA


  241 AAATATATAGTACGATCGGGAAGGCGGCCGAAAGATTTGCGGAGAGCGAAATTGGATCGG
                                        <<<<<<<<<<<<<<<<<<<

  301 CAGCAATTGATGGGCTTGTACAAGGAAGTGTACACTCGATATTAACAGGT


KEYS (in order of precedence):
>>>>>> left primer
<<<<<< right primer

ADDITIONAL OLIGOS
                   start  len      tm     gc%   any    3' seq

 1 LEFT PRIMER       128   21   59.27   33.33  4.00  1.00 CCGAAAGATTTGCGTTAAAAA
   RIGHT PRIMER      307   19   60.43   42.11  4.00  3.00 ATTGCTGCCGATCCAATTT
   PRODUCT SIZE: 180, PAIR ANY COMPL: 3.00, PAIR 3' COMPL: 3.00

 2 LEFT PRIMER       128   21   59.27   33.33  4.00  1.00 CCGAAAGATTTGCGTTAAAAA
   RIGHT PRIMER      308   20   61.68   40.00  5.00  3.00 AATTGCTGCCGATCCAATTT
   PRODUCT SIZE: 181, PAIR ANY COMPL: 3.00, PAIR 3' COMPL: 3.00

 3 LEFT PRIMER       128   21   59.27   33.33  4.00  1.00 CCGAAAGATTTGCGTTAAAAA
   RIGHT PRIMER      299   19   60.70   52.63  5.00  0.00 CGATCCAATTTCGCTCTCC
   PRODUCT SIZE: 172, PAIR ANY COMPL: 5.00, PAIR 3' COMPL: 0.00
```


Fig. 5 : Primer3 (http://frodo.wi.mit.edu/cgi-bin/primer3-web-cgi-bin-0.4.0/primer3_results.cgi)

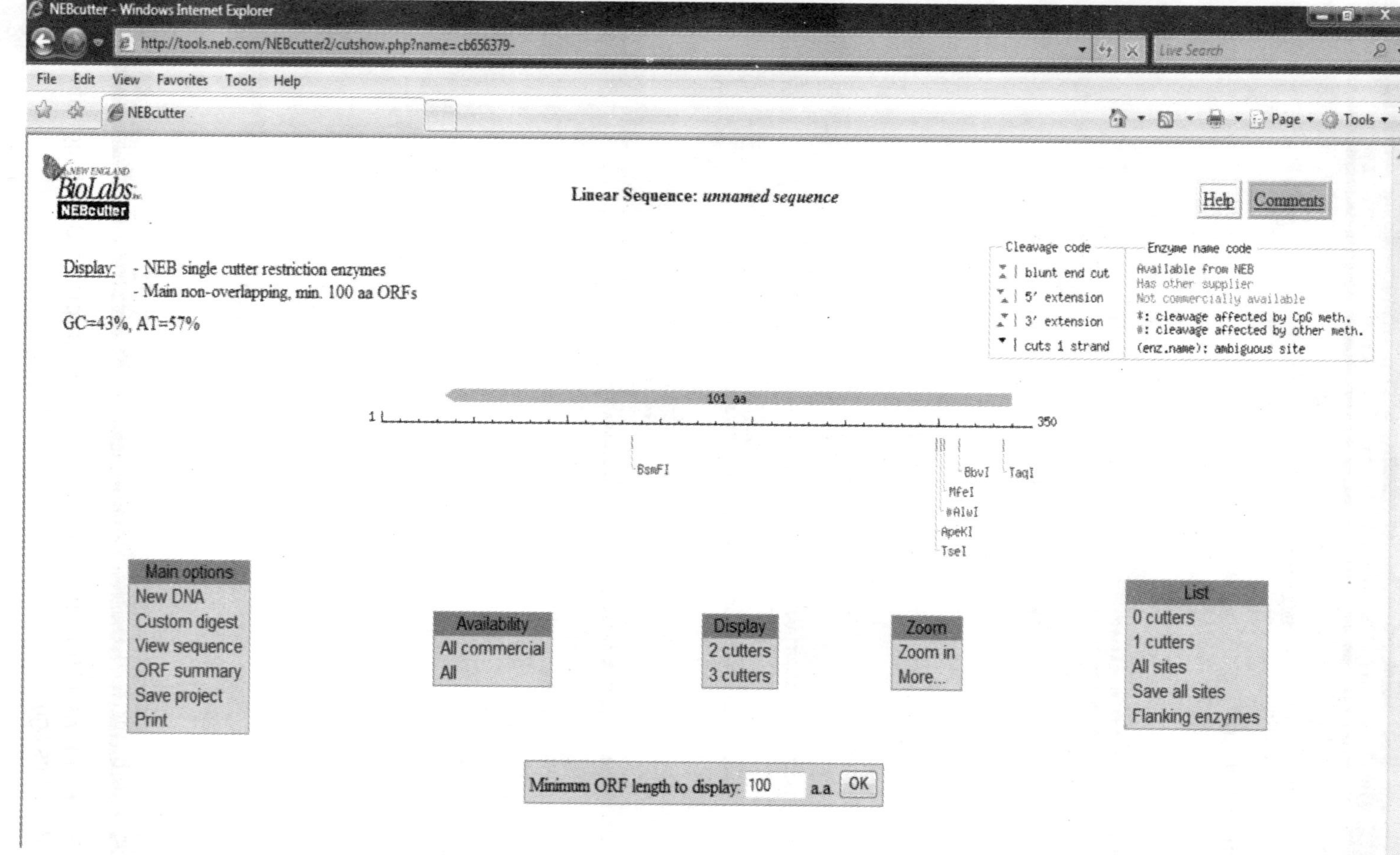

Fig. 6 : NEBcutter (http://tools.neb.com/NEBcutter2/cutshow.php? name=cb656379-)

3.7 ORF Finder

The ORF Finder (Open Reading Frame Finder) is a graphical analysis tool which finds all open reading frames of a selectable minimum size in a given sequence using the standard or alternative genetic codes. The deduced amino acid sequence can be saved in various formats and searched against the sequence database using the BLAST server (Fig. 7). The ORF Finder is helpful in preparing complete and accurate sequence submission.

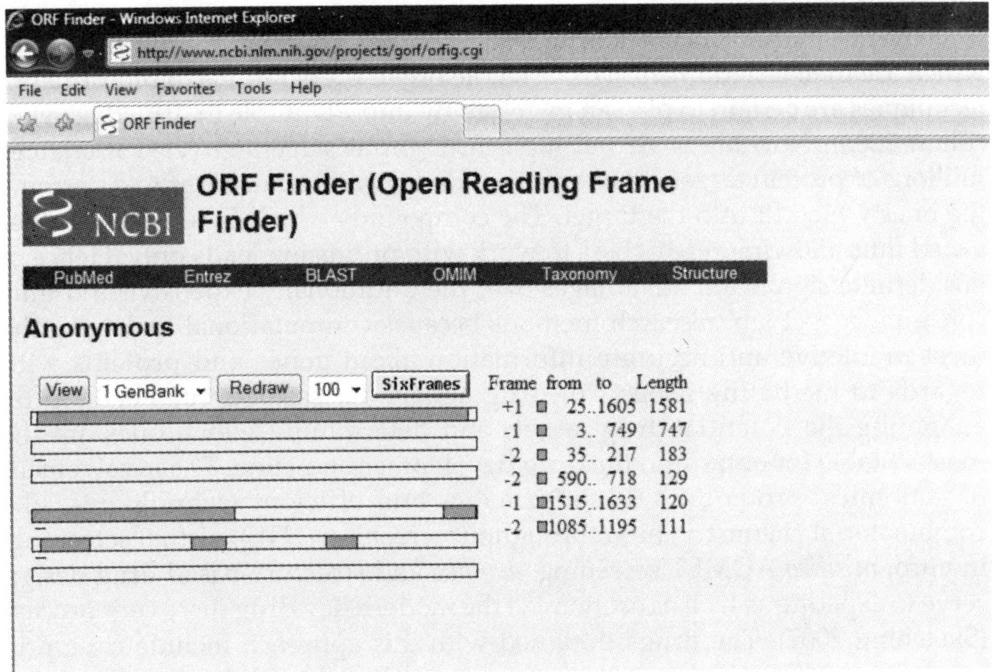

Fig. 7 : NCBI ORF Finder (http://www.ncbi.nlm.nih.gov/projects/gorf/orfig.cgi)

4. Applications in Livestock Health and Production

Bioinformatics has wide application in modern day biology and has made a dramatic impact on improving our understanding in areas like regulation of global gene expression, protein structure determination, comparative evolution, and drug discovery etc. It also holds great promise in identifying the mechanism of development, metabolic processes, and diseases. Some areas where bioinformatics tools and techniques are applicable are discussed below.

4.1 Identification of disease gene

Sequencing of human genome has marked impact on identification, isolation, and characterization of the genes involved in different diseases. Positional cloning is used to map the location of a human disease gene and to identify its function by using bioinformatics tools. The use of large-scale comparative analysis of genome sequence data from model organisms is emerging as the most important recent development in the application of bioinformatics methods for characterizing candidate disease genes (Rawlings and Searls 1997). It has become an important tool in making sense of genetic components of disease and is bound to make an even bigger impact through functional and structural genomics in the near future.

4.2 Drug discovery

The traditional process of drug discovery uses synthetic organic molecules which are then tested in animals or whole organ preparations. Bioinformatics techniques are certain to play an increasingly important role in drug discovery (Elkin 2003). Nowadays virtual high-throughput screening (vHTS) enables millions of protein targets to be screened daily against databases to determine the ones which fit into the target. The compounds which fit are then further tested thus allowing researchers to work with promising leads only. Hence, it has definite significant advantages over the traditionally expensive and time consuming 'wet lab' research methods because computational tools give the most predictive and accurate information about genes and proteins with regards to mediating aspects of drug action. These tools further help by validating the potential drug targets and determining which ones are the most suitable for entry into the drug development pipeline. The involvement of genomics, proteomics, bioinformatics and efficient technologies, like combinatorial chemistry, high throughput screening (HTS), virtual screening, in vitro, *in silico* ADMET screening, *de novo* and structure-based drug design serve to expedite as well as economize the modern day drug discovery process (Sketching 2007). The drugs designed with this approach include captopril, zanamivir, nelfinavir, amprenavir, lopinavir, dorzolamide and oseltamivir.

4.3 Systems biology

It is a multidisciplinary approach to integrate different levels of information to understand how biological system functions. It involves the study of the relationship and interactions between various parts of a biological system e.g. gene and protein networks involved in cell signaling, metabolic pathways, organelles, cells, physiological systems, organisms etc. (Chong and Ray 2002). This nascent field is expected to provide a prior knowledge about the whole system including its response to external perturbations at both individual and collective levels.

4.4 Reverse vaccinology

The conventional approach of vaccine development requires cultivation of the pathogenic microorganism and study of its characteristics using biochemical, immunological, and microbiological methods in order to identify the components important to vaccine development. Through successful in many cases, this approach failed to provide a solution for many of those pathogens for which a vaccine is not yet available. Today, the possibility of using genomic information allows us to design vaccine development *in silico*, without the need of cultivating the pathogen. The complete process includes antigen prediction to high-throughput purification, screening and selection of the vaccine composition (Bagnoli and Rappuoli 2006, Bagnoli *et al.* 2010). The 'reverse vaccinology' approach reduces the time required for the identification of vaccine candidates and provides alternative for those vaccines which have been difficult or impossible to develop by conventional approach. The potential of this new approach is illustrated by the development of a vaccine against serogroup *B. meningococcus* (Rappuoli 2000). It is based on genome-based antigen discovery. A number of vaccines are at the stage of preclinical studies now. Further improvement in this approach is possible with the support of proteomics, functional genomics and comparative genomics. It has the great advantage of being relatively rapid approach as no experimental work is needed once full sequence of the genome is available. Its drawbacks are: first, it is currently unable to predict if, when, and to what extent proteins are expressed and second is that its algorithm is not yet fully refined. Hence, *in silico* analysis has to be coupled with transcriptome analysis and proteome analysis (Grandi 2006) to fully utilize this approach for vaccine development.

4.5 Virology

Viruses are major factors of human and animal infectious diseases. To identify the potential anti-viral inhibitors and vaccine targets, understanding of the structure-function relation in viruses is important. Virus-related databases include viral sequences, homologous protein families, structures, taxonomy etc. These resources are useful for understanding viral diseases, as well as for the design and development of anti-viral agents (Yan 2008). To understand the relationships within complex datasets about viruses and host-virus interactions, virus-related databases and bioinformatics tools for the identification of open reading frames, gene prediction, homology searching, sequence alignment, and motif and epitope recognition are essential. The predictions of features like transmembrane domains, glycosylation sites, and protein secondary and tertiary structures are important for analyzing the structure-function relationship of proteins encoded in viral genomes. Microarray analysis provides methods for high throughput screening and gene expression profiling.

4.6 Parasitology

The availability of genome sequences and the associated transcriptome and proteome mapping projects has revolutionized research in the field of parasitology. As genome sequence information on more parasites are available, comparative and phylogenetic comparisons will improve the quality of gene prediction and annotation and help in understanding its biology, identifying new vaccine candidates and drug targets (Coppel and Black 2005). A modern concept for the development of novel antiparasitic drugs is the combination of bioinformatics and chemoinformatics approaches. It involves identification of target proteins serving as molecular points of attack for parasiticides. Krasky *et al.* (2007) identified potential target proteins in *Ascaris suum, Brugia malayi, Haemonchus contortus, Boophilus microplus* and *Rhipicephalus appendiculatus* using bioinformatics sequence comparison methods on expressed sequence tags. Interesting target proteins like S-adenosyl-L-methionine synthetase was also used to elucidate chemoinformatics approaches, like homology modeling and docking, for generating valuable data for the development of new drug candidates.

4.7 Public health

Epidemiologists are reformulating their classical approaches to diseases by considering various issues associated to "omics" disciplines. Public health and epidemiology are progressively looking forward to using methodologies and informatics tools for managing genomic for public health practice, research and education. The use of biomarkers, biobanks, and integrated genomic/ clinical databases provide great opportunities for informaticians to extract valuable information and knowledge for public health, biomedical research and healthcare. Integrated medical/biological ontologies and new semantic-based models for managing information have great role in research areas like genetic epidemiology and the "omics" (Maojo and Martin-Sanchez 2004). Molecular epidemiology and bioinformatics core is designed to bridge epidemiological, clinical, and bench research through collaborations and application of advanced methods in molecular biology, bioinformatics, biotechnology and population genetics. Its research focus is to elucidate the role of various factors like environmental/community, genetic and epigenetic, and gene-environment interactions in the development of complex diseases (Children's Memorial Research Center 2011).

4.8 Food industry

The rapid increase in useful knowledge due to the availability of complete genomic sequences of a number of organisms relevant to food industry, areas such as metabolic engineering, improvement of cells as microprocess factories and the development of novel preservation methods are being developed.

Genomic knowledge of microorganisms is set to revolutionize pre- and probiotic research to multi-species microbial ecology within the human host. Bioinformatics will hasten the development of novel risk assessment procedures and the development of foods with greater quality in all aspects. By utilizing the knowledge of bioinformatics, food products may be very different in coming time with considerable new values added to it as a result of availability of more biological and chemical data. Further, it will extend the already existing trend of personalized choice to enable consumers to match their food product choices with their own personal health. It will also contribute to an improved understanding of the molecular mechanisms underlying the relationships between food and health, the interactions between food microorganisms and immunocompetent cells, and the mechanisms underlying the interactions of the microbial community in the intestinal tract (Lee and Lee 2000).

4.9 Computational gene discovery

Methods for the prediction of gene structure are essential components in genome sequencing projects and provide the key to locating intron/exon junctions. Sequence comparison and database searching are the essential approaches for predicting the likely biochemical function of new genes. The most emerging recent development in the application of bioinformatics is for characterizing candidate disease genes by use of sequence database analysis for large-scale comparative analysis of genome sequence data from model organisms. The identification of putative genes in raw genomic DNA sequence is an important computational activity in support of disease gene analysis. The venerable GRAIL (gene recognition and analysis internet link) software remains one of the most-used systems for gene identification (Rawlings and Searls 1997). Expressed sequence tag (EST) technology has long been used for gene discovery. One of the fundamental components of large-scale gene discovery projects is that of clustering of expressed sequence tags (ESTs) from complementary DNA (cDNA) libraries. Another aspect of bioinformatics in sequence analysis is the automatic search for genes and regulatory sequences within a genome as not all of the nucleotides within a genome are genes. Within the genome of higher organisms, large parts of the DNA do not serve any obvious purpose. Bioinformatics helps to bridge the gap between genome and proteome, in the use of DNA sequences for protein identification. (http://www.biodatabases.com/whitepaper02.html).

4.10 Expression profiling

Gene expression information is important to the understanding of many aspects of cellular and organ function. The advent of microarray technology allows the analysis of the expression of thousands of genes simultaneously, thus creating a comprehensive expression profile of healthy and disease condition. It generates large amounts of data and analyse these using bioinformatics tools. These tools use computational methods to group (cluster) genes with similar profiles of changes in expression levels. The expression profile of an organism can be studied even by a single chip as in case of yeast. Comparing expression data of disease tissue and normal tissue provides a basis for explaining the different genes which are up or down regulated in a particular disease. Expression profiling experiments with microarray can be used to evaluate responses to pharmacological intervention; and to predict the toxicity of trial drugs. Drug-based treatments could be tailored specifically to the patient and disease, thus providing the most effective course of medication with minimal side effects (Ignacimuthu 2008). The National Cancer Institute is the major contributor of EST library relevant to cancer tissue. Such data help in understanding the changes in gene expression between healthy and diseased cells allowing to find *in silico* answers to biological questions (Buehler and Rashidi 2005).

4.11 Genomic revolution

The science of bioinformatics is increasingly being used to improve the quality of life. Massive DNA sequencing projects have evolved and added in the growth of the science of bioinformatics. It is variation in the genomic DNA which ultimately defines the likelihood of developing diseases resistance. The ultimate goal of bioinformatics is to uncover the wealth of biological information hidden in the mass of sequences, literature and other biological data and obtain a clear insight into the fundamental biology of organisms and to use this information to enhance the standard of life. It is being used now and in the foreseeable future in the areas of molecular medicine to help produce better and more customized medicines to prevent or cure diseases (EBI 2011). It has environmental benefits in identifying waste cleanup bacteria. In animal breeding it can be used for producing high yielding and disease resistance breeds. If bioinformatics is combined with experimental genomics, there may be a lot of advances to revolutionize the future healthcare programmes by postnatal genotyping to assess susceptibility from specific pathogens; prescription of a unique combination of vaccines; minimizing the healthcare costs and anticipating the onslaught of diseases later in life, which could lead to guidance for nutrition intake and early detections of diseases. Over the recent years, bioinformatics has rapidly developed into an essential aid for genomic data analysis.

4.12 Metagenomics

It is the study of metagenomes, the genetic material recovered directly from environmental samples. It may also be referred to as ecogenomics, environmental genomics, or community genomics. It enables the genomic study of uncultured microorganisms. This new field has proven to be rich and comprehensive and is making important contributions in areas like biodiversity, bioremediation, bioprospection of natural products, ecology and medicine. Faster, cheaper sequencing technologies and the ability to sequence uncultured microbes sampled directly from their habitats are expanding and transforming our view of the microbial world. Extracting meaningful information from the millions of new genomic sequences presents a serious challenge to bioinformaticians as the data come from heterogeneous microbial communities, with the sequence data being noisy and partial in comparison to cultured microbes, where the genomic data come from a single clone making sequence assembly and annotation easier. Further, bioinformatics faces new demands in interpreting voluminous, noisy, and often partial sequence data for gene calling and function prediction (Wooley *et al.* 2010). The ultimate goal of metagenomics is to generate sequence assemblies resulting in at least full-length genes and preferably complete genomes. Generating assemblies of the sequence reads is critical for characterizing full-length genes, discovering new genes and ultimately helping model microbial communities based upon sequence similarities (Harkins and Jarvie 2007). Metagenomics is a relatively new field and an explosion in computational methods applied to it has taken place in recent times.

4.13 Livestock improvement

The contribution of bioinformatics in livestock improvement has drastically changed with the advent of modern genome projects. Genomes of many livestock species have been sequenced (Table 1, 2). Bioinformatics in livestock sector is applicable to design tools to process and annotate livestock genome sequences, gene expression data, SNPs for breed identification, haplotype map development and genome-wide association analysis and quantitative trait loci (QTL) fine mapping to support genomic selection programme. The improved understanding of genetic control of milk production, feed utilization, meat quality, and litter size is leading to rapid genetic improvement. Current genome programmes generate large amounts of data that require processing, storage and distribution to the multinational research community. The data include not only sequence information, but also the information on mutations, markers, maps, functional discoveries etc. (Vassilev *et al.* 2005). Key objectives for animal bioinformatics are to encourage the submission of all sequence data into the public domain so as to understand the relationship of data within an animal, between animals, and with other organisms The Bioinformatics Group at the Roslin Institute provides access to appropriate bioinformatics tools and resources for farm animal genome analysis. Genome research in farm animals is largely concerned with mapping genes that influence economically important traits. Bioinformatics toolbox can be used for narrowing QTL which has already been demonstrated in mice (Burgess *et al.* 2008). Although QTL analysis has been a powerful tool for localizing the chromosomal regions underlying complex traits through systematically identifying the causal genes remains challenging.

Tools of bioinformatics are playing significant role in providing information about genes in the genome of different farm animal species and making it possible to predict the function of different genes and factors affecting these genes. The information about the genes makes the scientists to produce enhanced species of livestock which have disease resistance. Bioinformatics with the rapidly increasing whole genome sequences available are starting to change the old approach of livestock improvement. QTL largely depends on easy to detect genetic markers such as STSs, ESTs and SNPs. In the absence of whole genome sequences, marker density is usually low to detect QTL successfully. With genome projects, marker density has improved and novel gene targets can be identified comparatively with ease making possible the marker assisted breeding. With the help of whole genome sequence information, the use of model organism has accelerated gene discovery and the identification of promising gene candidates for genetic improvement of livestock (Buehler and Rashidi 2005). A number of genome wide association studies for candidate genes are reported in domestic animals. Illumna's SNP Biochips have been developed for cattle, horse, pig and sheep. These are commercially available and aid in selection for important economic traits (Fan *et al.* 2010).

Table 1 : Farm animal species genomes

Genomes	URL
Any species at NCBI	http://www.ncbi.nlm.gov/Genomes/index.html
Many species at Roslin Institute UK	http://www.thearkdb.org/
BovGBASE - bovine	http://www.genome.iastate.edu/
ChickGBASE - poultry	http://www.genome.iastate.edu/chickmap/dbase.html
PiGBASE - swine	http://www.genome.iastate.edu/maps/pigbase.html
SheepBASE - bovine	http://www.projects.roslin.ac.uk/sheepmap/front.html

Table 2 : List of sequenced whole genome of domestic animals

Species	Genome size (Gb)	Coverage (X)	No. of coding genes	Sequencing organization	Year of release	URL
Bos taurus	2.91	7.1	20684	Baylor HGSC	2009	http://www.ensembel.org/Bos_taurus/Info/Index/ http://www.hgsc.bcm.tmc.edu/projects-species-m-Bovine.hgsc?pageLocation=Bovine
Equus caballus	2.47	6.8	17254	Broad Institute/MIT Center for Genome Research	2009	http://www.ensembel.org/Equus caballus/Info/Index/ http://www.broadinstitute.org/mammals/horse
Ovis aries	2.78	3.0	-	AgResearch/ Baylor HGSC/CSIRO/ University of Otago	2008	http://www.sheepmap.org/ http://www.livestockgenomics.csiro.au.sheep/ https://isgcdata.agresearch.co.nz/
Gallus gallus	1.05	6.6	16450	Washington University Genome Sequencing Center	2004	http://genome.wustl.edu/genomes/view/gallus_gallus http://www.ensembel.org/Gallus gallus/Info/Index/
Meleagris gallopavo	1.08	-	11145	Virginia Bioinformatics Institute/USDA Beltsville/ University of Maryland	2009	http://www.ensembel.org/Meleagrisgallopavo/Info/Index/
Canis familiaris	2.38	7.5	15900	Broad Institute/MIT Center for Genome Research	2005	http://www.ensembel.org/Canis familiaris/Info/Index/ http://www.broadinstitute.org/mammals/dog
Sus scrofa	2.26	6.0	12678	Wecome Trust Sanger Institute	2009	http://www. piggenome.org/ http://www.ensembel.org/Sus scrofa/Info/Index/ http://www.sanger.ac.uk/Projects/Sscrofa/

4.14 Infectious disease control

The microbial profiling and biosurveillance focused text mining tools can facilitate integrated infectious disease outbreak detection and response environments based upon bioinformatics knowledge models and measured by outcomes including the accuracy and timeliness of outbreak detection (Sintchenko *et al.* 2009).

4.15 Comparative studies

Bioinformatics tools can be used to compare the genomes of different species to study the functions of different genes and the mechanisms of inherited diseases and species evolution. It can be used to make comparisons between the numbers, locations and functions of genes in different individuals and species. For example, mouse (human model) and human are very closely related (> 98%) and one to one correspondence between genes in the two species can be seen (Bioinformatics Web 2011). The detailed understanding of the mouse genome can help in finding the functions of human genes, elucidating the mechanisms of many human diseases and the evolutionary relationship between the two species by genome comparisons utilizing the tools of bioinformatics.

4.16 Phylogenetics

It is the study of the evolutionary history of living organisms using tree-like diagrams to represent pedigrees of these organisms. The advent of the genomic era with tremendous amounts of molecular sequence data has led to rapid development of molecular phylogenetics. It has made possible the study of evolutionary relationships of genes and other biological macromolecules by analyzing mutations at various positions and developing hypotheses about the evolutionary relatedness of the biomolecules. Based on the sequence similarity of the molecules, evolutionary relationships between the organisms can be inferred. Phylip (Phylogenetic inference package; by Joe Felsenstein) is a free multiplatform comprehensive package containing thirty-five subprogrammes for performing distance, parsimony, and likelihood analysis, as well as bootstrapping for both nucleotide and amino acid sequences. It is command-line based, but relatively easy to use for each single programme.

4.17 Proteomics

Bioinformatics has an enormous analytical and predictive potential in the area of proteomics. The prediction of three-dimensional structure of proteins from the linear amino acid sequence is the objective of bioinformatics. Protein folding alone is among the most significant and fundamental problems. Its understanding gives better insight into diseases and ways to fight them.

To utilize the data for healthcare and drug development, characteristics of proteomes of the entire species have to be understood first. Structure analysis and prediction, detection of specific regions, alignments, data mining, 2D PAGE analysis, or protein modeling benefit from the information stored in different databases and make use of different protein analysis tools to provide computational analysis of whole proteomes (Pruess and Apweiler 2003). There is a need of relevant methods for the prediction of immunome, with special emphasis on quantitative methods, and the sub-cellular localization of proteins within bacteria (Doytchinova *et al.* 2003).

5. Limitations and Challenges

Bioinformatics has a number of intrinsic limitations. Bioinformatics predictions are not formal proofs and do not replace the traditional experimental research methods. However, the quality of bioinformatics prediction depends on the data quality and sophistication of the software. The software lacking capability and sophistication often makes incorrect predictions that make no sense when placed in a biological context. Software with low computing power takes more time in computing. The limited availability of gene-functionality from the wet-lab data, protein-protein and protein-DNA interactions is another constraint.

Finding new and faster approaches to deal with the volume and complexity of data, and providing researchers with better access to computing tools is quite important for advancing the understanding of genetic information and its effect on phenotypes. The development of better tools and resources is, thus, the main challenge. In future, systems biology approach, the next wave of bioinformatics will be utilized which involves the integration of different 'omics and bioinformatics information to create a complete system view of a cell/tissue which is the ultimate objective of bioinformatics.

References

1. Bagnoli F, Norais N, Ferlenghi I, Scarselli M, Donati C, Savino S, Barocchi MA, Rappuoli R (2010). Designing vaccines in the era of genomics. In: Vaccine design: Innovative approaches and novel strategies (Ed. Rappuoli R, Bagnoli F, Caister Academic Press.
2. Bagnoli F, Rappuoli R (2006). Mechanisms of pathogenesis and prevention of meningococcal disease. Drug Discov Today Dis Mech 3:273-279.
3. Bioinformatics Web (2011). http://bioinformaticsweb.net/applications.html. Accessed 20 January 2011.
4. Buehler LK, Rashidi HH (2005). Bioinformatics basics, Taylor & Francis.
5. Burgess SL, Cox HA, Tsaih SW, Paigen B (2008). Practical applications of the bioinformatics toolbox for narrowing quantitative trait loci. Genetics 108:90-175.

6. Children's Memorial Research Center (2011). Molecular epidemiology and bioinformatics. http://www.childrensmrc.org/childhealthresearch/ bioinformatics/. Accessed 20 January 2011.
7. Chong L and Ray LB (2002). Whole-istic biology. Science 295:1661.
8. Clifford RJ, Edmonson MN, Nguyen C, Scherpbier T, Hu Y, Buetow KH (2006). Bioinformatics tools for single nucleotide polymorphism discovery and analysis. Annals New York Academy Sci 1020:101-109.
9. Coppel RL, Black CG (2005). Parasite genomes. International J Parasitol 35: 465-479.
10. Doytchinova IA, Taylor P, Flower R (2003). Proteomics in vaccinology and immunobiology: An informatics perspective of the immunone. J Biomed Biotech 5:267-290.
11. EBI (2011). European Bioinformatics Institute. www.ebi.ac.uk/2can/ bioinformatics.
12. Elkin PL (2003). Primer on medical genomics part V: bioinformatics mayo Clin Proc 78:57-64.
13. Fan B, Du ZQ, Gorbach DM, Rothschild MF (2010). Development and application of high density SNP arrays in genomic studies of domestic animals. Asian Aust J Anim Sci 23:833-847.
14. Goddard ME, Ben JH (2009). Mapping genes for complex traits in domestic animals and their use in breeding programmes. Nature Reviews Genetics 10:381-391.
15. Grandi G (2006). Genomics and proteomics in reverse vaccines. In: Microbial proteomics: Functional biology of whole organisms (Ed. Smith IH, Hecker M), John Wiley & Sons, Inc. New York.
16. Hamosh A, Scott AF, Amberger J, Bocchini C, Valle D, McKusick VA (2002). Online mendelian inheritance in man, a knowledgebase of human genes and genetic disorders. Nucleic Acids Research 30:52-55.
17. Harkins T, Jarvie T (2007). Metagenomics analysis using the Genome Sequencer™ FLX system. Nature Methods 4:iii-v.
18. Ignacimuthu S (2008). Bioinformatics an introduction. Narosa Publishing House, New Delhi.
19. Kaminsky N (2000). Bioinformatics- A user's perspective. Am J Respir Cell Mol Biol 23:705-711.
20. Krasky A, Rohwer A, Schroeder J, Selzer PM (2007). A combined bioinformatics and chemoinformatics approach for the development of new antiparasitic drugs. Genomics 89:36-43.
21. Lee PS, Lee KH (2000). Genomic analysis. Curr Opin Biotech 11:171-175.
22. Maojo V, Martin-Sanchez F (2004). Bioinformatics: towards new directions for public health. Methods Inf Med 43:208-214.

23. Pruess M, Apweiler R (2003). Bioinformatics resources for in silico proteome analysis. J Biomed Biotech 4: 31-236.

24. Rappuoli R (2000). Reverse vaccinology. Curr Opin Microbiol 3:445-450.

25. Rawlings CJ, Searls DB (1997). Computational gene discovery and human disease. Curr Opin Genet Dev 7:416-23.

26. Ricketts SL (2009). Bioinformatics- computer based approaches to genetic analysis in molecular diagnostics for the clinical laboratory. (Ed Coleman WB, Tsongalis GJ) Humana Press, Totowa, NJ.

27. Sintchenko V (2009). Infectious Disease Informatics. Springer Science.

28. Sketching A (2007). Physicochemical pathway for lead molecule design in silico. Curr Pharmaceutical Design 13:3454-3470.

29. Vassilev D, Leunissen J, Atanassov A, Nenov A, Dimov G (2005). Application of bioinformatics in plant breeding. Biotech Biotechnol Eq 19:139-152.

30. Vincze T, Posfai J, Roberts RJ (2003). NEBcutter: a programme to cleave DNA with restriction enzymes. Nucleic Acids Research 31:3688-3691.

31. Wooley JC, Godzik A, Friedberg I (2010). A primer on metagenomics PLoS Computational Biology 6:1-13.

32. Xiong J (2005). Essential bioinformatics. Cambridge University Press.

33. Yan Q (2008). Bioinformatics databases and tools in virology research: An overview. *In Silico* Biology 8:71-85.

□□□

Chapter 23

Applications of Geoinformatics in Animal Health

ARUN K. SANGWAN
Department of Veterinary Parasitology, College of Veterinary Sciences, Lala Lajpat Rai University of Veterinary and Animal Sciences, Hisar-125004

Contents

1. Introduction

Geoinformatics has gained momentum with the recent all-round development of Geographical Information Systems (GIS) and the improved earth observing satellites and sensors for remote sensing (RS). Applications of geoinformatics are increasing exponentially in newer fields including veterinary sciences. GIS and RS have greatly facilitated monitoring of the physical, biological, environmental and anthropogenic factors which influence the prevalence, incidence, spread and seasonality of diseases. Large landscape pattern analysis, combined with statistical analysis, allows the determination of landscape predictors of disease risk. This makes RS and GIS a powerful set of tools for disease surveillance, enabling the prediction of potential disease outbreaks and targeting intervention programmes. As evidenced by current publications, GIS and RS have become part of mainstream veterinary epidemiology and parasitology. Since this new discipline is still evolving, the terminology used in this field is also in the evolving phase. The discipline draws its strength from many traditional and newer technologies necessitating newer terms to represent this field. Geoinformatics is one such term that encompasses this emerging branch of science. It is also known as geomatics. Some people still like the term GIS for it but replace systems with science i.e. Geographic Information Science rather than Systems (Goodchild 2000, Kistemann *et al.* 2002) while others consider the Space-Time Information Science (STIS) as a better term (Kistemann *et al.* 2002, Hendrickx *et al.* 2004).

2. What is Geoinformatics?

Geoinformatics has emerged as a specialized branch of the modern information science to address issues related to spatial information in any branch of science, engineering or humanities. Spatial information basically consists of location specific attributes (non-spatial data e.g. census data) and the coordinates of the location (spatial data e.g. latitude and longitude) on the earth's surface. Geoinformatics combine geovisualization (in the form of maps), geospatial analysis (e.g. pattern detection), modeling (e.g. disease or vector prediction) and development of geospatial databases. With its varied applications geoinformatics is now playing a significant role in all walks of life as it facilitates creative problem solving and sound decision making and hence, it is a Decision Support System. Issues related to spatial information or spatial analysis in veterinary sciences include field data collection, data capture using remote sensing and information extraction from it; mapping and analysis for the development of descriptive disease maps; studying the environmental features that influence the distribution of diseases; predicting occurrence/ seasonality of diseases based on their environmental requirements and as decision support for disease intervention; and surveillance and monitoring of animal diseases. Geoinformatics tools also assist in locating distribution of health-relevant environmental factors via interpolation and modeling.

Branches of geoinformatics include Geographic Information Systems (GIS), Remote Sensing, Photogrammetry, Geodesy including Global Positioning System (GPS) and Cartography.

2.1 Geographical Information Systems (GIS)

GIS are interdisciplinary, multi-functional tools that combine computing, spatial analysis and mapping to provide new ways of dealing with the location based issues related to any discipline including animal health and husbandry. GIS is a generic term indicating the use of computers to create and depict digital representations of the earth surface. It is a major research, application and business area in the information technology (IT) sector. GIS technology integrates common database operations such as query and statistical analysis with the visualization and geographic analysis benefits offered by maps. These abilities distinguish GIS from other information systems and make it valuable for explaining events, predicting outcomes, and planning strategies for the location based issues.

2.2 Remote Sensing (RS)

RS is the science which deals with obtaining information about objects on the earth's surface by analysis of data received from a remote sensor onboard earth-orbiting satellite. The earth's features are identified by analysis of electromagnetic radiation, which is reflected/ emitted by the earth surface and captured by the satellite sensors as remotely sensed data (images). The identification of the earth's surface through remote sensing involves two steps: (1) Detection and measurement of variation in electromagnetic spectrum called data acquisition. (2) Correlation of measurements to know the Earth surface called data interpretation and analysis. The remotely sensed imageries are a major data source used in geoinformatics. These imageries help in characterization of land cover and thereby in predicting distribution of diseases.

2.3 Photogrammetry or aerial remote sensing

Aircraft is used with aerial cameras to record information in the form of photographs. Such aerial photography has applications in various fields like topographic mapping and various surveys for example urban planning. Its application in veterinary sciences is not common as it is not a cost effective way to analyze animal health and husbandry related issues.

2.4 Geodesy and Global Positioning System (GPS)

Geodesy is the discipline concerned with the measurement of the size and shape of the earth and positions on it. It is important to remote sensing and GIS as it underpins the essential process of georeferencing images (remotely sensed data) and associated vector features to earth surface locations. Global Positioning System (GPS) and several other such systems are being used to determine the exact location of the phenomena of interest on the surface of the Earth. GPS is a system of Earth-orbiting satellites transmitting precisely timed signals which provide direct measurement of position on the Earth's surface. Location is expressed in latitude/longitude or other standard system. Signals are received by special electronic devices which are becoming common and cheaper these days and the smaller versions are hand-held. GPS is U.S.A operated. A similar system deployed by the Russian Federation is called GLONASS (global navigation satellite system) and another such system called Galileo will soon be put in place by the European Space Agency. China's Compass and India's IRNSS (Indian Regional Navigation Satellite System) are also under development.

2.5 Cartography

The art and science of map making is cartography. With the advent of digital cartography map making has become much more dynamic, versatile and common. Cartography is an old technology that has been revolutionized by GIS.

2.6 Spatial analysis

Spatial analysis in relation to GIS, in broad terms, can be described as the ability to manipulate spatial data into different forms and extract additional meaning as a result. In a spatial epidemiology context, one can distinguish between three types of spatial analysis tasks, namely (1) visualization/ mapping, (2) exploratory data analysis, and (3) modeling (Bailey and Gatrell 1995). The development of spatial statistics has also contributed a lot in making geoinformatics directly useful to ecologists, parasitologists, epidemiologists, and infectious disease biologists among others.

Thus, GIS, RS and GPS are commonly used geoinformatics technologies in veterinary epidemiology for capture, storage, retrieval, update, analyses, mapping, display and rapid communication of data for the management of animal diseases. A variety of GIS, statistical and image processing software are available to visualize, explore and model disease and health data sets. The computer revolution since 1980s has fuelled the increasing use of

Geoinformatics. Large datasets and complicated algorithms can now be handled relatively quickly and efficiently by the modern computers. Geoinformatics enables us to take advantage of the unprecedented amount of digital geodata and computing power available through electronic networks. Geoinformatics also exploits the enormous potential of the World Wide Web and grid computing to link computing and data resources to allow users to turn observational and computational geodata into knowledge.

3. History of Geoinformatics Applications in Medical and Veterinary Sciences

Geoinformatics is an emerging, rapidly progressing and highly applied field without a long history. However, taking advantage of hindsight, researchers have linked it with the 4th century BC philosopher Hippocrates (Rinaldi *et al.* 2006). Essentially geoinformatics techniques like GIS and RS are contemporary techniques that flourished with advances in digital and information technology as well as simultaneous improvements in the Earth-observing satellites and sensors. However, the concept that geographic location can influence health and diseases is a very old one in medicine. It is a well recorded common knowledge since ancient times in all cultures that certain diseases are location specific. NASA pioneered the use of remote sensing data for human health in the early 1970s with the creation of the Health Applications Office at the Johnson Space Center (Fuller 1972). This initiative gave impetus to the application of RS to related disciplines like animal health. In 1985, NASA began the Global Monitoring and Human Health programmes for the applicability of RS and GIS technologies in human health research. In 1998, NASA created the Center for Health Applications of Aerospace Related Technologies, for evaluating current and planed satellite sensors systems, to determine if the data could be applied to human health research in the area of landscape epidemiology. Over 17 vector-borne diseases including malaria, Lyme and schistosomosis (http://geo.arc.nasa.gov/sge/health/bydisease.html) have been studied using a variety of satellite instruments. Recently, NASA has developed a new Earth science and public health programme, named the Healthy Planet (http://healthyplanet.gsfc.nasa.gov/). This programme is for developing new tools for health-related surveillance and early warning systems.

These NASA initiatives fuelled the publication of original research articles and reviews in veterinary and human health with an emphasis on GIS and/or RS in an exponential way. In addition, recent GIS/RS symposia organized at national and international conferences and several thematic issues on this topic published in the peer-reviewed international literature (e.g. special theme issues in Advances in Parasitology in 2000 and 2006, and Parassitologia in 2005) demonstrate the wide array of applications and benefits of these tools (Cringoli *et al.* 2005a, Rinaldi *et al.* 2006). Furthermore, the publication of thematic books pertaining to geoinformatics e.g. GIS and Spatial Analysis in Veterinary Science (Durr and Gatrell 2004a) and Spatial Analysis in Epidemiology (Pfeiffer *et al.* 2008), as well as international peer-reviewed journals e.g. *Geospatial Health* (www.geospatialhealth.unina.it) have essentially established these new technologies in veterinary and medical sciences. Some pioneering and landmark applications in epidemiology that had cascading effect (Linthicum *et al.* 1987, Lessard *et al.* 1990, Rogers and Randolph 1991) have been followed by rapid publications of research articles and reviews in this area (Hendrickx *et al.* 2004, Cringoli *et al.* 2005b, Rinaldi *et al.* 2006, Brooker *et al.* 2006, Bergquist and Rinaldi 2010) leading to the establishment of GIS and RS technologies as basic tools to study epidemiology of diseases. In addition, new websites have appeared recently to share opinions and experiences on GIS in animal and public health, e.g. www.gnosisgis.org and www.gisvet.org.

4. GIS as a Vital Component of the Epidemiologists' Tool Kit

The application of GIS in veterinary epidemiology involves firstly visualizing spatial patterns in the disease data, then describing these spatial patterns, and finally to explain the observed patterns. This further enables us to predict changes in the patterns and to use our explanations and predictions to guide decisions and policy formulations. The visualization, exploration and modeling capabilities of GIS are explained by Pfeiffer (2004). The integration of spatial dimension into epidemiological investigations provides an opportunity for conducting more informative descriptive analysis and gaining additional insights into the causal processes under investigation. A particular strength of spatial dimension is that special model outputs can be visualized through maps, greatly facilitating effective communication. Application of spatial analysis in epidemiological surveillance and research is increasing exponentially. Disease maps are useful for several purposes such as identification of areas with higher risk, formulation of hypothesis about disease aetiology, assessing needs for health-resource allocation and additionally facilitate effective communication. In addition, there has been an increasing demand for evidence based decision making which includes the need to produce spatially explicit inferences. Durr and Gatrell (2004b) discussed GIS as a tool for veterinary epidemiology. Pfeiffer *et al.* (2008) highlighted the vital importance of GIS and spatial analysis in veterinary epidemiology. The subject of spatial statistics is rapidly evolving with considerable progress made in recent years in the development of methodologies related to disease mapping and ecological analysis. With the increasing availability of data, analytical techniques, high speed computers and user friendly software it is likely that GIS will become a vital component of the epidemiologists' tool kit.

5. RS as a Vital Component of the Epidemiologists' Tool Kit

The links between remote sensing and diseases have been discussed by Curran *et al.* (2000). The application of remote sensing to epidemiology is based on the development of a logical sequence that links measures of radiation made by a sensor to measure of a disease and its vector. A basic sequence could be: (i) remotely sensed data can be used to provide information on land cover (e.g. different vegetation types or classes of vegetation amount) and thereby habitat (ii) the spatial distribution of a vector-borne disease is related to the habitat of that vector and (iii) therefore, remotely sensed data can be used to provide information on the spatial distribution of the vector-borne diseases. To begin with the use of remote sensing in epidemiology concentrated on the development of correlations between images and diseases and then the use of images to predict diseases. Curran *et al.* (2000) summarized the vital importance of RS in epidemiology. Land cover is central to the links between remote sensing and epidemiology. The accurate identification and quantification of land cover could be a useful part of prediction methodologies in epidemiology. Remotely sensed data contains spectral, spatial and temporal information that can be used to characterize the Earth's surface.

6. Applications of Geoinformatics in Veterinary Sciences

Applications of geoinformatics in veterinary sciences are a recent phenomenon which is still developing as evidenced by the progressively increasing number of publications. GIS and RS are being integrated as standard technologies in the investigations of the issues of animal health and decision making. Special theme issues in Advances in Parasitology in 2000 and 2006 provide the best descriptions of the applications of RS and GIS in veterinary and human health in single volumes. Parasites are the most investigated pathogens using these techniques compared to other pathogenic organisms. The most prominent parasitic groups investigated are tsetse and trypanosomosis, ticks and tick-borne diseases, mosquito and malaria, snails and snail-borne helminths, vector-borne filarial worms and soil transmitted helminths. Some pioneering applications in epidemiology include those by Linthicum *et al.* (1987), Lessard *et al.* (1990) and Rogers and Randolph (1991). High risk areas of Rift valley fever were detected using satellite imagery and published in Science by Linthicum *et al.* (1987). This is the earliest example of the effective use of RS in veterinary science. Lessard *et al.* (1990) mapped and analyzed the spatial patterns of theileriosis across the whole continent of Africa. Rogers and Randolph (1991) published a paper in Nature correlating abundance of tsetse flies with the satellite imageries through the use of spectral index NDVI (normalized difference vegetation index). This methodology has been expanded for a range of vector-borne diseases.

The control of 2001 epidemic of FMD in UK placed space-time simulation models at the centre of national disease control policy and decision support. The contribution of GIS to FMD management via disease modeling has been discussed by French and White (2004). Durr (2004) discussed applications of spatial epidemiology to animal diseases like bovine spongiform encephalopathy, bovine tuberculosis and multidrug-resistant *Salmonella* Newport. Pfeiffer *et al.* (2008) used bovine tuberculosis data (1986-1999) to illustrate various applications of GIS in veterinary sciences like visualization of the data, exploration of the data and modeling techniques.

Disease mapping, spatial statistics, ecological analyses and epidemiological surveillance of animal parasitic diseases are summarized by Rinaldi *et al.* (2004). Tsetse flies and African trypanosomosis is one such area where satellite data and GIS have been used for risk mapping in smaller regional areas as well as at the continental scale (Rogers 2000). Predicting the distribution of livestock ticks and tick-borne diseases using RS has been discussed and reviewed by Randolph (2000) and Daniel *et al.* (2004). Application of GIS and RS for assessing and monitoring malaria risk has been reviewed and discussed by Hay *et al.* (2000), Ceccato *et al.* (2005) and Guerra *et al.* (2006). It is shown that a useful early warning system can be developed with these techniques. Sudhakar *et al.* (2006) identified spatial distribution of indicator land cover classes for *Phlebotomus argentipes* and Kala-azar using RS and GIS techniques in India.

Rinaldi (2007) discussed applications of GIS/RS in parasitology with particular regard to filarial worms. These tools have also been used successfully to describe the environmental factors associated with patterns of soil transmitted helminth infection in selected geographical locations, and helped identify the relative importance of different environmental factors in determining geographic distributions (Brooker and Michael 2000, Brooker *et al.* 2006). Cringoli *et al.* (2004) used RS/GIS to identify environmental features that influence the distribution of paramphistomosis in sheep from the southern Italian Apennines. Sangwan (2007) used RS data to delineate snail habitats in parts of eastern Doon valley by digital image processing techniques and following the FAO framework of land evaluation. Sangwan *et al.* (2006) prepared a risk map of snail-borne diseases of livestock in the state of Haryana in India. GIS has been used in epidemiology to model the distribution of various parasites/ diseases, e.g. *Ixodes scapularis* that transmits Lyme disease (Nicholson and Mather 1996), malaria (Kleinschmidt *et al.* 2000), alveolar echinococcosis (Conraths *et al.* 2003, Pleydell *et al.* 2004), tsetse flies that transmit human African trypanosomosis (Sciarretta *et al.* 2005), *Calicophoron daubneyi,* the causative agent of paramphistomosis in ruminants (Biggeri *et al.* 2004), *Oncomelania hupensins,* the intermediate host snail of *Schistosoma japonicum* (Zhang *et al.* 2005), coinfection with *S. mansoni* and hookworm among schoolchildren in Côte d'Ivoire (Raso *et al.* 2006), human filariosis (Brooker and Micheal 2000) and canine filariosis (Genchi *et al.* 2005, Vezzani and Carbajo 2006).

Applications of GIS and RS in helminthology had been attempted for schistosomiasis (reviewed by Brooker 2002) and filariasis (reviewed by Brooker and Michael 2000); soil transmitted helminth infection (reviewed by Brooker *et al.* 2006), *Loa loa* (Thomson *et al.* 2004) and onchocerciasis (Carabin *et al.* 2003). These studies have focused on the use of RS data to identify ecological correlates of infection and develop statistical models of disease risk. Bergquist and Rinaldi (2010) have illustrated the possibilities of disease prediction based on the environmental characteristics of geographical area and specific requirements of the causative infectious agents.

The above examples have led the way in using GIS/RS for control programmes. An important emerging trend is that national governments are beginning to use this approach for designing and developing sustainable control programmes. It is likely that these techniques will get integrated with the livestock health programmes in near future.

7. A Worked Out Example of Application of Geoinformatics in Veterinary Sciences

Snail-borne trematode infections are restricted to areas that serve as habitat of fresh water snails. Such areas have water bodies and high moisture levels which are dependent on water availability, canals, ground water quality, soil physiography, rainfall, land use, flooding hazards, slope, relief, temperature, vegetation etc. Depending on all these environmental factors, some of the area is more suitable than others in supporting snail-borne diseases. If the disease transmitting snails' data is represented by point locations, we may model disease risk (presence or absence) as a function of the environmental covariates measured at those point locations. Thus, risk assessment of snail-borne trematode infections for a particular area can be done. In this example, the ecological units in various suitability classes as snail habitat were worked out using point data of snail recordings and five environmental covariates (distance from canal, rice cultivation, rainfall, flood proneness and soil physiography) in Rohtak and Jhajjar districts of Haryana state in India. The effects of these predictor variables on the presence or absence of snails were assessed using the logistic regression analysis.

Forty four locations found infested with either *Indoplanorbis* or *Lymnaea* snails and likewise 55 locations where snails were not found during field checks were identified in Rohtak and Jhajjar districts. GIS was used to visualize these point locations and a map (Fig. 1) was produced using latitude and longitude of snail infested village points. The 44 snail-infested locations were used as 'cases' while 55 snail-negative locations were used as 'controls' in a logistic regression model to predict the risk of snail infestation in the two districts. A GIS database using five sets of variables (land use i.e. whether the area is rice growing or not, soil physiography units, rainfall, flood prone areas or not based on historic data, and the Euclidean distance from canal) were used as a set of candidate environmental covariates (Fig. 2 to 6) derived through remote sensing and digital image processing. All the five sets of environmental variables depicted as maps (Fig. 2 to 6) were converted into raster data format. A risk model was generated combining GIS with logistic regression to predict *Lymnaea* and *Indoplanorbis* infestation risk in Rohtak and Jhajjar districts. This resulted into a risk map (Fig. 7). The final model included rice growing area ($P < 0.0001$) and distance from canal (P 0.02) as the most significant factors influencing snail infestation in this area. The model predicted that snails are more likely to be present in the areas growing rice than in the areas where rice is not grown (odds ratio = 9.24) and that snails are less likely to be present with every 1 km increase in the distance from a canal (odds ratio = 0.86). This model can be applied on larger areas having similar environment i.e. canal irrigated semi-arid areas.

8. Technology Scenario: Developed Nations versus India

Geoinformatics in animal health and husbandry is now being widely used in several developed countries and its applications are becoming more and more visible as high adaptability, affordability and utility of these technologies are being demonstrated. The readiness to use these technologies is partly because of the availability of veterinary spatial information in these countries. Policies and institutional arrangements exist to use these technologies for developmental purposes. Capacity building infrastructure, in general, is better

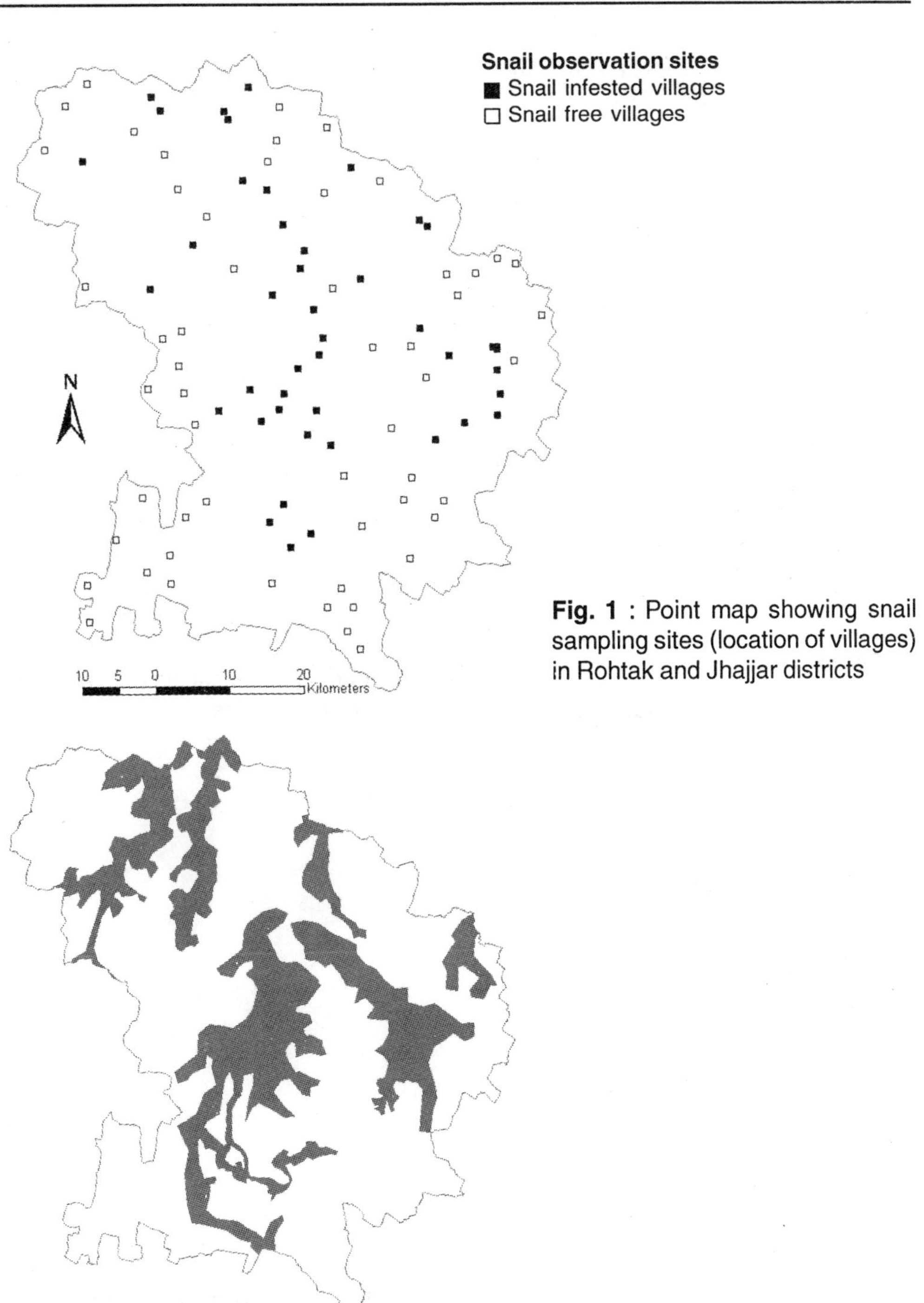

Fig. 1 : Point map showing snail sampling sites (location of villages) in Rohtak and Jhajjar districts

Fig. 2 : Rice growing areas in Rohtak and Jhajjar districts as derived from remotely sensed satellite imagery

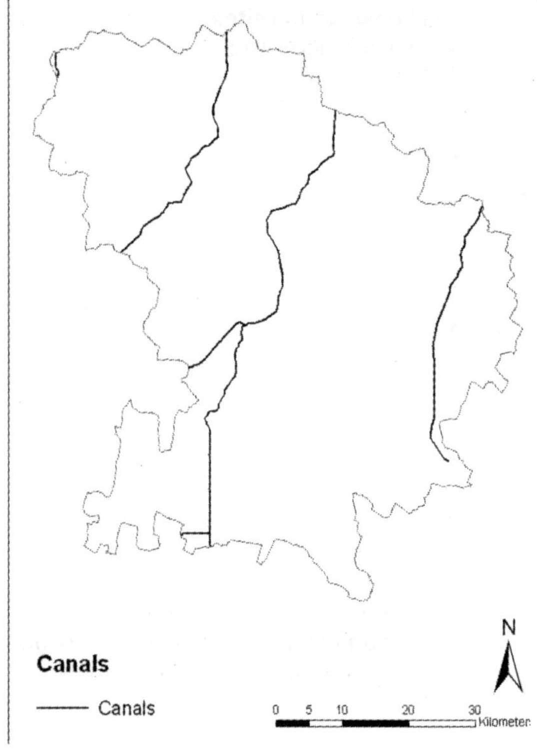

Fig. 3 : Major canals in Rohtak and Jhajjar districts

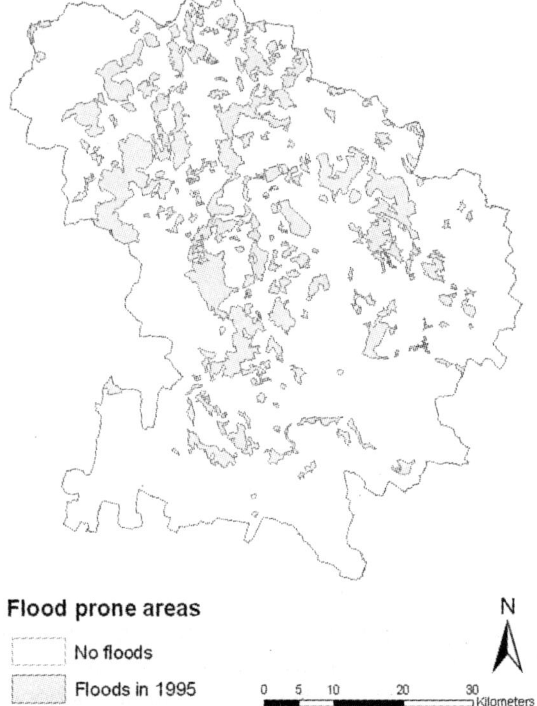

Fig. 4 : Flood prone areas in Rohtak and Jhajjar districts based on remotely sensed satellite imagery where water logging was observed in 1995 floods

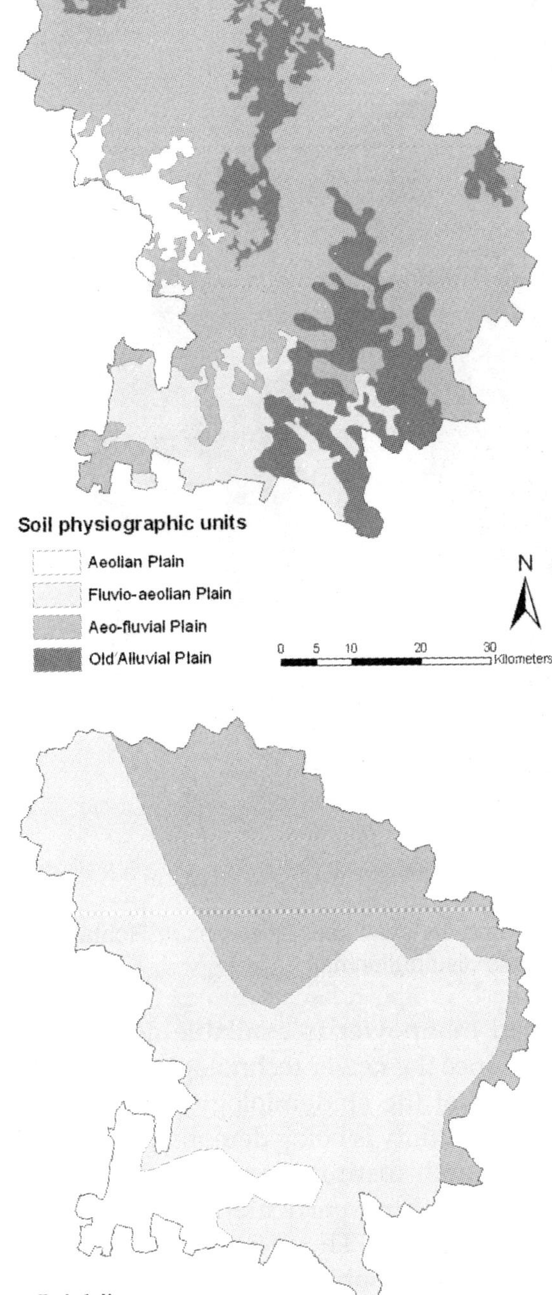

Fig. 5 : Soil physiographic units of Rohtak and Jhajjar districts showing aeolian, fluvio-aeolian, aeofluvial and old alluvial plains

Fig. 6 : Rainfall in Rohtak and Jhajjar districts based on average meteorological records

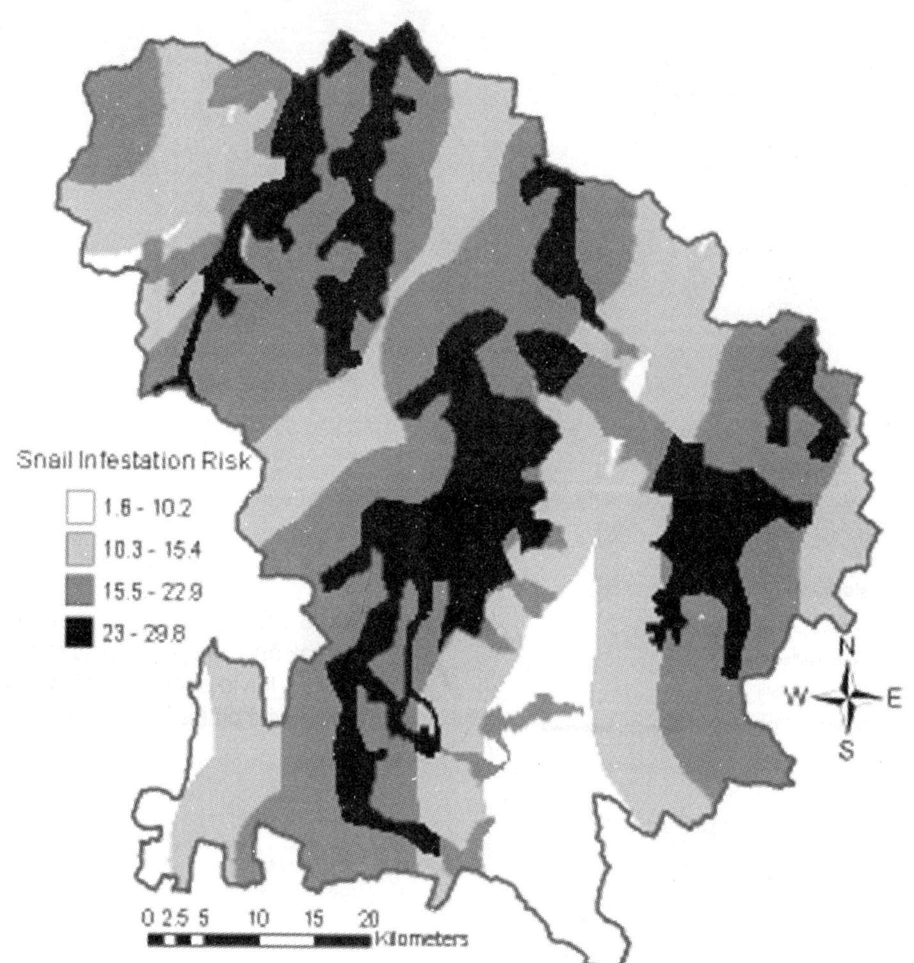

Fig. 7 : Prediction of *Lymnaea* and *Indoplanorbis* snail infestation risk in Rohtak and Jhajjar districts reflecting snail-borne disease distribution risk

placed in developed nations. Trained manpower is available as relevant trainings are organized and conducted once the newer technologies are found useful. GIS and remote sensing are part of the epidemiology postgraduate programmes at several universities. As the utility is being demonstrated, more and more veterinary teaching and research institutes are including these technologies as part of their course curriculum, particularly postgraduate programmes where geoinformatics is relevant. These trainings influence research work, its applications and further publications. However, the publications related to geoinformatics in veterinary science or its gainful applications in animal health are dominated by a few groups in the developed nations obviously due to the spirit of scientific innovation backed by the availability of the required facilities, trained manpower and availability of the spatial data related to animal health which is because of better disease reporting procedures in these countries. Almost all the contributors to the special issues of Advances in Parasitology (2000 and 2006) dedicated to applications of GIS and RS to human and animal health, described by the editors as a 'formidable array of talented research workers' belong to the UK or USA. Such is the dominance of a few advanced laboratories and workers in this area.

It is a technology and knowledge intensive area with a substantial input of training and infrastructure. The data, both remotely sensed and field-collected, are major prerequisite to take advantage of geoinformatics. Quality data from secondary sources related to veterinary science is generally not available in the developing countries while such data is generally available in the advanced nations. This advantage is being reflected in the number of publications from the developed nations and applications of geoinformatics as a decision support system related to animal health and public health. In several advanced countries, the application of geoinformatics has increasingly been used in facilitating epidemiological studies of animal disease outbreaks, disease reporting, monitoring, surveillance, prediction and intervention programmes over the last two decades.

8.1 Indian perspective

Application of geoinformatics in animal health and husbandry is at the initial stage in India. However, its applications in several other fields including agriculture have seen rapid progress. Geoinformatics is not a strong component of either the PD-ADMAS (Project Directorate on Animal Diseases Monitoring and Surveillance) or any of the ICAR research institutes dedicated to animal health and production. There is no unit or centre at national or state level for application of geoinformatics in veterinary sciences. The state space application centers throughout India and several other national centers working under ISRO or Department of Space, Government of India have no component related to veterinary sciences. The state Animal Husbandry Departments or the Commissioner Animal Husbandry, Government of India have no policy framework so far to use geoinformatics as decision support system related to animal health and husbandry.

Geoinformatics is not yet in the curricula of any of the Indian veterinary colleges at graduate level, neither is there as yet any center devoted to the application of RS/GIS to animal health and production. However, a new course on the applications of remote sensing and GIS tools in veterinary parasitology has been accepted in the new course curriculum approved by the ICAR for PhD and these techniques have also been added in Master's course in veterinary parasitology and a PhD course in veterinary epidemiology.

Some publications in this area, particularly in public health, epidemiology and vector-borne diseases, have appeared recently as some enthusiastic medical science workers managed to team up with the persons having required skills and facilities (Sudhakar *et al.* 2006, Bhunia *et al.* 2010) and some concerted efforts by the ICMR (Subbarao and Arora 2010). Publications in veterinary sciences are rare (Sangwan *et al.* 2006, Sangwan 2007). However, application possibilities of geoinformatics in animal health are immense.

The capabilities of the Indian earth-observing satellites to provide quality data at various spatial and temporal resolutions as well as the Indian competence in the information and communication technology (ICT) sector including GIS are well known. Robust spatial data infrastructure determines a country's ability to use geoinformatics effectively and fortunately NSDI (National Spatial Data Infrastructure) is well placed in India (India GeoPortal: www.nsdiindia.org.in). NSDI helps in access, interoperability, sharing and use of spatial data generated by various sources. These factors place India at an advantageous position, however, the link between geoinformatics and veterinary sciences is missing which can only be established by training veterinarians in these emerging fields.

8.2 Comparative analysis

Insufficient human and technical resources are important factors that undermine the ability of developing countries to use spatial information effectively in the planning and management. However, India is not constrained by these two factors. The factors that hinder the application of geoinformatics in animal husbandry sector in the country include apathy of veterinarians to learn and use these techniques, low stock of spatial data, inadequate data recording processes, uncertain data access and exchange mechanism, general lack of awareness in veterinarians and above all, lack of quality spatial data in the field of animal health and husbandry.

9. Constraints and Challenges

While geoinformatics has potential to become a significant component in disease control strategies, it makes substantial demand in terms of data quality, costs, training and development. It requires long-term commitment to data collection. It is demanding in terms of time and attention to familiarize with the tools, methods and concepts of this specialty. To creatively utilize these techniques, a good understanding of geographical and ecological concepts and advanced statistical skills are required. Since these are not taught in veterinary courses at any level, a veterinarian user would always be a late starter. This hinders the application of geoinformatics in veterinary sciences.

However, training and infrastructure development in geoinformatics alone will not be sufficient for the gainful application of these techniques unless we have quality data related to the issues we want to solve. Development of sufficient and relevant veterinary database is a great challenge. Quality data collection faces several constraints including: Inadequate and inconsistent disease reporting procedures, non-computerized (manual) disease recording techniques, disease recording not supported by standard diagnostic tests, poor information networking and poor awareness of the role of geoinformatics in veterinary field. Multidisciplinary and multi-institutional collaboration is often required to bring in all the relevant data to a single platform, which is difficult at times.

Another challenge relates to integration of disease mapping and prediction into disease prevention and control programmes and resource allocation plans. This can be achieved by demonstrating greater practical application of geoinformatics where tangible improvements in prevention and control of diseases are influenced by the spatial analysis of the diseases. Thus, the meaningful applications of geoinformatics in veterinary science depend in strengthening data collection systems and further demonstrating its applicability in real world decision making.

Lack of awareness of veterinary administrators regarding geoinformatics and specialized software requirements are other factors hindering promotion of the application of geoinformatics for disease surveillance, monitoring and control.

10. Developmental Guidelines

10.1 Capacity building

To promote increased awareness and use of RS/GIS in veterinary sciences, multilateral efforts will be required in the training of personnel and equipping of veterinary geoinformatics units. Stronger and closer collaboration between veterinarians and geoinformatics experts to develop expertise to address animal health issues is essential. The international organizations like the OIE, WHO or FAO with their collaborating centers can play a pivotal role in providing technical training and facilitating sharing of experiences and technical resources. Several institutes in India like the Indian Institute of Remote Sensing, Dehradun and the National Remote Sensing Centre, Hyderabad are playing a significant role in capacity building in several application areas of geoinformatics like agriculture, forestry, geology, oceanography, urban planning etc. However, animal health and husbandry has not found the required priority so far. Nevertheless, the same infrastructure for capacity building can be used to train veterinarians. Review of veterinary curriculum to incorporate veterinary geoinformatics at undergraduate and particularly at postgraduate level in epidemiology and parasitology is required. Applications of veterinary geoinformatics in supervised projects of undergraduate and research programmes of postgraduate students is a sure way to introduce geoinformatics expertise amongst veterinarians.

10.2 Improved disease reporting

As discussed earlier, development of sufficient and relevant veterinary database is required. To achieve this, inadequacies of the disease reporting procedures must be removed through evidence supported free and fair disease reporting, computerization, urgency in reporting and inclusion of spatial information in the disease reports. Unfortunately the reporting of contagious and infectious diseases is many times influenced by other factors than the reality about the disease. Such issues should be solved by the state animal husbandry departments to avoid improper reporting. To effectively use geoinformatics, it is vital to have a national veterinary spatial data infrastructure which can provide essential information generated by veterinarians as well as establish partnerships with other data providers to obtain population and environment information. With NSDI well placed in India and the availability of skeleton veterinary infrastructure throughout India, spatial disease reporting procedures should be standardized so that suitable data is available for analysis to make decisions. Incorporating GIS into state and national disease surveillance systems will result into better control strategies.

10.3 Infrastructure development

Sufficient funding for the acquisition of the relevant geoinformatics facilities, software and hardware for education, training and research is required. Funding and equipping a national centre for veterinary geoinformatics as a lead centre and training centre for veterinarians is needed to give directions and develop networks for collaboration. Additionally, promotion of awareness of the indispensable role of veterinary geoinformatics is also needed. Above all, a demonstration of the practical utility of this infrastructure and facilities in solving veterinary problems is needed to secure funding for the infrastructure development.

11. Conclusion

Geoinformatics is the synergy of multiple disciplines, namely, geographic information system (GIS), remote sensing, photogrammetry, cartography, spatial statistics, global positioning system (GPS) and geodesy. It is relevant to all the disciplines which use data identified by their locations. Geoinformatics represent new tools for the study of epidemiology of diseases. Spatial epidemiological studies will become increasingly common in the future, both because of the instant visual appeal in the form of maps and the wide availability of the new geoinformatics techniques for describing, exploring, analyzing and modeling the disease data for predictive purposes. With the ongoing improvements in the data and methodologies, the new techniques will play an increasingly important role in our understanding of the complex relationships between environment and health at scales varying from local to global. While geoinformatics has potential to become a significant component in disease control strategies, it makes substantial demand in terms of data quality, costs, training and development. The capability of the Indian Earth observing satellites to provide quality data at various spatial and temporal resolutions as well as the Indian competence in ICT sector including GIS place India at an advantageous position, however, the link between geoinformatics and veterinary sciences is missing which can only be established by training veterinarians in these emerging fields.To utilize the new techniques, development of a sufficient and relevant veterinary database is required. To achieve this, inadequacies of the disease reporting procedures must be addressed. Funding and equipping a national centre for veterinary geoinformatics for research and training of veterinarians is needed to give directions and develop networks for collaboration. Strengthening of data collection systems is required for meaningful applications of geoinformatics and further demonstrating its applicability in real world decision making in veterinary sciences.

References

1. Bailey TC, Gatrell AC (1995). Interactive Spatial Data Analysis. Longman, Harlow, UK.
2. Bergquist R, Rinaldi L (2010). Health research based on geospatial tools: a timely approach in changing environment. J Helminthol 84:1-11.
3. Bhunia GS, Kumar V, Kumar AJ, Das P, Kesari S (2010). The use of remote sensing in the identification of the eco-environmental factors associated with the risk of humanvisceral leishmaniasis (kala-azar) on the Gangetic plain in north-eastern India. Annals Trop Med Parasitol 104:35-53
4. Biggeri A, Catelan D, Dreassi E, Lagazio C, Cringoli G (2004). Statistical models for spatial analysis in parasitology. Parassitologia 46:75-78.
5. Brooker S (2002). Schistosomes, snails and satellites. Acta Tropica 82:209-216.
6. Brooker S, Clements ACA, Bundy DAP (2006). Global epidemiology, ecology and control of soil transmitted helminth infections. Adv Parasitol 62:221-261.
7. Brooker S, Michael E (2000). The potential of geographical information systems and remote sensing in the epidemiology and control of human helminth infections. Adv Parasitol 47:246-279.

8. Carabin H, Escalona M, Marshall C, Vivas-Martinez S, Botto C, Joseph L, Basanez MG (2003). Prediction of community prevalence of human onchocerciasis in the Amazonian onchocerciasis focus: Bayesian approach. Bull WHO 81:482-490.

9. Ceccato P, Connor SJ, Jeanne I, Thomson MC (2005). Application of Geographical Information Systems and Remote Sensing technologies for assessing and monitoring malaria risk. Parassitologia 47:81-96.

10. Conraths FJ, Staubach C, Tackmann K (2003). Statistics and sample design in epidemiological studies of *Echinococcus multilocularis* in fox populations. Acta Trop 85:183-189.

11. Cringoli G, Malone JB, Rinaldi L (2005a). Guest editors' preface. Parassitologia 47:3-4.

12. Cringoli G, Rinaldi L, Veneziano V, Musella V (2005b). Disease mapping and risk assessment in veterinary parasitology: some case studies. Parassitologia (Roma) 47:9-25.

13. Cringoli G, Taddei R, Rinaldi L, Veneziano V, Musella, V, Cascone C, Sibilio G, Malone JB (2004). Use of remote sensing and geographical information systems to identify environmental features that influence the distribution of paramphistomosis in sheep from the southern Italian Apennines. Vet Parasitol 122:15-26.

14. Curran PJ, Atkinson PM, Foody GM, Milton EJ (2000). Linking remote sensing, land cover and disease. Adv Parasitol 47:37-80.

15. Daniel M, Kolar J, Zeman P (2004). GIS tools for tick and tick-borne disease occurrence. Parasitol 129 (Suppl.):329-352.

16. Durr PA (2004). Spatial epidemiology and animal diseases: introduction and overview. In: Durr PA and Gatrell AC (eds) GIS and spatial analysis in veterinary science. CABI Publishing, UK, p. 35-67.

17. Durr PA, Gatrell AC (2004a). GIS and spatial analysis in veterinary science. CABI Publishing, UK, pp. 303.

18. Durr PA, Gatrell AC (2004b). The tools of spatial epidemiology: GIS, Spatial Analysis and Remote Sensing. In: Durr PA and Gatrell AC (eds) GIS and spatial analysis in veterinary science. CABI Publishing, UK, p. 1-33.

19. French NP, White PCL (2004). The use of GIS in modelling the spatial and temporal spread of animal diseases. In: Durr PA, Gatrell AC (eds) GIS and spatial analysis in veterinary science. CABI Publishing, p. 177-203.

20. Fuller CE (1972). Public Health Implications of Remote Sensing. Final Report, NASA contract NAS-9-11522.Houston, TX: University of Texas, School of Public Health.

21. Genchi C, Rinaldi L, Cascone C, Mortarino M, Cringoli G (2005). Is heartworm disease really spreading in Europe? Vet Parasitol 133:137-148.

22. Goodchild MF (2000). Communicating geographic information in a digital age. Ann Assoc Am Geogr 90:344-355.

23. Guerra CA, Snow RW, Hay SI (2006). Defining the Global Spatial Limits of Malaria Transmission in 2005. Adv Parasitol 62:157-179

24. Hay SI, Omumbo JA, Craig MH, Snow RW (2000). Earth observation, geographic information systems and *Plasmodium falciparum* malaria in sub-Saharan Africa. Adv Parasitol 47:173-215.

25. Hendrickx G, Biesemans J, de Deken R (2004). The use of GIS in veterinary parasitology. In: Durr PA, Gatrell AC (eds) GIS and spatial analysis in veterinary science. CABI Publishing. p. 145-176.

26. Kistemann T, Dangendorf F, Schweikart J (2002). New perspectives on the use of Geographical Information Systems (GIS) in environmental health sciences. Int J Hyg Environ Health 205:169-181.

27. Kleinschmidt I, Bagayoko M, Clarke GP, Craig M, Le Sueur D (2000). A spatial statistical approach to malaria mapping. Int J Epidemiol 29:355-361.

28. Lessard P, L'Eplattenier R, Norval RAI, Kundert K, Dolan TT, Croze H, Walker JB, Irvin AD, Perry BD (1990). Geographical information systems for studying the epidemiology of cattle diseases caused by *Theileria parva*. Vet Rec 126:255-262.

29. Linthicum KJ, Bailey CL, Glyn Davies F, Tucker CJ (1987). Detection of Rift Valley fever viral activity in Kenya by satellite remote sensing imagery. Science 235:1656-1659.

30. Nicholson MC, Mather TN (1996). Methods for evaluating Lyme disease risks using geographic information systems and geospatial analysis. J Med Entomol 33:711-720.

31. Pfeiffer DU (2004). Geographical information science and spatial analysis in animal health. In: Durr PA, Gatrell AC (eds). GIS and spatial analysis in veterinary science. CABI Publishing, UK. p. 119-144.

32. Pfeiffer DU, Robinson TP, Stevenson M, Stevens KB, Rogers DJ, Clements ACA (2008). Spatial analysis in epidemiology. Oxford University Press. p.140.

33. Pleydell DR, Raoul F, Tourneux F, Danson FM, Graham AJ, Craig PS, Giraudoux P (2004). Modelling the spatial distribution of *Echinococcus multilocularis* infection in foxes. Acta Trop 91:253-265.

34. Randolph SE (2000). Ticks and tick-borne disease systems in space and from space. Adv Parasitol 47: 130-173.

35. Raso G, Vounatsou P, Singer BH, N'Goran EK, Tanner M, Utzinger J (2006). An integrated approach for risk profiling and spatial prediction of *Schistosoma mansoni* - hookworm co-infection. Proc Natl Acad Sci USA 103:6934-6939.

36. Rinaldi L, Cascone C, Sibilio G, Musella V, Taddei R, Cringoli G (2004). Geographical information systems and remote sensing technologies in parasitological epidemiology. Parassitologia 46:71-74.

37. Rinaldi L, Musella V, Biggeri A, Cringoli G (2006). New insights into the application of geographical information systems and remote sensing in veterinary parasitology. Geospatial Health 1:33-47.

38. Rinaldi L, Musella V, Ghenchi C, Cringoli G (2007). Geographical information systems in health applications: Experience on filariosis. Mappe Parassitologiche 8:19-38.

39. Rogers DJ (2000). Satellite, space, time and African trypanosomosis. Adv Parasitol 47:130-173.

40. Rogers DJ, Randolph SE (1991). Mortality rates and population density of tsetse flies correlated with satellite imagery. Nature 351:739-741.

41. Sangwan AK (2007). Snail-borne parasitic diseases of livestock: Mapping of risk prone areas using RS and GIS techniques (A case study of a part of eastern Doon Valley). Project report, Indian Institute of Remote Sensing, Dehradoon, p. 24.

42. Sangwan AK, Prasad J, Siroha GP, Hooda RS (2006). Application of remote sensing and geographic information system (GIS) for mapping snail-borne livestock diseases in Haryana. Proc 17th Natl Cong Vet Parasitol, Pondicherry, p. 70-71.

43. Sciarretta A, Girma M, Tikubet G, Belayehun L, Ballo S, Baumgartner J (2005). Development of an adaptive tsetse population management scheme for the Luke community, Ethiopia. J Med Entomol 42:1006-1019.

44. Subbarao SK, Arora R (Eds.), (2010). Application of GIS and RS technologies in epidemiology and control of vector-borne diseases. ICMR, New Delhi. ISBN: 81-901-853-9-X

45. Sudhakar S, Srinivas T, Palit A, Kar SK, Bhattacharya SK (2006). Mapping risk prone areas of Kala-azar (visceral leishmaniasis) in parts of Bihar state, India: an RS and GIS approach. J Vector Borne Dis 43:115-122.

46. Thomson MC, Obsomer V, Kamgno J, Gardon J, Wanji S, Takougang I, Enyong P, Remme JH, Molyneux DH, Boussinesq M (2004). Mapping the distribution of Loa loa in Cameroon in support of the African Programme for Onchocerciasis Control. Filaria J 3:7.

47. Vezzani D, Carbajo AE (2006). Spatial and temporal transmission risk of *Dirofilaria immitis* in Argentina. Int J Parasitol 36:1463-1472.

48. Zhang ZY, Xu DZ, Zhou XN, Zhou Y, Liu SJ (2005). Remote sensing and spatial statistical analysis to predict the distribution of *Oncomelania hupensis* in the marshlands of China. Acta Trop 96:205-212.

□□□

Chapter 24

Ethnoveterinary Medicine

N. PUNNIAMURTHY
Ethnoveterinary Herbal Training and Research Unit, Veterinary University Training and Research Centre, Tamil Nadu Veterinary and Animal Sciences University, Thanjavur-613006

Contents

1. Introduction

Veterinary healthcare is not just a scientific matter; it is also an economic and social issue. Veterinary inspectors in British-India had then pointed out the expensive nature of 'European drugs' and the unavailability of the same in rural areas (Hirachandra 1924). Some earlier Indian veterinarians also expressed similar views (Krishnamurthi 1946, Krishnaswamy 1945, Parera 1941) and studied specific local treatments (Mushtaq 1926, Naidu 1933).

The core of the present day global medicine is based on traditional medicines. Plant species have been recorded as possessing medicinal properties and used for healing in traditional medical systems globally for the past at least 2500 years. These have been evaluated by modern scientific methods and found to possess the suggested medicinal properties in experimental models. Among the 300,000 plant species identified and listed, only 5 to 10% have been chemically investigated. Though a lot of indigenous knowledge is already well documented and subjected to evaluation, yet some of this knowledge exists only in folk traditions generally beyond the reach of the laboratory oriented academia.

According to the World Health Organisation (WHO), 'traditional medicine' constitutes a vague term used to distinguish any ancient or culture-based healthcare practice from the modern medicine. Traditional medicine involves those systems which are currently regarded as indigenous and includes popular and codified Asian systems that are well documented since ancient times, for example, Siddha, Ayurveda, Chinese, Unani and Tibb medical systems as well as the less widespread, largely orally transmitted practices (ethnomedicine) used by traditional communities.

Despite the worldwide importance of traditional medicine, attitudes have been largely skeptical towards these diverse, culture-based holistic systems of medicine.

2. Ancient Treatises on Animals

Animal healthcare has been an integral part of Indian tradition with rich indigenous knowledge. Many ancient treatises on upkeep of domestic animals are available. The Emperor Ashoka (300 BC) erected the first known veterinary hospitals of the world. It is a common knowledge that cultivation of herbal medicines for man and animals in his empire and adjoining kingdoms was ordered by him. Some of the common treatises on animals of ancient times include *Hastya Ayurveda, Agni Puran, Mutangalila, Asva Shastra, Gaja Shastra Sara, Krishi Sukti, Brihat Samhitha, Sarabendra Vaidya Muraikal, Maadugal Kuthiraikal, Paravaikal Lakshanamum, Vaithyamum* and *Pasu Vaidya Mattu Vagadam.* The term *mattu vagadam* (treatise on cattle medicine) refers to the compilation of various clinical practices employed for the prevention and treatment of diseases in cattle, originally recorded in palm scripts by traditional healers. Saraswathi Mahal Library in Thanjavur (Tamil Nadu) has brought into print the compilations collected by Raja Serfoji II (1798-1832), the then king of Thanjavur.

Though it is not fair to compare the traditional classification of diseases and their course in animals with the modern one on a word to word basis; it is there for everyone to see that there are many diseases described in such detail that they may be compared to modern day terms such as rinderpest, anthrax etc. *Mattu vagadams* contains information concerning recording of morbid conditions of cattle, horses, goats, sheep and fowls which is comparable to modern day classification of diseases in livestock (Parameswaran 1983).

3. Ethnoveterinary Medicine

Ethnoveterinary medicine includes the indigenous knowledge, skills, methods, and practices pertaining to the healthcare of animals. Indigenous knowledge systems have proven to be dynamic and adaptive with the qualities of simplicity, functionality, integrative holism and sustainability. The efforts by individuals and institutions in the recent past to revive the traditional systems of veterinary healthcare on scientific lines have been sporadic and ephemeral.

The desperate and resource-poor livestock farmers have kept alive and continue to use the vibrant and dynamic traditional medicine system. Use of indigenous/traditional veterinary medicine is a cost effective treatment alternative for livestock farmers who maintain only a few heads of livestock, especially in primary healthcare for sustainable livestock production. Ethnoveterinary medicine practices and preparations are apparently time tested, readily available, location specific, resource specific, species specific and environment friendly while the livestock farmers in many situations are self-reliant (Jain and Srivastava 1999, Ghotge *et al.* 2002, Punniamurthy 2009, Punniamurthy and Udayasurian 2010).

The resource constrained village farmers, who do not have access to either modern medicine or cost effective control measures, rely on ancestral indigenous knowledge to deal with the diseases of their livestock and poultry. Most ethnoveterinary practices employ natural products of plant origin for prevention and treatment of livestock diseases (Ghotge *et al.* 2002).

Not until the 1980s did many western-world researchers and developers begin to take a sustained scientific interest in traditional livestock healthcare systems and related management practices (McCorkle 1986), but in the last few years, efforts for pharmacological and clinical validation of herbal preparations have resulted in a number of scientific publications on ethnoveterinary medicine (Jain and Srivastava 1999, Mathias 2004, Nair and Punniamurthy 2010).

4. Choice of Treatment Alternatives for the Farmers

Characteristics of the disease, especially the frequency of a disease, can influence the choice of treatment. The need to search for the alternative drug formulations in the plant kingdom for therapeutic use in veterinary medicine is exemplified by the following fact. While the antimicrobial drugs are in use for the last sixty years, mastitis still exists as an enormous and difficult problem that continues to engage the attention of research workers throughout the world. In areas where there is improved sanitation and machine milking the focus has, however, shifted from streptococcal mastitis to staphylococcal mastitis. Antimicrobial chemotherapy is a prolonged and a costly practice.

The issue of widespread use of antimicrobials and the associated drug residues and antimicrobial resistance problems, looming large on the Indian horizon, there is an urgent need to look into herbal remedies for veterinary healthcare. Research to make available as many options as possible, including both traditional and modern knowledge is needed (Padmakumar 1997, Ghotge *et al.* 2002, Punniamurthy 2002, 2005).

5. Herbal Preparations for Clinical Situations

During the last few decades, there has been a resurgence of interest in plants as sources of medicines and of novel molecules for use in the elucidation of physiological/biochemical phenomena. There are a number of reasons for this. First, there is the genuine expectation in developing countries that their drug problems can be alleviated through a sensible scientific exploitation of medicinal plants, some of which have been used for generations by indigenous populations. All the major traditional medicine systems approach illness first by trying to support and induce the self-healing process of the person. If recovery can occur from this, the likelihood of adverse effect and the need for high-impact, high-cost intervention is reduced. It is this orientation towards self-healing and health promotion (salutogenesis rather than pathogenesis) that makes traditional medicine especially attractive.

Practicing veterinarians in the field have reported problems related to failures and untoward effects with antimicrobial chemotherapy especially in commercial poultry establishments and there are occasions when desperate farm owners resort to traditional remedies (Udayasurian 2004). The use of turmeric (*Curcuma longa*) powder administered in feed for broiler chicken as protection against mycotoxicoses-induced hepatotoxicity and fresh extract of the plant *Tridax procumbens* during beak trimming to stop bleeding in layer chicken are reported in large commercial poultry operations. Use of neem oil (*Azadirachta indica*) with camphor externally and the paste made of neem leaves, garlic, pepper, tulsi, turmeric powder internally help out small scale turkey farmers in outbreaks of pox of moderate nature in turkey poults. Several fresh herbal traditional remedies assessed for primary healthcare have helped in safeguarding the interests of the rural livestock holders and the society at large with safe animal products free from antimicrobial residues (Udayasurian and Punniamurthy 2004, Nair and Punniamurthy 2010).

6. Chemistry of Herbs

Within any traditional society, the range of plants used in the treatment of common ailments is generally extremely broad, the species used often representing a large number of plant families. The plant secondary metabolites used in traditional herbal medicine are chemically extremely diverse and are isolated from a wide range of plant taxa.

6.1 Terpenoids

The terpenoids, with more than 30,000 metabolites, is the most diverse class of plant secondary compounds. Simple molecules like isoprene or isopentane combine to form terpenes, containing multiples of the basic 5-carbon molecules, making up the volatile oils. As they are transported and distributed throughout the body, they act locally and on the whole system. When they are used internally or externally, they soon show up in the urinary system, the lungs and the bronchi, and in secretions like sweat, saliva, tears or the vaginal fluids and in milk or travel through the placenta to the foetus. Besides their direct antiseptic action, they stimulate the production of white blood cells, thereby augmenting the body's own natural defence system.

6.2 Phenolic compounds

Phenol is a basic building block of many important plant constituents. Phenolic compounds may be simple in structure, or a complex combination of a range of basic molecules. These are ubiquitous in plants which collectively synthesize several thousand different chemical structures characterized by hydroxylated aromatic ring(s). They represent a striking example of metabolic plasticity enabling plants to adapt to changing biotic and abiotic environments and provide to plant products colour, taste, technological properties and putative health promoting benefits. One of the simple phenolics is salicylic acid. This chemical has antiseptic, pain killing and anti-inflammatory properties. Eugenol, the pain-killing oil found in cloves, and thymol present in oil of thyme both have effects similar to salicylic acid.

6.3 Tannins

Tannins in herbs cause an astringent action. They act on proteins and some other chemicals and form a protective layer on the skin and the mucous membranes. Thus they can, for instance, bind the tissue of the gut and reduce diarrhoea or internal bleeding. Externally they are useful in the treatment of burns, for sealing wounds and to reduce inflammation. Tannins help in infections of the eye (conjunctivitis), mouth, vagina, cervix and rectum.

6.4 Flavonoids

Flavonoids are nearly ubiquitous in plants and are recognized as the pigments responsible for the colors of leaves. They are low molecular weight compounds composed of a three-ring structure with various substitutions. This basic structure is shared by tocopherols (vitamin E). Over 4000 structurally unique flavonoids have been identified in plant sources. The flavonoids are found in fruits, vegetables, nuts, seeds, herbs, spices, stems and flowers. They are usually subdivided according to their substituents into flavanols, anthocyanidins, and flavones, flavanones and chalcones. The flavonoids have long been recognized to possess anti-inflammatory, antioxidant, antiallergic, hepatoprotective, antithrombotic, antiviral and anticarcinogenic activities. The bioflavonoids are also essential for the complete absorption of vitamins and occur in nature wherever vitamin C is present.

6.5 Alkaloids

The important function of alkaloids in plants is possibly to discourage grazing by herbivores. The alkaloids are very diverse in structure and have a marked physiological activity upon the living system. There are alkaloids that act on the liver, nerves, lungs and digestive system. Many of the valued herbs contain these potent chemicals.

6.6 Bitter principles

The bitter principles chemically show a wide diversity of structure, with most bitters belonging to the iridoids, some to the terpenes and some to other groups. The bitter principles have been shown to have valuable therapeutic effects. Through a reflex action via the taste buds, they stimulate the secretion of digestive juices and also stimulate the activity of the liver, aiding hepatic elimination.

6.7 Synergy of phytochemicals

There are significant synergetic effects in plant extracts and, therefore, under field conditions, it is justifiable to use the crude plant extract rather than a single purified chemical (Wagner 2004). The biological diversity that synergistically constitutes the living world is complex beyond understanding and valuable beyond our ability to measure. Indigenous concepts recognize that environmental sustainability and diversity are ecologically linked. This is because diversity offers a multiplicity and synergism of interactions, which can safeguard and if necessary, heal any part of the system. The synergy of phytochemicals has proved to be effective in the clinical management of livestock diseases (Nair and Punniamurthy 2010).

7. Conservation and Development of Ethnoveterinary Knowledge

Loss of ethnoveterinary knowledge must be curtailed through increased research within the logic of local strategies while dissemination of the results in local language should be taken up. For example, thesis research on traditional livestock systems and ethnoveterinary knowledge can be undertaken. Ethnomanagement and ethnoveterinary medicine should become regular courses in academic curricula. This however does not mean abandoning western thought process altogether. A pragrnatic approach lies in rationalising the indigenous knowledge in the social and cultural milieu where the livestock production system, if it exists, means subsistence rather than imitating western standards (Punniamurthy 2002, Nair and Punniamurthy 2010).

The study of ethnoveterinary medicine may be broadly divided into four main approaches:

- Understanding traditional concepts of livestock health, disease and management practices
- Ethnobotany, identification and application of plants used in traditional ethnoveterinary medicine practices
- Ethnopharmacology/toxicology of traditional remedies and pre-clinical assessment
- Use of natural products of plant origin in livestock health, production and protection

8. Constraints

A major issue to be sorted out in ethnoveterinary medicine related healthcare is diagnosis, particularly differential diagnosis. By nature, veterinary disease diagnosis is a challenging area with little scope for objective clinical signs especially under field conditions. The practice of herbal medicine in livestock diseases without the support of modern veterinary diagnostics would complicate the treatment.

Another major reason that has put the traditional system of medicine on the defensive is that a number of genuine practices which have apparently stood the test of time for centuries have been tarnished by a flurry of unqualified claims by persons not properly trained in the traditional system of medicine. It is quite common to encounter such herbal preparations falsely claiming to be effective against a variety of clinical conditions in commercial livestock and poultry farming. Despite their logical and clinical success, EVM preparations are often shown in poor light for want of an effective regulatory system to ensure quality and efficacy of the poly herbal preparations.

9. Conclusion

Ethnoveterinary medicine practices and preparations are time tested, readily available, location specific, resource specific, species specific, environment friendly and suitable for the poor livestock farmers. Conditions like wounds and inflammation, gastroenteritis, rumen disorders, endoparasitisms, ectoparasitism, reproductive disorders, mastitis, dermatitis and other infectious conditions of livestock in the rural area respond to traditional approaches using local herbs, for which, preparations have been validated with varying levels of success under field conditions. Disseminating ethnoveterinary medicine will help to conserve biological diversity of the precious herbs and to propagate the knowledge on herbal medicine, which will empower farmers in primary animal healthcare in rural India. Ethnoveterinary medicine is a cost effective, culturally acceptable, scientifically valid and environmentally sound idea for sustainable livestock production. Yet there is a continued loss of invaluable ethnoveterinary knowledge.

It is essential to save and use the age-old wisdom on animal production and healthcare by open-minded inquiry and not lose it by indifferent attitude. Efforts are required to revitalize the traditional veterinary healthcare systems at local and regional levels. It has been observed that veterinarians show interest in the medicinal plants employed in ethnoveterinary medicine. This trend in favour of herbs is partly due to the antimicrobial drug resistance and partly due to the demand for safe (organic) foods of animal origin. Under Indian conditions, largely the rural scenario today has many similarities with the past, for good, where livestock production is by and large organic in the villages. The future of Indian farming system needs 'moderate inputs and reasonable outputs' approach to conserve natural resources. The 'one world one health' concept is now advocated globally. It is high time that we learnt the positive aspects of the traditional/ancient systems of medicine and make them integrated into the mainstream medicine.

References

1. Ghotge NS, Ramdas SR, Ashalata S, Mathur NP, Broome VG, Sanyasi Rao ML (2002). A social approach to the validation of traditional veterinary remedies -The Anthra Project. Trop Animal Health Prod 34(2):121-143.
2. Hirachandra (1924). Indigenous drugs of certain ailments of livestock. Indian Vet J 1(1):100-103.
3. Jain SK, Srivastava S (1999). Dictionary of ethnoveterinary plants of India. Deep Publications, New Delhi.
4. Krishnamurthi A (1946). Indigenous drugs of India, their veterinary and economic aspects. Indian Vet J 23(2): 375-385.
5. Krishnaswamy A (1945). What a veterinarian can learn from the ancient Indian veterinarian. Indian Vet J 22(4):388-410.
6. Mathias E (2004). Ethnoveterinary medicine: Harnessing its potential. Vet Bull 74(8):27N-37N.
7. McCorkle CM (1986). An introduction to ethnoveterinary research and development. J Ethnobiology 6(1):129-149.
8. Mushtaq A (1926). Asafoetida in the treatment of wounds. Indian Vet J 13(1): 35-45.
9. Naidu NK (1933). How sheep pox vaccination is conducted by a quack. Indian Vet J 10(3): 278.
10. Nair MNB, Punniamurthy N (2010). (Eds) Proceedings International Conference on Ethnoveterinary Practices, 4-6 January 2010, Thanjavur.
11. Padmakumar V (1997). Ethnoveterinary medicine in Kerala (South India) Proceedings International Conference Vol. 1, 4-6 November 1997, Pune.
12. Paramsewaran K (1983). Siddha medicine for cattle diseases. In: Siddha Medicine. International Institute of Tamil Studies, Chennai.
13. Parera HC (1941). Indigenous drugs in the treatment of livestock. Indian Vet J 17:261-265.
14. Punniamurthy N (2002). Ethno-veterinary medicine practices for primary healthcare of livestock: Issues and strategies. Siddha International Congress, Gandeepam, Tamil Nadu.
15. Punniamurthy N (2005). Ethno-veterinary medicine: Use of fresh herbal extracts under field conditions for primary veterinary health care in India. Proceedings Fourth International Congress of Ethnobotany, 21-26 August 2005, Istanbul, Turkey, pp 249-255.
16. Punniamurthy N (2009). Ethnoveterinary medicine - Using fresh herbals for livestock health care at farmers' level. Proceedings World Conference on Medicinal and Aromatic Plants, November 2008, Capetown, South Africa.

17. Punniamurthy N, Udayasurian K (2010). Ethnoveterinary medicine for veterinary primary health care. International Conference on Ethnoveterinary Practices, 4-6 January 2010, Thanjavur.

18. Udayasurian K (2004). Problems in chemotherapy with commercial flocks of chicken. Personal communication.

19. Udayasurian K, Punniamurthy N (2004). Resurgence of indigenous practices in commercial chicken establishments. Field Report.

20. Wagner H (2004). Natural products chemistry and phytomedicine research in the new millennium: New developments and challenges. ARKIVOC 2004(vii):277-284.

□□□

Chapter 25

Surveillance in Veterinary Medicine

L. GUNASEELAN
Department of Veterinary Public Health and Epidemiology, Madras Veterinary College, Tamil Nadu Veterinary and Animal Sciences University, Chennai-600007

Contents

1. Introduction

Surveillance is simply an observation of a situation and refers to the observation of diseases and disease processes. The purpose of surveillance is, therefore, basically to define the presence or absence of a disease in population. This can also include the location, category or type of the affected population, and season. Although surveillance initially focused on infectious diseases, recently it has gone on to add noninfectious conditions too which include both surgical and medical disorders. Surveillance systems thus consist of continuous and systematic use of the routinely collected data to guide action in a timely manner. Besides this, surveillance can also watch for health events (e.g. deaths from a disease or new cases of a disease) and health services (e.g. visits to a veterinarian, hospital admissions, vaccination, surgery, provision of prescribed drugs) as they occur.

Some systems collect information on risk factors related to various diseases, including food, water supply and drug use, while other systems measure environmental factors (e.g. air, food, or water quality) independently. It must be borne in mind that surveillance differs from occasional surveys for diseases and planned research programmes.

2. History of Surveillance Activities

Prevailing governments have assumed the responsibility over the years to identify, control and prevent diseases in populations. Though the understanding of these disease processes were incomplete at times, the illnesses were closely monitored, regulations were passed for recommended operations such as safe burials, food handling, protected water supplies and preventing pollution of public areas.

The first known use of the word surveillance was in 1802 and it was derived from the French word - *surveiller*, meaning to *watch over*. The first health surveillance activity was attributed to John Gaunt, who first summarized causes of death in London in 1662. The modern concepts of surveillance were however developed by William Farr in Great Britain who was responsible for possibly the first comprehensive mortality and morbidity statistics the public in England.

In the twentieth century, there were significant gains in global health as a result of immunization, which was made possible because of routine surveillance of infectious diseases. The continued surveillance after the introduction of vaccines monitored the effectiveness of immunization programmes. Perhaps the most impressive example of this was the World

Health Organization (WHO) programme for the elimination of smallpox. This programme involved intensive worldwide surveillance to identify all suspected cases of smallpox. Specialized teams then confirmed the diagnosis and instituted immunization programmes in the population surrounding each case. Surveillance data were also used by many countries to justify elimination of routine smallpox vaccination programmes as the number of new cases diminished. This public health programme directed by surveillance led to the eventual elimination of smallpox in 1977.

Most countries publish national data on a weekly or monthly basis for communicable diseases, and annually for causes of death. In these ways, health surveillance provides health departments and related agencies with ongoing measurements of health of populations. These are some examples concerning human health management.

In veterinary medicine, surveillance means at a minimum that veterinarians and diagnostic laboratories report every instance of certain disease or pathogens they detect. Emerging animal and zoonotic diseases and increasing international trade have resulted in an increased demand for veterinary surveillance systems.

3. Veterinary Surveillance

Veterinary surveillance describes everything that is to be done to collect information on diseases affecting animals and arrange to get the information to concerned agencies. It is to be understood that it is not just to do with farm animals, but pets and wildlife too. Veterinary surveillance is not just about the diseases caused by bacteria and viruses but the animal welfare problems and poisonings also form a part of the veterinary surveillance activities. Animals can also carry infections that can be a threat to humans too (zoonoses).

Surveillance has been defined by major world organizations as given below.

- The continuous investigation of a given population to detect the occurrence of disease for control purposes, which may involve testing of a part of the population - World Organization for Animal Health (OIE, Office International des Epizooties)
- Systematic ongoing collection, collation and analysis of data and the timely dissemination of information to those who need to know so that action can be taken - World Health Organization (WHO)

- The ongoing systematic collection, analysis and interpretation of health data, essential to the planning, implementation and evaluation of public health practice, closely integrated with timely dissemination of these data to those who need to know - US Centers for Disease Control and Prevention (CDC)

Veterinary surveillance involves a combination of all the efforts listed below.

- Collection of data
- Analysis of the data
- Interpretation
- Dissemination
- Initiating action

No single action can provide the desired results.

4. Role of Veterinary Surveillance

Surveillance is an epidemiological practice which can serve to be a sentinel or watch dog for natural infectious disease epidemics. The main role includes:

4.1 Predict

Normally we get the information about the disease when it has occurred in the population. However, we can predict the disease in advance when there are conditions suitable for a particular disease to occur. For example, an abundant snail population, conducive moisture for their survival, susceptible sheep is more than likely to result in liver fluke problem.

4.2 Observe

To predict we need to observe the prevailing situation, the susceptible population and the risk factors for the disease.

4.3 Minimize

Following prediction of a possible disease event and observing the factors that are likely to be responsible, action plan may be devised to minimize or totally prevent the event.

4.4. Increase awareness

The increased awareness prepares the veterinarian for overcoming the upcoming problems or planning for action to prevent and control the disease.

For example, in case of an outbreak of salmonellosis in a dairy herd, it can be predicted that the food poisoning organism *Salmonella* may get into milk. So, preventive measures can be taken well in time. Similarly detection of a disease such as foot and mouth disease (FMD) at an early stage helps to stop its spread and eliminate it from the herd. Likewise, early detection of any unusual or a new disease such as spongiform encephalopathy, SARS, Nipah virus etc. require active surveillance set ups in veterinary medicine. We may also need to carryout research urgently in such conditions to evaluate the extent of threat they may cause to animals and human beings.

We, therefore, need to conduct surveillance activities in populations so that we can detect important or unusual conditions as quickly as possible. This is to make sure that we can take any action that may be needed. Some diseases may confirm contamination of the animal's feed or water. This could alert us to an environmental problem. The countries to which we export animals or animal products may want us to prove that certain diseases are absent to rule out the risk of bringing a disease into their own country by importing animals or products from us. Similarly, other countries may have certain diseases that are not present here. The import of animals from such countries may result in the entry of new infectious agents into our geographical area. Dogs and cats taken abroad may also bring back some new infections. Our quarantine stations play role in preventing entry of such exotic diseases.

Diseases or infections in the wildlife also highlight possible threat to farm animals. It is also, therefore, an important facet of veterinary surveillance. Certain animal infections may pose risk of contaminants getting into human food. Monitoring diseases also helps us to detect situations where changes in the way animals are kept cause deterioration in animal welfare.

Veterinary surveillance covers other areas too. For example, there is growing concern about the development and spread of resistance to drugs that are used to treat infections in both animals and people (antimicrobial resistance or AMR). The classical example can be the recent NDM-1 gene i.e. New Delhi metallo-beta-lactamase bacteria which are found to be resistant to carbapenems that are used as a last resort antibiotic in emergencies. It means that surveillance of AMR is a high priority.

The use of veterinary medicines may occasionally cause unexpected reactions in the treated animals. These 'suspected adverse reactions' are monitored and reported. Some medicines that are used to treat food producing animals or fish may leave residues if the correct withdrawal period (the time elapsing between treatment and slaughter) is not followed. Surveillance is carried out to detect possible residues in meat, fish, eggs, honey and milk.

5. Veterinary Surveillance in India

In view of the increasing concern in the above areas, a $100 million World Bank project was launched in India in 2004 to form the backbone for a surveillance system in the same scale as the US Centers for Disease Control and Prevention (CDC). This now covers 600 districts with a rapid response team in each district and 24/7 satellite communication links with the capital.

Some Institutions in India whose priorities include surveillance are listed below.

- Indian Veterinary Research Institute (IVRI), Mukteswar, Izatnagar and Bangalore
- National Dairy Research Institute (NDRI), Karnal
- Central Avian Research Institute (CARI), Izatnagar
- Project Directorate on Animal Disease Monitoring and Surveillance (PD_ADMAS), Bangalore
- High Security Animal Disease Laboratory, Bhopal
- Biotechnology Laboratory, National Dairy Development Board (NDDB), Anand

Surveillance programmes have been launched in India against rinderpest, FMD, avian influenza, tuberculosis, Johne's disease, brucellosis, infectious bovine rhinotracheitis and bluetongue. Some of these diseases of economic and public health importance are also notifiable. The surveillance programme includes:

1. Rapid and reliable diagnosis of disease
2. Data collection, analysis, interpretation
3. Formulation of recommendations
4. Dissemination/publication of conclusions

There are basically 4 categories of animals that we need to consider in a surveillance programme in Indian context. These include companion animals; farm animals like dairy cows, sheep, goats, pigs, poultry, fish; wildlife; and captive animals.

The surveillance activities concentrate efforts through the network explained below.

6. Veterinary Surveillance Network

The animal owner is likely to be the first person to notice something wrong among the animals, hence constitutes the first link in the chain. Hikers or trekkers or tribals may notice problems in wildlife or grazing farm animals in the wildlife interface. Volunteer groups such as birdwatchers may report observations they have on wildlife. Veterinary surgeons inspect animals on farms, at markets, at agricultural shows or at slaughterhouses for signs of disease. Veterinary practitioners know a lot about diseases in their practice and can use this knowledge to advise their clients and help us watch out for anything new. Veterinarians may send samples for testing, or dead animals for postmortem examination to government laboratories. Private laboratories may also collect useful information. A simple surveillance network is depicted in Fig. 1.

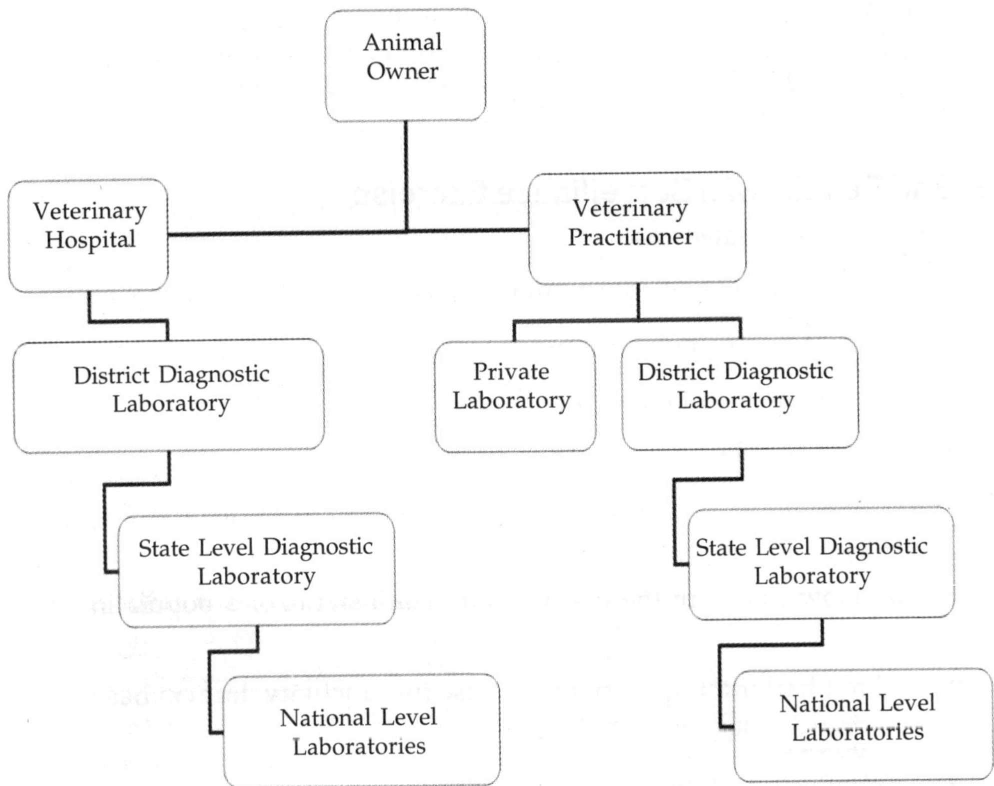

Fig. 1 : A simple surveillance network

7. Importance of Surveillance

Livestock is important in supporting the livelihood of poor farmers, consumers, traders and labourers throughout the developing world. The greatest impact of livestock in sustainable development designed to help the poor is enhancement of the livestock production systems, while animal diseases are crucial constraints in this. From the above highlights it is obvious that surveillance identifies:

1. Presence of a disease
2. Factors contributing to the disease
3. Relationships (seasons, trends, populations and other biological events)

In addition, there are two specific reasons why animal surveillance may be important.

First, the direct impact on human health and well being, immediately meaning zoonotic diseases that are in plenty. Besides this, antimicrobial resistance can arise in both the animals as well as humans consuming animal proteins as a result of antimicrobial overuse in animals. Secondly, the economic impact is at times very heavy as in the case of FMD outbreaks which can result in 20 to 25% loss in production, or in case of mastitis that can lead to losses anywhere from 10 to 20%.

8. End Results of a Surveillance Exercise

Surveillance enables us:

- To enhance our knowledge and understanding of livestock diseases
- To detect and respond to epidemics
- To detect new and emerging diseases
- To identify risks
- To facilitate planning and implementation of control strategies to manage disease
- To follow trends in the disease and health status of a population over time
- To limit harmful impact of the disease (productivity, human health risk, veterinary costs)
- To establish priorities
- To evaluate the effectiveness of programmes and services

9. Surveillance Activities – Mode of Operation

Surveillance activities can be regarded as Active or Passive or in-between.

9.1 Active surveillance

This is also termed as targeted surveillance. Specific surveys are undertaken for particular issues. We have done the following animal disease surveys:

- Bluetongue virus exposure in sheep since 1997
- Rinderpest which was eradicated from the country in 2004 and surveillance continues
- Antibiotic resistance in microbes
- Canine rabies occurrences in Chennai city (Fig. 2)

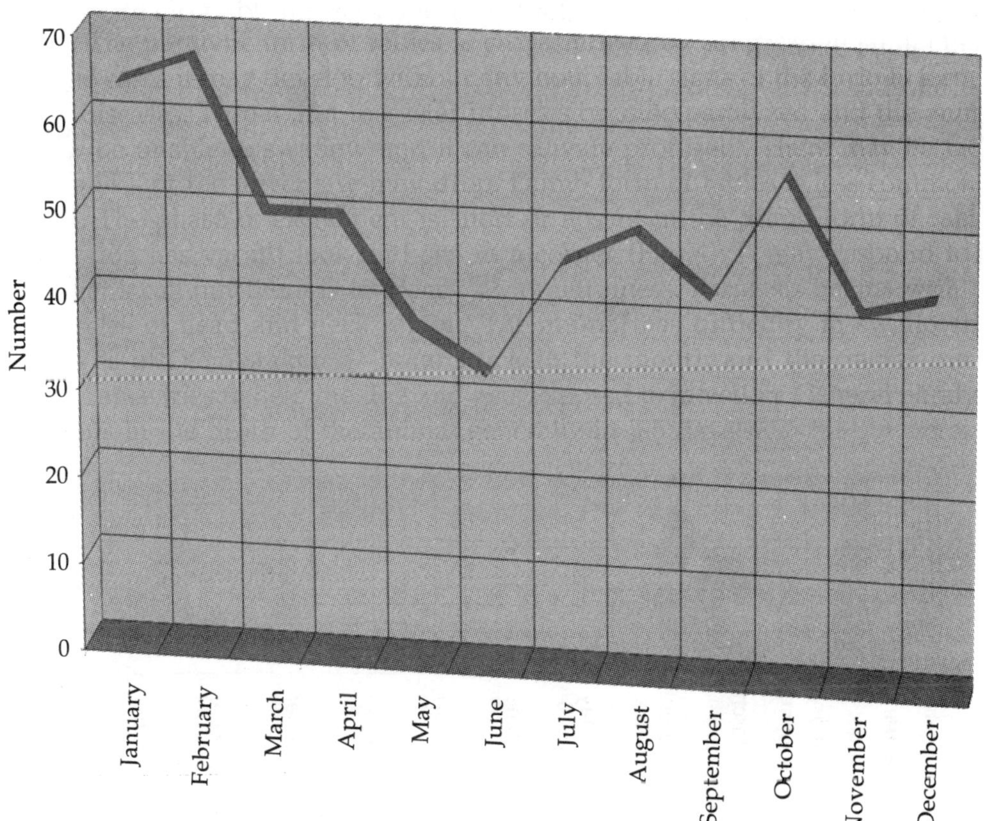

Fig. 2 : Pattern of canine rabies in Chennai (1993-2002)

9.2 Passive surveillance

This is also termed general surveillance. Here the data is collected for a routine purpose of knowing the disease occurrences in a locality following a report by a livestock producer or an animal owner. Veterinarians examine sick animals, collect samples, decide upon a diagnosis and provide advice about the condition. The information collected is entered into a database that can be queried at a later date, and provides a valuable source of knowledge over time.

For example, the rainfall in an area is often assessed to predict a liver fluke outbreak in a region by the following formula.

$M = n \times (r - p) + 5$

Where M represents month, 'n' is the number of wet days in the month, 'r' is the rainfall in inches, and 'p' represents the evapotranspiration in inches in that month.

When the value crosses 100, the conditions are suitable for liver fluke infection. Now if this formula is done over one year, this kind of surveillance will tell us the action we could initiate for liver fluke.

Another leading example of the results of general surveillance is given below in the graphical representation which highlights the likely periods of FMD outbreaks in Tamil Nadu (Fig. 3). This is a result of a surveillance reporting system by local and state level veterinarians.

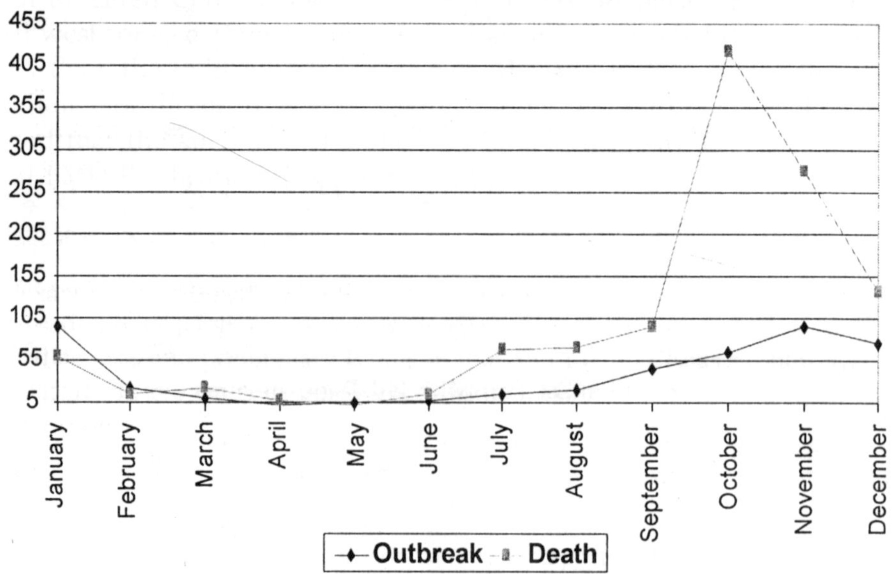

Fig. 3 : Pattern of occurrence of FMD in Tamil Nadu

On analysis, the outbreaks seem to appear more during July and the identified risk factors include windy conditions and cattle markets during this period which provide the greatest source of infection and spread. So, this is a classical example of the end result of a surveillance network team action.

10. Steps in the Surveillance Programme

Surveillance involves many integrated steps carried out by many people as described below.

10.1 Reporting

Reporting of the event or the disease is the primary step. This is usually done by veterinarians, animal owners, livestock producers and village level workers. They complete a form recording various bits of information.

10.2 Data accumulation

It involves collecting the data from all the reports and assembling it in order. This is often done by someone higher up at the district headquarters who sorts out the reports to gather the following information

1. Date animal affected
2. Addresses/contact person
3. Species of animal
4. Number
5. Age and sex
6. Location and area involved
7. Clinical status of the animals
8. Signs observed before death
9. History of earlier events in the area
10. Treatment, if any, given

10.3 Data analysis

The data so assembled should be analysed to calculate the rates of disease, changes in disease rates etc. This often requires an epidemiologist with specific data analysis and computer skills.

10.4 Judgment and action

This is often done by the authorities at the state or national level. In emergencies, it is often a collective opinion of state and national authorities as local experience is a must in formulating policies. Hence, coordination is necessary.

If any of these steps breaks down or is unavailable, it will not be possible to have usable information for taking appropriate action.

11. Prerequisites for Surveillance

Surveillance is done when

- We need continuous data to make immediate decisions
- The basic infrastructure and people are available to gather, transmit, and analyze the data
- Resources for action based on the data are available

12. Comparison with Other Data Collection Methods

Besides surveillance, survey is another method of data collection. However, surveys or other methods of rapid assessment cannot meet some of the objectives of data collection (Table 1). Data collection should be frequent enough so that rapid decisions can be taken to redirect or revised programmes quickly.

Table 1 : Differentiating surveillance and survey

Surveillance	Survey
Collects quantitative data	Collects quantitative data
Collects limited data	Collects a wide variety
Collects data on each case of sickness	Usually collects data on a sample of the population
Collects data over present and prospective time period	Collects data at any particular point in time
Collects data only for the numerator of incidence and prevalence rates	Collects data for numerator and denominator to calculate prevalence or incidence rates

13. The Attributes of a Surveillance System

13.1 Sensitivity

To what extent does the system identify all or most cases in a target population? This may be assessed by an efficient diagnostic tool or any standard method that allows for a near accurate way of finding the disease status in a population.

13.2 Timeliness

This refers to how rapidly reports are received, evaluated, and analyzed and the information provided to those in a position to intervene. This may be critical to control an outbreak of an acute disease such as the recent episodes of H_1N_1 or the innumerable diseases that breakout in animal populations in India.

13.3 Representativeness

This refers to whether the likelihood of reporting a disease is the same within subgroups of the population or in different populations. If surveillance reports are not representative, this could affect the application of control efforts.

13.4 Positive Predictive Value

This refers to the specificity of the case report. To what extent are the reported cases really diseased? This is an important attribute of a surveillance system in most situations.

13.5 Simplicity

This refers to the network and user friendly attributes for ease of operation. It would be expensive and burdensome to collect data and not be able to understand its applications for use.

13.6 Acceptability

This refers to the willingness of field level personnel to participate in the surveillance system which indicates the success of its acceptability. This is very critical for a surveillance programme to go on.

13.7 Flexibility

There should always be room for change in a later stage to suit a situation such as the emergence of a new disease. Generally, simple systems are more flexible.

14. Surveillance as a Tool

Besides providing useful and current information on important infectious diseases to epidemiologist for developing methods for their prevention, routine surveillance is often a critical component of other prevention programmes too.

14.1 Surveillance as a tool for evaluating vaccines

After a vaccine is licensed, it is important to continue surveillance to measure its effectiveness in controlling the disease in the population and the extent of its use. Some examples are given here.

- *Any modification of dosing schedule* - Immunity provided by a vaccine can be assessed by surveillance to decide if any modification in the dosing schedule is required.
- *Modification of vaccine components* - Changes in virus types makes it important to add or delete the vaccine components. It would also help to assess whether a live or inactivated component is necessary.
- *Monitoring vaccine administration* - All vaccinations are not immunisations but all immunisations are vaccinations. This means that vaccines to be able to immunise or protect need to be administered properly which includes proper route, proper storage, proper age etc.
- *Calculating vaccine effectiveness* - Vaccine effectiveness can be measured by comparing the rates of disease in vaccinates (V) and non-vaccinates (NV). The standard formula for calculating vaccine efficacy (VE) compares the attack rates for disease in NV with the disease in the V as follows.

$$VE\ (\%) = \frac{(NV - V)}{NV} \times 100$$

14.2 Surveillance as a tool to eradicate disease

The National Project for Rinderpest Eradication (NPRE) Campaign showed that an active and aggressive surveillance programme would be the best of means of containing or eradicating a disease. The eradication programme relied not only on the reports of rinderpest cases in the susceptible population but also had intensive surveillance of villages where cases had occurred. This highly active surveillance system was coupled with vaccination of contacts and preventing their contact with additional susceptible populations during the infectious period.

14.3 Surveillance as a tool to prevent disease spread

Surveillance may also be used to prevent spread of the disease to others. When a case of active bovine tuberculosis is identified, the report is usually followed by an investigation of the contacts. The contacts are then monitored and action initiated to prevent further spread.

15. International Involvement in Surveillance Activities

15.1 Office International des Epizooties (OIE)

The Office International des Epizooties (Paris, France) is an independent intergovernmental world organization to protect animal health. It currently has 158 member countries. The OIE collects, analyses, and disseminates information on animal disease control in an effort to guarantee the sanitary safety of international trade in animals and animal products. The OIE sets international standards but does not have the power of legal enforcement.

15.2 The World Trade Organization (WTO)

The WTO has a series of Agreements on Agriculture (AOA) and Agreements on Sanitary and Phytosanitary (SPS) Measures which apply to certifying animals and animal products for international trade.

16. Animal Disease Classification Systems and Resources

There are several classification systems for animal diseases. A system used most commonly in surveillance is that defined by the OIE. It categorises diseases into three lists, A, B, and C, based on the contagiousness and the pathogenicity. However, for reporting standards there are currently no veterinary diagnostic codes. OIE uses a numeric code for reporting diseases but it is not used universally.

Although there are very detailed guides to the diagnosis of animal diseases in OIE documents such as the International Animal Health Code, most of the diagnoses depend on a positive laboratory test, performed according to the OIE's Manual of Standards for Diagnostic Tests and Vaccines.

16.1 OIE diseases list A, B and C

OIE List A diseases are transmissible diseases with potential for widespread and rapid transmission. These may have serious socioeconomic or public health consequences, and are of major importance in international trade of animals and animal products.

OIE List B diseases are transmissible diseases which are of socioeconomic, and/or public health importance within individual countries and are significant in international trade of animals and animal products. This list includes about 90 diseases, categorised by animal species.

OIE List C diseases are transmissible diseases with important socioeconomic and/or sanitary influence at the local level.

For a complete list of the categorized diseases, one can refer to the latest version of the OIE's Manual of Standards for Diagnostic Tests and Vaccines.

16.2. Current software systems in animal disease information management

In today's advancing communication scenario and information technology, animal health information systems are quite important. These are similar to human health information systems. These include VADDS, VetCare, VETECH and VetSoft. A most comprehensive listing of commercial veterinary information systems can be found at http://netvet.wustl.edu/infor.htm.

16.3 Professional continuing education

There have been aggressive efforts to educate animal health professionals and the state veterinarians about their role in identifying animal disease outbreaks through programmes sponsored by the state and central governments such as the ASCAD (Assistance to States for Control of Animal Diseases) and TNIAMWARM (Tamil Nadu Irrigated Agricultural Modernisation and Water Resource Management). This is a mandatory exercise which is a form of continuing education to keep the professionals abreast of the advances in animal diseases surveillance.

16.4 Important organizations and websites

- American Association of Public Health Veterinarians: www.avma.org/aaphv/default.htm
- American Association of Wildlife Veterinarians: www.aawv.net
- American Association of Zoo Veterinarians: www.aazv.org
- Animal Health Association: www.usaha.org
- Centre for Epidemiology and Animal Health: www.aphis.uda.gov/vs/ceah
- Office International des Epizooties (OIE): www.oie.int
- World Health organization (WHO): www.who.int

17. Conclusion

Infectious diseases globally are estimated to cause 13 million deaths annually. Approximately 75% of the emerging diseases are zoonotic in nature. This coupled with increasing international trade has resulted in an increased demand for veterinary surveillance systems. Surveillance is a systematic collection, analysis, interpretation, and dissemination of data and risk factors. Epidemiologists can use these data to detect outbreaks, describe patterns of disease transmission, evaluate prevention and control programmes, and prioritize on future needs for animal health activities.

Traditionally, veterinary disease surveillance and monitoring programmes have focused on control and eradication of diseases. Today, animal disease surveillance and monitoring is largely focused towards establishing national and regional disease status to support international trade in animals and animal products. Hence the responsibility to engage actively in identifying risk factors in preventing and controlling animal diseases is clear.

Whether it is to define the burden of disease in a population to inform policymakers or to evaluate the success of a vaccine or other prevention programmes, monitor intentional or unintentional emerging diseases, or to provide insight into underlying health and risk behaviours in a population, surveillance is one of the cornerstones of veterinary medicine and public health.

References

1. Nelson KE, Sifakis F (2007). Surveillance. In: Infectious Disease Epidemiology - Theory and Practice, second edition, Jones and Bartlett Publishers, Massachusetts.
2. Pappaioanou M (2004). Veterinary medicine protecting and promoting the public's health and well-being. Preventive Veterinary Medicine 62:153-163.
3. Rebecca MS, Michael L, Popovich MS (2002). Animal Disease surveillance: A frame work for supporting disease detection in public health. White paper: Animal Disease Surveillance, WHPO27-A Scientific Technologies Corporation. p 1 -7.
4. Thrusfield M (2005). Veterinary Epidemiology. 3rd Edition, Blackwell, London.
5. Urquhart GM *et al.* (1996). Veterinary Parasitology 2nd Edition, Blackwell.

□□□

Chapter 26

Essentials of Necropsy and Diagnostic Material Collection

R. P. GUPTA, DEEPIKA LATHER AND VIKAS NEHRA
Department of Veterinary Pathology, College of Veterinary Sciences, Lala Lajpat Rai University of Veterinary and Animal Sciences, Hisar-125004

Contents

1. Introduction

Necropsy (post-mortem examination) is a systematic and critical examination of a dead animal/cadaver to determine the cause and manner of death and to evaluate any disease or pathological change that may be present. The term autopsy (Greek *autopsia* - seeing with one's own eyes) is preferred in human medicine for post-mortem examination whereas necropsy (Greek *nekros* - corpse + *opsis* - view) is used in veterinary practice. Post-mortem examination is generally performed by a veterinary pathologist/ veterinarian. It is important that veterinary professionals are knowledgeable of the importance and systematic procedure of conducting necropsy for the purpose of diagnosis or collecting diagnostic material.

2. Objectives of Necropsy

Necropsy is regarded as a valuable diagnostic procedure particularly in case of herd problems/outbreaks. Making a diagnosis is much easier in dead animal than in a living animal. Many of the diagnostic tests (radiographs, blood/serum tests etc.) that we perform on living animals are attempts to find out what is happening inside the animal but these tests may not provide precise answers to the problem. However, post-mortem examination is extremely valuable because it provides an opportunity to examine everything, both inside and outside. Post-mortem examination is far more common in veterinary medicine than in human medicine. In fact, a skilfully conducted and intelligently interpreted post-mortem examination usually helps in making doubtless diagnosis of a disease.

Necropsy is also performed to gain more insight into pathological processes of disease. It plays a vital role in research, teaching and in understanding pathogenesis of diseases of unknown aetiology. Moreover, post-mortem examination provides valuable material for subsequent laboratory studies. In addition, post-mortem examination affords an excellent opportunity for the pathologist/veterinarian to distinguish between normal and abnormal tissues.

Necropsy also provides an opportunity to the pathologist/veterinarian to further educate themselves. By trying to fully appreciate and understand the changes that have occurred during the disease and comparing the gross pathology with the clinical signs, they are more likely to diagnose that disease early in future leading to better prognosis.

In vetero-legal cases, necropsy helps to determine the cause and manner of death.

3. Pre-Necropsy Guidelines

The essential points which should be borne in mind prior to post-mortem examination are given below:

i. A proper written requisition/authority for conducting the necropsy should be secured before beginning it. In case of vetero-legal/forensic cases, request from the local police is necessary. State laws may prohibit or place some restrictions on the post-mortem examination of animals suspected to be dead due to certain communicable diseases. Some animal owners may also object to the necropsy of their pet animals.

ii. The necropsy should be performed in day light as far as possible since colour differentiation may not be proper in artificial light. The necropsy should be performed as soon as possible after death, because decomposition sets in quickly especially in hot weather and particularly in animals with thick layer of fat and insulating wool. Advanced decomposition of the carcass by putrefactive organisms may alter the appearance of organs and tissues rendering the final decision inaccurate. One should carefully compare the time and date of death or destruction with that of necropsy as it may aid in determining the cause of certain tissue changes. However, certain conditions (abscess, neoplasm, exudate, thrombi, granulomas, valvular defects and many other lesions) may be recognized even in advanced stages of decomposition. At places where cold room facilities are available, post-mortem decomposition of carcases can be delayed, if not prevented.

iii. It is preferred that the dead animal is brought without undue delay to a veterinary institution. The smaller animals should be readily transported to a suitably equipped laboratory/post-mortem hall. The laboratory/ post-mortem hall should have provisions for cadaver disposal and lowering the chances of environmental contamination (Cabana 1999). Usually, a clinical diagnosis will aid in deciding the site for necropsy, for example, a clinical diagnosis of anthrax does not warrant necropsy at all as the potential of contamination is great. Animals that have died of suspected transmissible, zoonotic or exotic diseases require that the post-mortem examination always be done in a laboratory/post-mortem hall.

iv. Site for the post-mortem examination is selected taking into account the proximity to other facilities and environmental implications. Extreme care should be exercised in selecting the possible site for necropsy, especially in the field, to avoid transmission of infection. The selected site should be away from the sources of feed, forage and water. The sites that are frequented by other animals in the herd should be avoided. Insects, predators and other biological vectors of diseases should be warded off from the examination site. The site to be used for the post-mortem is prepared by cleaning and in such a way that blood and fluids do not contaminate the surrounding areas or facilities. It would be better to perform the necropsy in a place which can be fenced off or otherwise isolated from animals and human beings for some time. If the necropsy is to be performed near the farm building or on the ground, it will be advantageous to have a deep (thick) bed of straw below the carcass. The straw will absorb the fluid and can be burnt or buried afterwards.

v. Proper personal protection is must. Every animal assigned to necropsy should be considered as a potential source of transmissible infection, either zoonotic or highly contagious to animals. Full protective clothing must be worn when performing necropsy which includes double gloves, cap, disposable gown/apron, shoe covers/rubber gum boots, mask (or respirator if required), and eye protection (Fig. 1). A one-piece garment is preferred to two pieces since it avoids the hanging flaps of the coat which are likely to touch the contaminated material as the operator bends over his work.

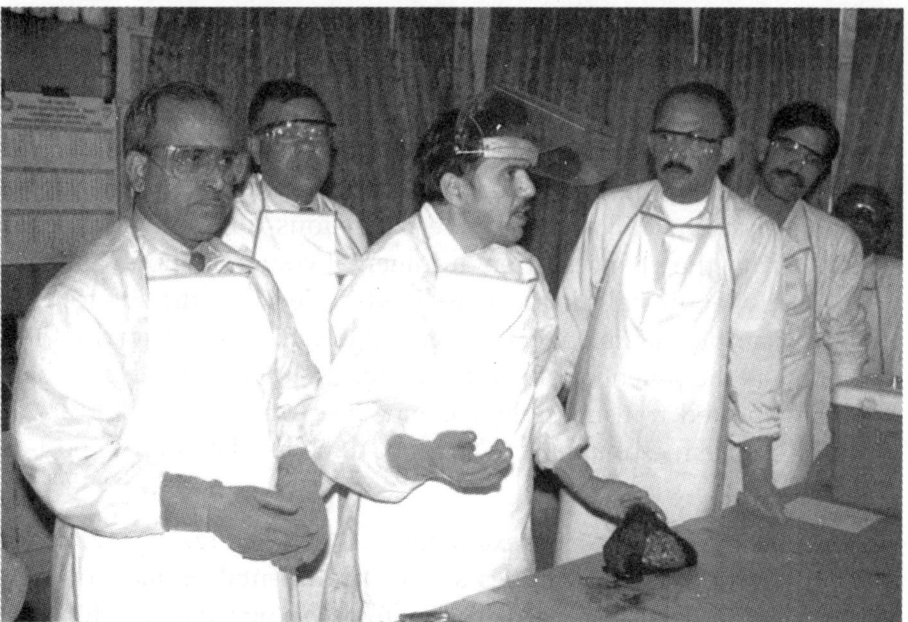

Fig. 1 : The author explaining necropsy procedures to the field Veterinary Officers

4. Basic Infrastructure, Instruments and Material Requirements for Necropsy

4.1 Basic infrastructure facility

The post-mortem examination should be done in a post-mortem hall or laboratory as far as possible, preferably in veterinary institutions. Main infrastructural facility requirements in the post-mortem building are mentioned below.

- A big post-mortem hall with raised floor area for large animals and steel top tables for small animals
- Adequate natural light, water, ventilation, drainage and provisions for lowering the chances of contaminating the surroundings
- Provision for artificial lighting, preferably flood lights, in the post-mortem hall for proper examination of lesions in visceral organs
- An efficient wide cold room to preserve the carcasses brought for necropsy till post-mortem examination
- At least two hand-washing sinks with running water inside the hall
- A separated room/access area with facilities for changing clothes, footwear and protective articles; hand-washing and showering, if possible, and a locker for personal items near the entrance
- A store room for equipments and supplies
- Room for decontamination of used equipments should be present
- A separate area for incinerator for hygienic disposal of carcasses after necropsy
- Water-resistant walls, floors, and ceiling surfaces to facilitate cleaning and disinfecting, any holes or penetrations in these surfaces should be sealed or sealable to facilitate fumigation or space decontamination
- Hygienically constructed floor drains with drain traps filled with water or a suitable disinfectant
- Self closing wide doors that open outwards, windows closed and sealed unless situated sufficiently away from other areas, well-separated and fenced
- Ventilation system if the windows are closed and sealed, arrangement of filtration of exhausted air with dispersal of exhausted air away from the building and other occupied areas after filtration
- Effective rodent, feral animal and insect control arrangement
- Telephone facility

Telephone numbers of the contact persons responsible for conducting necropsy and safety instructions for entering the necropsy area should be displayed at the entry gate. Where adequate infrastructure is not available, necropsy can be performed with the available facilities taking necessary precautions for biosafety.

4.2 Instruments and materials

Major instruments and materials required for necropsy on large and small animals are depicted in Table 1 and Fig. 2 and 3.

Table 1 : List of instruments/material required for necropsy

Instruments/material	Use
Butcher's knife with a convexity curved or straight cutting edge (about 18 cm long)	General purpose knife for cutting skin and organs
Forceps-20 cm long, blunt anatomical type	For holding delicate tissue structures
Small and large scissors with either pointed or round ends	For cutting skin and organs
Enterotome	For examination of intestinal tract.
Chisel and hammer - Chisel 18 cm long, 2 cm wide, hammer with metallic handle	For bone cutting
Surgical saw or hack saw	For bone cutting
Chopper	For cutting hard tissue in small pieces
Scalpel and blades	For fine work and for cutting nerves when removing brain or spinal cord
Bone cutter or castotome	For cutting ribs
Ruler - preferably of metal	For measuring the length of organs
Metal probe	For testing the patency of ducts, fistulas and other openings
Specimen bottles - half-filled with 10% neutral buffered formalin	For sample collection for histopathological examination
Specimen bottles - half-filled with 50% buffered glycerine	For sample collection for virus isolation
Sterile swabs and petri dishes	For collecting organs/tissues for bacteriological examination
Sterile syringes, needles and Pasteur pipettes	For collecting body fluids/heart blood for laboratory examination
Glass slides	For making impression smears for diagnosis
Ordinary fishing twine or thread	For tying up hollow organs

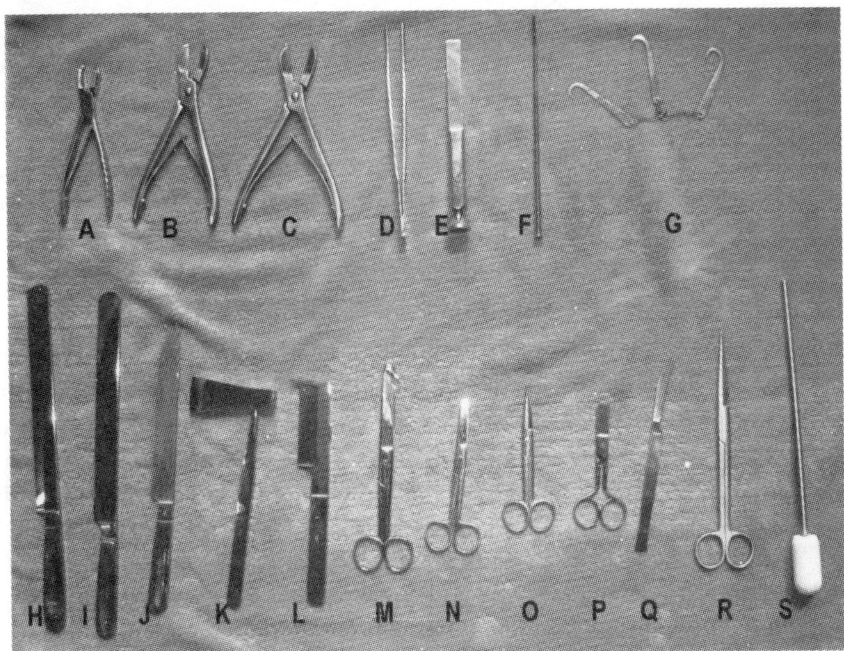

Fig. 2 : Major instruments for necropsy: (A-C) Bone cutters, (D) Forceps, (E) Chisel, (F) Blower, (G) Hooks, (H-J) Butcher's knife, (K) Axe, (L) Sharpening steel, (M-P) Scissors, (Q) Scalpel, (R) Scissors, (S) Probe

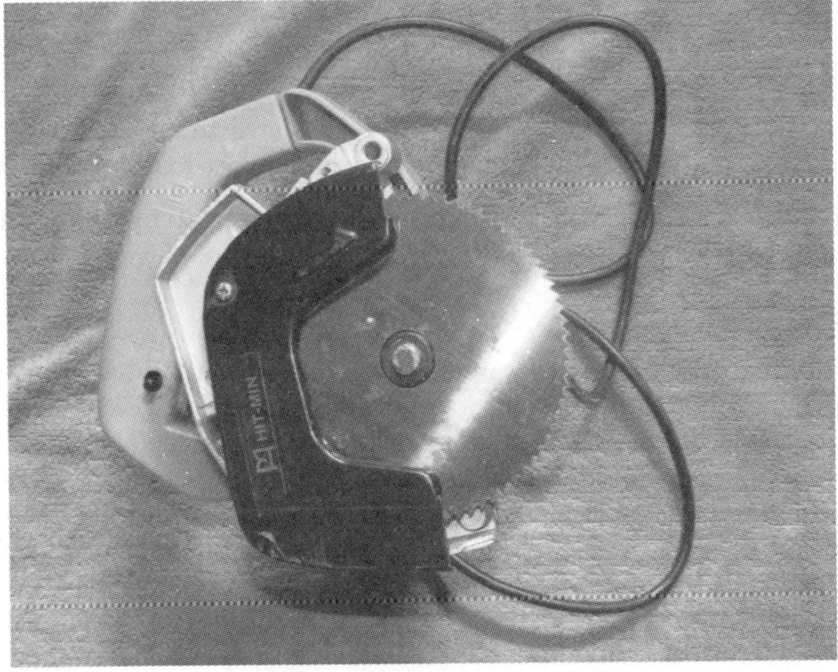

Fig. 3 : Electric saw (Bone cutter)

For most purposes, two sharp knives, a pair each of scissors and forceps, a metal probe, and an ordinary mechanical hacksaw are sufficient. Preference for the size of the knives depends on the size of the cadaver, ease of handling and safety. A steel rod or sharpening stone to keep the knives sharp is essential. The instruments should be sharp and arranged in an easy-to-handle manner. After finishing the work, instruments, clothes and other materials should be cleaned, disinfected or disposed of.

5. General Procedure for Post-Mortem Examination

Post-mortem examination begins with the review of preliminary information and clinical history of the animal provided in the requisition form. A complete history of the animal is extremely important because it provides pertinent background information which increases the chances of finding the true cause of death. Any information the owner can provide is valuable. The requisition form (Stahl 1996) should include the following points.

i. Age and identification number of animal
ii. Date of death of animal/date on which animal was found dead
iii. Husbandry practices (feeding, housing, vaccination etc.)
iv. Previous clinical problems and treatments
v. Current clinical problems, period of ill health and treatments
vi. Health of other livestock

It is often observed that animal owners may not disclose complete information. They should be motivated to share this information with veterinarian/pathologist for better inference of the post-mortem observations.

The systematic process of conducting post-mortem examination is described below.

5.1 External examination

External examination of carcass takes only few minutes but can give valuable information. It includes identification of the carcass (species, breed, age, sex, colour and special features such as brand mark, tag No., tattoo marks or ear, wing or leg band number etc., if any), recording of nutritional status/ body condition as good, fair, poor, emaciated/cachectic or hide bound, and looking for the type of discharge, if any from natural body openings. External examination further involves recording of post-mortem changes such as extent of rigor mortis, post-mortem autolysis and putrefactive signs; stained blood vessels, greenish discoloration, odour, softening of eye balls, exudation from nose and mouth, ova or flies, moving maggots, blebs over body, peeling of cuticle, loosening of hair, thorax and abdomen burst, eye changes, adipocere and mummification.

Visible mucous membrane should be observed for colour, congestion and haemorrhages. Skin should be checked for abnormal pigmentation, traumatic (abrasions, lacerations, perforations) and other lesions (swellings, abscess, and tumour), ectoparasites etc. Umblicus in young animals and mammary glands and external genitalia in adults should also be examined for lesions.

5.2 Internal examination

After careful examination of exterior, the carcass is placed in suitable position. In case of horses, mules, asses and donkeys, the carcass is placed on the right side. The position is reverse (left side) in case of adult ruminants and very large swine. Dogs, cats, rabbits, small sized swine and calves are placed in the dorsal position (back facing the ground/table). The skin is incised along the ventral midline from the mandibular to pelvic symphysis and separated from upper part of body as far as possible towards the back bone, cutting the pectoral muscles between the fore leg and thorax. This brings into view subcutaneous, muscle tissue and superficial lymph nodes. Hip joint is disarticulated through incision in the medial muscles of hind leg to turn the hind legs away from the body (King *et al.* 2006).

5.2.1 Subcutaneous tissue and musculature

After removal of skin, subcutaneous tissue and musculature may be examined for the presence of various types of lesions such as congestion, haemorrhages, oedema, exudates, abnormal growth, anaemia, discoloration, pigmentation and necrosis of musculature. Normally blood in subcutaneous tissue of dead animals is dark red and coagulated. The variations in colour of blood may be of diagnostic significance, for instance pale colour in leukemia, cherry red in carbon-monoxide poisoning, brownish due to methemoglobinemia in nitrate, nitrite, chlorate poisoning, black tar like in anthrax and insufficient coagulation in suffocation and oxalate poisoning.

5.2.2 Thoracic cavity

The thoracic cavity is opened by cutting the ribs along the sternum and the vertebrae with the bone cutter. If bone cutters are not available, a saw, a chopper or an axe may be used. Alternately, the ribs may be separated from each other with knife and broken one by one from vertebrae, starting from the posterior end. This facilitates the examination of pleura, heart and lungs (Fig. 4). One should also observe for adhesions and fluid/hydrothorax in the thoracic cavity.

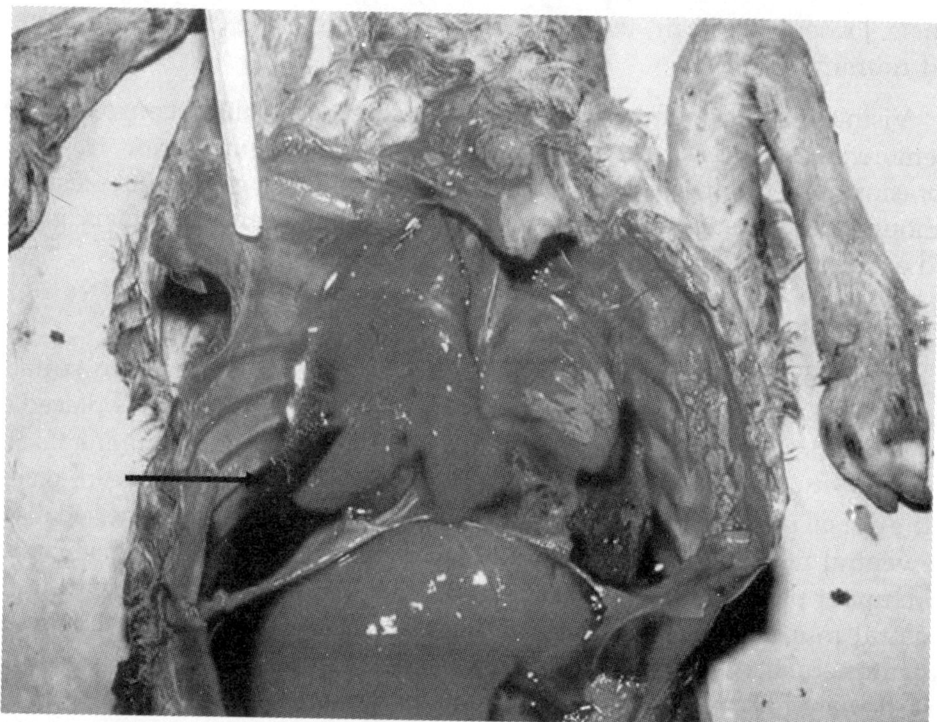

Fig. 4 : Thoracic cavity showing heart, congested lungs and fluid mixed blood (arrow)

5.2.3 Respiratory system

Discharge and abnormal growth such as polyp may be noticed in nasal passage. Trachea and bronchi should be examined for haemorrhages, fluid or froth content, foreign bodies and broken cartilage rings. Animals that died from lung oedema may show a stable froth in the trachea. The surface of the lungs and pleura should be examined for congestion (Fig. 5), haemorrhages, consistency of individual lobes, collapsed or dilated lobes, abnormal tissue masses, nodules, emphysema and necrosis. Areas of consolidations should be characterised as to location and degree of involvement of lung parenchyma and its distribution. Mediastinal lymph nodes should be examined for enlargement, hardening, congestion and haemorrhages.

5.2.4 Cardiovascular system

It is convenient to examine the heart that is still attached to the lungs. Pericardial sac is examined for colour, turbidity, amount and quality of pericardial fluid, haemorrhages and any type of exudates; endocardium and myocardium for areas of haemorrhages, degeneration/necrosis, fibrosis and any other lesions.

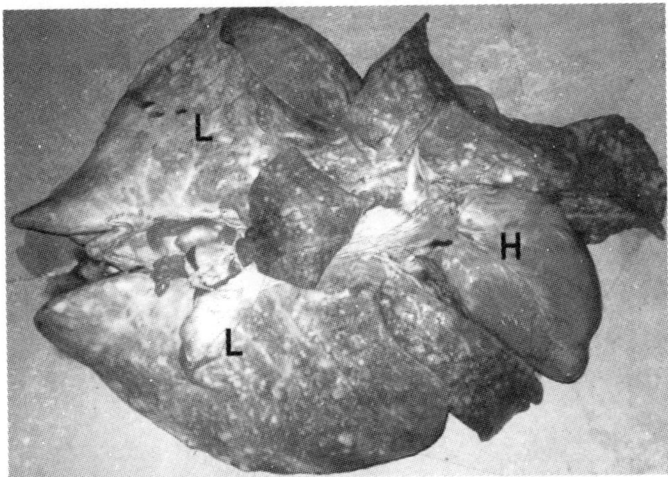

Fig. 5 : Congestion in heart (H) and lungs (L)

5.2.5 Abdominal cavity

Abdominal cavity is exposed by cutting away the abdominal wall along the last rib, linea alba and the vertebral column, thus exposing the peritoneum, stomach and intestines (Fig. 6). Their removal exposes the liver, uterus, urinary, bladder, rectum, spleen and kidneys. In order to have thorough information, first of all the organs should be examined *in situ* i.e. before they are displaced

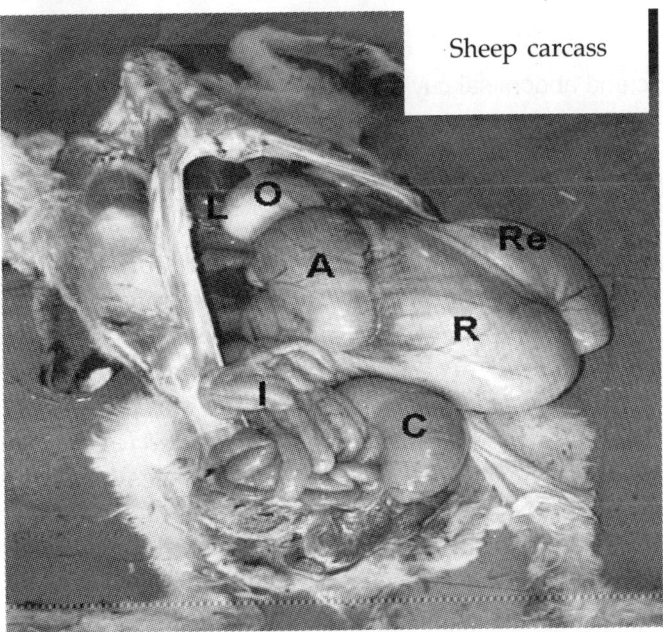

Fig. 6 : Organs in the abdominal cavity *in situ* (R- rumen, Re- reticulum, O- omasum, A- abomasum, I- small intestine, C- caecum, L- liver)

or cut out. All important organs and parts are removed and the intact and cut surfaces examined carefully. One should also observe for lesions in the abdominal cavity, displacement of organs, accumulation of serous fluid (ascites), serosanguinous fluid (Fig. 7), blood, adhesions, parasites, tumour growth etc.

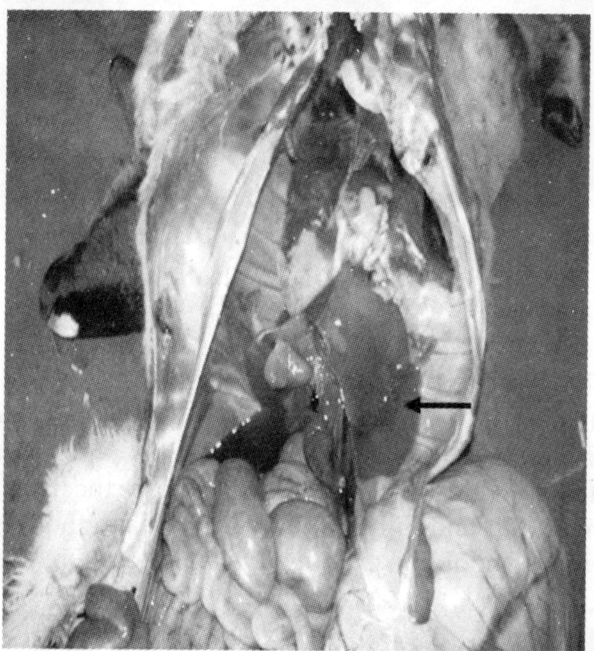

Fig. 7 : Thoracic and abdominal cavity showing lesions in organs and serosanguinous fluid (arrow)

5.2.6 Digestive system

Dorsal and ventral surfaces of the tongue are looked for the presence of ulcers, suppurative foci, wounds and nodules or abnormal masses. Whole length of the oesophagus is opened to examine the mucosa for the presence of ulcers, strictures and abnormal tissue masses. Gastrointestinal tract should be examined for erosions, ulcers, congestion, haemorrhage, oedema, necrosis, abnormal pigmentation, abscess, pus, perforation and parasites. In ruminants, fore stomach, particularly reticulum must be inspected for any foreign needles, and abomasum for congestion (Fig. 8), haemorrhages and ulcers. Intestines should be examined for intussusception, torsion, volvulus and parasites. Intestine should also be examined by giving longitudinal cut to note the lesions such as thickness of the walls, presence of ulcers and strictures, foreign bodies, exudates, contents in the lumen and congestion or haemorrhages (Fig. 9). The surface of liver should be examined for necrotic areas (Fig. 10), tumour growth, haemorrhages, congestion etc.

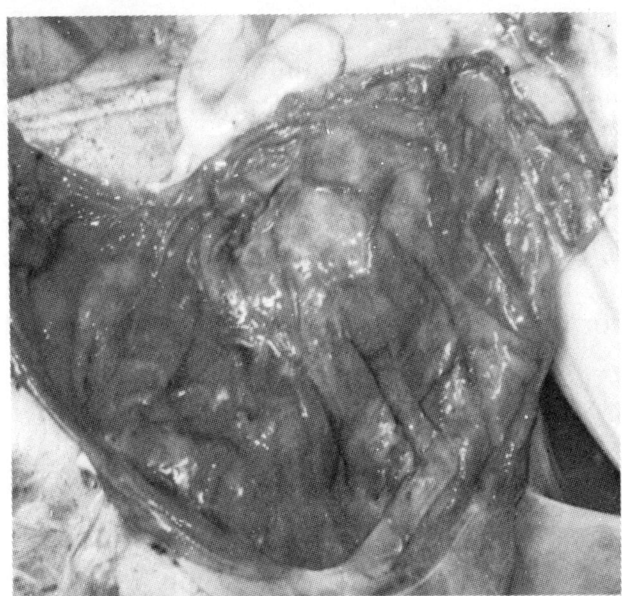

Fig. 8 : Abomasum mucosal folds showing thickening and congestion

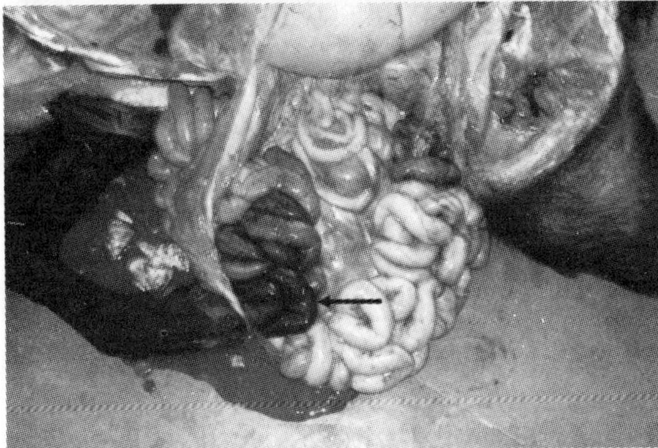

Fig. 9 : Intestine showing dark red colour due to severe haemorrhages and blood in the lumen (arrow)

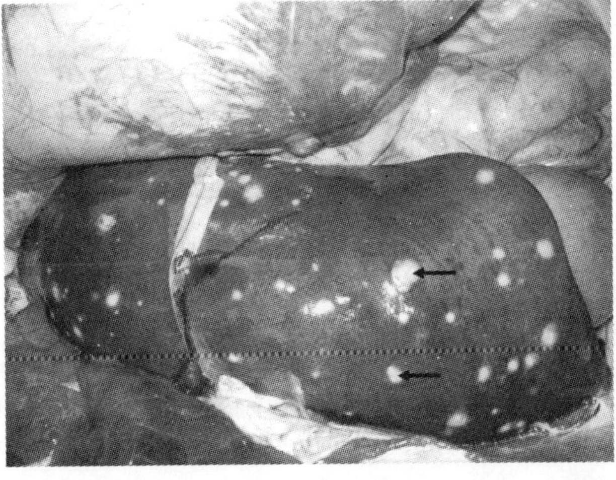

Fig. 10 : Liver showing necrotic areas (arrows)

5.2.7 Urinary system

Kidneys, urinary bladder and urethra are examined for congestion, haemorrhage and oedema. Both kidneys are also examined for infraction necrosis, nodules, calculi, obstruction and pus in the pelvis.

5.2.8 Genital system

Ovaries, oviduct, uterus, cervix and vagina in females, and testicles, epididymus, penis and prepuce in males are examined for different types of lesions. Uterus is examined for foetal abnormalities, pus or abnormal fluid material.

5.2.9 Nervous system

Head is examined separately. To open the vault of the cranium and expose the brain, a hack saw may be used to saw off the overlying bones. Alternatively, a chisel may be used but care must be taken not to penetrate the cavity and damage the brain. Before removing the whole brain from the cavity, the surface of the brain is examined to look for the evidence of oedema such as cerebellar coning and flattening of the gyri and sulci. Clinical history of sudden and/or progressive paralysis warrants the examination of spinal cord, nerve plexus, and associated ganglia. The spinal cord should be removed by opening the spinal column. Two approaches may be used to do this. First, the spinal column may be split with a saw, cutting about one third of the vertebra and second, by removal of the dorsal arches.

5.2.10 Musculoskeletal system

Bones and joints are seldom examined unless the clinical history suggests lameness. However, by doing it, samples of bone marrow, which often reveal some clues on the haemopoeitic status of the animal, can be collected for laboratory examination.

5.2.11 Sensory organs

It includes the examination of eyes and organs of hearing. The eyes should be examined first. Since the eyes often do not allow easy handling, it is best to have them fixed in formalin. To examine the middle ears, external ear canal is opened.

6. Post-Mortem Changes

It is important to differentiate between alterations that occur in the body before death and those which take place after death, known as post-mortem changes. Post-mortem changes result from degradation of tissues associated with the release of proteolytic lysosomal enzymes from the cells and putrefaction by the bacteria. Animals died of bacterial diseases usually show post-mortem changes more rapidly than those died of other causes.

6.1 Terminology associated with post-mortem changes

There are certain scientific terms that indicate post-mortem changes but these changes are not due to any pathological condition. These changes are of significance to ascertain approximate time of death.

6.1.1 Rigor mortis

It is the stiffness which rapidly sets in after death due to hardening of muscular tissue in consequence of the coagulation of myosinogen and paramyosinogen. Rigor mortis occurs first in the heart muscles but the earliest superficial evidence of it is usually found in the eyelids and masseter muscles which gradually spreads backwards over the entire cadaver. The normal sequence of the occurrence and disappearance of rigor mortis is heart, respiratory muscles, masticatory muscles, neck, fore limbs and hind limbs. Rigor mortis begins immediately after death and may last from half hour to 24 hours or more. Classically, rigor mortis begin from 1-6 hours after death and passes off in 24-48 hours. However, the onset of rigor mortis is influenced by several factors including nutritional status of the animal, environmental temperature, body temperature of the cadaver, and the cause of death.

As a rule, the earlier it sets in, the sooner it passes off and vice versa. In the case of an animal that has died suddenly without any serious illness or by accident, the rigor mortis is considerably delayed. Well-fed animals have large glycogen reserves and may show a delay in the onset of rigor, while cachectic animals may develop rigor quickly. Animal cadavers that are exposed to hot temperatures may develop and pass off rigor mortis quickly. Those died of septicaemic diseases may not develop rigor mortis at all. Once a part of the animal body that has passed into rigor is moved, it passes off the rigor mortis.

6.1.2 Algor mortis

It is the gradual cooling of the animal body after death, and is associated with a fall in energy source (ATP).

6.1.3 Livor mortis or post-mortem lividity

It is the settling of blood to the down side of the animal body. Gravitational force and hydrostatic pressure of blood due to stoppage of cardiac activity cause blood to settle to the lowest points within the body (depending on the body position of the animal). Livor mortis begins at or very soon after death since it is a function of cardiac activity. The area where the blood has settled is generally dark blue or purple in colour.

6.1.4 Bile imbibition

It means golden yellow colouration imparted on tissues following the seepage of bile. Discolouration is most evident on the surfaces of the organs in contact with gall bladder and on duodenal mucosa.

6.1.5 Haemoglobin imbibition

It represents pinkish to reddish colouration imparted to tissues due to the lysis of red blood cells. This is most evident on the surfaces of large arteries and on outer surfaces of visceral organs.

6.1.6 Chicken fat clot

It is an old term referring to the gelatinous mass formed by separation and coagulation of plasma proteins from the component of blood. This is usually seen inside the major blood vessels and the heart. They sometimes give a cast of the ramifications of the vessels. To prevent misconceptions, the use of this term should be avoided.

6.1.7 Putrefaction

It usually begins in 3-36 hours depending upon the condition of animal and the atmospheric conditions (aided by warmth and moisture and excess of putrefactive organisms). The bacteria which are always present in the intestinal tract produce great quantities of gas by fermentation of ingesta and distend the intestines which exert a great force against the diaphragm and abdominal walls. The abdomen appears round and greatly bloated, the skin is tight and a reasonable sound is produced by tapping upon the belly wall. The pressure may be so great as to evert or protrude the rectum. Putrid odours are given off by the cadaver.

6.2 Post-mortem changes in main organs

Post-mortem changes including the colour and consistency alterations in various organs are described below.

6.2.1 Heart

At death, the heart stops in diastole. Within the first hour, rigor mortis develops beginning with the left ventricle. As a consequence, the left ventricle becomes almost empty and the right ventricle only about half full. If the myocardium is degenerated, rigor mortis may not appear. Under usual condition, rigor mortis disappears in 20-30 hours (1-1½ days). Necropsy at this time shows a flabby heart with an empty left ventricle. However, if at this time the heart is flabby and the left ventricle is filled with coagulated blood, it is an indication that there is myocardial degeneration and rigor mortis did not occur at all or only slightly. On the other hand, if the heart is flabby and filled with uncoagulated blood, rigor mortis may have occurred but the fluid blood returned to the ventricles (asphyxia, haemolysis). Usual post-mortem coagulation occurs slowly with separation of the clot into two portions, upper "chicken fat" clot and lower "current jelly" clot. Predominance of the former indicates slow death. Post-mortem granular coagulation of the sarcoplasm of the cardiac muscle cells resembles cloudy swelling in colour. The endocardium is frequently blood stained (imbibition of blood). Occasionally, gas vesicles appear in the myocardium as a result of post-mortem decomposition.

6.2.2 Lungs

Normal lungs are pale pink in colour. After death, post-mortem congestion becomes evident apart from livor mortis. Blood and fluid may ooze when the surface is cut. The airways may contain considerable quantities of froth and fluid. The organ becomes soft, collapsed, discoloured red to gray, and gas bubbles may appear on the parenchyma as time progresses.

6.2.3 Forestomach of ruminants

Post-mortem tympany is produced by continued fermentation after death. It is differentiated from ante-mortem tympany by lack of passive hyperemia of the thoracic and abdominal organs and absence of ecchymoses in the serous membranes. Extreme distension may cause rupture of the rumen or diaphragm. This can be differentiated from ante-mortem rupture by the absence of haemorrhagic infiltration and swelling of the border of the rupture. Another change which is frequently noted by veterinarians is loosening of the epithelium by maceration. It occurs within a few hours after death and is noticed particularly in the omasum.

6.2.4 Stomach

Hypostatic congestion is observed, wherein, the lowermost portions of mucosa and serosa have bluish red colour. There is perivascular diffusion of haemoglobin (imbibition of blood) leading to the formation of sulphmethemoglobin and iron sulphide and eventually the colour becomes grayish-blue or grayish-green (pseudomelanosis). A yellowish discolouration can be seen in the mucosa and on the serous coat in the vicinity of gall bladder (imbibition of bile). Because of autolytic changes, the mucosa becomes soft, transparent and strips off easily leaving the submucosa bare. Fermentative and decomposition changes after death produce gas which distends the stomach and may produce rupture of stomach and diaphragm. Like ante-mortem rupture, it occurs on the greater curvature and, therefore, should be differentiated from it.

6.2.5 Intestines

Post-mortem changes in the intestines are quite similar to those of stomach. The additional change that can be noted is post-mortem displacements such as torsion and invagination. Absence of hyperemia, oedema and haemorrhage in the displaced intestines marks the difference between post-mortem and ante-mortem displacements. As time progresses, gaseous distensions occur invariably resulting in stripping of the mucosa, perforation and rupture.

6.2.6 Liver

Haemoglobin imbibition imparts a shiny reddish discolouration on the surface of the liver or bluish-black discolouration due to the formation of sulphmethemoglobin and iron sulphide. The liver parenchyma close to the gall bladder may be stained yellowish or greenish because of bile imbibition. As time progresses, the liver may lose its turgidity, become soft, pulpy and clay-like in colour. The presence of gas-distended bubbles on the parenchyma usually suggests a more advanced stage of post-mortem decomposition.

6.2.7 Pancreas

Post-mortem change occurs rapidly in the pancreas. It may be discoloured red from haemoglobin imbibition, loose its lobular pattern, become soft and translucent. The portion that is facing the gall bladder may show bile imbibition. In advanced stages of post-mortem degradation, the pancreas turns into a sac-like structure containing red-tinged fluid and may even disappear leaving a flimsy membranous structure.

6.2.8 Kidneys

The kidneys may be discoloured red from haemoglobin imbibition, and later discoloured black (pseudomelanosis). The demarcation between cortex and medulla becomes not apparent. As time progresses, the organ becomes soft and gas bubbles form at the peri-renal tissues.

6.2.9 Spleen and Lymph Nodes

The spleen may be discoloured gray to black, becomes soft and mushy. Advanced stages of post-mortem degradation usually turn the spleen into a sac-like structure containing liquefied parenchyma that oozes when cut. The lymph nodes may be discoloured, become soft and pulpy.

6.2.10 Brain

The brain, being located farther from the gut shows delayed post-mortem changes. Vacuolation of the brain parenchyma due to seepage of cerebrospinal fluid may be observed. With advanced stages of post-mortem degradation, the brain turns into a soft mushy mass. Later, the brain liquefies and will ooze when the calvarium and meninges are opened.

6.2.11 Muscles

Discolouration of the muscles, fascia and tendon sheath occurs after death because of seepage of myoglobin. Intense colouration of the muscles may be seen at the down side of the animal. Air pockets demarcating muscle groups and fascial places occur in advanced stages of degradation.

6.2.12 Eye

The cornea of the eyes turns opaque due to absorption of the aqueous humour. The globe may either protrude or collapse. When opened, detached retina may be noted.

6.2.13 Body cavities and orifices

Surfaces of body cavities may show discolouration following haemoglobin imbibition and pseudomelanosis. The cavities may contain red-tinged fluid and may be copious in its amount. Gaseous distensions render the carcass to appear bloated. It is not uncommon to find post-mortem rectal or vaginal prolapse because of the developing internal pressure. Straw-coloured fluid may be seen oozing from the body opening in advance stages of post-mortem decomposition.

7. Collection of Diagnostic Specimens for Laboratory Examination

Collection of morbid materials during necropsy is important task since an exact diagnosis can be determined only by laboratory diagnostic procedures (Wobeser *et al.* 1980). The value of specimens for laboratory diagnosis depends on the adequacy and correctness of the collection, preservation and dispatch procedures. Many a times, the samples reaching the laboratory are useless, though the veterinarians may blame the laboratory for not providing complete and correct diagnosis. The specimens should be appropriately collected, preserved, labelled for proper identification and dispatched keeping in view the nature of material and the type of the tests envisaged. In case of any doubt, it would be useful to contact the concerned laboratory for advice. The following information should be sent along with the specimen to aid in diagnosis.

i) Species identification

ii) Clinical history

iii) Relevant necropsy findings

iv) Nature of the sample and the mode of collection and preservation

v) Type of examination requested

It is the responsibility of the examiner to notify relevant government offices when the specimen is collected from suspected cases of highly contagious, zoonotic or exotic diseases. Such samples should be adequately labelled to warn others about the potential of spread of infection or danger to the biological system, or risk to the courier of the specimen due to improper handling. The methods of collection and preservation of specimens for different purposes are briefly described below.

7.1 Collection of tissues for histopathological examination

For histopathological examination, the pieces of organs or tissues particularly showing lesions should be collected in 10% neutral buffered formalin immediately during the post-mortem examination and these pieces should not be more than 0.5 cm in thickness. The specimen should include both the normal and abnormal portion (lesion) of the organ or tissue. The tissue is collected using a sharp knife or scissors taking care not to crush or allow the tissue to dry; otherwise it may cause undue distortion in the morphology of the tissue cells. The collected tissue is immediately fixed in 10 times the tissue volume of 10% neutral buffered formalin. It is advisable to wash the specimen in physiological saline solution before fixing it in formalin if it is heavily soiled with debris or blood. In case of brain, the whole brain may be immersed in a large volume of the fixative, allowing it to harden for 24 hours, and then slicing the brain and taking desired sections. For gastrointestinal tract specimens, a segment is cut open longitudinally before putting the segment in the fixative to ensure adequate and prompt preservation of the mucosal lining and to increase the surface area for the penetration of the fixative.

7.2 Collection of specimens for microbiological examination

The specimens intended for microbiological examination are collected aseptically. The instruments are flamed every time before collecting each specimen or separate pre-sterilized instruments are used for each specimen. The samples from the gut or intestine, which are highly contaminated, should be collected in the end. It is recommended to sear the surface of the organ or tissue with a hot spatula followed by incision and collection of the required material from the deeper portion of solid organs, abscess, or coagulated masses. Heart blood should be collected in sterilized syringes for bacteriological isolations in septicaemic diseases (Fig. 11). Sterile swabs, tissue fragments and aspirates may be taken and placed in special transport media, especially if the suspect organism is a fastidious one. The choice of transport media depends largely on the microorganism suspected to be present in the specimen. If sterile swabs are to be taken from the body cavities or openings, the swabs should be taken immediately before fully opening such part of the animal cadaver. Hollow organs such as segments of the gastrointestinal tract are best handled by obtaining a loop tied at both ends and placed in a sterile petri dish. For bacteriological examination, samples should be collected in complete sterile conditions without using any chemical preservative and should be dispatched in ice box. For viral examination, 5-10 volumes of 50% buffered glycerine is used as preservative. For mycological studies, skin scrapings are collected in 20% potassium hydroxide solution.

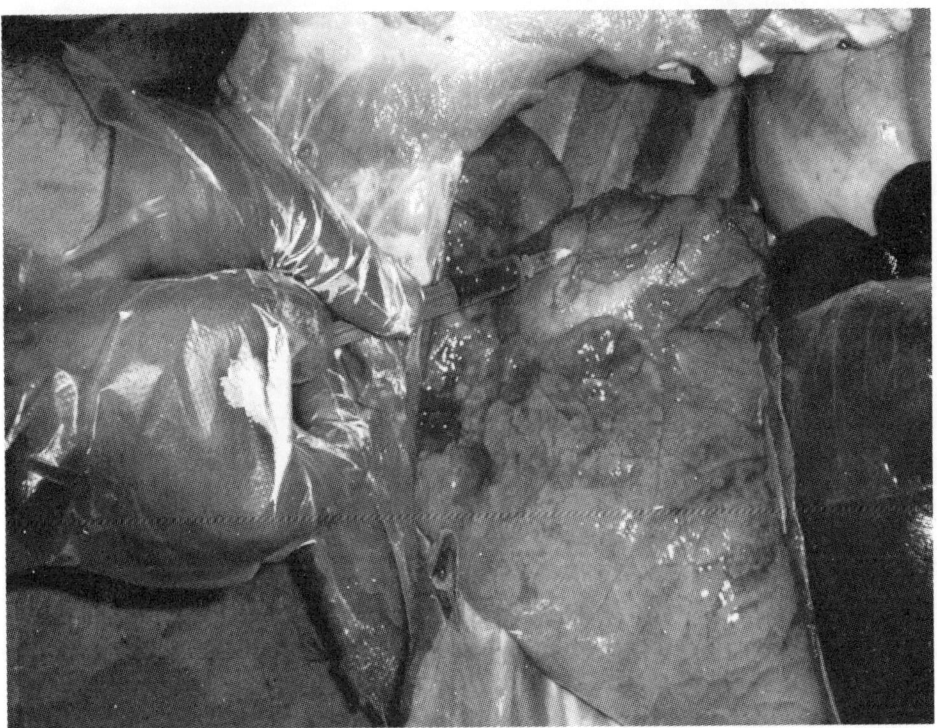

Fig. 11 : Collection of heart blood for bacteriological studies

7.3 Collection of tissue for toxicological examination

The material for toxicological examination should be free from any contaminating chemicals being used during necropsy. Chemicals that may contaminate the specimen include fixatives, detergents and disinfectants routinely used during necropsy. The sample is collected in clean wide mouthed glass or plastic bottles with stoppers of capacity one liter. Separate bottles are taken for each material. Rectified spirit is used normally as preservative but it is contraindicated in cases of suspected poisoning by alcohol, phosphorous, paraldehyde, acetic acid, carbolic acid and other drugs of phenol groups. The amount of spirit added to each bottle should be measured and the amount so added should be written on the label affixed to the container. Saturated solution of common salt is employed where rectified spirit is contraindicated. The material required for laboratory examination in the cases of poisoning is indicated in Table 2.

Table 2 : Diagnostic materials in suspected cases of poisoning

Material	Amount	Indications
Stomach and its contents	500-1000 g in large animals, and all available contents in small animals	Suspicion of mycotoxins and certain plant poisonings
Upper part of small intestine with its contents, any suspicious substance in stomach and intestine	500-1000 g in large animals, and all available contents in small animals	Suspicion of mycotoxins and certain plant poisonings
Liver	500-1000 g in large animals, and whole liver in small animals	Suspicion of mycotoxins like aflatoxin present in feed, confirmation of toxic conditions like cyanide, organophosphates, selenium, arsenic, carbamates and certain plant poisonings
Kidney	One complete kidney	Suspicion of mycotoxins like ochratoxin, other toxic conditions, plant poisonings
Spleen	Complete or portion , if large	Confirmation of toxic conditions like cyanide, organophosphates, selenium, arsenic, carbamates and certain plant poisonings
Urine (all available) and faeces in preservative kept separately	Sufficient quantity, thymol used for preserving if rectified spirit is contraindicated	Confirmation of toxic conditions like cyanide, organophosphates, selenium, arsenic, carbamates and certain plant poisonings such as Senecio, Astragalus, Crotolaria etc.
Heart and portion of brain	Sufficient portion	Suspicion of strychnine poisoning

Lung tissue and heart blood without adding preservative	Sufficient portion	Suspicion of poisoning of carbon monoxide, coal gas, hydrocyanic acid, alcohol or chloroform
Portion of skin and subcutaneous tissue	Sufficient portion	Suspicion of poisoning by subcutaneous injection
Hair	5 to 10 g	Suspicion of subacute or chronic poisoning by mineral especially arsenic or lead etc. (Most minerals are eliminated through hair).
Portion of long bones	Sufficient portion	Suspicion of subacute or chronic poisoning by arsenic and antimony (especially in case of extreme putrefaction or when body is exhumed after long burial)

7.4. Collection of specimens for parasitological examination

Occasionally, ectoparasites and endoparasites are collected during necropsy for identification. Collection of samples of ectoparasites is done before the cadaver is cut open for examination. Ticks, fleas and lice should be carefully brushed off from the fur or feather and fixed in 10% formalin. Wetting the fur or feather of the animal with a detergent solution may be done to disable these organisms. While collecting ticks, damage to the mouthparts should be prevented by wiping the body part of the tick with ether. It kills the tick and allows it to drop. The collected specimens are fixed in 70% ethyl alcohol or in 10% formalin. Information about the degree of ectoparasite infestation should be provided along with the submission. Mange mites are collected by scrapping the affected skin deeply and putting the scrappings on a glass slide with a drop of mineral oil. Roundworms collected from intestinal segments may be fixed in 10% formalin immediately after collection. It is advisable to allow the worms to relax by dipping in menthol solution or lukewarm water before fixation to prevent curling of the specimen. Tapeworm segment collection should include both mature and immature segments, with the scolex still intact. The tapeworm should never be lifted from its attachment because it may break the scolex. The scolex is important in species identification. The part where the scolex is attached is excised and fixed in formalin. The specimens of cestodes are pressed between two glass slides held together by a rubber band, a piece of twine or paper clips before immersion in the fixative. For total worm count in ruminants, the abomasum is tied at both ends and all its contents are saved. Scrapping from the deep mucosa of the affected intestinal segment and examining the scrappings as a wet smear may do the diagnosis of coccidial infection. Coccidial oocysts faeces are collected in 2.5% dichromate solution.

7.5 Collection of specimens for cytological examination

Smears from the tumour tissues are prepared occasionally for cytological evaluation. It is often possible to have a diagnosis by preparing and examining smears (from cut surfaces of the tumour) and aspirates even before tissue blocks of the tumour tissues are processed by conventional paraffin embedding technique. The smears should be allowed to dry immediately after collection to preserve the cell architecture. Fixation may be done by heat treatment or by dipping in absolute methanol. Some workers suggest the use of hair spray, which presumably contains alcohol in a concentration that is sufficient to fix the cells in the smears. Smears may be prepared from body fluids by putting a few drops onto the glass slide. The fluid may be collected and centrifuged and the cell pellet at the bottom of the tube fixed in formalin or methanol and the smears prepared. Alternatively, gelatin or albumin may be used to suspend the cell pellet and then fixing the mixture in formalin. This preparation may then be submitted for routine paraffin embedding technique similar to a tissue block.

7.6 Collection of body fluids

The general rule in collecting body fluid is to obtain samples free from contaminants. Body fluids should be collected as the examination progresses if it is anticipated that such examination is required. Urine may be collected directly from the urinary bladder by aspiration. Pleural, pericardial, synovial or cerebrospinal fluid should be collected by aspirating the fluid with syringe and needle. In case of abortion, particularly in brucellosis, stomach content from aborted foetus may be collected with the help of sterilized syringe or Pasteur pipette.

8. Submission or Dispatch of Specimens to Diagnostic Laboratory

The transport of diagnostic specimens from place of post-mortem to diagnostic laboratory is required to be meticulous. The diagnostic specimens must be handled as infectious substances; therefore the material should not have any possibility of escaping from the package. The brief account of the labelling, sealing and packing of specimens is as under.

8.1 Labelling

Labelling should be secure that cannot be lost or easily destroyed. For example adhesive tape should go entirely around the vial so that it will not be dislodged by moisture. Writing should be with pencil or waterproof ink. It is advisable to put labelled paper inside the specimen bottle and a similar label pasted on the outside of the specimen bottle. The label should carry the following information: (a) case number, (b) species, and (c) name of the organ.

A piece of absorbent cotton should invariably be placed to keep the tissues moist particularly for floating tissues and in case the bottle breaks during transit.

8.2 Sealing

Enough care should be taken to seal the mouth of the bottle with paraffin wax so as to make it water tight. It is better to use plastic screw-cap containers instead of glass containers where practical. Electrical tape should be wound around the cap in the same direction as the screw cap is applied.

8.3 Packing

Sealed and labelled receptacles containing specimens should be placed in a suitable container along with the history sheet and/or post-mortem report having clinical/post-mortem diagnosis. Enough packing material should be provided to ensure safe delivery of the contents in the laboratory.

8.4 Precautions while forwarding the diagnostic material

The following methods are erroneous and must be avoided:

- Sending large pieces of tissues such as whole organ - In this case only the surface of the tissues is preserved and the interior undergoes autolysis, rendering the tissues unfit for correct histopathological examinations.
- Forcing large pieces of tissues or whole organ in small receptacles - With the hardening effect of fixative like formalin, it is impossible to remove the material without breaking the bottle. Moreover the tissues are mutilated.
- Sending material from the centre of an extensive lesion like suppuration/ tumour which does not give the maximum information.

9. Writing of Post-Mortem Report

It is highly desirable to make a true and complete record of the post-mortem findings and so far as possible it should be made immediately after the completion of necropsy. The findings may be dictated to another person while conducting necropsy because even the best memory is not always trustworthy. The availability of complete record is very essential when animals are examined for research purpose and in vetero-legal disputes. The style and type of post-mortem forms may vary from institute to institute, however, the form should include the following basic entries in general.

General information

1. Species of animal
2. Date
3. Case No.
4. Breed
5. Age/Birth date
6. Sex
7. Identification No.
8. Owner's name, address and phone No.
9. Referred by
10. Clinical history of the case
11. Reported date & time of death
12. Date and time of post-mortem examination
13. Type of specimen and preservative used

Post-mortem findings

Post-mortem changes
External examination
Subcutaneous tissue and musculature
Respiratory system
Cardiovascular system
Digestive system
Urinary system
Genital system
Immune system
Nervous system
Miscellaneous observations
Results of laboratory examination

Diagnosis

Date

Place

Signature

Name and designation

10. Post-Necropsy Guidelines

Proper disposal of the carcass after post-mortem and thorough cleaning and disinfection of the area and instruments are very important post-necropsy tasks. Depending upon the facilities, the carcass may be either buried (with a layer of lime) or incinerated. The site must also be cleaned after post-mortem examination. Incineration is the best method for the disposal of small animal cadaver, though it may not be practically very suitable for large animals. The amount of time involved in the incineration and the amount of fuel required turning the large heap of flesh and bones into ash preclude this procedure. For both small and large animals, burying deep into the ground may be practical. However, the pit should be dug deep enough so that stray animals and other predators cannot have easy access to the disposed cadaver. The site should be away from the sources of feed or where underground water is being pumped. All dead animal cadavers should be considered possible sources of infection that should be disposed of responsibly. Lastly, the protective clothing worn during necropsy such as gloves, cap, disposable gown/apron, shoe covers/rubber gum boots, mask etc. should be removed in the post-mortem room and disinfected before disposal.

11. Vetero-Legal Necropsy

Vetero-legal necropsy is the detailed and systematic examination of a dead animal to ascertain the time since the death and the cause of death, when a crime is involved (Sriraman 2006). Some major examples which involve vetero-legal necropsy are listed below.

- Unauthorized killing of wild animals
- Accidental death due to electric shock when fault is not of the animal owner
- Death due to feed toxicity and environmental pollution with toxic chemicals
- Death of animals due to intentional poisoning, shooting, or other means due to rivalry

11.1 Major considerations in vetero-legal cases

i. For vetero-legal cases, post-mortem request should be signed by a police officer not below the rank of an inspector or by magistrate; without which no post-mortem examination should be done.

ii. Maximum information should be collected on history, date and time of death of animal and treatment given.

iii. Animal identification including species, breed, age and number or mark must be clearly established before conduct of post-mortem examination. It is particularly necessary in insured animals as well as in cases of religious disputes.

iv. All the lesions present on skin surface should be clearly defined as laceration, wound, trauma, incision, erosion, vesicle, and ulcer. If there is suspected sharp edge wound or bullet injury, its depth and width should be recorded. The side on which the animal is lying down (e.g. ventral portion touching earth) should also be noted.

v. In case of dispute over stillbirth or calf having born alive, a piece of lung should be placed in water. The lung piece sinks in water in case of atelectasis neonatum (stillbirth) while it floats if the calf was born alive.

vi. If the case is suspected for toxic condition/poisoning, it is advisable to mention the type of suspected poison in the report. It helps the police authorities to establish/confirm the type of toxin/poison in forensic laboratory.

vii. The post-mortem examination of wild animals should be conducted as a special case. One should conduct the post-mortem examination only when an authorized officer makes request for post-mortem examination. It should be noted on the report that all the viscera including skin, bones teeth etc. are returned to the person who requested for the necropsy and no item should be left behind.

viii. The post-mortem report should be prepared clearly in neat handwriting and clear language avoiding ambiguity. Writing general sentences should be avoided and only specific findings and conclusions should be given. The report should be signed with date and a copy of it should be kept for record and future evidence in the court of law.

ix. Post-mortem examination should be conducted in day light. Where the pathologist is not able to recognize the lesion due to darkness, the post-mortem examination should not be conducted.

x. At the time of post-mortem examination, entry of the outsiders should not be allowed. Post-mortem examination should be done in closed premises to avoid wild birds and animals.

xi. In case of poisoning, a sample of preservative used should be kept separately.

xii. The sample bottles should be placed in a cardboard box. All the bottles and packets should be carefully sealed and closed in such a manner that they can not be opened without destroying the seal.

xiii. The covering letter should include details of material collected, railway receipt (if sent by railway parcel), post-mortem report along with history, details of seal (sample seals to be affixed on the covering letter) and copy of the request and report from police should be sent separately by registered post to the chemical examiner.

12. Vetero-Legal Wounds

Vetero-legal wounds occur due to shooting, malicious injury by sharp objects or other means generally due to rivalry between people, commonly neighbours. The knowledge of the characteristic features of the wounds caused by different objects is essential to arrive at final diagnosis in such cases.

12.1 Types of vetero-legal wounds

The vetero-legal wounds may be of the following types.

12.1.1 Incised wounds

These are produced by sharp cutting weapon (e.g. razors, knives, sword, axes etc.). The edges of these wounds are smooth, even, clean cut, well defined and are characterized by 'gaping' from retraction of the divided skin and tissues. The point of commencement of such a wound is deeper and gradually becomes shallower. There may be severe haemorrhage, if a main artery is cut. While describing these wounds, it is important to mention the location, depth and direction.

12.1.2 Lacerated wounds

These are caused by tearing of the tissues. The edges are torn and irregular and are generally produced by barbed wire and the claws, teeth or horns of animals. These are also common in street vehicle accidents. Lacerated wounds are often associated with injuries to internal organs and fractures of bones. These wounds usually show some loss of substance.

12.1.3 Punctured/penetrating wounds

These are caused by pointed bodies such as knives, daggers and spears or any pointed instruments. The external opening is small but the object may penetrate deep into tissues or may enter body cavity and injure vital organs. External haemorrhage is less but internal may be profuse. The depth of the punctured wound should be noted as it gives a clue to the length of the weapon.

12.1.4 Gun shot wounds

The appearance of these wounds depends upon the kind of weapon, nature and velocity of projectile, nature of powder, range at which the weapon is fired, the part of the body struck and direction of fire. However, the study of fire arms and ammunition is complex and demands specialisation. The veterinarian is expected to say whether the given weapon could have caused the wounds.

12.1.5 Contused wounds

These are injuries produced by blunt weapons. The weapons leave their outline on the bruise (e.g. whipping, spurring and blows from stones and sticks). It can be accompanied by rupture of internal organs or extensive crushing of the tissue. In most cases, there is little haemorrhage, but an extravasation of serum on to the surface of skin producing a scab is seen.

12.2 Major considerations while examining vetero-legal wounds

- Vetero-legal wounds (ante-mortem wounds) must be differentiated from post-mortem wounds. In ante-mortem wounds, there will be arterial haemorrhages and inflammatory reaction.
- The description of wounds should include the number, position, direction and type of wounds, condition of their edges and ends, presence of foreign bodies, nature of weapon, signs of inflammatory reaction (swelling, pus etc.) and the presence of clotted/unclotted blood.
- The death from wounds may be due to external or internal haemorrhages, injury to vital organs such as lungs, heart, brain etc., necrosis of internal organs, or infection in the wound such as tetanus.

13. Conclusion

Necropsy plays a vital role in diagnosis of diseases and ultimately in their control as well as in research, teaching and in understanding pathogenesis of diseases of unknown aetiology. It should be performed in a very systematic manner simultaneously recording the findings to arrive at an accurate diagnosis. It is quite essential to be well versed with the post-mortem changes that occur after death so as to differentiate between the alterations that occur in the body before death and those which take place after death. Collection of the morbid material, its preservation and dispatch to the laboratory in a correct manner is another important aspect of the necropsy procedure for correct diagnosis. Post-mortem examination assumes even greater significance in vetero-legal cases and animal welfare issues.

References

1. Cabana EM (1999). Necropsy Procedures: General Considerations. http://www2.mozcom.com/~emcdvm.
2. King JM, Dodd DC, Roth L (2006). The Necropsy Book, 4th ed. Charles Louis Davis, DVM Foundation, Gurnee, FL.
3. Sriraman PK (2006). A guide to post-mortem examination of animals. Jaypee Brothers Medical Publishers (P) Ltd., New Delhi.
4. Wobeser GA, Spraker TR, Harms VL (1980). Collection and field preservation of biological materials. In: Wildlife management techniques manual, 4th edition, SD Schemnitz (ed.). The Wildlife Society, Washington DC, p. 537-551.

❑❑❑

Chapter 27

Intersectoral Coordination for Control of Zoonotic Infections

B. R. SINGH[1], VIDYA SINGH[2] AND S. R. GARG[3]
[1]Centre for Animal Disease Research and Diagnosis, Indian Veterinary Research Institute, Izatnagar-243122, [2] National Research Centre on Mithun, Jharnapani-797106, [3] Department of Veterinary Public Health and Epidemiology, College of Veterinary Sciences, Hisar-125004

Contents

1. Introduction

The concept of intersectoral cooperation for health of human race and other creatures of our mighty planet is not new. More than several thousand years ago since the times of Veda, the oldest Hindu scriptures, verses have been recited for happiness of all creatures so that humanity can also prosper (*Sarve bhavantu sukhinah, sarve santu niramaya......*). However, the scientific advancements and development of human race subsequently created a concept of human supremacy. By virtue of his mental superiority and innovative ability, man has been trying to tame the nature including all its living and nonliving components for his greed and necessities of civilization. Human race probably first met its needs with hunting and then through domestication of animals and farming for obtaining a variety of goods and services e.g. food, clothing, fibres and transport etc. Taming the nature brought humans in a relation of intimacy and frequent interaction with nonhuman life forms, leading to many transformations in the human animal environment. The ever innovative human minds evolved several branches of science for the ease of study. However, the egoistic attitudes of the scientists created compartments, spheres, and inner spheres, often impermeable to others.

Not long ago, the field of medicine was considered one for whole of the world but last few centuries saw its sectorization into human medicine, veterinary medicine, plant health, environmental health etc. even though it is still difficult to differentiate between human medicine and veterinary medicine in *Ayurveda, Unani,* Chinese herbal and homeopathic systems. Narration of several surgeries and medicines is cited in the ancient Indian epics. Lord *Ganesha*, the elephant god with the head of an elephant and body of the human, is one of the many examples of chimera created through surgery by the greatest surgeon, Lord *Shiva*, who must be well versed in human and animal anatomy, surgery and medicine. In modern civilization, the first successful caesarean section was performed in the 1580s, in Siegershausen, Switzerland by Lacob Nufer, a veterinarian, a pig doctor (Conner 2005). Prior to it, caesarean section usually resulted in the death of the mother. Most of the surgical and medical methods are first perfected on animals and then brought to human practice even now, pointing to the relevance of the intersectoral coordination to relieve humanity from pain and suffering.

Due to the intensification and convergence of the people, animals, plants, aquatic life and the environment, the health of each group is now inextricably interconnected. There are predictions for animal based protein to increase by 50% by 2020 but the survival of many animal species is threatened and loss of biodiversity is speeding at alarming pace (Delgado *et al.* 1999). Due to the loss in biodiversity, there have been paradigm shift in the number and nature of infectious diseases in both animals and human beings. The infectious agents are diversifying their host range and are crossing from their natural hosts to others. More than 60% of 1,461 diseases now recognized in humans are zoonotic (Torrey and Yolken 2005) while most of the emerging and reemerging human infectious diseases (about 75%) have been recognized as zoonotic (Taylor *et al.* 2001). Studies in the recent past have revealed transmission of infectious agents even from plants to human beings (pepper mild mottle virus). Several plants can host human infectious agents like typhoid bacillus (Siddiqui *et al.* 2006, 2008, Singh *et al.* 2004, 2005, 2007a,b,c) and can transmit them to consumers. Many noninfectious ailments also get transmitted from animals, aquatic or aerial life forms and plants to human beings and vice versa, the most common being the toxins and poisons of various organisms. Our increasing interdependence and association with other life forms due to shrinking niche may well be the single most critical risk factor to our health and well being with regard to infectious diseases. It has led to an increase in the frequency and severity of various diseases. These threats also have the potential to affect regional and global economies.

Further, if the world has shrunken for human race through faster means of transport, increased movement of the people, real time communication systems and globalization of trade, it has shrunken at much faster pace for pathogens. The change has contributed to the emergence of new diseases and serious consequences. Most of the current emerging diseases are zoonoses either of food origin (e.g. salmonellosis and campylobacteriosis) or the classic ones including tuberculosis, anthrax, Ebola, transmissible spongiform encephalopathies or more recently severe acute respiratory syndrome (SARS), and highly pathogenic avian influenza (HPAI) posing real threat of global pandemics. These also have the potential to affect the regional and global economies. Another major concern is the potential of the pathogens of zoonotic importance in bioterrorism acts.

As evident, the issue of infectious agents frequently crossing the species barriers is very alarming and needs to be addressed sincerely and urgently. Professionals from various sectors such as medical, veterinary, aquaculture, ecology, agriculture, toxicology, pharmacology etc. have to play their role individually as well as collectively. The episodes of major global health threats in the recent past have amply emphasized the need for application of the principles of 'One Health' to address the problems in a holistic and more effective manner.

2. Imminent Threats to Animal and Human Domains

2.1 Emerging and reemerging zoonoses

The spread of Ebola, West Nile, SARS and monkey pox viruses in virgin areas has permanently changed the landscape of human and animal medicine.

Foodborne bovine spongiform encephalopathy (BSE) in cattle and its probable association with Creudtzfeldt Jakob disease (CJD) in humans has changed the global agricultural practices and trade. HIV-AIDS transmitted from nonhuman primates to humans has severely impaired the life expectancy and health of humans. Conditions like foot and mouth disease (FMD), rinderpest (RP) and Peste des Petits Ruminants (PPR) though do not affect human health but cause huge economic losses and have major consequences on the food supply chain. Rough estimates reveal that water and foodborne enteric diseases are causing more than 1.5 million human deaths annually. In USA (one of the most developed countries and holding only about 300 million people) alone, 47.8 million foodborne illnesses result in around 4000 deaths every year (Scallan *et al.* 2011a,b). The grim situation in the global perspective can very well be visualized.

Regrettably, despite the vast knowledge, dramatic achievements in science, and the emergence of diseases such as Ebola virus, Lyme disease, SARS, avian influenza and swine influenza, veterinary medicine and public health remain in quite separate domains. Schools and other training institutions, healthcare facilities, nongovernmental organizations (NGOs), public health agencies at all administrative levels, professional and scientific organizations, and scientific journals nearly all remain segregated by their interest in either human medicine or animal health or plant protection etc. Several health problems in the recent past have left permanent scars on the humanity which necessitates an urgent need of cooperation among different disciplines to safeguard the health of all.

Many non-communicable conditions and factors are also affecting both animal and human health adversely. In fact, these factors are likely to accelerate in intensity and complexity that may surely create consequences and implications of unprecedented scope and scale. The resulting global economic devastation may thus be of much greater consequences than those encountered previously. In such a situation, only integrated strategies based on the tenets of One Health can be of help to sail through the rough sea ahead.

2.2 Transmission of fish diseases to humans

The ever increasing urbanization, rapid industrialization and shrinking water bodies have created pressure on the aquatic environment. There have been reports of increase in the number of zoonotic organisms, especially enteric pathogens. Since 1972, the number of enteric genera affecting human and animals has doubled and the species have tripled (Shotts 1987).

After deciphering the close association of BSE and CJD and the impact of use of animal by-products (bone meal) in BSE outbreak in the European countries, it has been proposed that fish might play role in transmission of prions from BSE affected cattle to humans causing variant CJD as fishes are fed with animal by-products.

Fishes and other aquatic organisms such as oysters, mussels and clams can bioaccumulate pathogens and toxicants from polluted waters. The consumption of contaminated shellfish has caused gastroenteritis, respiratory illness, fever, hepatitis and toxicity in man. Fishes even act as vector or intermediate host for many human and animal diseases and have been reported to transmit bacterial diseases like skin tuberculosis, salmonellosis, vibriosis, edwardsielosis and erysepalothrix causing illnesses of varying degrees. Apart from these, fish nematodes such as cod worm (*Phocanema decipiens*), *Anisakis* sp., *Dioctophyme renale* and *Gnathostoma hispidium* can infect man causing larva-migrans (visceral/ cutaneous) and allergic response (Myers 1970). Several organisms earlier considered only as fish pathogens (*Edwardsiella tarda)* have emerged as important organisms affecting not only human beings but also the animals and birds (Singh and Tiwari 1996). It all points towards the need of disease control strategies seeking coordination between aquatic, veterinary, avian and human medical experts.

2.3 Disease transmission from plant to humans

A group of pathogens have been proposed as Phytonoses that includes pathogens which either inadvertently or opportunistically may get transmitted to man or animals. There are several outbreaks of salmonellosis on record after consumption of foods of vegetable origin in different parts of the world. Recently, it has been proved that not only *Salmonella* but other human pathogens including *Klebsiella* and *Escherichia coli* can colonize in plant tissues and cause pathology, particularly in seedlings. Seedlings infected in their infancy may carry these notorious pathogens for their life in growing parts with some effect on overall growth (Singh *et al.* 2004, 2005, 2007a,b,c). There is evidence to suggest that pepper mild mottle virus, a virus common in pepper causing mottling of leaves, may have moved on to infect humans causing fever, abdominal pain, and itching. This may be attributed to species jump of the virus due to any drastic changes in the genotype or the attempt of the virus to broaden its host range by changing its cell binding receptors (Colson *et al.* 2010).

Very high degree of homology has been reported between the genome of human uveitis mycoplasma-like organisms (MLO) and that of plant MLO, which indicates the probability of cross infection of MLO between plants and man. The probability of prion/prion-like elements and viroids has also been proposed under this group. Though there are no evidences to support this yet, it cannot be ruled out completely.

There is significant homology between the genomes of circoviruses and nanoviruses infecting animals and plants, respectively. They have similarity in the genes and encoding proteins. It has been proposed that during the course of evolution, the virus shifted from plants to animals and has acquired subsequent changes to adapt in the vertebrates.

3. Multidisciplinary approach for healthy world

The multidisciplinary approach for healthy world through 'One Health' initiative is a paradigmatic shift from the traditional viewpoint to expand interdisciplinary collaborations and communications in all aspects of healthcare for humans, animals and the environment. It involves collaborative effort of professionals from multiple disciplines, working at local, national, and global level with a common objective. It promotes the concept of total health by integration of all biotic and abiotic components of the system through communication and collaboration among physicians, veterinarians, wildlife professionals, environmental and public health experts, ecologists, ornithologists, biomedical engineers, physicists, biochemists, plant pathologists as well as political and administrative personnel. It helps to understand and address the contemporary health issues created by the convergence of human, animal, and environmental domains. The multidisciplinary approach is of great importance as it facilitates better understanding of the disease processes through a comparative medicine approach, involving public health, environmental health, biomedical research (including laboratory animal science), and clinical medicine and surgery.

4. History of the One Health concept

The interaction between man and animals has been recognized since ancient times. Animals have made a very strong contribution to the rise of modern medicine and to the development of public health. The concept that human and animal health is linked is not new. Rudolph Virchow asserted that between animal and human medicine there are no dividing lines, nor should there be (Kahn *et al.* 2007). He also coined the term 'zoonosis' for a disease transmissible from animals to humans. Most of the early clinicians, researchers and great souls who relieved humanity from pain had only one concept of health. Father of modern medicine, Sir William Osler (1849-1919) conducted research on several animal diseases (e.g. hog cholera, verminous bronchitis in dogs) in collaboration with his veterinary medical student.

Salmonellosis, a foodborne illness, was named after Daniel E. Salmon (1850-1914), a veterinarian, who hired physicians to work for him. They jointly discovered that heat-killed pathogens can immunize against live pathogens and also reported the tick transmission of babesiosis in cattle. John McFadyean

(1853-1941), a veterinarian, proved that bovine tuberculosis can be transmitted to humans through milk. He also developed a McFadyean's methylene blue stain for the diagnosis of anthrax. Karl F. Meyer (1884-1974), a medico turned veterinarian, made enormous contributions to the field of infectious diseases and epidemiology, working on human and animal diseases, including typhoid fever, malaria, influenza, brucellosis, anthrax, plague, equine encephalomyelitis, coccidioidomycosis and *Yersinia pestis*. Calvin W. Schwabe (1927-2006), a veterinarian by training, a noted epidemiologist and parasitologist, pioneered the use of human disease tracking techniques in the study of animal illnesses. In the recent past Murphy, a veterinarian, worked in association with Karl Johnson, a physician and unraveled the mystery of Ebola haemorrhagic fever outbreak (Kahn *et al.* 2009).

In 1996, a landmark was created, when the collaboration between veterinary and human medicine was recognized at the highest level of science by awarding the prestigious Nobel Prize jointly to a physician, Rolf M. Zinkernagel, and a veterinarian, Peter C. Doherty, who worked together and discovered how the body's immune system distinguishes normal cells from virus-infected cells. The emergence of West Nile virus in New York City in 1999 was a seminal event. A veterinarian played key role in recognizing that the disease in humans and animals was linked by a newly emerged virus, emphasizing the critical role for One Health principles in public health.

One Health concept is, thus, not entirely new; it persisted even thousands of years ago in the Vedic era, though its revival in the modern science is not very old. Dr. Calvin W. Schwabe coined the phrase 'One Medicine' in 1960s and called for a unified approach between veterinary and human medicine to combat zoonotic diseases. The concept got major emphasis in the last decade of 20th century due to continuous efforts of the Society for Tropical Veterinary Medicine which organized conferences with the banner "working together to promote global health." It has been advocating the need for a multidisciplinary approach to meet the challenges of the 21st century. Inspired by this, the Wildlife Conservation Society (WCS) and Rockefeller University initiated the mission One World-One Health in 2004 (WCS 2009, STVM 2009). The phrase "One World, One Health and One Medicine" was evolved by the World Veterinary Congress and the expressions 'One Medicine', 'One Health' and 'One World - One Health - One Medicine' are now often used interchangeably. In recent years, a number of like-minded individuals across professional spectrums have begun recognizing the concept as an essential element for advancing research progress for human and animal health (Kahn *et al.* 2007, 2009).

5. Aims of One Health concept

One Health seeks to promote, improve and defend the health and well being of all species by enhancing cooperation and collaboration between physicians, veterinarians, and the other scientific, health and environmental professionals and by promoting strengths in leadership and management to achieve these goals. The One Health initiative and growing international collaboration in response to pandemic threats, coupled with the developments in the fields of informatics and genomics, hold promise for improved sentinel event coordination in order to detect and reduce environmental health threats shared between species. To summarize, the goals of intersectoral cooperation towards one health can be outlined as under:

1. To revive the integration of animal, human and environmental health for the mutual benefit of all
2. To increase communication and collaboration between human, animal and ecosystem health professionals
3. To bring integration of educational systems within and between medical colleges, veterinary colleges and public health institutions
4. To promote and improve the health of humans, animals and the environment, individually and collectively, by encouraging and ensuring the acceptance and adoption of One Health and its associated activities

6. Holistic Collaborative Approach

One Health has now become a rallying call due to the emergence of new diseases pointing to the urgent need of a holistic approach to human, animal and ecosystem health for a sustainable future. Pollution and contamination of the environment has drastically impaired the health and sustainability of our environment, thereby creating conditions conducive for the spread of infectious as well as an increasing number of acute and chronic noninfectious conditions detrimental to both human and animal health. Noninfectious threats also include toxins and chemical contaminants, such as endocrine-disrupting chemicals in the environment (Colborn *et al.* 1996). Climate change and increasing human populations will definitely increase the need for multidisciplinary, collaborative programmes. The study of virulence mechanism and host-pathogen interactions of zoonotic and animal pathogens calls for multidisciplinary collaborative efforts of scientists. Further, in the modern globalized world, pathogens travel very fast and a single microbe may wash over the entire humankind, animal and environmental domains (Brundtland 2001).

Increasing interdependence with animals and their products has also spurred the medical and veterinarian professions to readdress holistic collaborative approach locally, nationally, and globally to attain optimal health for people, animals and the environment. The disease triangle is a conceptual model that shows the interactions between the environment, the host and an infectious (or abiotic) agent. This model can be used to predict epidemiological outcomes in plant health and public health, both in local and global communities.

6.1 Applicability of One Health approach

There is similarity among all living beings in the basic molecules of life, nucleic acids/proteins and biochemical and metabolic mechanisms, which have revealed closer relationship and provide a scope for new insight for applicability of common medicine in one health perspective. Molecular biology studies by sequencing genetic codes have confirmed a remarkable similarity between all mammalian species with highly conserved genetic sequences. The similarities have even been among all life forms in their receptors on/within the cell as routes for invasion and tools for defense.

These similarities at basic level can be exploited to develop and adopt universal measures which can be applicable to all life forms to achieve the goal of one health. Further, we need to identify the areas where the integration of human, animal, and environmental health exists and to identify the areas where the concept and operation of One Health are especially needed.

As many as 335 events of emerging diseases have been reported since 1940 and these have gradually increased over the decades (Scholthof 2007). Most of the these diseases have originated in the developing world and the pattern is likely to continue in the future at much faster pace because the antimicrobials, antivirals, anthelmintics, insecticides, pesticides and thousands of other ecology modulating chemicals are available everywhere now including the developed and developing countries. The threat is much more serious in developing and less developed countries primarily due to the indiscriminate use of drugs in human beings, aquaculture, agriculture and animals and secondly due to inadequate diagnostic facilities that provides every chance to an emerging pathogen to fully bloom.

In the past few decades, emerging and re-emerging diseases such as Hanta virus, plague, leptospirosis, West Nile virus, Lyme disease, and schistosomiasis have all been associated and impacted by changing pattern of the weather, floods, land use and host-vector dynamics. A collaborative effort is required if they are to be detected and contained.

6.2 Collaboration at the local, national and global levels

The inclusion of a variety of health professionals in local, national, and international organizations is the key to develop feasible plans to control most of the emerging and re-emerging diseases. Human and veterinary medical associations could meet more frequently to discuss topics of mutual interest in their communities. Despite the fact that most of the emerging diseases have emerged in developing world, our surveillance systems have been developed and implemented with a bias towards the richer and developed countries. Thus, the areas with high risk and probability get overlooked and are left for incubation of another emerging disease. The efforts to create and establish good surveillance and monitoring systems in the developing countries as an integrated strategy and across domains are lacking where we need them the most.

A strong leadership is required to embrace the One Health concept, to execute a change over programme on global level and to change the healthcare professionals' mindset from therapeutic to prophylactic one.

Internationally, the collaboration should occur among different agencies and organizations such as the World Health Organization (WHO), Food and Agriculture Organization of the United Nations (FAO), United Nations Children's Fund (UNICEF), Office International des Epizooties (OIE), World Wildlife Fund (WWF), Wildlife Conservation Society (WCS), International Union for Conservation of Nature (IUCN) and the advanced research organizations and laboratories, including those of the Consultative Group on International Agriculture Research (CGIAR) system. Regionally, this would include different organizations such as the Association of Southeast Asian Nations (ASEAN), Asia-Pacific Economic Cooperation (APEC), South Asian Association for Regional Cooperation (SAARC) and African Union - Inter-African Bureau for Animal Resources (AU-IBAR) among others. The regional organizations are playing key roles increasingly in managing diseases with transboundary potential.

In addition, public-private alliance and partnerships with NGOs can help to provide long-term sustainability of emerging infectious disease control. The mechanisms for regular information-sharing and collaboration across sectors need to be established at national, regional and international levels for successful alliances and partnerships.

7. Initiatives in Action

In 2004, the Wildlife Conservation Society in an international symposium on the current and potential movement of diseases among human, domestic animals and wildlife delineated priorities for an international, interdisciplinary approach for combating threats to the health of life on earth as 'Manhattan Principles' with twelve recommendations for establishing a more holistic approach to prevent epidemic/epizootic diseases and for maintaining ecosystem integrity for the benefit of humans, their domesticated animals, and the foundational biodiversity that supports us all. The meeting was attended by professionals and agencies belonging to all sectors.

Further, One Health Initiative Task Force has been set up and is being promoted jointly by the American Medical Association and American Veterinary Medical Association in USA. The task force has proposed 12 recommendations for the accomplishment of the objectives of 'One World, One Health, One Medicine'. The success of these recommendations will depend heavily on the collaboration of various health science professions, academic institutions, governmental agencies, and private industries. The recommendations are as follows:

1. Create and fund a One Health Joint Steering Committee to begin the execution of the other recommendations and associated actions.
2. Complete a One Health Proposal for donors as well as a business plan and continue the process of engaging potential donors and sponsors.
3. Create and implement initial components of a One Health communication effort.
4. Engage an all-inclusive communication firm to develop and implement a communication plan and coordinate ongoing media relations, public relations, publicity, marketing and advertising.
5. Plan a study on One Health to be conducted by the National Academy of Sciences (NAS) and secure necessary funding to underwrite this effort.
6. Develop, charter and form a National One Health Commission (to replace the Steering Committee) and recruit fulltime staff in key positions to support the goals and mission of the Commission and complete the recommendations within this report.
7. Appoint a national/global One Health Advisory Team to help and support the National One Health Commission, and give it direction, counsel and wisdom.
8. Plan and hold a One Health National Summit.
9. Convene several panels and a national meeting to establish a national research agenda for One Health.
10. Work towards the inclusion of key One Health outcomes for listing in the strategies for Healthy People 2020 and Healthy Animals 2010.
11. Inform, engage, and solicit the support of medical, veterinary and public health students and their respective organizations.
12. Create a guiding coalition of liaisons, champions and key supporters to promote the One Health concept.

In Israel, a new course, Middle East Programme for Interventional Epidemiology Training (MEPIET) has been initiated to bring all the health professionals at one platform to teach the value of 'One World - One Health' in meeting the challenge of emerging diseases.

In India, the High Security Animal Disease Laboratory (HSADL) and the National Institute of Virology (NIV) are world class research laboratories and are engaged in research on the emerging, reemerging and exotic diseases of the livestock and humans, respectively. They both are working in synergy and collaboration with each other sharing their resources, expertise and information. It became quite evident recently when these worked together in monitoring, surveillance, diagnostic and vaccine development programmes during the episodes of bird flu and swine flu in the country.

Kahn-Kaplan-Monath-Woodall One Health team has created a One Health Initiative website (www.onehealthinitiative.com) which is getting huge response. In India too, very recently, one of the coauthors, S.R. Garg, has launched the Scientific Consortium for Health Without Borders (www.health-without-borders.blogpot.com) which is also drawing worldwide attention.

8. Strategies for Intersectoral Cooperation for One Health

Partnership is critical to success; so the outcome of the One Health movement relies on the commitment of all health professionals, each contributing valuable skills and perspectives that will ultimately advance the cause. Intersectoral cooperation may be evolved with the following strategies.

1. Joint educational efforts between human medicine and veterinary medicine colleges, and making study of zoonotic diseases mandatory in all institutions of public health
2. Cross-disciplinary communication in journals and conferences, and via allied health networks
3. Joint efforts in clinical care through the assessment, treatment and prevention of cross-species disease transmission
4. Cross-species disease surveillance and control efforts in public health
5. Efforts for better understanding of cross-species disease transmission through comparative medicine research
6. Joint development and evaluation of new diagnostic methods
7. Comparative medicine approach to health and use of medicines and vaccines for the control and prevention of diseases across the species
8. Joint efforts to inform and educate political leaders and the public sector through media publications (newspapers, magazines) and health talks

9. An online One Health newsletter, a blockbuster health book and movie for widespread education
10. Continual efforts in all the above directions

This will need synergistic strategies and actions of the authorities and scientists concerned; in other words, a strong demand for a one health concept and policy.

9. Examples of Successful Intersectoral Cooperation in Control of Zoonoses

9.1 Development of humanized animal models for the study of zoonotic diseases

A multidisciplinary group of Nahum Shpigel, a veterinarian, Ilan Rosenshine, a molecular microbiologist and Simcha Yagel, a gynaecologist worked together, made a human bovine intestinal graft in mice and using it they unraveled the close association of *Mycobacterium avium paratuberculosis* to Crohn's diseases as an etiological agent (Greenstein and Collins 2004). The humanized and bovinised mice model enabled to understand the virulence mechanism of enterohaemorrhagic *E. coli* (EHEC) in human and bovine gut. It will help to develop the therapeutics and prophylactics.

9.2 Control of relapsing fever

The etiology, vector transmission and epidemiology of relapsing fever was established by a group of workers that included veterinarians, physicians, epidemiologists and molecular microbiologists. The knowledge evolved by them can be used for prophylactic measures against the disease (Barbour 1999).

9.3 Harnessing avian influenza

The recent episodes of avian influenza outbreak are a classic example where a multidisciplinary group of professionals worked together at all levels and across the state and political borders to contain the disease and develop prophylactic measures, Further, differentiating infected from vaccinated animals (DIVA) strategy for the disease was developed by common sharing of the information and data across different diagnostic agencies for epidemiological investigation and vaccine development.

Ilaria Capua has promoted and advocated an open access to the scientific data for epidemiological investigation and vaccine development which has been widely accepted for attainment of 'One Health'. Through this approach, the disease has been contained and controlled, thereby succeeding in saving millions of lives till now. Any flaws in collaboration may repeat the history of Spanish Flu when more than 50 million people died with a strain which was 25 times less fatal than the current strain of the virus (Taubenberger and Morens 2006).

The continual global circulation of human, swine, and avian influenza viruses via interspecies transmission calls for better trans-disciplinary influenza surveillance in pigs, birds, and other animals to aid in monitoring and assessing the mounting risk of future pandemic viruses.

9.4 Nipping in the bud of haemorrhagic fevers caused by Marburg and Ebola viruses

The etiology, vector, reservoir host and epidemiology of the haemorrhagic fever epidemic in Uganda in 2007-08 were established by a group of multidisciplinary workers Fred Murphy (veterinarian), Karl Johnson and Pat Webb (both physicians). Several agencies including Afrinet, WHO, Red Cross, UNICEF, Centers for Disease Control and Prevention (CDC) and public health colleagues from Uganda supported the work. Marburg and Ebola viruses have been established as the etiological agent and bats as the reservoir host.

9.5 Restricting enterohaemorrhagic *Escherichia coli*

EHEC are illustrative of the One Health concept as they embody the complex ecology of agricultural animals, wildlife, and the environment in zoonotic transmission of EHEC O157. They present a strong case that zoonotic disease is not associated with simple transmission from a reservoir host, but instead is involved with a complex environmental-host ecology that directly affects the likelihood of zoonotic transmission (Monath *et al.* 2010).

9.6 Containing Methicillin-resistant *Staphylococcus aureus*

Methicillin-resistant *Staphylococcus aureus* can reciprocally infect human and animal populations (Weese 2010). The success in containing the problem in recent years is testimony to collaboration between physicians, veterinarians, wildlife experts, ecologists, and healthcare workers; providing a true example of team work and the spirit of One Health in action.

9.7 Banning of diclofenac

In a campaign by the Bombay Natural History Society (BNHS), cooperation between the environmentalists, avian disease experts, drug research department, veterinarians and several others led to the ban of diclofenac (a pain killer anti-inflammatory medicine known as 'vulture killer drug'). The drug causes mortality in slender-billed vultures (*Gyps tenuirostris*),

Indian vultures (*G. indicus*) and white-rumped vultures (*G. bengalensis*) due to kidney failure after eating the flesh of cattle and buffaloes treated with diclofenac (http://www.birdlife.org/news/news/2006/05/vulture_update.html).

10. Application of One Health Principles for Control of Zoonotic Infections

A large number of zoonotic agents require One Health approach for their effective surveillance, detection, and treatment. For hantaviruses and arenaviruses, rodents act as reservoir host and transmit the viruses to humans through contaminated urine, causing haemorrhagic fever with renal syndrome and hantavirus pulmonary syndrome (CDC 2010).

Influenza viruses have been isolated from a variety of animals in addition to humans, pigs, horses, wild birds, domestic birds and sea mammals (Kruse *et al.* 2004). Nipah virus is a newly discovered virus of fruit bats, responsible for encephalitis outbreaks in Southeast Asia (WHO 2009). West Nile virus, a virus of birds, invaded the United States in 1999 and is now endemic (CDC 2009). The list of emerging bacterial disease agents transmitted by food animals is long and continues to expand (Hansen *et al.* 2001). It includes *E. coli* O157:H7, *Salmonella* species, *Campylobacter* species and *Streptococcus iniae* (from farmed fish). Zoonotic diseases from companion (pet) animals are of low incidence in humans but can cause serious health problems.

10.1 Role of veterinary medical practice

Veterinarians accomplish an important job of educating the animal owners about zoonotic diseases and help in reducing the risk of disease transmission by advising regular deworming and vaccination of the animals as prophylactic measure.

Veterinary medicine has responsibility in individual human health, public health, and research. The veterinary professionals are responsible for the care of companion animals, food animals, and exotic animals and wildlife as well as making significant contributions to biomedical research, ecosystem management, public health, food and agricultural systems safety, and biosecurity (Phillips *et al.* 2009).

10.2 Role of laboratory animal research

Laboratory animal experimentation serves as the common gateway for human medicine, veterinary medicine and other health science researchers. Laboratory animals are used as models for various diseases of human and animals. The areas of common interest where maximum collaborations have happened among veterinarians, physicians and health science researchers include cancer (Thamm and Dow 2009), obesity, diabetes, cardiovascular diseases, biomechanical devices such as orthopedic joint replacements (Bian *et al.* 2008), flexible coil balloon expandable intracoronary stent development, heart valve advances, and vaccine development.

10.3 Role of mainstreaming animal-assisted therapy

One health principle can be used as a treatment modality for emotional and possibly physical well being of humans. The animal-assisted therapy (AAT) interventions would not only facilitate the execution and reproducibility of clinical studies but also enable the interpretation of results across studies and the eventual integration of AAT into medical practice (Palley *et al.* 2010).

10.4 Use of comparative oncology for drug development

Conventional drug development pathways are relatively unidirectional; drugs are first considered in preclinical (*in vitro* and *in vivo*) models followed by clinical trials. Translational studies in pet dogs may provide an opportunity to answer questions in a more appropriate and predictive model system. In other words, the application of One Health principles may change the status quo of conventional drug development and speed efficacy rates for cancer therapies (Withrow and Wilkins 2010).

10.5 Improving public perception of wildlife

One Health may affect public acceptance of wildlife and support for wildlife conservation. Public perceptions play a critical role in the continued support of wildlife conservation as a component of the global ecosystem. Association with media and communication experts to incorporate the articulation of wildlife health and management will have great impact on mass awareness (Decker *et al.* 2010).

10.6 Human and animal sentinels for shared health risks

Segregation of human and veterinary medicine has prevented timely recognition, interpretation and action based on the important sentinel surveillance data. Under One Health principles, sentinel events can be used to identify and prevent health risks to man and animals. Sentinel events include preventable disease, disability, or untimely death whose occurrence serves as a warning signal suggesting the need to improve the preventive and therapeutic measures (Rutstein *et al.* 1983). Sentinels may be animals, human or both and these help in forecasting the future disease conditions. Animals can be used as sentinel for many disease conditions in humans and vice versa. Animal health professionals routinely track disease events in sentinel animal colonies and sentinel herds. The use of animals as sentinels for human health threats, or humans as sentinels for animal disease risk dates back at least to the era when coalminers took caged canaries into mines to provide early warning of toxic gases. A slaughterhouse worker diagnosed with brucellosis could serve as a sentinel for an outbreak of brucellosis in cattle that has escaped detection by the animal health authorities and farmers. Identification of sentinel cases of significant travel related illness can be used to indicate widespread risk to other travelers and residents in a particular region (Davis *et al.* 2008).

Sentinel events can be of great use in toxicity cases. Recently, massive die offs in birds were found to be associated with the increased use of pesticides including DDT and other organochlorine compounds. They caused widespread toxicity in the environment that could also be a threat to human health. Besides, zoonotic disease agents may also be detected more easily and prevented more effectively through employing the concept of animal sentinels.

The incidences of Minamata disease due to mercury poisoning in Japan in 1956 (Harada 1995), regular reports of lead poisoning cases in pet animals and painters, outbreak of anthrax in animals, dying crows with neurological signs due to West Nile virus in 1999 in New York (Mostashari *et al.* 2003) are some more examples of sentinel events.

Marine mammals not only are important sentinels for health, they are charismatic too, and thus can help to trigger helpful behavioral responses among humans, including paying closer attention to ocean health issues. Therefore, tracking marine organisms as sentinels provides a valuable way of evaluating the well being of aquatic ecosystems and identifying damaging environmental trends. In turn, these warnings can help the experts in characterizing and managing health risks (Gregory 2007).

11. One Health Approach - Advantages and Challenges

For cross-sectoral approaches, addressing global linkages and multiple perceptions (from farmers to policy makers of developing and developed countries), it is important to outline the advantages of the One Health approach and the challenges in its practicability.

11.1 Advantages

- The risk of global spread of many emerging zoonotic diseases can be managed only by aiming to prevent disease emergence, spread and persistence, rather than trying to cure the symptoms.
- Cooperation across sectors and disciplines will provide better understanding of the epidemiology of diseases and will enable early detection and prompt actions. It will build cooperation front line (e.g. farmers, veterinarians and local governments) who are dealing with

multiple diseases and public health issues, which will support faster and better coordination in crisis.

- Intersectoral coordination will lead to efficient and economic utilization of resources while dealing with many diseases through coherent and common approach for therapeutic and prophylactic measures.
- The collective effort of different international agencies (WHO, FAO, UNDP, UNICEF and OIE) to deal with root causes will create sense of shared responsibility and act as models and source of encouragement at all levels.
- The concept will help in meeting new global challenges head-on through collaboration among multiple professions viz. veterinary medicine, human medicine, and environmental, wildlife and public health sectors.
- The collective efforts will help in developing centres of excellence for education and training in specific areas through enhanced collaboration among colleges and schools of veterinary medicine, human medicine, and public health.

11.2 Challenges

- Countering the sectarian attitude of the specialists, educationists, policymakers and administrators etc. is the major challenge in the way to 'One Health'.
- There are many uncertainties that need to be assessed such as time, money, entry points for action and priorities.
- There is an enormous challenge in assessing benefit - cost ratios where there are little comparable measures (different economists) for benefits across the health domains.
- There is lack of total political and bureaucratic will for interaction and cooperation between different governments, public and private sectors and between countries.
- The joint activities incur a high transaction cost for collaboration (e.g. for different ministries to come together for discussion and planning).
- There may also be cultural and perception issues to overcome. It needs very concrete actions to make any change in a large bureaucratic system. Further, it needs cultural shifts within agencies and change in attitudinal relationship between professions (veterinarians, doctors, extension workers, biologists, ecologists and sociologists etc.)

12. Barriers in the Implementation of One Health concept

12.1 Professional segregation

Separation of professional training of health professionals despite many interrelated health related issues is a major barrier. There are no significant channels of communication between them and they adopt 'us versus them' attitude. They neglect the fact that both animals and humans may in fact be facing similar 'shared risks' of disease emergence from changing environmental conditions (Rabinowitz *et al.* 2008a,b).

12.2 Data separation

The links between human and animal disease surveillance data are limited because of separation of surveillance efforts. Except few diseases like rabies and some potential bioterrorism agents, there are few mandates for direct communication between human and animal health authorities. As a result, many disease events in animals that are reported to the department of animal husbandry and have sentinel implication for the public health professionals may never come to their attention while the reverse is also true as sentinel reports in humans may not be available to the animal health agencies (Rabinowitz *et al.* 2009).

12.3 Evidence gaps

As a result of limited comparison of human and animal surveillance data, there is paucity of evidences on sentinel events which can be used to effectively predict and mitigate health risks for animals and humans for many infectious and toxic hazards in the environment. The relevance of a particular disease of humans in animals and vice versa is not clear (Rabinowitz *et al.* 2009).

13. Conclusion

In fact, we are living in an era dominated by the emergence and reemergence of zoonotic diseases as out of 1,461 diseases now recognized in humans, about 60% are due to multihost pathogens characterized by their movement across species lines (Torrey and Yolken 2005). Over the last three decades, about 75% of new emerging human infectious diseases have been zoonotic (Taylor *et al.* 2001). Therefore, cooperation of all different sectors including human medicine, veterinary medicine, plant health, environment protection and biodiversity preservation agencies have to come together to protect the human and animal health on this mighty planet.

The last few decades in medical history have seen eradication of a few devastating diseases and emergence and reemergence of many more diseases revealing that working in isolation is not a wise strategy. Therefore, the concept of One World-One Health-One Medicine came into reemergence to have control over the emerging, reemerging and existing zoonotic infections. The infectious agents find their niche and hiding place to live in peace for years together either in wild, in soil, in plants or in animals and wait for the opportunity to attack or to be attacked. Human beings and their pets often contract diseases by invading to the silent niche of the pathogens or through creating favourable circumstances for the pathogen. Human beings may also enhance the risk by providing a crossbreeding ground for pathogens of different lineages either in laboratory or in integrated farming systems. Collaborative efforts, concerted intersectoral research and a unidirectional multifaceted attack on the pathogen are essential to control such infections. Efforts are already on to bring together different spheres and sectors of health (human, animals, birds and plants) research; it is the matter of few opportunities to unite them in to a fist which can land a blow at the face of zoonoses.

References

1. Barbour AG (1999). Relapsing fever and other *Borrelia* infections. In: Guerrant RL, Walker DH and Weller PF (eds) Tropical infectious diseases: principles, pathogens and practice. Churchil Livingstone, Philadelphia, p. 535-546.
2. Bian L, Lima EG, Angione SL *et al.* (2008). Mechanical and biochemical characterization of cartilage explants in serum-free culture. J Biomechan 41: 1153-1159.
3. Brundtland GH (2001). United Nations Association's Global Leadership Awards. www.who.int/director-general/speeches/2001/english/20010419_UNAawardsdinnernewyork.en.html.
4. CDC (2009). Final 2009 West Nile Virus Activity in the United States. Division of Vector-Borne Infectious Diseases. Centers for Disease Control and Prevention. www.cdc.gov/ncidod/dvbid/westnile/index.htm. Accessed May 25, 2010.
5. CDC (2010). All About Hantaviruses. National Center for Infectious Diseases, Special Pathogens Branch. Centers for Disease Control and Prevention. www.cdc.gov/ncidod/diseases/hanta/hps/index.htm. Accessed May 25, 2010.
6. Colborn T, Dumanoski D, Meyers JP (1996). Our stolen future: how we are threatening our fertility, intelligence and survival. Dutton, Penguin Books, New York.
7. Colson P, Richet H, Desnues C *et al.* (2010). Pepper Mild Mottle Virus, a plant virus associated with specific immune responses, fever, abdominal pains, and pruritus in humans. PloS One 5: e10041.
8. Conner CD (2005). A people's history of science: miners, midwives, and "low mechanicks". p. 3. Cited from: http://en.wikipedia.org/wiki/Caesarean_section.
9. Davis XM, MacDonald S, Borwein S *et al.* (2008). Health risks in travelers to China: the GeoSentinel experience and implications for the 2008 Beijing Olympics. Am J Trop Med Hyg 79:4-8.

10. Decker DJ, Evensen DTN, Siemer WF *et al.* (2010). Understanding risk perception to enhance communication about human wildlife interactions and the impact of zoonotic diseases. ILAR J 51:255-261.

11. Delgado C, Rosegrant M, Steinfeld H *et al.* (1999). Livestock to 2020: the next food revolution. Food, Agriculture, and the Environment discussion paper 28. Washington, DC: International Food Policy Research Institute.

12. Greenstein RJ, Collins MT (2004). Emerging pathogens: is *Mycobacterium avium* subspecies *paratuberculosis* zoonotic? Lancet 364:396-397.

13. Gregory DB (2007). Emerging Diseases in Marine mammals: from Dolphins to Manatees. Microbe 2:544-549.

14. Hansen GR, Woodall J, Brown C *et al.* (2001). Emerging zoonotic diseases. Emerg Infect Dis 7 (Suppl):537. www.cdc.gov/ncidod/eid/vol7no3_supp/hansen.htm. Accessed May 25, 2010.

15. Harada M (1995). Minamata disease: methylmercury poisoning in Japan caused by environmental pollution. Crit Rev Toxicol 25:1-24.

16. Kahn LH, Kaplan B, Monath TP (2009). One Health in Action No. 7. Vet Ital 45: 204-206.

17. Kahn LH, Kaplan B, Steele JH (2007). Confronting zoonoses through closer collaboration between medicine and veterinary medicine (as 'one medicine'). Vet Ital 43:5-19.

18. Kruse H, Kirkemo AM, Handeland K (2004). Wildlife as source of zoonotic infections: Factors influencing the epidemiology of zoonoses with a wildlife reservoir. Emerg Infect Dis 10. www.medscape.com/viewarticle/496311_4. Accessed May 25, 2010.

19. Monath PT, Kahn LH, Kaplan B (2010). Introduction: One Health perspective. ILAR J 51:193-198.

20. Mostashari F, Kulldorff M, Hartman JJ *et al.* (2003). Dead bird clusters as an early warning system for West Nile virus activity. Emerg Infect Dis 9:641-646.

21. Myers BJ (1970). Nematodes transmitted to man by fish and aquatic mammals. J Wildl Dis 6:266-271.

22. Palley LS, O'Rourke PP, Niemi SM (2010). Mainstreaming animal-assisted therapy. ILAR J 51:199-207.

23. Phillips CJ, Harrington AM, Yates TL *et al.* (2009). Global Disease Surveillance, Emergent Disease Preparedness, and National Security. Lubbock: Museum of Texas Tech University. www.nsrl.ttu.edu/publications/miscpubs/global%20disease.pdf. Accessed May 19, 2010.

24. Rabinowitz P, Scotch M, Conti L (2009). Human and animal sentinels for shared health risks. Vet Italiana 45:23-34.

25. Rabinowitz P, Wiley J, Odofin L *et al.* (2008a). Animals as sentinels of chemical terrorism agents: an evidence-based review. Clin Toxicol (Phila) 46:93-100.

26. Rabinowitz PM, Odofin L, Dein FJ (2008b). From 'us vs them' to shared risk: can animals help link environmental factors to human health? Ecohealth. 5: 224-229.

27. Rutstein DD, Mulan RJ, Frazier TM *et al.* (1983). Sentinel health events (occupational): a basis for physician recognition and public health surveillance. Am J Public Health 73:1054-1062.

28. Scallan E, Griffin PM, Angulo FJ *et al.* (2011a). Foodborne illness acquired in the United States- unspecified agents. Emerg Infect Dis 17:16-22. doi:10.3201/eid1701.p21101.

29. Scallan E, Hoekstra RM, Angulo FJ *et al.* (2011b). Foodborne illness acquired in the United States- major pathogens. Emerg Infect Dis 17:7-12. doi:10.3201/eid1701.p11101.

30. Scholthof KBG (2007). The disease triangle: pathogens, the environment and society. Nature Rev Microbiol 5:152-156.

31. Shotts EB (1987). Bacterial diseases of fish associated with human health. Vet Clin North Am Small Anim Pract 17:241-247.

32. Siddiqui MZ, Singh BR, Agrawal RK *et al.* (2006). An in vitro seed model for determination of *Salmonella* serovars toxicity. Indian J Comp Microbiol Immunol Infect Dis 27:42-43.

33. Siddiqui MZ, Singh BR, Chandra M *et al.* (2008). Detection and partial purification of *Salmonella* serovar Typhimurium cytotoxic protein affecting seed germination. J Appl Anim Res 33:77-79.

34. Singh BR, Agrawal RK, Chandra M (2004). Pathogenic effects of *Salmonella enterica* subspecies enterica serovar Typhimurium on sprouting and growth of maize. Indian J Exp Biol 42:1100-1106.

35. Singh BR, Chandra M, Agrawal RK (2005). Interaction of *Salmonella enterica* subspecies *enterica* serovar Typhimurium and mung bean (*Phaseolus aureus*) plants. J Food Protection 68 (3):476-481.

36. Singh BR, Chandra M, Agrawal RK *et al.* (2007a). Interactions between *Salmonella enterica* subspecies *enterica* serovar Typhimurium and cowpea (*Vigna unguiculata* variety Sinensis) seeds, plants, and persistence in hay. J Food Safety 28:169-187.

37. Singh BR, Chandra M, Agrawal RK *et al.* (2007b). Effect of *Salmonella* contamination on soil fertility. Res Crops 8:136-140.

38. Singh BR, Kumar A, Agrawal S *et al.* (2007c). Effect of *Salmonella* Typhimurium and *Serratia fonticola* on germination of seeds of common crops. J Infect Developing Ctri 1:67-71.

39. Singh BR, Tiwari AK (1996). Toxigenicity of *Edwardsiella tarda* isolates of fish and pig origin in experimental models. Indian J Exp Biol 34:1254-1256.

40. STVM (2009). Society for Tropical Veterinary Medicine. STVM, Stillwater, Oklahoma, www.soctropvetmed.org/. Accessed February 24, 2009.

41. Taubenberger JK, Morens DM (2006). 1918 Influenza: the mother of all pandemics. Emerg Infect Dis 12:15-22.

42. Taylor LH, Latham SM, Woolhouse ME (2001). Risk factors for human disease emergence. Philos Trans R Soc Lond B Biol Sci 356:983-989.

43. Thamm D, Dow S (2009). How companion animals contribute to the fight against cancer in humans. Vet Italiana 45:111-120.

44. Torrey EF, Yolken RH (2005). Beasts of the Earth. New Brunswick, NJ: Rutgers University Press.

45. WCS (2009). One World, One Health. Wildlife Conservation Society, New York, www.oneworld onehealth.org/. Accessed February 24, 2009.

46. Weese JS (2010). Methicillin resistant *Staphylococcus aureus* in animals. ILAR J 51: 233-244.

47. WHO (2009). Fact Sheet No. 262: Nipah virus. World Health Organization. www.who.int/mediacentre/factsheets/fs262/en/. Accessed May 25, 2010.

48. Withrow SJ, Wilkins RM (2010). Crosstalk from pets to people: Translational osteosarcoma treatments. ILAR J 51:208-213.

❑❑❑

Chapter 28

Occupational Risk Alleviation in Livestock Sector

B. SUNIL AND K. VRINDA MENON
Department of Veterinary Public Health, College of Veterinary and Animal Sciences, Mannuthy, Thrissur-680651

Contents

1. Introduction

The knowledge that one's health can be intimately connected with one's occupation must have become apparent at an early stage of social evolution. The first occupational disease was probably silicosis occurring in the makers of flint tools and the next most ancient occupational disease might have been farmer's lung which followed the advent of man engaging in agricultural activities. Since 1950, the International Labour Organization (ILO) and the World Health Organization (WHO) have shared a common definition of occupational health. It was adopted by the Joint ILO/WHO Committee on Occupational Health at its first session in 1950 and revised at its twelfth session in 1995. The definition reads: "Occupational health should aim at: the promotion and maintenance of the highest degree of physical, mental and social well-being of workers in all occupations; the prevention amongst workers of departures from health caused by their working conditions; the protection of workers in their employment from risks resulting from factors adverse to health; the placing and maintenance of the worker in an occupational environment adapted to his physiological and psychological capabilities; and, to summarize, the adaptation of work to man and of each man to his job" (WHO 2005).

India is an agrarian society with the highest livestock population in the world where, as much as 70% of the livestock is owned by 67% of small and marginal farmers and by landless people. Majority of poultry in India are still reared in the backyards, where birds produce eggs and meat by scavenging around their habitation. The close proximity with the animals makes the people rearing them prone to various forms of diseases.

The occupational hazards among the people engaged in animal husbandry sector including veterinarians can be classified as physical hazards, chemical hazards and biological hazards. Additionally, some ergonomic, psychological and social factors may also affect the occupational safety of the workers.

2. Physical Hazards

Veterinary practice settings and other facilities that handle animals have a unique set of occupational health and safety issues and the workers are prone to a wide range of physical injuries and trauma as shown in Table 1.

2.1 Trauma

Trauma can result either from the attack by an animal or due to other reasons.

Table 1 : Physical hazards

Occupational physical hazards
Slips, trips and falls
Cuts and pricks caused by sharp objects, broken glass and syringes
Bites, goring and/or attack by domestic or wild animals
Kicks, bites, scratches and stings caused by laboratory animals
Fall from horses and other riding animals
Road accidents while transporting animals
Accidental injury caused by firearms while hunting animals (in zoos etc.)
Fire hazard at animal-waste rendering plants
Eye injury caused by metallic splinters (e.g. in farriers while horseshoeing or while branding)
Burns from hot metal objects (e.g. in farriers while horseshoeing)
Electric shocks caused by defective or incorrectly operated electric and electromechanical equipment
Exposure to ionizing radiation emitted by veterinary X-ray equipment and by laboratory animals investigated or treated with radioisotopes
Exposure of skin and eyes to ultraviolet radiation used for sterilization
Exposure to excessive noise, heat stress and hand-arm mechanical shocks and vibrations during forging and related operations (in farriers)
Hearing impairment

2.1.1 Trauma due to animal related attacks

This includes mainly animal kick, bite and scratch, crushing, goring, head butting, and running over by the animal (Fig. 1).

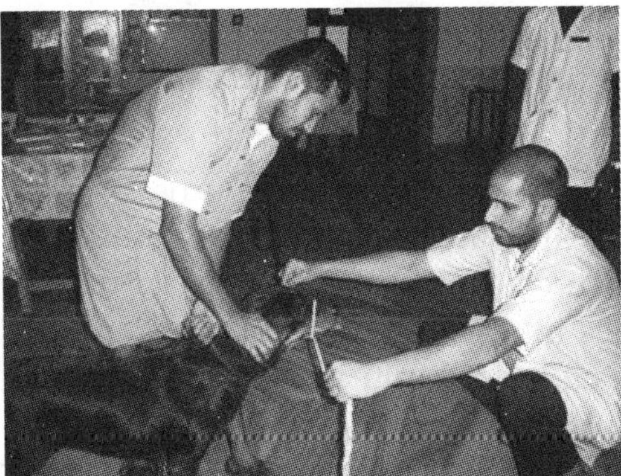

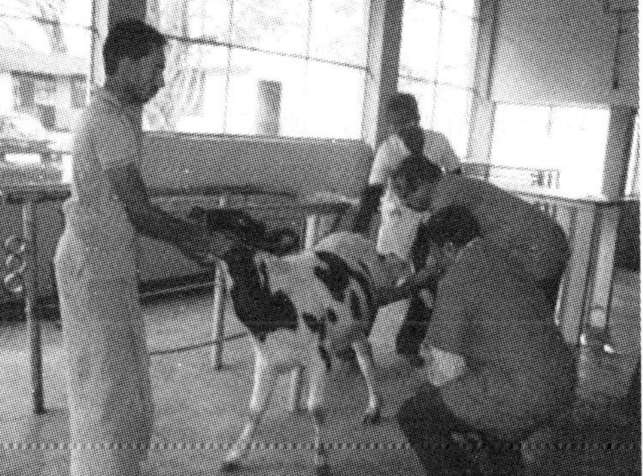

Fig. 1 : Risk of occupational physical injury (Photo courtesy: Dr Shyam K Venugopal, Mannuthy)

2.1.2 Trauma not related to attack by animal

This includes trauma due to lifting and turning large and heavy animals, restraining animals, awkward postures while performing procedures e.g. needle stitch, traveling long distances in vehicles leading to muscular aches, spondylitis, back pain etc.

The animal attacks leading to trauma vary in severity and are common in veterinarians and personnels engaged in raising animals. The outcome of the attacks related to animals includes strains, dislocations, bruising, contusions and fractures. The records of 134 general patients admitted to a hospital as a result of trauma caused by cattle or horses showed that fall from horses was the most common cause of admission (33%). Other causes included cow kick (21%), attack by a cow (19%), equine attack (13%) and horse kick (8%). Only three (2%) of the patients were identified as veterinarians, two of whom sustained facial injuries while examining cows for mastitis (Schnurarenberger 1977). According to another report, 66% of the reported accidents are due to scratches, bites or kicks from animals and incidence of accidents in veterinarians is 2.9 times higher than that in the general practitioners (Nienhaus *et al.* 2005).

2.2 Injuries caused by equipments and instruments

Needles, scalpels and other instruments often cause injury in veterinary practice. In a survey of 99 Wisconsin veterinarians on the frequency and severity of accidental self inoculation and other forms of exposure to vaccine of *Mycobacterium paratuberculosis* (Johne's bacterin), 11% of the veterinarians reported one or more exposures including 19 needle-stick injuries (Patterson *et al.* 1988). It is unlikely that needles and scalpels cause severe injuries alone. Other equipment used in veterinary practice such as nose tongs for cattle, halters, calf pulling equipments, metal cattle chutes, restraining equipment and even ophthalmoscopes may cause injury especially to fingers, wrists and hands. Veterinarians are at risk because they pull, push and lift animals, some of which are very heavy.

Other physical injuries include burns from heat or ice. Burns are more likely to occur from excess heat from steam valves such as from autoclaves and radiators, and from liquid nitrogen or cryogens. There is no data on occurrence of such injuries. Two studies in the USA reported 14% and 31% of veterinarians experiencing cold or heat related injuries, respectively, such as from climatic temperature extremes. Male veterinarians were significantly more commonly affected than females (Hafer 1996). Injuries among the abattoir and meat plant workers are also not uncommon (Fig. 2-3).

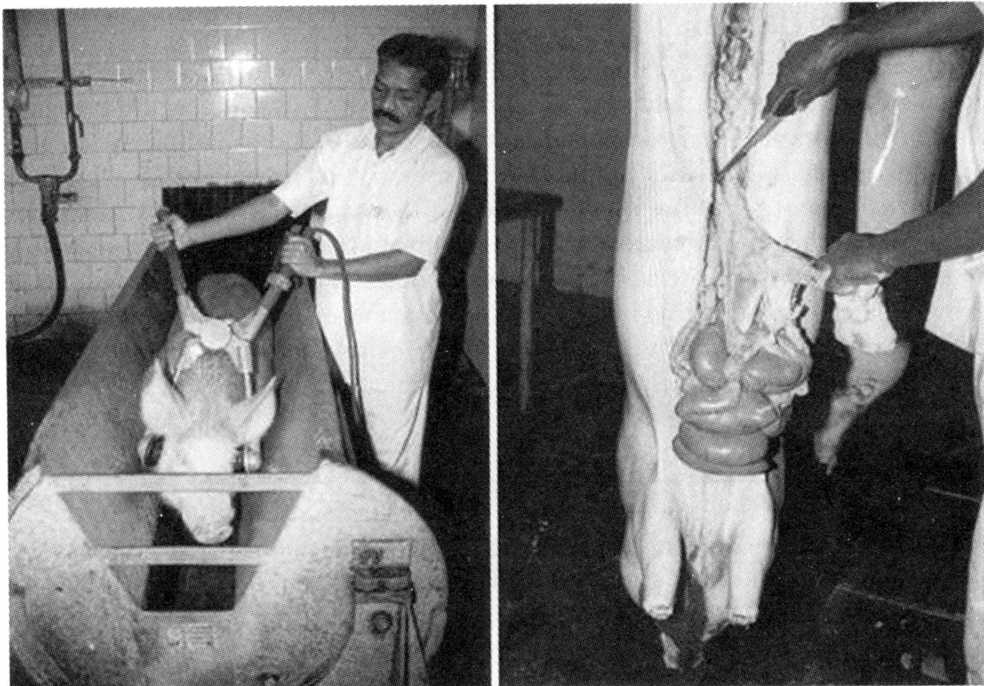

Fig. 2 : Physical and biological occupational risk

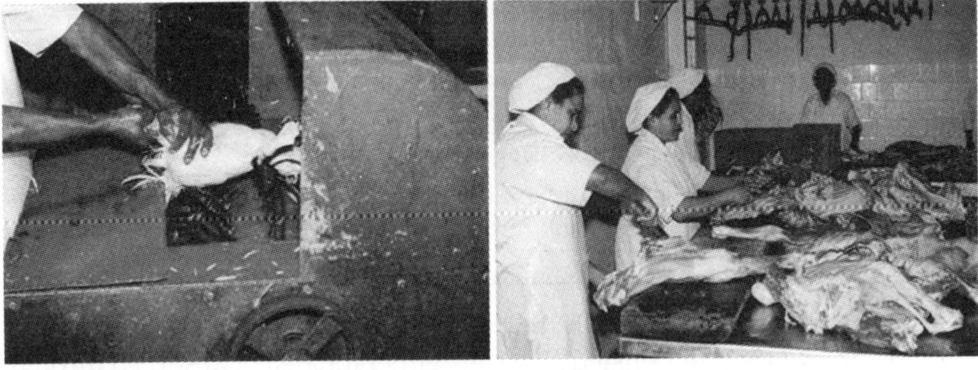

Fig. 3 : Physical and biological hazards among abattoir and meat plant workers

2.3 Assault and drug abuse

Assault is a physical injury reported by veterinary staff as they are at risk from drug addicts because veterinary practitioners stock drugs that drug-abusers desire viz. pethidine, ketamine, barbiturates and many analgesics. Veterinarians who respond to emergency calls after their working hours are particularly susceptible to assault and need to take preventive measures to ensure their safety.

3. Chemical Hazards

Many chemicals used in veterinary practice can cause hazardous effects, which include mutagenicity, teratogenicity, carcinogenicity, acute toxicity, flammability, explosiveness, skin irritation, allergic reactions, and lung damage. The hazardous chemicals commonly used in veterinary practice include disinfectants (ethylene oxide, hexachlorophene, glutaraldehyde, formaldehyde), inhalant anaesthetic gases (nitrous oxide, halothane), injectable anaesthetic agents, pesticides (organophosphates, pyrethrins), antineoplastic drugs, analgesics (including narcotics like pethidine and morphine), therapeutic agents (antibiotics), diethylstilboestrol (DES), non-DES hormones, solvents like xylene, and heavy metals. The list of chemical hazards is cited in Table 2.

Table 2 : Chemical hazards

Occupational chemical hazards

- Intoxication or dermatoses due to contact with chemicals, such as pesticides, rodenticides, solvents, strong acids and alkalis, detergents, animal medication
- Allergies due to contact with formaldehyde and other synthetic or natural allergenic substances
- Health hazards caused by exposure to metallic, solvent and other fumes during forging, shoeing and other hoof-care operations (especially in farriers)
- Systemic and gastrointestinal effects caused by exposure to cytotoxic agents (especially in laboratory animal handlers)
- Exposure to various carcinogenic, mutagenic and teratogenic agents (especially in laboratory animal handlers)
- Mercury poisoning (in fur-processing workers)
- Exposure to anesthetic gases, pharmaceuticals, including antineoplastic agents, disinfectants such as phenol and formaldehyde, and sterilants such as ethylene oxide.

Chemicals may accidentally be spilt on the skin, inhaled, ingested or injected. Most of the agents listed above are either inhaled or absorbed through skin or mucous membranes. Apart from physical damage caused by needle-stick injuries, there is also the possibility of introducing chemicals and biological agents causing disease. An accidental self-injection could have serious consequences for veterinarians and their staff. Veterinarians have accidentally injected themselves with animal preparations and been hospitalised. Female veterinarians of childbearing age could be at risk from some of these chemicals. An analysis of data from a survey of female veterinarians in the USA pertaining to preterm delivery showed no strong associations between occupational factors including exposure to chemicals commonly used in veterinary practice, and abnormal births (Gold and Berin 1983).

As far back as the 19th century, anaesthetic gases were known to be a health hazard to health professionals. Exposure to waste anaesthetic gases has been associated with renal and hepatic disease, spontaneous abortion, congenital malformations, cancer, neurological and psychological disorders. The effects of gaseous anaesthetics on human reproduction are inconclusive. A study showed that exposure to X-rays in veterinary practice was associated with increased occurrence of spontaneous abortion. Euthanasia hazard among animal handlers and veterinarians is also an area of concern because euthanasia of an animal involves a lethal agent, hence inherently dangerous for operators too.

The pesticides commonly used in veterinary practice include organophosphates, carbamates and pyrethrins. These are either directly used on animals or applied in cattle sheds or cages. The administration of certain drugs poses a risk of exposure to the veterinary staff through direct contact or inhalation. Other sources of exposure are contact with body fluids or effluent during chemotherapy treatments. Anticancer drugs have been found to be carcinogenic, teratogenic and/or mutagenic. It has been noticed that prostaglandins, widely used in large animal practice for control of oestrus cycles in cattle, sheep and horses, could cause adverse respiratory conditions or abortion. Formaldehyde is often used by veterinarians to sterilise tissues or as a preservative for pathological specimens. It is mutagenic and teratogenic in animals and considered to be carcinogenic in humans. It also causes adverse health effects such as dermatitis and irritation of the eyes and respiratory tract. Sensitisation to formaldehyde may lead to asthma. Hence personal protective equipment should be used during preparation, administration and disposal of these drugs.

4. Biological Hazards

Veterinary personnel and animal handlers are exposed to numerous pathogenic organisms during their careers. According to a report, approximately 3% to 18% of dog bites and 28% to 80% of cat bites become infected. Most infected dog bite and cat bite wounds contain mixed aerobic and anaerobic bacteria. The most commonly isolated aerobes are *Pasteurella multocida* (cats), *Pasteurella canis* (dogs), *Streptococcus* spp, *Staphylococcus* spp, *Moraxella* spp and *Neisseria weaveri*. The most commonly isolated anaerobes are various species of *Fusobacterium, Bacteroides, Porphyromonas,* and *Prevotella* (Talon and Citron 1999). In addition, rare but serious systemic infections with invasive pathogens such as *Capnocytophaga canimorsus, Bergeyella zoohelcum* and *Bartonella henselae* have also been reported. Needle stick injuries are also among the most frequent accidents in the veterinary workplace. For example, self-injected vaccines containing live *Brucella* organisms can cause infection. Postmortem examination of animals also carries a great risk (Fig. 4).

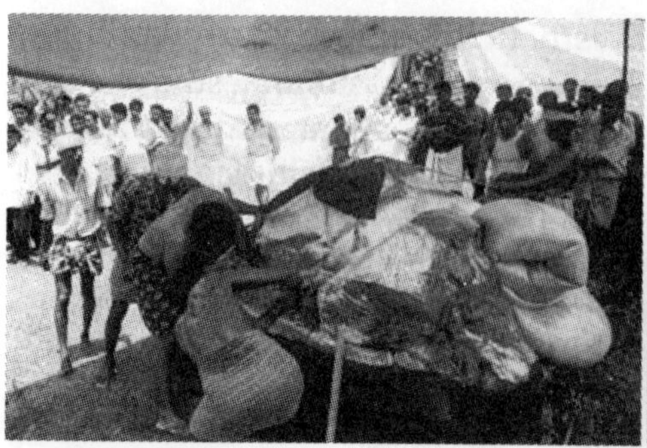
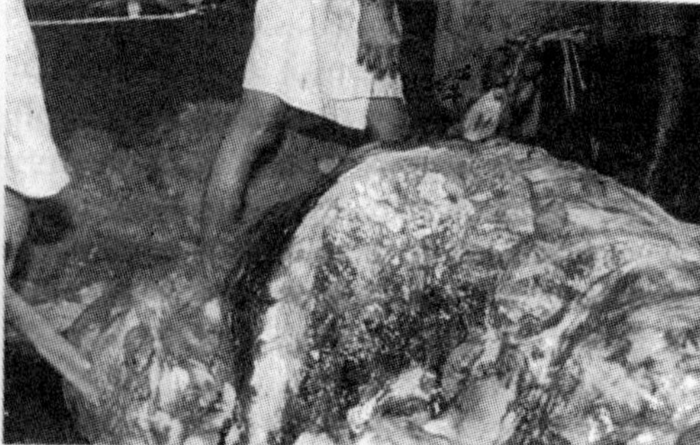

Fig. 4 : Postmortem of elephant and TB lesions (Photo courtesy Dr. N. Vijayan, Mannuthy)

4.1 Occupational activities leading to biological risks

- Farms, animal trade, fairs, markets, exhibitions
- Transportation of animals
- Semen banks
- Kennels, catteries, animal housing
- Surgeries and other clinical activities
- Diagnostic laboratories (collection and analysis of biological samples, organs, carcasses)
- Slaughtering
- Meat processing
- Milk collection and transportation
- Production of cheeses, dairy and egg products
- Collection, transportation and processing of carcasses, wastes of animal origin, slaughter by-products (hides, hooves, hair, feathers), manure and guano
- Maintenance of the animal waste treatment plants or recycling plants (biological refuse from farms, abattoirs, meat processing industries)

The list of biological hazards in handling of animals is given in Table 3.

Table 3 : Biological hazards

Occupational biological hazards
❑ Infection due to contact with sick or carrier animals or due to exposure to pathogens of zoonotic importance (bacterial, viral, fungal, parasitic and rickettsial organisms)
❑ Laboratory animal allergies (occupational asthma, allergic alveolitis, bronchitis, pneumonitis, rhinitis, skin rashes etc.)
❑ Airborne diseases due to inhalation of contaminated animal products and dust carrying microorganisms and their spores, animal hair (causing furrier's lung), bird droppings residues (causing pigeon- breeder's lung) etc.

4.2 Allergens

Veterinarians may be allergic both to the animals they treat and the therapeutic agents they use. Cats and birds are known to produce the greatest number of reported allergies in zoo veterinarians. Veterinarians are frequently exposed to the animals and allergens from animal hair, dander, urine, saliva and other body fluids as well as chemicals that can cause irritation or allergic reactions. Contact with vaginal secretions and amniotic fluid of animals and handling of intestines, pancreas, and blood have been reported to cause dermatitis in veterinarians. Frequent exposures to allergens of animal origin including blood proteins, ascarid worms and ectoparasites increase the probability of veterinarians developing occupational allergic respiratory diseases.

4.3 Zoonotic diseases

Veterinary practices are unique environments that bring humans into close contact with many species of animals. Whether in a clinic or in field settings, veterinary personnel are routinely exposed to infectious pathogens, many of which are zoonotic. The risk of acquiring a zoonotic infection can be high for veterinarians and livestock farmers because of their close occupational contact with animals. Bacteria, dermatophytes, viruses, *Chlamydia*, *Rickettsia*, and parasites carried by animals or in the surrounding environment can infect the veterinarian. Exposure to these organisms occurs through abraded skin, mucosal tissues, ingestion, inhalation, and injection. Often it is difficult to quantify the occurrence of these infections because many are self-limiting or can be mistaken for a cold or flu without proper diagnosis. Zoonotic diseases can be mild or serious for male and female veterinarians and staff. Since they are directly exposed to the infectious agents, large animal practitioners and public health veterinarians are more at risk of developing zoonotic diseases.

4.3.1 Routes of transmission

The transmission of biological agents is mainly through contact, aerosol or vectors.

4.3.1.1 Contact Transmission

Contact transmission occurs when pathogens from animals or their environments enter the human host through ingestion, cutaneous or percutaneous exposure, or mucous membrane exposure. Direct transmission may occur during examination, bathing, and general handling of animals or during administration of treatment. Common zoonotic agents like *Brucella* spp., *Coxiella burnetii* and *Listeria monocytogenes* may be found in high concentration in the birth fluids of aborting or parturient animals and in stillborn foetuses and neonates. Necropsy is a high-risk procedure because of potential contact with infectious agents in body fluids and aerosols and on contaminated sharp instruments. Indirect transmission involves contact with a contaminated intermediate object, such as during cleaning of cages and equipment.

4.3.1.2 Aerosol transmission

Aerosol transmission occurs when pathogens travel through the air to enter the host. Aerosols may be large droplets that are deposited on the mucous membranes or smaller particles that are inhaled. In general, risk of aerosol transmission increases with proximity to the source and duration of exposure. Large droplets are created by coughing, sneezing, and vocalization and by procedures such as lancing abscesses and dentistry. Particles that can be inhaled may be generated through procedures such as suction, bronchoscopy, sweeping, vacuuming, and high-pressure spraying. Certain aerosolized pathogens may remain infective over long distances, depending on particle size, nature of the pathogen, and environmental factors e.g. *Coxiella burnetii* and *Mycobacterium bovis*.

4.3.1.3 Vector-borne transmission

Vector-borne transmission occurs when vectors such as mosquitoes, fleas and ticks transmit pathogens. Animals may bring flea and tick vectors into contact with veterinary personnels and animal handlers. Working in the outdoor settings may increase the risk of exposure to arthropods and other biological vectors.

The list of zoonotic diseases along with the occupational groups at higher risk is cited in Table 4.

Short description of some major zoonotic diseases presenting occupational risk is given below.

Anthrax has been known since antiquity. Naturally occurring anthrax in humans is acquired from contact with anthrax-infected animals or anthrax-contaminated animal products, which allows one to distinguish agricultural anthrax, among veterinarians, agricultural workers and butchers, from industrial anthrax, resulting from exposure to contaminated sheep wool or goat hair that are processed into yarns used in the textile and carpet industry, as well as cattle hides that are processed into leather goods, or bones used for the manufacture of gelatin and/or fertilizer. The disease can be contracted through the skin (cutaneous), lungs (pulmonary), or gastrointestinal routes. The commonest occupational presentation of the disease is the cutaneous anthrax. It is contracted from exposure to bones from ruminant animals. This type of lesion called a malignant pustule.

Table 4 : Occupational zoonoses

S. No	Disease	Causative agent	Principal animal host	Occupational groups at risk
1.	Anthrax	*Bacillus anthracis*	Cattle, sheep, goat, horses, wild and other herbivores	Wool sorters, knacker-man, veterinarians, abattoir workers, farm workers
2.	Brucellosis	*Brucella meletensis, B. abortus, B. suis*	Goat, cattle, pig	Veterinarians, farmers, dairymen, meat packers, laboratory workers
3.	Campylobacteriosis	*Campylobacter jejuni, C. fetus subsp fetus*	Poultry birds, cattle, sheep, goat, swine	Poultry farm workers, livestock farmers, veterinarians
4.	Erysipeloid or Swine erysipelas	*Erysipelothrix insidiosa*	Swine, sheep, poultry	Pig farmers, Abattoir workers
5.	Listeriosis	*Listeria monocytogenes*	Mammals and birds	Immunosuppressed persons engaged in livestock rearing and handling e.g pregnant women, diabetic persons etc.
6.	Leptospirosis	*Leptospira interrogans*	Domestic and wild animals, rodents, dogs	Rice field workers, sewage workers, abattoir workers, veterinarians, dairy farmers
7.	Salmonellosis or paratyphoid fever	*S. typhimurium, S. enteritidis, S. cholarae suis, S. arizonae, S. dublin, S. typhi, S.paratyphi*	Farm animals, poultry	Farmers, al[illegible]toi. workers, veterinarians
8.	Streptococcal meningitis	*Steptococcus suis* (type 2)	Pigs	Abattoir workers, meat plant processing operators, pig farmers, veterinarians
9.	Tuberculosis	*Mycobacterium bovis, M. tuberculosis, M. avium*	Cattle, poultry	Dairy farmers, abattoir workers, poultry processing and zoo workers,

contd...

10	Tularaemia	*Francisella tularensis*	Wild animals, hare, rabbit, sheep	Ranchers, sheep rearers and handlers, rabbit fur processing workers
11.	Yersiniosis or pseudoappendicitis	*Yersinia pseudotuberculosis, Y. enterocolytica*	Mammals mainly pigs, dogs, cats, birds	Farm workers, abattoir workers
12.	Glanders	*Burkholderia mallei*	Equines	Horse handlers, veterinarians
13.	Psittacosis and ornithosis	*Chlamydia psittacii*	Parrots, parakeets (Psittacosis); Pigeon, turkeys ducks geese (Ornithosis)	Poultry farmers, pet shop owners and breeders, zoo workers, veterinarians
14.	Q fever	*Coxiella burnetii*	Cattle, sheep, goat, rabbit and other domestic and wild animals	Abattoir workers, dairy farmers, veterinarians, laboratory workers, workers in meat processing plant, hide, fat and rendering industries
15.	Ringworm	*Trichophyton* spp, *Microsporum* spp, *Epidermophyton* spp	All domestic and wild animals	Farm and laboratory workers, pet owners, veterinarians
16.	Bird flu and swine flu	*Orthomyxovirus* (Influenza A virus)	Poultry , wild birds, pigs	Poultry and pig farmers, abattoir workers, veterinarians
17.	Louping ill	*Flavivirus*	Sheep, goat , small rodents	Farm and laboratory workers
18.	Orf or contagious papular dermatitis	*Parapox virus*	Sheep , goat	Farm workers
19.	Newcastle disease	*Paramyxovirus*	Poultry and wild birds	Poultry farm workers
20.	Rabies	*Lyssa virus*	Wild and domestic canids, vampire bats	Pet owners, veterinarians, kennel workers

contd...

21. FMD	*Apthovirus*	Cattle, swine and other cloven hoofed animals	Animal farm workers, veterinarians
22. Herpes B virus disease	*Herpes virus*	Old world monkeys	Laboratory workers
23. Milkers nodules	*Pseudocowpox virus*	Cattle	Milkers
24. Monkey pox	*Monkey pox virus*	Nonhuman primates, other African rodents, prairie dogs, other pet rodents	Laboratory workers
25. Nipah virus disease	*Nipah virus*	Swine, dogs, fruit bats	Animal handlers
26. Capnocytophaga infection	*Capnocytophaga canimorsus, C. cynodegmi*	Dogs, cats	Animal handlers
27. Rat bite fever	*Streptobacillus moniliformis*	Rodents	Animal handlers
28. Dermatophilosis	*Dermatoph ilus congolensis*	Cattle, horses, deer, sheep, other mammmals	Animal handlers
29. Histoplasmosis	*Histoplasma capsulatum*	Dogs, chickens	Poultry house workers
30. Sporotrichosis	*Sporothrix schenchii*	Horses, other domestic and laboratory animals, birds	Animal handlers and laboratory workers
31. Hanta virus infection	*Bunya virus*	Rodents	Laboratory workers, field biologists
32. *Baylisascaris procyonis* infection	*Baylisascaris procyonis*	Racoons	Veterinarians and animal handlers

Rabies is considered one of the most important occupational hazards to veterinarians and persons working with pet animals and is usually transmitted by bite and scratches by dogs. It is the tenth leading cause of death due to infectious disease on a worldwide basis. Unfortunately, on a global scale, there are at least 50,000 reported deaths per year due to rabies, which is a grossly underreported disease. This is due to the reservoir of infected dogs in developing countries, lack of resources to accomplish control or mass vaccination of dogs and the unavailability of post exposure prophylaxis in poor or remote regions. It is a viral disease that causes acute encephalitis in warm-blooded animals. It is transmitted most commonly by a bite from an infected animal but occasionally by other forms of contact. Rabies is almost invariably fatal if post-exposure prophylaxis is not administered promptly. The pre-exposure vaccination among veterinarians in India is not common though recommended in high risk groups.

Brucellosis is another disease which causes the greatest morbidity in this occupational group. The serological testing of cattle for brucellosis has to be concentrated at the centres where automated equipment reduces the exposure of the laboratory staff, who themselves are regularly examined at intervals for antibodies to *Brucella abortus.* In India, Ajay Kumar (1998) reported that 21.76% serum samples from slaughtered pigs were positive for brucellosis and the incidence of the disease in humans was 1.6%. Ajithkumar *et al.* (2009) revealed the seroprevalence of brucellosis in goats to be 3.13% in Ernakulam district in Kerala state and the incidence of the disease in farmers was 2.78%

Ringworm is among the commonest reported zoonoses among veterinary surgeons which is usually contracted early in their careers and seldom recurring.

Leptospirosis is also a risk to veterinarians and they should take measures to decrease the potential exposure to infectious agent. A case of a veterinarian in Washington State developing leptospirosis after an occupational exposure has been reported recently (Baer *et al.* 2009). Diagnostic tests for leptospirosis should be considered when veterinarians have febrile illnesses of unknown origin.

Cutaneous listeriosis in persons associated with livestock sector has been documented. (McLauchlin and Low 1994). The condition appears as papular or pustular lesions on the arms or hands, and is most often acquired as an occupational hazard from infected animals. Listeric infections are potentially fatal, and as the initial cause of the lesion may be unknown, it is recommended that veterinarians and farmers should have suspect lesions examined microbiologically.

Toxoplasmosis has been found in virtually all warm-blooded animals including most pets, livestock, and human beings. Individuals become infected by eating raw meat or ingesting the oocyst (egg) that is excreted in cat faeces. Ingestion of the oocyst from cat faeces is the primary hazard to the personnel working in laboratory animal facilities. Since it takes several days for the oocyst to become infective after faecal excretion, daily routine cage sanitation greatly decreases the chance of transmission (Tester *et al.* 2000). However, every effort should be made to arrange a temporary job re-assignment while a susceptible employee is pregnant.

Q fever is a zoonotic disease associated primarily with sheep (and other ruminants). Q fever is a highly infectious rickettsial infection caused by *Coxiella burnetii*. Infection usually causes flu-like symptoms, and in some cases, these symptoms can be severe. Chronic endocarditis may develop, particularly in persons with preexisting valvular disease and is seen in persons rearing sheep.

The concept of zoonotic *mycoplasmosis* is new So far eight species in the genus *Mycoplasma* and two species of the genus *Acholeplasma* can be claimed as zoonotic. The importance of mycoplasmas in human and animal infections has accentuated with recent reporting of instances of human infections (Garg and Singh 2008) with animal mycoplasmas and vice-versa leading to recognition of zoonotic mycoplasmosis. The slow reporting of zoonotic mycoplasmosis can be attributed mainly to difficulty in measuring zoonotic potential of mycoplasmosis as in some other diseases viz. multiple sclerosis, rheumatoid arthritis, leukaemia, atherosclerosis, chronic fatigue syndrome, CJD, Crohn's colitis etc.

The highest rate of infection with *tuberculosis* is occurring within the age group (15-59) that constitute the workforce of every country. The zoonotic serotypes of tuberculosis are *M. bovis* and *M. avium* which are acquired mainly from cattle and birds, respectively. The infection occurs via inhalation or via an infected carcass. *M. marinum* is the serotype that infects fish but it can be acquired from fish bite or consumption or swimming in infected water (Worell 2003). Transmission of tuberculosis between humans and elephants has been documented in an exotic animal farm in Illinois, California (1996) where a number of elephants had died. When the animal handlers on the farm were tested for tuberculosis via purified protein derivative (PPD) skin prick tests, 50% of the handlers were PPD positive indicating that they had tuberculosis. Chest X-rays and sputum samples confirmed the disease (Michalak *et al.* 1998).

5. Ergonomics, Psychological and Social Factors Associated Hazards

The value of ergonomics is easily understood by anyone who has tried to do a job using the wrong tools. The increased difficulty causes the job to take longer, leading to frustration and loss of temper. International Labour Organization defines ergonomics as the application of the human biological sciences in conjunction with the engineering sciences to the worker and his working environment so as to obtain maximum satisfaction for the worker which at the same time enhances productivity. This definition emphasizes the important triad of ergonomic elements viz. comfort, health and productivity. Various ergonomic, psychological and social factors leading to occupation health risk are shown in Table 5.

Table 5 : Ergonomic, psychological and social factors leading to occupation health risk

Ergonomic, psychological and social factors
▫ Musculoskeletal problems (particularly of back and knees) in animal handlers engaged in lengthy horse riding and/or leaning on their knees (especially on concrete floors) during work (e.g. in farriers)
▫ Job dissatisfaction related to the working environment (dirt, smells etc.) and mainly physical character of work
▫ Danger of developing drug addiction facilitated by easy availability of animal medications
▫ Psychological stress due to responsibility for high economic values and animal welfare, working alone, unexpected events (sick animal, machinery breakdown), fast paced work in milking stations and bad working conditions (noise, lifting heavy loads, bad working postures, dust, drafts)
▫ Discomfort, decreasing work efficiency and safety resulting from poor illumination and exposure to noxious smells from manure, urine and gases.

5.1 Activities leading to musculoskeletal injuries

In veterinary practice, there are a lot of activities that lead to musculoskeletal injuries (Fig. 5). The risk factors which may result in injuries are given below.

5.1.1 Awkward postures and highly repetitive motion

Working with the hand above the head, or the elbow above the shoulder, working with the neck, back or wrist bent more than 30 degrees, squatting or kneeling, sustained position for extended time periods cause muscle fatigue and injury. The activities that may lead to such awkward postures include rectal palpations, dystocias, prolapse repair, stocking shelves, colic surgeries, palpations, floating teeth, venipuncture, grooming, kennel and stall cleaning; data entry, surgeries performed while kneeling, driving a vehicle etc.

5.1.2 High hand force

Pinching an object and applying more than two pounds of force per hand or gripping an object and applying more than 10 pounds of force per hand for extended time periods can cause muscle fatigue and injury. The examples include large animal abdominal surgeries, ear tagging and restrain of animals.

5.1.3 Heavy, awkward lifting

Repeatedly or infrequently lifting heavy objects causes muscle fatigue which could lead to musculoskeletal injuries. The activities that lead to it are patient lifting, restraining, and positioning; carrying equipment; large animal foot and leg work; carrying feed and other products; dystocias etc.

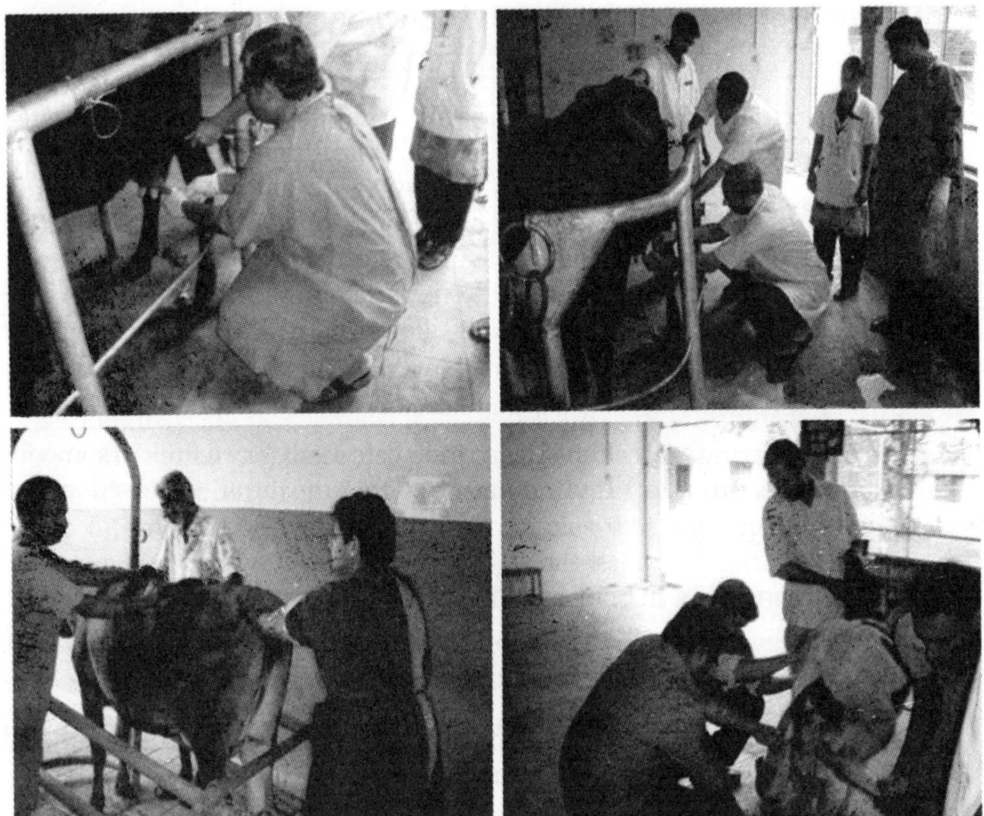

Fig. 5 : Ergonomics related occupational health risk (Photo courtesy: Dr. Metilda Joseph, Dr. Shyam K. Venugopal and Dr. S. Anoop, Mannuthy)

6. Prevention and Control of Occupational Risks

Workers can reduce their occupational risk by taking the following measures.

6.1 Sanitation and hygiene

1. Washing hands frequently with soap and water before and after handling animals; after coming into contact with animal saliva, urine, faeces, or blood; after cleaning cages or equipment; before eating, drinking, smoking, taking breaks, or leaving work and after removing gloves
2. Using alcohol-based hand sanitizers for cleaning hands when soap and water are not available
3. Wearing clean clothing/ uniform
4. Changing into clean clothing before leaving the workplace

6.2 Personal protective clothing and equipment

1. Wearing medical examination gloves that provide the skin with a protective barrier when handling animals, animal waste, cages, equipment, and pesticides; wearing two pairs of gloves if one pair alone might tear; powder-free gloves to reduce exposure to allergy causing proteins; and wearing cotton or leather work gloves as the outer pair when heavy work gloves are needed
2. Wearing protective eyewear (safety glasses with side shields) or face shields if there is a risk of spitting or splashing of contaminated material
3. Wearing sturdy clothing and protective footwear with non-slip soles to provide protection from bite, puncture or crushing injuries
4. Wearing hearing protection if you must raise your voice to talk to someone an arm's length away (for example, when working in enclosed spaces with barking dogs).

6.3 Safety measures against animal bites and scratches

1. Rabies pre-exposure vaccination before directly handling dogs, cats, ferrets, or other mammals that may be infected with rabies
2. Thoroughly cleaning all bite wounds and scratches with soap and water
3. Reporting any bite injury to your supervisor
4. Immediate medical evaluation of any bite wound and the need for possible rabies post-exposure vaccination and treatment

6.4 Protection against asthma in animal handlers

1. Modifying ventilation and filtration systems; increasing the ventilation rate and humidity in animal housing areas; separating ventilation of animal-housing and handling areas from the rest of the facility; and directing the airflow away from workers and towards the backs of the animal cages
2. Performing animal manipulations within ventilated hoods or safety cabinets when possible
3. Decreasing animal density (number of animals per cubic meter or room volume)
4. Avoiding wearing street clothes while working with animals
5. Keeping cages and stables clean and taking care to control exposures during cleaning
6. Using absorbent pads for bedding

7. Keeping a pet animal species that is less allergenic than others
8. Reducing contact with animal products such as dander, serum, and urine by using gloves, lab coats, and approved particulate respirators with face-shields
9. Educating workers about animal allergies and steps for risk reduction
10. Providing health monitoring and appropriate counseling and medical follow up for workers becoming sensitized or having developed allergy symptoms.

6.5 Protection against injuries

1. Taking precautions when using scalpels, forceps, and other sharp instruments; dispose of sharp devices in labeled, puncture-resistant, leak proof sharps disposal containers immediately after use; avoiding recapping, bending, or removing contaminated needles and sharps; and avoiding shearing or breaking contaminated needles
2. Taking precautions when lifting heavy or awkward loads; using proper lifting techniques; reducing the weight of loads when possible; and working together to lift loads that are unsafe for one person to handle
3. Pregnant or immunocompromised workers avoiding contact with cat faeces and pet rodents to reduce risk of zoonotic disease

6.6 Safe work practice guidelines for laboratory workers

1. Adhere to the biosafety level indicated for specific research protocol.
2. Adhere to standard operating procedures in order to decrease transmission of diseases.
3. Complete laboratory safety training and follow laboratory safety guidelines.
4. Decontaminate spills or splatters of potentially infectious blood, and/or body fluids with a 1:10 dilution of bleach (1 part bleach to 10 parts water).
5. Keep doors closed and limit access to appropriate personnel.
6. Practice frequent hand washing and good housekeeping.
7. Dispose of needles and sharps in an appropriate sharps container.
8. Avoid touching mouth, nose, and eyes while performing research duties.
9. Wear protective gloves, lab coat/gown, mask, goggles, hair bonnets, and shoe covers when handling infectious agents and/or animals.
10. Decontaminate infectious waste before disposal.

7. Occupational Health Regulation in India

Article 21 of the Indian Constitution guarantees the protection of life and personal liberty of a person. Various Supreme Court judgments have, under this "right to life" upheld the right to employees' health. The Constitution of India has also specified provisions for ensuring occupational health and safety for workers in the form of three Articles i.e. 24, 39 (e and f) and 42. The regulation of labour and safety in mines and oil fields is under the Union list. While the welfare of labour including conditions of work, provident funds, employers' invalidity and old age pension and maternity benefit are in the Concurrent list. The Ministry of Labour, Government of India and Labour Departments of the States and Union Territories are responsible for safety and health of workers.

The Factories Act, 1948, the Mines Act, 1952, The Dock Workers (Safety, Health & Welfare) Act, 1986 are some of the laws, which contain provisions regulating the health of workers in an establishment. Whereas the Employees State Insurance Act, 1948 and the Workmen's Compensation Act, 1923 are compensatory in nature.

7.1 Health provisions under the Factories Act, 1948

The Factories Act, 1948 was enacted with the object of protecting workers from subjecting to unduly long hours of bodily strain or manual labour. It lays down that employees should work in healthy and sanitary conditions so far as the manufacturing will allow and that precautions should be taken for their safety.

7.2 The Employees' State Insurance (ESI) Act, 1948

It is a social security legislation enacted with the object of ameliorating various risks and contingencies sustained by workers while serving in a factory or establishment. It is designed to provide cash benefit in the case of sickness, maternity and employment injury, payment in the form of pension to the dependents of workers who dies of employment injury and medical benefit to workers. The Act does not cover 'seasonal employments'. It defines 'employment injury' as personal injury to employees, caused by accident or occupational diseases, in an insurable employment.

The Act lays down provisions to set up an ESI Corporation, to promote measures to improve health and welfare of insured persons and a Medical Benefit Council to advise the Corporation on medical benefits, certification etc. Section 39 of the Act makes the employer primarily liable for the payment of contribution on behalf of himself and his employees towards the ESI Fund. In case of misuse of the contribution by employer, the employee can sue the employer in the Employees' State Insurance Court set up by the respective State Government.

Under the Workmen's Compensation Act, 1923, there exists a legal obligation on the employer to pay compensation to workmen involved in accidents arising during the course of their employment. Compensation is decided on the nature of injury caused.

There is no comprehensive law on occupational health, though the Central Government has in its various policies stressed the need to effectively implement the existing laws. A broad insight into the existing occupational health laws in India explicably brings out the verity of non-implementation of such laws. There is a need to develop Occupational Safety and Health Administration (OSHA) regulations as in the United States, which will help to preserve the good health of workmen by ensuring safe and healthy working conditions and provide prompt compensation on account of injury or occupational disease.

References

1. Ajay Kumar VJ (1998). Public health significance of brucellosis in pigs. MVSc thesis Kerala Agricultural University, Thrissur. p. 69.

2. Ajithkumar S, Chattopadyay UK, Nanu E, Bishor VJ (2009). Seroprevalence of brucellosis in bovines, goats and human contacts in Ernakulam district of Kerala. Proceedings of National Seminar on recent trends in diagnosis and control of animal diseases with special reference to public health, Ernakulam. p. 10-17.

3. Baer R, Turnberg W, Yu D, Wohrle R (2009). Leptospirosis in a Small Animal Veterinarian: Reminder to Follow Standardized Infection Control Procedures. Zoonoses and Public Health 57 (4):281-284. Published online 17 Jun 2009.

4. Decostere A, Hermans K, Heasebrouck F (2004). Piscine mycobacteriosis: a literature review covering the agent and the disease it causes in fish and humans. Vet Microbiol 99:159-166.

5. Garg DN, Singh Y (2009). Zoonotic mycoplasmosis: Waiting to happen In: Singh SP, Funk J *et al.* (Eds) Food safety quality assurance and global trade: Concerns and strategies. International Book Distributing Co, Lucknow, India. p. 167-172.

6. Gold C, Beran G (1983). Occupational hazards to pregnant veterinarians. Iowa State Vet J 45: 55-60.

7. Hafer A, Langley R, Morrow W, Tulis J (1996). Occupational hazards reported by swine veterinarians in the United States. Swine Health Prod 4:128-141.

8. Kazacos KR (1997). Visceral, ocular and neural larva migrans. In: Connor DH, Chandler FW, Schwartz DA (eds) Pathology of Infectious Diseases, Appleton and Lange, Stamford, Connecticut.

9. McLauchlin J, Low JC (1994). Primary cutaneous listeriosis in adults: an occupational disease of veterinarians and farmers. Vet Rec 135(26):615-617.

10. Michalak K., Austin C, Diesel S, Bacon JM, Zimmerman P, Maslow JN (1998). *Mycobacterium tuberculosis* Infection as a zoonotic disease: Transmission between humans and elephants. Emerg Infect Dis 4 (2):283-387.

11. Nienhaus A, Skudlik C, Seidler A (2005). Work related accidents and occupational diseases in veterinarians and their staff. Int Arch Occup Enviorn Health 78: 230-236.

12. Patterson C, LaVenture M, Hurley S, Davis J (1988). Accidental self-inoculation with *Mycobacterium paratuberculosis* bacterin (Johne's bacterin) by veterinarians in Wisconsin. J Am Vet Med Assoc 192:1197-1199.

13. Schnurrenberger P, Martin R. (1977). Mortality in Illinois veterinarians. J Am Vet Med Assoc 170:1071-1075.

14. Talan DA, Citron DM, Abrahamian FM *et al.* (1999). Bacteriologic analysis of infected dog and cat bites. N Engl J Med 340:85-92.

15. Tenter AM, Heckeroth AR, Weiss LM (2000). *Toxoplasma gondii*: from animals to humans. Int J Parasitol 30:1217-1258.

16. WHO (2005). Future trends in veterinary public health: Report of a WHO study group technical report series No 907. World Health Organisation, Geneva.

□□□

Chapter 29

Capacity Building of Veterinarians for Disaster Response

S. R. GARG AND V. J. JADHAV
Department of Veterinary Public Health & Epidemiology, College of Veterinary Sciences,
Lala Lajpat Rai University of Veterinary and Animal Sciences, Hisar-125004

Contents

1. Introduction

A disaster is a serious disruption of the functioning of a society that causes widespread damage, economic destruction, loss of human life and deterioration in health and health services on a scale which exceeds the ability of the affected society to cope using only its own resources and, thus, warrants an extraordinary response from outside the affected community or area. Disasters may be sudden (e.g. earthquake, cyclone) or slow (e.g. drought). Millions of people are affected by natural catastrophe from floods, cyclones and tsunami, earthquakes, landslides and volcanic eruptions across the world. Apart from the loss of human life, disasters cause great loss to the economy. The countries worldwide are estimated to have lost an average of 2-5 per cent of their GDP from natural calamities in the recent past (Goel 2007).

The global picture of natural disasters that occurred during the years 1976 to 2005 and their impact is shown in Fig. 1-2. The occurrence of natural disasters in the year 2009 and the damage caused by them worldwide is depicted in Fig. 3-6.

2. Types of Disasters

Disasters are classified broadly as natural disasters, man-made disasters and other disasters. These may either be major disasters or minor disasters. Depending upon the cause, disasters may be grouped as given in Table 1.

Table 1 : Classification of disasters based on the cause

1.	Water and climate related disasters	Floods and drainage management, cyclones, tornadoes and hurricanes, hailstorm, cloud burst, heat wave and cold wave, snow avalanches, droughts, sea erosion, thunder and lightning
2.	Geology related disasters	Landslides and mudflows, earthquakes, dam failures/ bursts, mine fires
3.	Chemical, industry and nuclear related disasters	Chemical and industrial disasters, nuclear disasters
4.	Accident related disasters	Forest fires, urban fires, village fires, mine flooding, oil spill, major building collapse, bomb blasts, festival disasters and fires, electrical disasters and fires, and air, road, rail and waterway accidents
5.	Biology related disasters	Biological disasters and epidemics, pest attacks, cattle epidemics and food poisoning

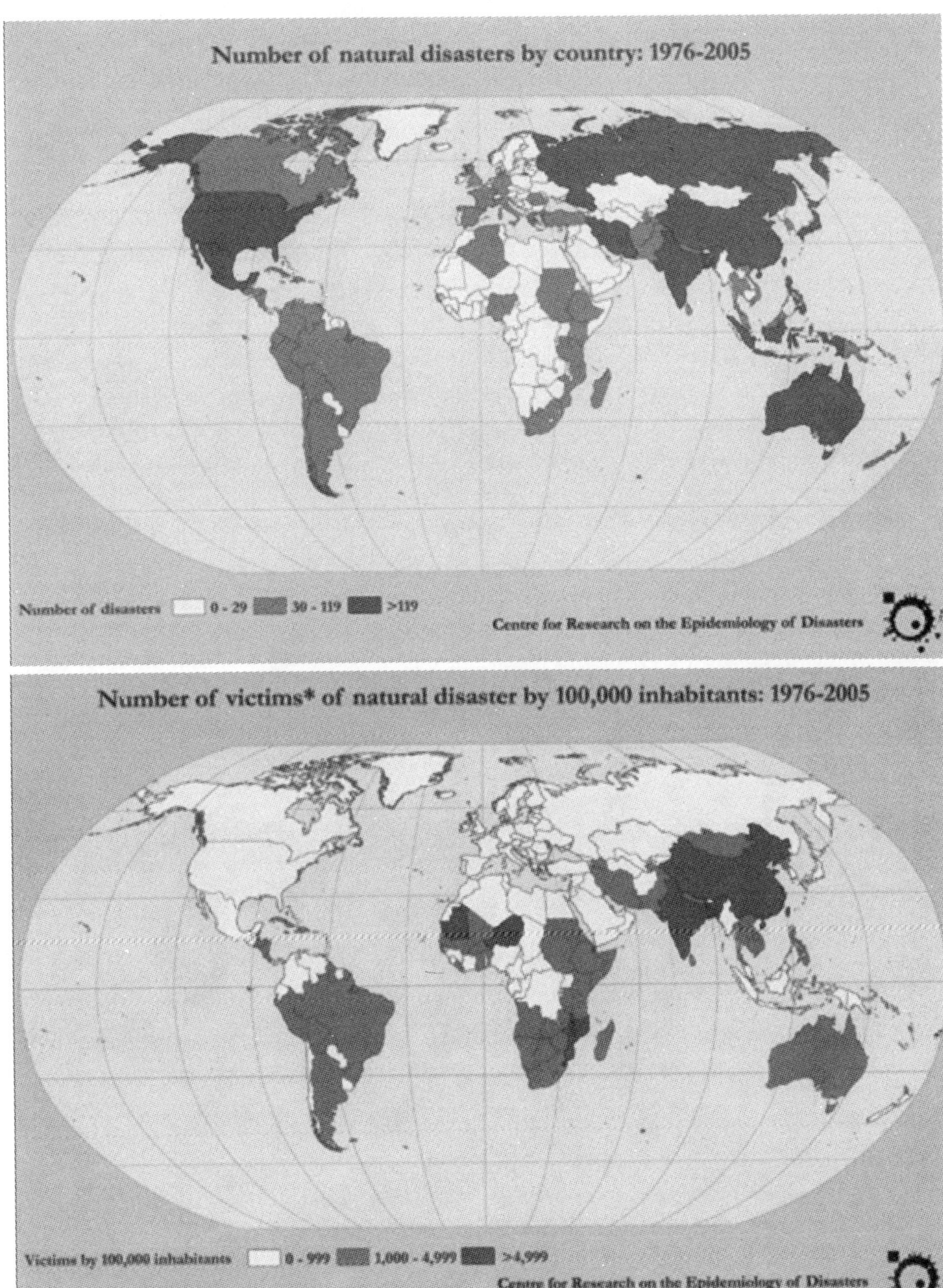

Fig. 1-2 : Number of natural disasters and number of victims during 1976-2005

Source: EM-DAT: The OFDA/CRED International Disaster Database www.emdat.be - Université Catholique de Louvain - Brussels – Belgium. Accessed 11 January 2011.

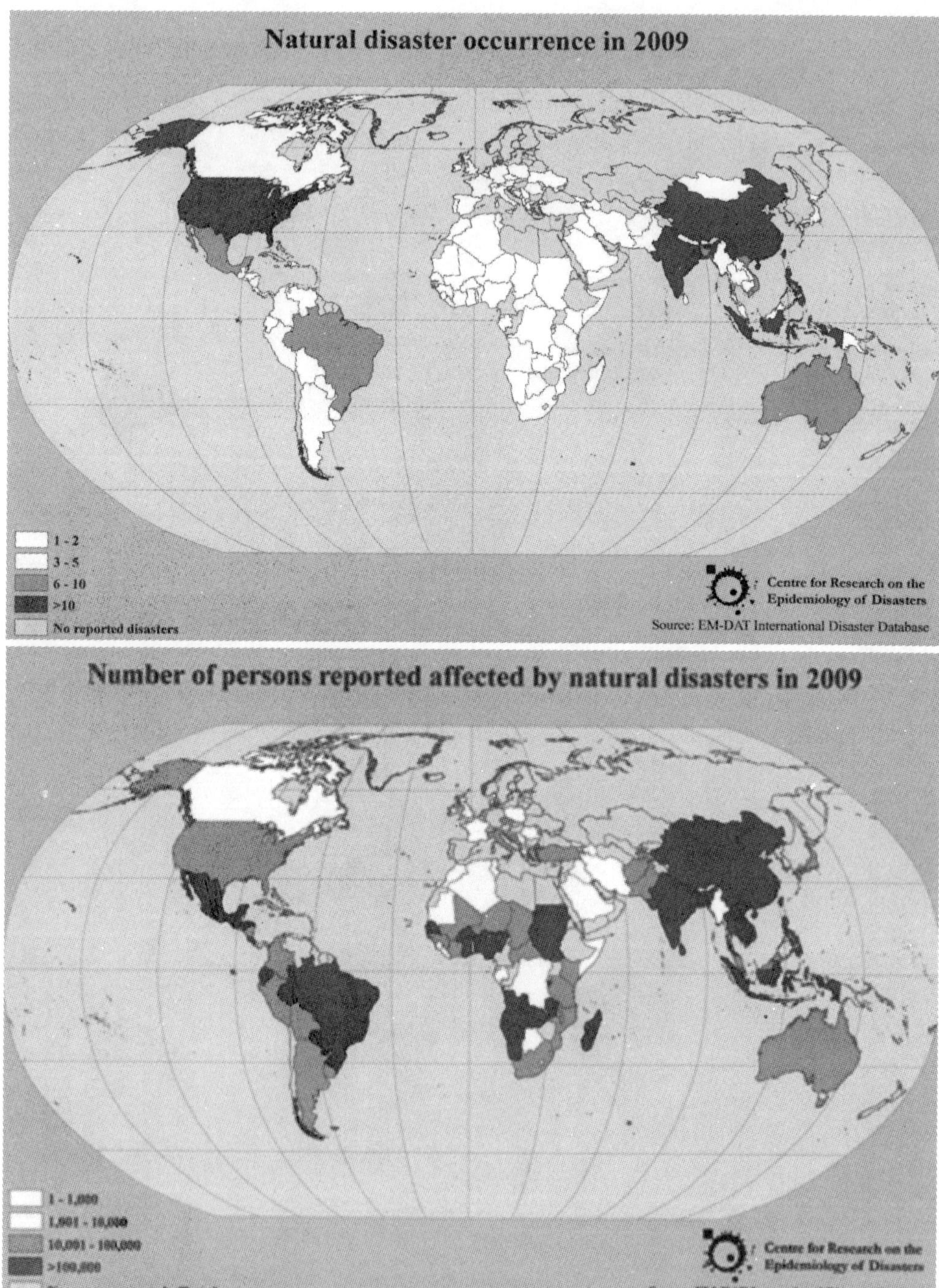

Fig. 3-4 : Natural disaster occurrence and persons affected during 2009

Source: EM-DAT: The OFDA/CRED International Disaster Database www.emdat.be - Université Catholique de Louvain - Brussels – Belgium. Accessed 11 January 2011.

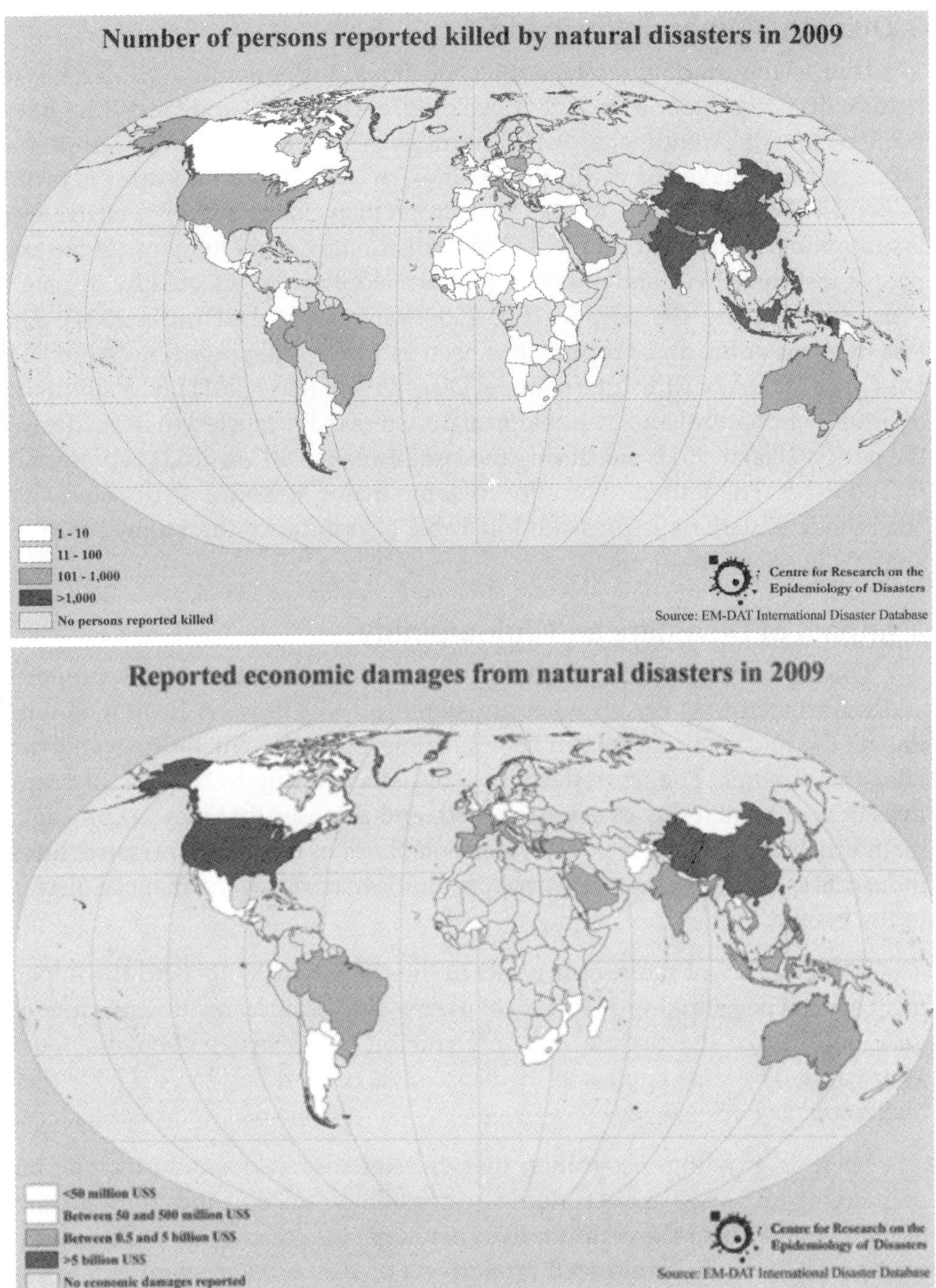

Fig. 5-6 : Human fatallty and economic damage from natural disasters during 2009

Source: EM-DAT: The OFDA/CRED International Disaster Database www.emdat.be - Université Catholique de Louvain - Brussels – Belgium. Accessed 11 January 2011.

3. Disaster Vulnerability in India

Due to the unique geo-climatic conditions, India is quite vulnerable to natural disasters. Floods, droughts, cyclones, earthquakes and landslides have been recurrent phenomena in the country. About 60% of the landmass is prone to earthquakes of various intensities; over 40 million hectares is prone to floods; about 8% of the total area is prone to cyclones and 68% of the area is susceptible to drought. According to the estimates, more than four thousand people lost their lives and about 30 million people were affected by disasters every year during the decade 1990-2000 (Government of India 2004). The loss in terms of life and property has been astronomical according to the EM-DAT: The OFDA/CRED International Disaster Database (2011). The summary of prominent natural and technological disasters that occurred in India during the period 1900 to 2011 and during the last 10 years (2002 to 2011) is presented in Table 2-5. The animal mortality in some major episodes of disasters and emergency situations is presented in Table 6 to indicate the vulnerability of animals in such situations.

4. Impact of Disasters and Vulnerability

The direct devastating impact in terms of loss of human life, property and infrastructure is not all what disasters lead to. Disasters have long term impact too and their effects can be felt for months and sometimes even years after the disaster. The aftereffects of a disaster are due to the loss of crops, livestock, unavailability of essential food, and diseases that may occur due to malnourishment, hunger, poor hygiene etc. Loss of farmland infrastructures, industrial set up, and employment opportunities causes severe financial distress to the people.

Vulnerability of the people refers to their ability to withstand the impact of an emergency situation. The loss of means of livelihood results in increased vulnerability of the people not only during the disaster event but even afterwards. This also applies to the people who depend on livestock for their livelihood.

There is growing recognition that disaster response should include not only saving human lives but should also consider protection and strengthening of the livelihoods of the community. This helps in reducing the vulnerability of the people to the prolonged aftereffects of the disaster event (Livestock Emergency Guidelines and Standards 2009). This is particularly important for countries like India where livestock play great role in the livelihoods of major chunk of the population.

Table 2 : Summarized table of natural disasters in India from 1900 to 2011

Disaster	Type of event	No. of events	Killed persons	Total affected	Damage (000 US$)
Drought	Drought	14	4250320	1061841000	2441122
	average per event		303594.3	75845785.7	174365.9
Earthquake (seismic activity)	Earthquake (ground	25	61705	27265183	4079900
	shaking)		2468.2	1090607.3	163196
	average per event	1	16389	654512	1022800
	Tsunami		16389	654512	1022800
	average per event				
Epidemic	Unspecified	6	293	95997	-
	average per event		48.8	15999.5	-
	Bacterial infectious diseases	24	4103948	70856	-
	average per event		170997.8	2952.3	-
	Parasitic infectious diseases	5	3411	57135	-
	average per event		682.2	11427	-
	Viral infectious diseases	33	436222	197485	-
	average per event		13218.8	5984.4	-
Extreme temperature	Cold wave	23	4752	25	144000
	average per event		206.6	1.1	6260.9
	Extreme winter conditions	1	180	-	-
	average per event		180	-	-
	Heat wave	23	8869	225	400000
	average per event		385.6	9.8	17391.3
Flood	Unspecified	95	30860	455269954	11673059
	average per event		324.8	4792315.3	122874.3
	Flash flood	22	7419	23431026	416200
	average per event		337.2	1065046.6	18918.2
	General flood	111	21370	307705877	19631929
	average per event		192.5	2772125	176864.2
	Storm surge/coastal flood	4	569	11500000	275000
	average per event		142.3	2875000	68750
Insect infestation	Locust	1	-	-	-
	average per event		-	-	-

contd...

Mass movement dry	Landslide	1	45	-	-
	average per event		45	-	-
Mass movement wet	Avalanche	7	878	10456	50000
	average per event		125.4	1493.7	7142.9
	Landslide	35	3934	3828660	4500
	average per event		112.4	109390.3	128.6
Storm	Unspecified	32	2702	5337261	225000
	average per event		84.4	166789.4	7031.3
	Local storm	22	2280	558095	2226000
	average per event		103.6	25368	101181.8
	Tropical cyclone	97	159130	87392126	8600900
	average per event		1640.5	900949.8	88669.1
Wildfire	Forest fire	2	6	-	2000
	average per event		3	-	1000

Source: EM-DAT: The OFDA/CRED International Disaster Database www.emdat.be - Université Catholique de Louvain - Brussels – Belgium. Accessed 11 January 2011.

Table 3 : Summarized table of natural disasters in India from 2002 to 2011

Disaster	Type of event	No. of events	Killed persons	Total affected	Damage (000 US$)
Drought	Drought	2	-	300000000	910722
	average per event		-	150000000	455361
Earthquake (seismic activity)	Earthquake (ground shaking)	2	1311	156822	1000000
			655.5	78411	500000
	average per event	1	16389	654512	1022800
	Tsunami		16389	654512	1022800
	average per event				
Epidemic	Unspecified	1	44	-	-
	average per event		44	-	-
	Bacterial infectious diseases	2	114	405	-
	average per event		57	202.5	-
	Parasitic infectious diseases	1	50	4950	-
	average per event		50	4950	-
	Viral infectious diseases	8	989	159317	-
	average per event		123.6	19914.6	-

contd...

Extreme temperature	Cold wave	6	1583	25	-
	average per event		263.8	4.2	-
	Extreme winter conditions	1	180	-	-
	average per event		180	-	-
	Heat wave	7	3058	25	400000
	average per event		436.9	3.6	57142.9
Flood	Unspecified	3	97	10486	2000
	average per event		32.3	3495.3	666.7
	Flash flood	13	1942	9819010	123000
	average per event		149.4	755308.5	9461.5
	General flood	68	9221	160295807	15130923
	average per event		135.6	2357291.3	222513.6
	Storm surge/coastal flood	1	80	7200000	275000
	average per event		80	7200000	275000
Mass movement wet	Avalanche	3	289	5000	50000
	average per event		96.3	1666.7	16666.7
	Landslide	4	104	20	-
	average per event		26	5	
Storm	Unspecified	6	116	68794	-
	average per event		19.3	11465.7	-
	Local storm	10	382	505295	16000
	average per event		38.2	50529.5	1600
	Tropical cyclone	12	609	5800550	328416
	average per event		50.8	483379.2	27368

Source: EM-DAT: The OFDA/CRED International Disaster Database www.emdat.be - Université Catholique de Louvain - Brussels – Belgium. Accessed 11 January 2011.

Table 4 : Summarized table of technological disasters in India from 1900 to 2011

Disaster	Event	No. of events	Killed persons	Total affected	Damage (000 US$)
Industrial accident	Chemical spill	2	2	100460	-
	average per event		1	50230	-
	Collapse	9	203	11	-
	average per event		22.6	1.2	-
	Explosion	39	2075	4913	228000
	average per event		53.2	126	5846.2

contd...

	Fire	17	360	126577	470900
	average per event		21.2	7445.7	27700
	Gas leak	3	2500	300751	-
	average per event		833.3	100250.3	-
	Other	6	149	-	-
	average per event		24.8	-	-
	Poisoning	14	980	1743	-
	average per event		70	124.5	-
Miscellaneous accident	Collapse	38	2666	150998	10000
	average per event		70.2	3973.6	263.2
	Explosion	10	301	214	-
	average per event		30.1	21.4	-
	Fire	30	1518	63527	-
	average per event		50.6	2117.6	-
	Other	23	1607	6051	-
	average per event		69.9	263.1	-
Transport accident	Air	20	1387	96	36000
	average per event		69.4	4.8	1800
	Rail	108	4602	6482	-
	average per event		42.6	60	-
	Road	239	8156	3510	-
	average per event		34.1	14.7	-
	Water	76	4573	204	-
	average per event		60.2	2.7	-

Source: EM-DAT: The OFDA/CRED International Disaster Database www.emdat.be - Université Catholique de Louvain - Brussels – Belgium. Accessed 11 January 2011.

Table 5 : Summarized table of technological disasters in India from 2002 to 2011

Disaster	Event	No. of events	Killed persons	Total affected	Damage (000 US$)
Industrial accident	Collapse	5	136	11	-
	average per event		27.2	2.2	-
	Explosion	7	180	2243	200000
	average per event		25.7	320.4	28571.4
	Fire	6	141	456	410000
	average per event		23.5	76	68333.3
	Other	1	17	-	-
	average per event		17	-	-
	Poisoning	1	66	97	-
	average per event		66	97	-
Miscellaneous accident	Collapse	13	383	284	-
	average per event		29.5	21.8	-
	Explosion	4	70	81	-
	average per event		17.5	20.3	-
	Fire	11	282	26178	-
	average per event		25.6	2379.8	-
	Other	10	851	767	-
	average per event		85.1	76.7	-
Transport accident	Air	3	200	27	-
	average per event		66.7	9	-
	Rail	25	832	1482	-
	average per event		33.3	59.3	-
	Road	70	2151	1316	-
	average per event		30.7	18.8	-
	Water	21	785	129	-
	average per event		37.4	6.1	-

Source: EM-DAT: The OFDA/CRED International Disaster Database www.emdat.be - Université Catholique de Louvain - Brussels – Belgium. Accessed 11 January 2011.

Table 6 : Animal mortalities in some major natural disasters

Year	Cause and animal mortalities	Reference
1977	Cyclone in Andhra Pradesh, mortality of 574212 animals	Kerala Veterinary Council (2011)
1982	Cyclone in Orissa, loss of 11468 cattle	Kerala Veterinary Council (2011)
1990	Cyclonic storm in Andhra Pradesh, loss of 23728 cattle and 91764 sheep and goats	Reddy (1991)
1991	Earthquake in Uttarkashi, death of 3096 cattle	Department of Animal Husbandry, Uttarkashi (2011)
1993	Earthquake in Latur district of Maharashtra, death of 14845 cattle	Goel (2007)
1995	3750 cattle mortality due to intense heat in USA	USDA (2002)
1997	Heavy snowfall in USA, mortality of 13700 animals	Friez (1997)
1998-99	Floods in Texas in 1998, livestock losses of about $11 million	Ellis (2001)
	Hurricane Floyd in North Carolina in 1999, loss of 2 million chickens, 750000 turkeys, 28000 hogs, and over 1100 cattle	
2004	Flood in Bihar, 2497 farm animals dead	Goel (2007)

The disaster-hit animals may also have serious public health consequences, such as threat to food supply, water contamination and transmission of zoonotic diseases, making human population more vulnerable to the impact of the event. Due to emotional attachment with the pets or livestock, the animal owners are unwilling to leave them behind in the situations of emergency which makes the task of evacuation of people more difficult. Separation from their animals affects the people's mental health too making their rehabilitation difficult (Sen and Chander 2003).

5. Disaster Management System

Disasters may be of different kinds but all of them have typical similarities regarding unpredictability, speed, urgency, uncertainty and threat. These features make the possibility of prevention of disasters very bleak. Therefore, the problem of disasters is addressed through a management system that helps to cope up with the aftereffects and minimize the losses.

The world over it has been experienced that a prompt, well-coordinated and effective response not only minimizes the loss of life and property but also facilitates early recovery. The important ingredients of an effective response system are integrated institutional arrangements, state of the art forecasting and early warning systems, failsafe communication system, rapid evacuation of threatened communities, quick deployment of specialized response forces and coordination and synergy among various agencies at all levels in dealing with any disaster (Government of India 2010).

Disaster management is, thus, a complex process that requires a system to be in place at the national, state, district and local level, comprising of different components and participating stakeholders, with most of the coordination being done by the disaster management department. It requires collective and participative action of many people from various government departments, NGOs, community based organizations, *panchayats*, paramilitary organizations, military services, media and even common people. It is important that all the agencies and their functionaries must clearly understand their roles and responsibilities and specific actions they have to take for responding to disaster or threatening disaster situations. Management system is in place in many countries including India.

6. Disaster Management Institutional Structure in India

The National Disaster Management Authority (NDMA), headed by the Prime Minister of India, is the Apex Body for Disaster Management in India. The Disaster Management Act, 2005 lays down a three tier institutional structure for disaster management at the national, state and district levels, respectively. The primary responsibility for undertaking the rescue, relief and rehabilitation measures rests with the concerned state governments. The role of the central government is supportive in terms of physical and financial resources and complementary in sectors such as transport, early warning systems etc. National Policy on Disaster Management (NPDM) has further specified the roles and responsibilities of various organizations for disaster response (Government of India 2010).

6.1 National level institutional structure

6.1.1 National Crisis Management Committee (NCMC)

At the national level, the command, control and coordination of the disaster response is overseen by the NCMC under the Cabinet Secretary. NCMC issues guidelines from time to time as required for effective response to natural disasters. All ministries/departments/agencies at the national level comply with the instructions of NCMC. The NPDM prescribes that NCMC shall deal with major disasters that have serious or national ramifications.

6.1.2 Ministry of Home Affairs (MHA)

MHA is the nodal agency at the national level for coordination of response and relief in the wake of natural disasters (except drought, pest attack and hailstorm). It is MHA's responsibility to provide financial and logistic support to the state governments, keeping in view their resources, the severity of the natural disaster and the capacity of the state governments to respond in a particular situation.

6.1.3 National Executive Committee (NEC)

NEC under the Union Home Secretary is responsible to coordinate response in the event of any threatening disaster situation or disaster. NEC may give directions to the concerned ministries/departments of the Government of India, the state governments and the state authorities regarding measures to be taken by them in response to any specific threatening disaster situation or disaster.

6.1.4 Other central ministries/departments

The other concerned central ministries/departments/organisations are meant to render Emergency Support Functions (ESF) wherever central intervention and support are needed by the state governments.

6.2 State level institutional structure

6.2.1 State Executive Committee (SEC)

It is the primary responsibility of the state government to respond to natural disasters and provide relief to the affected people. The SEC under the State Chief Secretary is required to coordinate response in the event of any threatening disaster situation or disaster. SEC may give directions to any department of the state government or any other authority or body in the state regarding actions to be taken in response to any disaster. Department of Relief/Disaster Management is the nodal department for disaster management and Secretary of the Department/Relief Commissioner is the authority to implement the decisions of the SEC pertaining to state level response to natural disasters.

Disaster response being a multi-agency function, other departments of the state governments are responsible to provide emergency support in their relevant domains at the state/district levels.

6.3 District level institutional structure

6.3.1 District Disaster Management Authority (DDMA)

DDMA under the chair of the Collector or District Magistrate or Deputy Commissioner, as the case may be, and the co-chair of the elected representative of the local authority is the authority to coordinate response to any threatening disaster situation or disaster. The Collector/District Magistrate/Deputy Commissioner, as the head of administration at the district, is the focal point in the command and control for disaster response at the district level, in accordance with the policies/guidelines/instructions from the national and state levels. Depending on the nature of disaster and response, he may act as the Incident Commander himself or delegate the responsibility to some other officer.

All the departments/agencies of the central and state governments in the district/city involved in response and relief work in accordance with the directions of the Incident Commander. The lower administrative units of districts viz. subdivisions under the administrative control of a Sub-divisional Magistrate/Officer and Blocks and *Tehsils* under the administrative control of the Block Development Officers/Tehsildars coordinate the functioning of various departments in their respective jurisdiction. The Incident Command Teams at subdivision and block levels under SDO/SDM or BDO/Tehsildar, as the case be, are responsible for all response and relief works.

7. Phases of Disaster Management

There are four generally recognized phases of emergency management (FEMA 1998) as shown below.

(i) *Mitigation*: Mitigation phase involves preventing future emergencies or minimizing their effects. This includes any activities that prevent an emergency, reduce the chances of an emergency or reduce the damage due to unpreventable disasters. Mitigation activities take place before and after the emergency.

(ii) *Preparedness*: Preparedness includes plans or preparation to handle an emergency and to save lives. Preparedness related activities take place before an emergency occurs and it helps in responding appropriately in emergency.

(iii) *Response*: The response phase includes the actions taken to save life and prevent further property damage in an emergency situation. It involves putting preparedness plans into action. The response activities take place during an emergency.

(iv) *Recovery*: The last phase is recovery phase which includes action taken for recovering from an emergency. It helps to return to a normal or an even safer situation following an emergency. Recovery activities take place after an emergency.

The same phases also apply to the management of animals, both livestock and pets, during disasters (FEMA 1998, Sen and Chander 2003). Humans and animals share the same vulnerability to disasters, but no doubt, the first priority of disaster relief is protecting and saving human lives. Protection of human property and animals is generally of secondary concern (Heath *et al.* 1997a).

8. Responsibilities of Veterinarians in Disaster Management

In disaster management, the basic responsibility of the veterinarians is to protect the livestock and animal food products, however, besides the animal related responsibilities, they can help in several direct public health actions (Box 1).

Box 1 : *Responsibilities of Veterinarians*

Animal related responsibilities

Before and during the event

- Protection of livestock and animal food products - indirectly protection of human health
- Major role in promoting local pre-disaster planning for timely and safe evacuation of livestock and pet animals - indirect facilitation of evacuation of people
- During relief efforts - Crucial role in increasing survivability of animals that are victims and those deployed in relief operations
- Inputs at the time of preparation of disaster management plan at state and local level
- Assistance in developing the animal evacuation and care plans during emergencies, e.g. planning evacuation routes, safe destination sites, alternate shelters
- Carcass management and disposal strategies in advance to avoid environmental and public health crisis

After the disaster event

- Search and rescue operation of all domestic and stray animals
- Transportation of rescued animals to safe places and treatment
- Immunization of surviving animal populations
- Restoration of animals to the claimants

Direct public health actions

- Emergency care and treatment of humans
- Sanitary supervision
- Food inspection
- Prevention and control of diseases

Veterinarians have a role to play in all stages of disaster mitigation and management. They can play major role in promoting local pre-disaster planning at community level for timely and safe evacuation of livestock and pet animals (Heath 2000a). This will facilitate the evacuation of people who otherwise may be reluctant to leave their animals behind. During relief efforts, veterinarians can play crucial role in increasing the survivability of animals that are victims, and of those that are deployed in relief operations. The contribution of veterinarians will be most effective if they integrate their expertise with other local, national and international groups and agencies involved in disaster management (Heath 2000b).

Veterinarians should provide their inputs at the time of preparation of disaster management plan at state and local level. They should assist the planning committees in developing the animal evacuation and care plans during emergencies. They should help in the development of action plans concerning evacuation routes that do not conflict with human evacuation routes, safe destination sites and alternate shelters for the animals. As animal mortality is an expected sequel to disaster, veterinarians should prepare the carcass management and disposal strategies in advance to avoid environmental and public health crisis.

After disaster, the veterinarians should carryout search and rescue operation of all animals including domestic and stray animals. Rescued animals should be transported to safe places and should be treated. The surviving animal populations should be immunized against epidemic outbreaks. Veterinarians should also help in restoration of animals to the claimants.

Apart from these animal related relief measures, veterinarians can also contribute directly to public health through emergency care and treatment of humans, sanitary supervision, food inspection and prevention and control of diseases. Veterinarians are familiar with medical emergencies and they are professionally trained to respond in situations with limited resources (Heath *et al.* 1997b). Their proximity to rural folks makes their task easier.

9. Veterinarian's Unique Qualities for Effective Disaster Response

Veterinarians by virtue of their educational training and place of their work have the following unique qualities which bring them to the fore for a quick and effective response during an emergency situation.

- Familiarity with medical emergencies
- Training to respond in situations with limited resources
- Proximity to rural folks

- Knowledge of epidemiology, hygiene, sanitation, water quality management, nutrition, livestock health and zoonotic diseases - Useful in improving the quality of life of both humans and animals in the post-disaster scenario.

10. Organizational Models for Veterinarians' Disaster Response

Several countries, particularly developed ones, have put in place the organized modern disaster response systems during the last two decades. The systems vary from country to country according to different political and administrative features of each country. The countries like USA, France and Italy have considered and vividly described the veterinarians' response in emergency situations. These models are being described below in short to facilitate an insight to the comparative situation in India.

10.1 USA model

In USA, the major role in disaster response is played by the American Veterinary Medical Association (AVMA). It has recently released a revised version of the Emergency Preparedness and Response guide in the year 2010 (AVMA 2010), the first version of which was published in the year 1994. It includes AVMA's Emergency Management Programme which aims to encourage and foster veterinary leadership and guidance in local, state and federal efforts within the United States in preparation for disasters and emergencies involving animals, animal and public health, and other veterinary issues.

The guide includes model veterinary service and animal care plan to function at state level. Its purpose is to provide guidelines for rapid response to disasters affecting the health, safety, and welfare of human beings and animals. Veterinary medicine and animal care resources in emergency preparedness, response, and recovery include, but are not limited to, small and large animal care, facility usage, and displaced pet/livestock assistance. Its concept of operation during different stages of a disaster event is presented below (AVMA 2010).

A. Mitigation

1. Zoological and wildlife parks, marine animal aquariums, laboratory animal research facilities, animal shelters, and university veterinary medical and animal science centers are encouraged/required to develop emergency procedures and evacuation plan for the animals in their care and to provide copies of the plans to the (state) Emergency Management Agency.

2. Veterinary services, permit applications to maintain a wild/exotic animal, recommend or require applicants to file an emergency procedure and evacuation plan with the (state) Emergency Management Agency and to maintain possession of a suitable container to transport the animal during evacuations.

B. Preparedness

1. The state Veterinary Medical Association (VMA) assists the State Emergency Management Agency (EMA) in developing an organizational structure and chain of command, and an outline of the duties and responsibilities of veterinarians involved in implementation of the response to a disaster or major emergency following Incident Command System (ICS).
2. Coordinating with the state and/or the state animal response team, the state VMA provides the names of current state and county Veterinary Liaison Officers to the Coordinator of Emergency Preparedness and Response for the AVMA.
3. Coordinating with applicable county animal response teams and county emergency boards, the state VMA provides a current directory of county Veterinary Liaison Officers (county veterinary coordinators) and member licensed veterinarians residing in the county/city to the local Emergency Management Agency (EMA) Coordinator.
4. The state VMA works with state policymakers to develop and enact state laws modeled after the Uniform Emergency Volunteers Health Practitioners Act.
5. Veterinary personnel, previously credentialed and certified as required by state law, participate in emergency exercises and training.
6. Directories of humane society and private animal holding facilities are provided to the county.
7. Humane society and animal control personnel participate in emergency exercises and training.
8. Veterinary services and animal care activities are incorporated into local Emergency Operations Plans (EOP).
9. Copies of animal-escape/evacuations plans for zoologic, wildlife, and aquarium parks; laboratory animal research facilities; animal shelters; and university veterinary medical and animal science centers are provided to the (state) Emergency Management Agency.

C. Response

Veterinarians involved in emergency management will:

a. First seek appropriate credentialing and certification as required by the State.

b. Coordinate with governmental authorities in establishment of emergency aid stations and staging of emergency relief.

c. Coordinate with governmental authorities in matters of evacuation.

d. Cooperate with governmental authorities in matters of equipment use and provision of transportation.

e. Cooperate with mutual aid operatives.

f. Cooperate in matters of salvage and restoration of community order.

g. Maintain security of veterinary medical facilities and supplies.

h. Coordinate with public information operations, specifically the Public Information Officer, to communicate alert status, volunteer mobilization, and casualty and damage information.

i. Temporarily arrange for or provide food, water, and shelter for small and large animals.

j. Provide care for sick/injured animals.

k. Assist in the coordination of efforts with animal control officials to apprehend animals that have escaped their confinement as recommended within the ICS structure of the incident at hand.

l. Recommend methods of proper disposal of dead animals; coordinate with (state) Departments of Agriculture, Health, Wildlife and (state) Environmental Protection Agency.

m. Recommend methods and supervise prevention and control of zoonotic diseases.

n. When medical facilities are unavailable, and when directed by state authorities, permit use of veterinary facilities and equipment for temporary human medical care during extreme emergencies involving mass casualties.

D. Recovery

Provide documentation of injuries and deaths of animals for insurance and reimbursement purposes.

10.2 France model

In France, emergency response is envisaged at municipal, departmental, zonal and central (national) levels. At each level, a veterinarian coordinates activities connected with animal health and food hygiene. Most of the operational response is by Fire Brigades, which include a medical and health service, and an organised corps of veterinarians (*Vétérinaires Sapeur Pompier*-VSP). VSP supports the Medical disaster manager when animals, food and environment are involved during rescue operations (Leonardi *et al.* 2006).

10.2.1 Tasks of VSP

Leonardi *et al.* (2006) have enlisted the tasks of VSP as follows.

- Prevention and response against technological and biological risks
- Inspection and control of live animals and foodstuffs
- Veterinary support to rescue operations
- Training and follow-up of rescue dog teams
- Management of means and materials for veterinary action and management of animals
- Health and hygiene education
- Advice on dead animals
- Advice to the Command of Sapeur Pompier on environment and food chain in disasters
- Advice to the Command of Sapeur Pompier on risk forecasting and prevention

10.3 Italy model

In Italy, veterinary services belong to the National Health Service and Department of Preventive Medicine, together with Public Hygiene, Food and Nutrition, Occupational Medicine Services. Veterinary services are an operational component of Civil Protection Service in the country. In emergency situations, local health agencies including veterinary services are activated by the local civil protection authority in Italy (Leonardi *et al.* 2006).

10.3.1 Veterinary actions in emergencies

In Italian model, the veterinary actions in non-epidemic emergencies are as given below (Dipartimento della Protezione Civile 1998, Mantovani *et al.* 1998, Leonardi *et al.* 2006).

A. Natural disasters

Immediate action

- Arrangement of safe food resources
- Care and slaughter of injured animals
- Disposal of carcasses and other animal waste
- Shelter, food and water for dispersed animals
- Zoonoses control
- Pest control
- Food safety

Successive action

- Resumption of normal activities of slaughtering, meat inspection, milk collection and storage
- Providing drugs, vaccines, disinfectants
- Disinfection of areas and premises at risk
- Establishing epidemiologic surveillance
- Evacuation of animals from the area at risk

B. Manmade disasters (chemical and radio-nuclear)

- Recognising the origin of hazardous contaminant
- Moving or keeping the animals indoors (away from the polluted zone)
- Avoiding feeding animals with contaminated material
- Monitoring contaminants in animal products
- Toxicological surveillance

11. Indian Perspective

The Standard Operating Procedure for Responding to Natural Disasters (Government of India 2010) in India includes Department of Animal Husbandry, Dairying & Fisheries and Veterinary Services as important functionaries in the disaster response teams. The following points relating to animals have been mentioned in it.

- *Animal care*: Animals, both domestic as well as wild, are exposed to the effects of natural and man-made disasters. It is necessary to devise appropriate measures to protect animals and find means to shelter and feed them during disasters and their aftermath, through a community effort, to the extent possible. It is pertinent to note that many communities have shown compassion to animals during disasters, and these efforts need to be formalized in the preparedness plans of the Departments of Animal Husbandry at the centre and the states.

- *Disposal of carcasses*: The state government/district authorities shall earmark authorities responsible for disposal of carcasses in the event of mass destruction. The process to be followed for mass disposal of carcasses shall be decided by Department of Animal Husbandry.

12. Capacity Building of Veterinarians for Disaster Response

Veterinary education is aimed at enhancing quality of life in society through animal welfare and livestock resource. Because of the educational background, training and experience, veterinarians constitute a resourceful workforce in emergency situations, however, specialized training of disaster response among the veterinarians is quite inadequate in the country. The persons without some training become liabilities rather than assets in emergency situations. Such persons may not be appropriate to work in disaster situations despite their eagerness to provide selfless dedicated service (Heath and Linnabary 1993).

Disaster management is not all about heroic rescue of humans and animals during the immediate response phase of an event, it also includes hazard analysis, mitigation, planning, continuing education of the personnel, staging mock drills, reviewing effectiveness of the strategies and intervention modalities, and public education. Disaster preparedness involves integrating all of these issues through a proactive, continual, cyclic process (Heath *et al.* 1997a). Thus, there is tremendous deficit in the number of qualified veterinarians to deal with disaster medicine.

The current situation needs to be corrected so that veterinarians are able to take leading role in emergency situations and can provide much required service to the local community and the state in the periods of distress. This will involve training and retraining of veterinarians. Veterinary colleges and research institutions need to play a definite role in improving the situation as elaborated below (Heath and Linnabary 1993).

13. Potential Role of Veterinary Colleges

Veterinary colleges require implementing steps for arming the graduates with unique skills of disaster medicine and disaster response. It is paramount that veterinary education creates a series of compatible global education programmes and training opportunities in the four areas of disaster and emergency response namely, mitigation, preparedness, response and recovery so that the graduates are trained to contribute meaningfully and effectively at all stages in emergency situation. Templates for veterinary disaster education programmes and certification at various levels of emergency training should be standardised/harmonised to assess capabilities at the regional, state and national level (Wingfield *et al.* 2009).

13.1 Disaster response education to veterinary students

As early as in the year 1993, Heath and Linnabary (1993) emphasised the need of education of veterinary graduates in emergency and disaster management. They suggested the following courses for certification of veterinarians in emergency response management.

Courses

- Classification and staging of disasters
- Organization of disaster responses
- Chain of command structures
- Regulatory and legal aspects of disasters
- Foodborne and zoonotic diseases that result from disasters
- Dealing with hazardous materials
- Historical data gathering
- Importance of maintaining a continual food supply for human beings
- Capture, handling, placing and rehabilitation of feral animals
- Search and rescue dog training and use in emergencies
- Evacuation psychology of animal owners
- Pathological sample collection

Workshops

- Case problem solving
- Organizing, selecting and motivating volunteers
- First aid training
- Staging exercises

Madigan and Dacre (2009) suggested that the essential components to prepare veterinary graduates for useful participation in a disaster include:

a) Core knowledge of the health and husbandry needs of a wide variety of species

b) Comprehensive knowledge of emergency procedures including surgery, medical management of infections, wounds, burns and shock, health consequences of floods, treating exposure to toxic or hazardous substances, nutritional needs of animals, the criteria for euthanasia and humane methods of euthanasia, and training in the Incident Command System of operations (incident management concept)

Many veterinary institutions in developed countries have already initiated acquainting their students with disaster management. College of Veterinary Medicine in the University of Florida is already providing training in disaster medicine to veterinary students via a series of courses, laboratories, and field exercises. Similarly, Purdue University offers a Web-based Graduate Certificate in Veterinary Homeland Security. The programme is a collaborative effort among the Purdue University School of Veterinary Medicine, the Purdue Homeland Security Institute, the Indiana State Board of Animal Health, the Indiana State Police, and others with the overall goal of increasing capacity and preparedness to manage animal-related emergencies.

13.2 Continuing veterinary education

Veterinary colleges can help in providing continuing education to veterinarians who may be deficient in handling the emergency situations (Heath and Linnabary 1993). Madigan and Dacre (2009) have suggested the following training areas for disaster and emergency response:

- Leadership
- Incident Command System, incident management concept
- Animal care
- Epidemiology
- Bioterrorism – zoonoses
- Decontamination methods and principles
- Search and rescue
- Human care
- Sources of veterinary medical equipment and supplies
- Community planning, outreach and education
- Animal vaccination methodologies
- Mental health

13.3 Facilities and personnel support in disaster response

Besides the availability of adequate space and treatment facilities, veterinary colleges have vast resources of faculty with expertise in clinical medicine, microbiology, epidemiology, pathology, toxicology, veterinary public health and other disciplines. These can, therefore, help by providing first response during emergency situations. The faculty can also contribute in planning for mitigation and resolution of disaster situations (Heath and Linnabary 1993).

College of Veterinary Medicine in University of Florida provides an excellent example of this. The College is a leader in disaster management and response in the state of Florida. The College deployed veterinary care teams to hurricanes Charlie, Frances, and Jeanne during the 2004 hurricane season, deployed a team to Hurricane Wilma in 2005, and operated a shelter for evacuated Hurricane Katrina animals at the College. During the wildfires of 2007, College response teams assisted in animal evacuation and managed several patients.

13.4 Research

Research in various aspects of disaster management is another important component where veterinary institutions can contribute. Some examples of multidisciplinary and collaborative projects that can be taken up by veterinary institutions are listed below (Heath and Linnabary 1993).

- Minimization of stress to animals during emergencies
- Nutritional, behavioural and environmental needs of animals and their modifications during emergency situations
- Development of new technology to facilitate emergency relief
- Selection and training of search and rescue dogs
- Prediction of timing, course and direction of spread of emergencies attributable to natural causes
- Animals as sentinels
- Epidemiological data collection, analysis and interpretation
- Risks, costs and implications of public health disruption attributable to animals in disasters
- Risk factor identification and prevention of crises
- Study of populations at risk
- Behaviour responses of pet owners during evacuations
- Evacuation attitudes of animal owners

14. Conclusion

Natural disaster management has emerged as a high priority area. Going beyond the age-old method of attempting relief and rehabilitation after the event, we now have to look ahead and plan for disaster preparedness and mitigation to minimize the loss. Though the threat to human life is a prime concern in emergency situations, the consequences of disasters on animals should not be ignored. The mortality of livestock not only gives a severe financial blow to the farming community, the innumerable dead animals also pose a major threat to the environmental health of man and animals. Veterinarians can provide considerable relief in such situations. Their proximity to the rural folks makes their task easier. Veterinarians can be helpful in all stages of disaster response including the rescue operations and crisis management as well as in mitigating the aftereffects of disasters. With their knowledge and training, they can contribute vastly in improving the quality of life of both humans as well as animals during and after the disaster event. The well defined and elaborate roles of veterinarians in disaster response in developed nations and the comparative analysis of Indian perspective reveal that there is urgent need to strengthen the integration of the veterinary services in the disaster response strategies of the country requiring multi-sectoral and multi-hazard prevention based approach. Veterinary institutions and animal husbandry departments should make concerted efforts towards capacity building of veterinarians to enable them make exemplary contribution in mitigating sufferings and loss in such situations.

References

1. AVMA (2010). Emergency Preparedness and Response. American Veterinary Medical Association. http://www.avma.org/disaster/emerg_prep_resp_guide.pdf.
2. Department of Animal Husbandry, Uttarkashi (2011). Disaster management action plan. http://uttarkashi.nic.in/Dept/animal_husbandry/Disaster_Management.pdf. Accessed 17 January 2011.
3. Dipartimento della Protezione Civile (1998). Linee guida per l'azione veterinaria nelle emergenze non epidemiche. Roma, DPC.
4. Ellis D (2001). Carcass disposal issues in recent disasters, accepted methods, and suggested plan to mitigate future events. Applied research project for Master of Public Administration. Texas State University-San Marcos.
5. EM-DAT:The OFDA/CRED International Disaster Database (2011). Université Catholique de Louvain, Brussels. www.emdat.be. Accessed 11 January 2011.
6. FEMA (1998). Animals in disaster (Module A): Awareness and Preparedness. Federal Emergency Management Agency, Emergency Management Institute (EMI) Independent study course. EMI, Emmitsburg, Maryland.

7. Friez DC (1997). Emergency Management in North Dakota, Situation Report No. 43, Incident No. 97-015. http://www.state.nd.us/dem/reports/docs/sitrep/1997/sr43-015.pdf. Accessed 17 May 2009.

8. Goel SL (2007). Disaster administration and management. Deep and Deep Publications Pvt. Ltd, New Delhi, India.

9. Government of India (2004). Disaster Management in India - A status report. National Disaster Management Division, Ministry of Home Affairs, Government of India. www.unisdr.org/eng/country-inform/reports/India-report.pdf

10. Government of India (2010). Standard operating procedure for responding to natural disasters 2010. Ministry of Home Affairs, Disaster Management Division, Government of India.

11. Heath SE (2000a). The role of veterinarians in disasters. World Veterinary Association Press Release, Washington, DC. Cited from Sen and Chander (2003).

12. Heath SE (2000b). Building an animal disaster program. In: Proceedings of Outbreak Symposium at AVMA, Schaumburg, USA. Cited from Sen and Chander (2003).

13. Heath SE, Dorn R, Linnabary RD, Hooks J, Casper J, Marshall K (1997a). An overview of disaster preparedness for veterinarians. JAVMA 210 (3):345-348.

14. Heath SE, Hooks J, Marshall K, Dorn R, Linnabary RD, Casper J (1997b). Participation of veterinarians in disaster management. JAVMA 210 (3):325-328.

15. Heath SE, Linnabary R (1993). Potential roles of veterinary schools in emergency and disaster management. JAVMA 203:953-956.

16. Kerala Veterinary Council (2011). Public information. http://keralaveterinary council.org/html/animal_resource.html. Accessed 17 January 2011.

17. Leonardi M, Borroni R, di Gennaro M (2006). Veterinary medicine in disasters. Ann Ist Super Santa 42:417-421.

18. Livestock Emergency Guidelines and Standards (2009). Practical Action Publishing, Warwickshire, UK.

19. Madigan J, Dacre I (2009). Preparing for veterinary emergencies: disaster management and the Incident Command System. Rev sci tech Off int Epiz 28:627-633.

20. Mantovani A, Leonardi M, Luini M, Volpini A (1998). Veterinary public health in emergencies. Europ J Emergency Medicine 5:108-109.

21. Reddy AVS (1991). The concept of cyclone shelters for livestock. Livestock Research for Rural Development 3:1-5.

22. Sen A, Chander M (2003). Disaster management in India: The case of livestock and poultry. Rev sci tech Off int Epiz 22 (3):915-930.

23. USDA (2002). Animal health hazards of concern during natural disasters. Washington, DC: United States Department of Agriculture Animal and Plant Health Inspection Service, Veterinary Services Unit. http://www.aphis.usda.gov/vs/ceah/cei/taf/emerginganimalhealthissues_files/hazards.PDF. Accessed 18 December 2009.

24. Wingfield WE, Nash SL, Palmer SB, Upp JJ (2009). Veterinary disaster medicine: working animals. Wiley-Blackwell, Ames, Iowa.

□□□

Chapter 30

Role of Financial Institutions in Livestock Development

D.V. DESHPANDE*
National Bank for Agriculture and Rural Development, Mumbai-400051

* The views expressed are author's personal views.

Contents

1. Livestock Sector: An Overview

Animal husbandry in a general sense includes sectors like dairy, poultry, sheep, goat and rabbits etc. At the macroeconomic level, the term 'allied sectors' (as part of 'agriculture and allied sector') also includes fisheries. India is blessed with substantial livestock resources as it is the biggest milk producer with 100.9 million ton and third biggest in egg production with 50.7 billion eggs produced in the year 2007 (GOI 2008). In terms of livestock numbers also, India ranks first in the world in respect of buffalo, second in cattle and goats, third in sheep, fourth in ducks, and seventh in poultry (GOI 2007).

Livestock sector plays a crucial role in the national economy and socioeconomic development of the country. It is also significant in supplementing family incomes and generating gainful employment in the rural sector especially among the landless, small and marginal farmers and women besides providing cheap nutritional food to millions of people (GOI 2007). There have been efforts to quantify the contribution of livestock sector to the Indian economy and the latest available data from the Central Statistical Organisation (CSO) indicate that the value of the output from livestock and allied sectors was Rs. 2,50,761 crore during 2006-07 (livestock sector Rs. 2,10,629 crore, fisheries sector Rs. 40,132 crore) which worked out to 31.7% of the total value of the output from agriculture and allied sector at Rs. 7,90,979 crore during 2006-07. The contribution of these sectors to the overall Gross Domestic Product (GDP) worked out to 5.26% in 2006-07. The share of livestock sector alone works out to 26.6% of the value of the output of agriculture and allied sectors (GOI 2007).

2. Livestock Census Data

As mentioned earlier, India is blessed with sizeable livestock population. The latest livestock data relate to 17th Livestock Census conducted in 2003. The data indicate that with 485 million total livestock consisting of cattle, buffaloes, sheep, goat, pigs, camels, horses, donkeys as well as yaks and mithun, but excluding poultry, the livestock population has marginally declined from 485.4 million in 1997. A significant finding of the census was that the number of crossbred cattle increased by 22.8% from 20.1 million in 1997 to 24.7 million in 2003. At the same time, the number of indigenous cattle declined by 10.2% from 178.8 million in 1997 to 160.5 million in 2007.

However, it is a matter of great concern that although the livestock population in the country is huge, the productivity of the animals is low. The livestock census has brought out the break up and certain details of the milch animals in the country. The same are presented below in Table 1.

Table 1 : Number and growth of milch animals

Particulars	1997	2003	% increase
Crossbred cattle (million)	8.356	11.231	34.4%
Indigenous cattle (million)	49.874	46.856	-6.1%
Buffaloes (million)	42.732	47.224	10.5%
Total (million)	100.962	105.311	4.3%
Milk production (million ton)	72.1	88.1	22.2%
Average milk production per animal (ton)	0.71	0.84	18.3%
Average productivity (litre/day/milch animal)	2.4	2.8	16.7%

Source : GOI (2005)

Thus, it may be seen from the above table that although the population of milch animals is quite huge, the average productivity is low at 2.8 litre per day. Although disaggregated data are not available, it is generally true that the productivity of crossbred cattle and buffaloes is much more than indigenous cows.

3. Constraints in Reaching the Potential

It is obvious that India is blessed with a variety of agroclimatic regions with vast potential in animal husbandry sector. However, there are several problems and constraints in reaching the potential. Low productivity of our livestock is the key constraint hindering the growth of the sector. Based on the field level feedback of the author of this chapter, it is learnt that the main reasons for the low productivity are:

- Lack of good quality/good breed animals as indicated in Table 1, despite the increase in recent years, the crossbred cattle are only 19% of the total milch cattle. This is despite the wide network of artificial insemination (AI) centres for cows and buffaloes.
- Lack of appropriate feeding and management.
- Lack of adequate and hygienic housing and veterinary care.
- Lack of awareness among the livestock farmers about scientific breeding, feeding and management.
- Non-availability of adequate, timely and affordable credit.

4. Role of Finance and Financial Institutions in Animal Husbandry

The question is whether finance and financial institutions could play any role in the root cause of these issues, that is, lack of awareness among the farmers and unavailability of financial resources for carrying out these activities. While awareness creation and capacity building is the task of the state animal husbandry departments and the agricultural universities, provision of financial resources is a matter which is of the concern of the policy makers. Therefore, Government of India, state governments, financial institutions like National Bank for Agriculture and Rural Development (NABARD), banks, foreign funding agencies, certain NGOs etc. have launched schemes and facilities for financial support for animal husbandry activities. Government schemes mainly provide for grants and interest subsidies for taking up certain activities as per the priorities of the government.

At a conceptual level, the financial support can be seen as a continuum ranging from 100% grant/subsidies on one extreme to 100% own capital (equity) on the other extreme. Credit is the third dimension of this continuum. Thus, most of the projects or activities of the livestock sector would be financed through a combination of farmer/ entrepreneur's own capital (or equity), credit and subsidy/grants from central or state government.

In several cases, the 'credit' component may be the most significant in the total funds requirement for the activity. However, it is important to understand that there are several sources of credit like, traditional money lenders, feed suppliers (including cooperative dairies), food grain/feed ingredient dealers, animal supplier/ sellers etc., besides the banks.

Although, credit plays a crucial role in animal husbandry activities, like other economic activities, the data about the total credit from various sources to animal husbandry is not readily available. However, data on credit from institutional sources/banks has been compiled by NABARD (2010) which is presented in Table 2.

Table 2 : Credit flow for agriculture and allied activities and the share of animal husbandry

Sector/Sub-sector	2005-06 (Rs. Crore)	2006-07 (Rs. Crore)	2007-08 (Rs. Crore)	2008-09 (Rs. Crore)	Growth rate (%) 2005-09*
Animal husbandry	7341	8045	9034	10398	12.3
Ground level credit flow for agriculture & allied activities	180486	229400	254658	301908	17.9
Share of animal husbandry in total credit flow to agriculture and allied activities (%)	4.1%	3.5%	3.5%	3.4%	Negligible

Source: NABARD (2010) *Compounded annual growth rate

Thus, the share of credit flow to animal husbandry sector is very low and stagnant for the last 4 years at only 3-4%. The share of agricultural credit is also lower than the sector's contribution to the GDP, which was 5.26% in 2006-07. This clearly brings out the need and scope for more credit flow to the sector. Nonetheless, the amount in absolute terms around Rs. 10398 (say Rs. 10000 crore) is sizeable and has shown a compounded annual growth rate of 12.3% which, although lower than that of credit to agriculture, can be considered healthy.

The institutional support to the sector can broadly be classified into two levels:

- *Small holder units* - mainly comprising of 2-5 milch animals or 100-200 poultry birds which are reared by an individual, often a poor farmer, and
- *Commercial units* - the size of these units generally larger than that of small holder and the scale of operation of the entrepreneur involving heavy investment.

5. Categories of Financial Assistance

The financial assistance/sources of funds can broadly be classified into the following categories, which are briefly discussed here.

5.1 Owner's funds - Equity, seed capital, venture capital etc.

As indicated earlier, equity can be considered as an ideal way of financing as in such a case the entrepreneur will be fully responsible for the decisions and will have full freedom to use the funds as he would like to do. Further, all the profits will be the returns to him as there will be no interest cost, loan servicing etc. However, in developing country like ours, the entrepreneurs, who are generally of small scale, are short of equity capital. Many times the entrepreneurs invest their own savings and borrowings from family members and relatives which is called Seed capital. In this context, a term called Venture capital (also known as VC or Venture) is often come across. Venture capital is also like seed capital to new companies who are not able to raise funds from banks etc. But the difference is that venture capital investor does it as his business i.e. for profit. In this process, the VCs also help the company in management processes, developing marketing plans and adding skill sets required to compete in the industry. Another term in this context is 'angel investor' who is generally an individual or a group who provides capital for starting a business for converting his funds into equity.

In case of animal husbandry activities, depending on the factors like size of investment, type of entrepreneur etc., the need for venture capital can be examined but in most of the animal husbandry projects, this kind of VC or formal angel investors are generally not involved at present. But from a futuristic point of view, this funding source needs to be looked at by prospective investors/entrepreneurs.

In case of small holder schemes, the equity or simply put, the margin money to be invested by the entrepreneur, is as low as 5% and it can be 'zero' if some subsidy/grant is available, which is considered in most cases as 'in lieu of margin money'. However, in case of commercial projects, the proportion of entrepreneurs' contribution can be as high as 15-50%. In case of big projects of companies, this is expressed as a ratio – 'debt equity ratio' expressed as debt : equity. For example, if an entity has Rs. 100 as debt (loan) and Rs. 50 as equity, the debt equity ratio will be 2:1. Normally 2:1 is the upper limit for considering loan support by any bank.

5.2 Term loans

For most of the economic activities, the financial requirement can be classified as term loans for the items which last long and keep on generating income. For example a cow or buffalo lasts for several years (5-6 years). Besides such assets, other items like buildings, equipments, etc. also are part of the term loans. Land is required for most of the activities but purchase of land is generally not financed by the banks. The entrepreneur is expected to acquire land from his own resources. However, in some cases land cost can be taken towards margin money (upto 10% of the total project cost).

The term of the loan or repayment period can vary depending on the cash flow or income but is generally upto 5 years in case of livestock activities. Some of the activities take some time to generate income or the cash flow is such that cash is not available for repayment. In such cases, grace period or 'gestation period' is provided during which no amount needs to be repaid. In general, during the gestation period, interest is repaid by the borrower but in certain projects where it is not possible to repay interest also (besides principal), 'interest moratorium' can also be provided

The interest rate on the loans varies from time to time, bank to bank and based on the purpose. These terms should be clearly understood by the entrepreneur before taking loan.

5.3 Working capital

Working capital is required for day to day operations of any economic activity. This includes, in case of animal husbandry activities, feed and fodder, veterinary care, labour payments, maintenance requirements, etc. In several cases, not the investment items but the working capital is responsible for failure of the project. Traditional sources of working capital for animal husbandry schemes are from informal sources like *halwais* (sweet shops), buy back arrangements from poultry marketing firms, etc. In case of cooperatives set up for dairy or poultry development, these institutions provide these facilities to their members and deduct the cost in the payments to be made which reduces cash requirement and interest burden on small holders.

5.4 Subsidies and grants

Government of India and the state governments have launched several schemes/programmes for promoting animal husbandry schemes which include grant/subsidy component to improve viability of the units. Integrated Rural Development Programme (IRDP) was the first large scale effort of the Government of India for reducing poverty in rural areas. It was launched throughout the country in the year 1980 with the objective of helping the rural families cross the 'poverty line' by providing them income generating assets. Although the scheme was not meant for animal husbandry activities alone, large number of poor families were assisted under the scheme through the animal husbandry activities.

In the year 1999-2000, the scheme was merged with some other schemes into a new programme named *Swarnjayanti Gram Swarozgar Yojana* (SGSY) wherein the emphasis was put on enterprise promotion through developing the poor beneficiaries into entrepreneurs - called as *'Swarozgaris'*. The proportion of poor people assisted under the programme through animal husbandry was quite high; for example during 2009-10, about 7.70 lakh people out of a total of 16.61 lakh were assisted under SGSY through animal husbandry which works out to 46% (GOI Ministry of Rural Development, http://rural.nic.in/sgsy/sgsyframetop.asp?id=08). The primary mode of implementation was proposed to be 'groups' like Self Help Groups (SHGs). An average subsidy of 30% has been provided under the programme while the subsidy level is 50% of the project cost for Scheduled Castes/Scheduled Tribes (SC/ST) to a maximum of Rs. 10,000. For groups of *Swarozgaris* (SHGs), the subsidy is provided at 50% of the cost of the project, subject to a ceiling of Rs. 1.25 lakhs (Ministry of Rural Development, Government of India, SGSY Guidelines, http://www.drd.nic.in/Guide/sgsy.htm). In the year 2011, SGSY has been revised and a new programme named 'National Rural Livelihood Mission' (NRLM) has been launched for covering these areas.

6. Value Chain Concept and its Finance

The concept of 'Value addition chain' or simply the **'value chain'** is a concept from business management that was popularized by Porter (1985). The concept is relevant not only for industrial products but also for agricultural and animal husbandry. Conceptually, a value chain is a chain of activities or processes through which the product passes before reaching the customer. At each stage, some 'value addition' is there to the product. The concept can be depicted in a generic way as presented in Fig. 1.

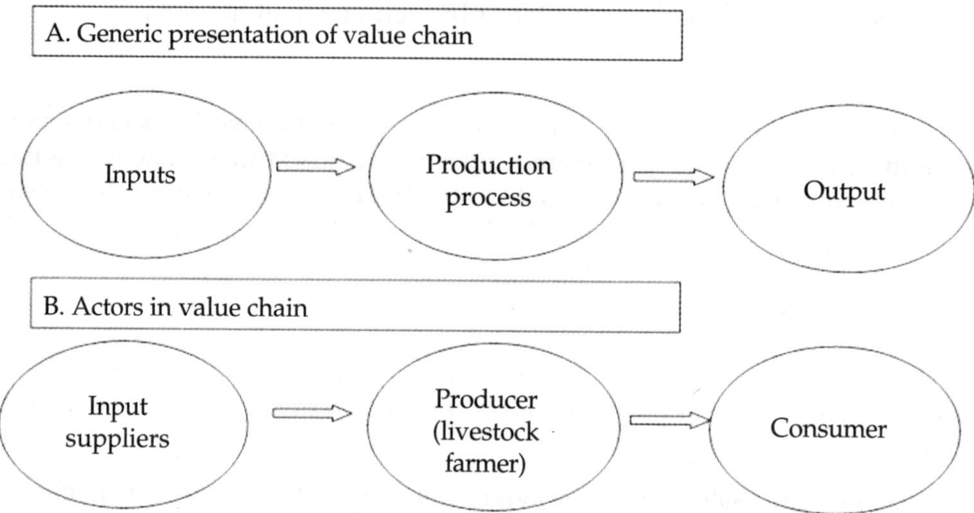

Fig. 1 : Value addition – a generic presentation

The above depiction may look a simplistic presentation but from animal husbandry point of view, each of the input (e.g. feed, fodder, mineral mixture etc.) is a separate and huge industry with several players. Similarly, the process of production and outputs also are different for different products and offer huge business potential. Hence financing of each element of value chain also has its own dynamics and system where institutional (like banks) and non-institutional (like traders) provide the finance.

7. Institutional Set up in India for Financial Assistance

There are several institutions involved in financial support. The present set up is briefly described below.

7.1 National Bank for Agriculture and Rural Development (NABARD)

NABARD was set up in 1982 as an apex Development Bank with a mandate of facilitating credit flow for promotion and development of agriculture, small-scale industries, cottage and village industries, handicrafts and other rural crafts. It also has the mandate to support all other allied economic activities in rural areas, promote integrated and sustainable rural development and secure prosperity of rural areas. It has supported development of animal husbandry sector through financial support and for several model animal husbandry schemes have been placed on its website (www.nabard.org) for the use of prospective borrowers/entrepreneurs. However, as a general policy, NABARD does not finance the farmers directly. It provides 'refinance support' to banks for supporting eligible activities, including animal husbandry activities.

7.2 Banks

Banks play the most crucial role in financing agriculture including animal husbandry. India has a multiple banking system comprising of commercial banks, Cooperative banks, Regional Rural Banks (RRBs), and Agriculture and Rural Development Banks (ARDBs). The commercial banks can again be classified as public sector, private sector and foreign banks. As on 31st March 2009, there were 80547 bank branches in the country of which almost 40% (31667 branches) were in rural areas and another 23% (18969 branches) in semi-urban branches. These numbers are excluding cooperative and ARDBs (RBI 2010). Thus, India has vast network of bank branches and almost every 20 villages have a commercial bank branch. Nonetheless, rural borrowers, especially those who are in remote areas, are still facing several problems in accessing credit from mainstream banks.

7.3 Other financial organisations

Besides the banks, there are several institutions which support, *inter-alia*, livestock development like women development corporations, National Scheduled Castes and Scheduled Tribes Finance and Development Corporation (NSFDC), Rashtriya Mahila Kosh, Livestock Development Corporations etc. which are set up for enabling specific target groups. Many of them have counterparts at state level. These corporations provide direct funding (often as a soft loan or as a combination of loan and grant) or along with commercial banks.

Now a sizeable network of Microfinance Institutions (MFIs) is also functioning in the country which provides financial support for small loans which include animal husbandry activities. Often these MFIs route their finance through groups of rural people (especially women) known as Self Help Groups (SHG). Although these MFIs and SHGs charge higher interest rates (from 2% per month i.e. equal to 24% per annum to almost 40% per annum), still there is heavy demand as these loans are available without much hassle.

7.4 Role of insurance in livestock farming

No discussion on finance for animal husbandry can be complete without a mention of insurance of the livestock. Every farmer or entrepreneur as a general precaution should insure the assets especially the animals as there can be mortality due to several reasons not in his control. Now besides the public sector insurance companies, some private sector companies are also offering the livestock insurance products.

7.5 Venture capital scheme of GOI

Government of India started a scheme termed 'Venture Capital Fund' for dairy and poultry in 2004-05 to bring about structural changes in these activities and to promote measures like milk processing, quality upgradation of traditional technology, value addition etc. Initially the scheme covered both dairy and poultry but since 2009-10 it has been split into two separate schemes - one for dairy and another for poultry.

Under the scheme, financial assistance is provided as loan through bankable projects which may include items like milk chilling centres, cold chain, refrigerated vans, feed godown for poultry etc. A unique feature of the scheme is that it does not give capital subsidy but provides interest free loan to the extent of 50% of total cost. Out of the remaining half, 10% is contributed by the entrepreneur and the remaining 40% is provided as loan by the bank at normal interest rate. Further, for regular repayments, interest paid on the bank loan is reimbursed to an extent of 50%. The fund is routed through NABARD. From 2005-06 to 2009-10, a total of 15368 units have been assisted under this scheme involving financial support of Rs. 147 crore. The details of the scheme are available at Government of India website (GOI 2010).

8. Action Plan for Boosting the Role of Financial Institutions

There is need to involve the financial institutions in the development projects meant for animal husbandry right from the beginning so that there is perspective of financial institutions in the projects. There is serious need also for increasing the capacity of the livestock farmers about technical aspects of the projects/animal husbandry activities (like breed selection, feeding and management of the animals) as well as economic and financial aspects so that they are able to repay the loans in time and do not become defaulters. This can broadly be covered under what is known as 'financial literacy.'

There is also a need for exposure and interface of financial institutions to the new technologies developed in the field of animal husbandry so that they feel more comfortable in financing the activities involving new technologies. Further, there could be involvement of development financial institutions like NABARD in supporting research institutions and universities in developing new technologies as a development project.

9. Conclusion

Finance is a crucial component of any economic activity and unless adequate, timely and reasonably priced finance is available to the entrepreneurs/farmers, animal husbandry activities will not be sustainable. Financial institutions play a crucial role in this regard. The main features and issues discussed above should be considered by the prospective entrepreneurs while considering taking up the activity. These aspects need to be considered by the policy makers and researchers as well, while considering policy changes or designing new schemes for animal husbandry promotion.

References

1. GOI (2005). 17th Indian Livestock Census- All India Summary Report 2005. Ministry of Agriculture, Department of Animal Husbandry and Dairying, Government of India, New Delhi.
2. GOI (2007). Annual report 2006-07. Department of Animal Husbandry, Dairying and Fisheries, Government of India, New Delhi.
3. GOI (2008). Agricultural statistics at a glance 2008. Directorate of Economics and Statistics, Department of Agriculture and Cooperation, Government of India, New Delhi.
4. GOI (2010). Department of Animal Husbandry, Dairying & Fisheries, Ministry of Agriculture, Government of India, http://dahd.nic.in/IDDP/guidelinesdavp.htm. Accessed 14 October 2010.
5. NABARD (2010). Annual Report 2009-10. National Bank for Agriculture and Rural Development, Mumbai, p 24.
6. Porter ME (1985). Competitive Advantage: Creating and Sustaining Superior Performance, Free Press.
7. RBI (2010). Reserve Bank of India website: http://www.rbi.org.in/scripts/PublicationsView.aspx?id=12485. Accessed 14 October 2010.

□□□

Chapter 31

Veterinary Legislations for Good Governance

RENU GUPTA[1], SANDEEP KUMAR[2] AND S. R. GARG[1]
[1]Department of Veterinary Public Health and Epidemiology, [2]Department of Veterinary Physiology and Biochemistry, College of Veterinary Sciences, Lala Lajpat Rai University of Veterinary and Animal Sciences, Hisar-125004

Contents

1. Introduction

Veterinary legislation is a key component of the national infrastructure that enables Veterinary Services to perform efficiently in carrying out the assigned functions that include preserving and improving animal health and welfare; epidemiological surveillance, early detection and reporting of animal diseases including zoonoses; food safety; certification of animals and animal products for export; environmental risk assessment and mitigation; rapid response in emergencies; animal resource and wildlife conservation; biomedical research and development and many others. Good governance in veterinary services is becoming more and more important and critical in the current global scenario of the emergence and re-emergence of animal diseases, of which some 75% are transmissible to humans; the growing threat of transboundary animal diseases; the impact of environmental changes and of the globalization of commodities and movement of people; as well as the growing consumer concern and demand for food security, food safety, health and animal welfare.

India has a rich culture and heritage where kindness and compassion for all living beings have been the foundation of society. Animals always had a respect and a special place in society in the country's traditions and culture. This is quite apparent from the mythological images of Hindu gods and goddesses who always had animals around them. Lord Krishna considered as protector of cows is always seen with cows around, Lord Rama with monkeys, Lord Vishnu with an eagle and snake '*Sheshnaag*', Lord Shiva with a snake around his neck and the bull '*Nandi*' at his feet, and Lord Ganesha with a mouse. The goddess of wisdom and literacy, Saraswati, is seen with a swan while the goddess of power, Durga, is seen riding a tiger. The great Hindu epic Mahabharata finds mention of a dog providing unfailing company to Pandava brothers during their last journey to heaven.

The most ancient law about animal rights originated in India. It was proclaimed by Ashoka, the great Emperor of India (269-232 BC). However, in the current period of population explosion, urbanization and consumerism, animals may fall prey to human greed and exploitation. This is a global challenge and requires attention worldwide. According to the World Organisation for Animal Health (OIE) recommendations, veterinary legislation is a critical infrastructure element for all countries. The Government of India has enacted several laws and has been constantly striving to update these legislative provisions concerning animal health, welfare and conservation and the related public health issues in line with the demand of modern times. Some of these provisions are discussed below in brief to assist the veterinary professionals to act proficiently and judiciously.

2. Infectious and Contagious Diseases Legislations

The Prevention and Control of Infectious and Contagious Diseases in Animals Act, 2009 (GOI 2009a) was made recognizing the fact that economic losses due to infectious and contagious diseases of animals are enormous in the country, with some of these diseases constituting a serious threat to the public and that many of such animal diseases are largely preventable by judicious implementation of vaccination programmes or by taking other appropriate and timely measures on scientific lines. Appropriate measures are necessary to facilitate the import and export of animals and animal products and to keep in tune with international practices. India being member of the OIE, it is necessary to implement the general obligations, decisions and recommendations of the organization and abide by the international Animal Health Code.

On the commencement of this Act, the Glanders and Farcy Act, 1899; the Dourine Act, 1910 and any other corresponding law of any state, so far as it is inconsistent with the provisions of this Act stand repealed.

2.1 The Prevention and Control of Infectious and Contagious Diseases in Animals Act, 2009

The salient provisions of this Act (GOI 2009a) are briefly given below.

2.1.1 Control of scheduled diseases

a) *Reporting scheduled diseases obligatory*: Every owner, or any other person, non-governmental organisation, public bodies or the village panchayat, in charge of any animal which he or it has reason to believe to be infective of a Scheduled disease (Table 1) has to report the fact to the Village Officer or village panchayat in-charge, who may report the same in writing to the nearest available Veterinarian who subsequently reports it to higher authorities.

Table 1 : Scheduled diseases

Multiple species diseases

1. Anthrax
2. Aujeszky's disease
3. Bluetongue
4. Brucellosis
5. Crimean Congo haemorrhagic fever
6. Echinococcosis/ hydatidosis
7. Foot and mouth disease

8. Heartwater
9. Japanese encephalitis
10. Leptospirosis
11. New world screwworm (*Cochliomyia hominivorax*)
12. Old world screwworm (*Chrysomya bezziana*)
13. Paratuberculosis
14. Q fever
15. Rabies
16. Rift Valley fever
17. Rinderpest
18. Trichinellosis
19. Tularemia
20. Vesicular stomatitis
21. West Nile fever

Cattle diseases

1. Bovine anaplasmosis
2. Bovine babesiosis
3. Bovine genital campylobacteriosis
4. Bovine spongiform encephalopathy
5. Bovine tuberculosis
6. Bovine viral diarrhoea
7. Contagious bovine pleuropneumonia
8. Enzootic bovine leucosis
9. Haemorrhagic septicaemia
10. Infectious bovine rhinotracheitis/ infectious pustular vulvovaginitis
11. Lumpy skin disease
12. Malignant catarrhal fever
13. Theileriosis
14. Trichomonosis
15. Trypanosomosis

Sheep and goat diseases

1. Caprine arthritis/encephalitis
2. Contagious agalactia
3. Contagious caprine pleuropneumonia
4. Enzootic abortion of ewes (ovine chlamydiosis)
5. Maedi-visna
6. Nairobi sheep disease
7. Ovine epididymitis (*Brucella ovis*)
8. Peste des petits ruminants
9. Salmonellosis (*S. abortusovis*)
10. Scrapie
11. Sheep pox and goat pox

Equine diseases

1. African horse sickness
2. Contagious equine metritis
3. Dourine
4. Equine encephalomyelitis (Eastern)
5. Equine encephalomyelitis (Western)
6. Equine infectious anaemia
7. Equine influenza
8. Equine piroplasmosis
9. Equine rhinopneumonitis
10. Equine viral arteritis
11. Glanders
12. Surra (*Trypanosoma evansi*)
13. Venezuelan equine encephalomyelitis

Swine diseases

1. African swine fever
2. Classical swine fever
3. Nipah virus encephalitis
4. Porcine cysticercosis
5. Porcine reproductive and respiratory syndrome
6. Swine vesicular disease
7. Transmissible gastroenteritis

Avian diseases

1. Avian chlamydiosis
2. Avian infectious bronchitis
3. Avian infectious laryngotracheitis
4. Avian mycoplasmosis (*M. gallisepticum*)
5. Avian mycoplasmosis (*M. synoviae*)
6. Duck virus hepatitis
7. Fowl cholera
8. Fowl typhoid
9. Highly pathogenic avian influenza and low pathogenic avian influenza in poultry
10. Infectious bursal disease (Gumboro disease)
11. Marek's disease
12. Newcastle disease
13. Pullorum disease
14. Turkey rhinotracheitis

Lagomorph diseases

1. Myxomatosis
2. Rabbit haemorrhagic disease

Bee diseases

1. Acarapisosis of honey bees
2. American foulbrood of honey bees
3. European foulbrood of honey bees
4. Small hive bettle infestation (*Aethina tumida*)
5. Tropilaelaps infestation of honey bees
6. Varroosis of honey bees

Fish diseases

1. Epizootic haematopoietic necrosis
2. Infectious haematopoietic necrosis
3. Spring viraemia of carp
4. Viral haemorrhagic septicaemia
5. Infectious pancreatic necrosis
6. Infectious salmon anaemia
7. Epizootic ulcerative syndrome
8. Bacterial kidney disease (*Renibacterium salmoninarum*)
9. Gyrodactylosis (*Gyrodactylus salaris*)
10. Red sea bream iridoviral disease

Mollusc diseases

1. Infection with *Bonamia ostreae*
2. Infection with *Bonamia exitiosa*
3. Infection with *Marteilia refringens*
4. Infection with *Mikrocytos mackini*
5. Infection with *Perkinsus marinus*
6. Infection with *Perkinsus olseni*
7. Infection with *Xenohaliotis californiensis*

Crustacean diseases

1. Crayfish plague (*Aphanomyces astaci*)
2. Infectious hypodermal and haematopoietic necrosis
3. Spherical baculovirosis (*Penaeus monodon*-type baculovirus)
4. Taura syndrome
5. Tetrahedral baculovirosis (*Baculovirus penaei*)
6. Yellowhead disease
7. White spot disease

Other diseases

1. Camelpox
2. Leishmaniosis

b) *Duty to segregate infected animals*: Every owner or person in charge of an animal, which he has reason to believe is infective of a scheduled disease, would segregate such animal and have it kept in a place away from all other animals which are healthy, and take all possible steps to prevent the infected animal from coming in contact with any other animal i.e. confine that animal and prevent it from grazing in a common place or to drink water from any common source including a vessel, pond, lake or river.

c) *Notification of controlled areas and free areas*: The State Government may, with the object of preventing, controlling or eradicating any scheduled disease, by notification, declare any area to be a controlled area in respect of any scheduled disease affecting any species of animal and any other species that may be susceptible to the disease specified. In such areas:

- All animals of the species in the controlled area are to be subjected to compulsory vaccination against that disease, and be subjected to such other measures against the disease, in such manner and within such time as the State Government, may, by public notice, direct.
- The State Government would make available necessary vaccine and it would be obligatory on the part of every owner, or the person in charge of an animal which is required to be vaccinated, to get the animal compulsorily vaccinated.

Where the State Government is satisfied, on a report received from the Director or otherwise, that, in any controlled area, any of the scheduled diseases affecting any species of animal is no longer prevalent, it may, by notification, declare the area to be a **free area** in respect of that disease in relation to the particular species of animal and in such area no animal of the species or of any other susceptible species with regard to which it is a free area would be allowed to enter the free area unless duly immunized by vaccination against that particular disease.

d) *Prohibition of movement of animals from controlled area*: No animal belonging to that species is allowed to be moved from the place where it is kept. The movement of all animals belonging to any species specified in the specific notification may be prohibited, from the place where it is kept, to any other place with some exceptions.

e) *Vaccination, marking and issue of vaccination certificate*: The competent person has to administer the vaccine to an animal and issue a certificate of administration of vaccination and put a mark by branding, tattooing or ear tagging, or in such other manner as directed and it would not be removed. The certificate of vaccination has to specify the date of vaccination, dates of manufacture and expiry of the vaccine, and the date upto which the vaccination of the animal with the particular vaccine would be valid.

f) *Entry and exit of animals into controlled area and free area*: Where any area has been declared as a controlled area in respect of any disease affecting any species of animals, no animal belonging to that species would be taken out of, or brought into that area. No carrier of goods or animal would carry any animal from or out of a controlled area, free area or infected area by land, sea or air unless it complies with the provisions of the Act.

g) *Precautionary measures in relation to controlled areas*: No person is allowed to take out of the controlled area, the following:

- Any animal, alive or dead, which is infected with, or reasonably suspected to have been infected with, any scheduled disease in relation to which the area has been declared to be controlled area.
- Any kind of fodder, bedding or other material which has come into contact with any animal infected with such disease or could, in any manner, carry the infection of the notified disease, or
- The carcass, skin or any other part or product of such animal.

h) *Prohibition of markets, fairs, exhibition etc. in the controlled areas*: No person, organisation or institution is to be allowed to hold any animal market, animal fair, animal exhibition and carry on any other activity which involves grouping or gathering of any species of animals within a controlled area with some exemptions in a case where animals belonging to that species are not susceptible to that scheduled disease and are incapable of carrying it.

i) *Prohibition of bringing of infected animals into market and other places*: No person is allowed to bring or attempt to bring into market, fair, exhibition or other congregation of animals or to any public place, any animal which is known to be infected with a scheduled disease.

j) *Check Posts and Quarantine Camps*: As many as required Quarantine Camps and Check Posts within the State may be established by the authorities which are meant:-

- For the detention of animals suffering from any scheduled disease or of animals which have come into contact with or have been kept in the proximity of any such infected animal;
- For ensuring the prevention of entry into or exit from any controlled area or infected area or free area, of any animal belonging to the species of animals in respect of which the notification regarding such area is in force.
- Any animal which is required to be detained, inspected, vaccinated, or marked, may be kept in the Quarantine Camp for such period as the Competent Officer may direct.
- Every animal detained at a Quarantine Camp will be under the custody of the person in charge of the camp, and the animal would be vaccinated and marked.

k) *Inspection and detention of animals at Check Posts and Quarantine Camps*: The person in charge of any Check Post or Quarantine Camp will inspect any animal stopped at the Check Post, or detained therein or at the Quarantine Camp.

l) *Entry and exit of vaccinated animals into controlled and free areas*: An animal belonging to the species of animals in respect of which an area has been declared as a controlled or free area in relation to any scheduled disease, which has been duly vaccinated against that disease, would be allowed to enter into or be taken out of the controlled area or free area, or to be taken out of any other place on the production of a certificate to the effect that vaccine against that disease has been administered and a period of not less than twenty-one days has elapsed thereafter.

m) *Cleaning and disinfection of carriers*: Every common carrier whether a vessel or vehicle would be cleaned and disinfected immediately before and after the transportation of any animal in that vessel or vehicle, and so also any other place where the animal has been kept in transit.

2.1.2 Actions concerning infected areas

a) *Declaration of infected areas*: If the Veterinary Officer, upon receipt of a report from a veterinarian or otherwise, is satisfied that, in any place or premises falling within his jurisdiction, an animal has been infected with any scheduled disease, or that an animal, which he has reason to believe has been so infected, is kept, may, by notification and publication in at least one local newspaper in the vernacular language and by declaration in loud voice and by beating drums, declare such area as he may deem fit (including the place or premises aforesaid) to be an infected area.

Following provisions apply in relation to an infected area, namely:

- In respect of every animal in that area which is infected or reasonably believed to be infected, with any scheduled disease, the owner or other person in charge of the animal would get it treated by a veterinarian
- All articles, which are likely to have come into contact with any such animal have to be treated or disposed of in such a manner as the veterinarian may direct.
- The owner or any other person in charge of the animal would keep the animal in isolation forthwith, and also take such other measures as may be necessary for the prevention, treatment and control of the disease as the veterinarian may direct.

b) *Denotification of infected area:* If the Veterinary Officer, after such enquiry as he/she may deem fit, is satisfied that there is no longer the threat or danger of any animal being infected with the scheduled disease in any infected area, by notification and publication in a local newspaper in vernacular language, declare that the area is no longer an infected area as aforesaid, whereupon all the restrictions referred to such areas would cease to apply.

2.1.3 Actions concerning infected animals

a) Segregation, examination and treatment of infected animals

i) Where the Veterinarian has, on receipt of a report or otherwise, reason to believe that any animal is infected with a scheduled disease, he/she may, by order in writing, direct the owner or any other person in charge of such animal

- To keep it segregated from other apparently healthy animals; or
- To subject it to such treatment as may be required under the circumstances

ii) On receipt of a report from the Veterinarian, the Veterinary Officer shall, as soon as possible, examine that animal as well as any other animal which could have come in contact with it, and for that purpose, submit the animal to such test and medical examination as may be required under the circumstances

If, after such test and examination, the Veterinary Officer is of the opinion that an animal is not infected with any of the scheduled diseases, he shall issue a certificate in writing that the animal is not infected with any such disease.

b) Drawing samples from animals

Where the Veterinary Officer considers it necessary for the purpose of ascertaining whether the animal which is suspected to have been infected with any scheduled disease or susceptible to such infection is actually infected, or for the purpose of ascertaining the nature of the scheduled disease with which an animal is infected, he may draw such samples, as may be required, from the animal for the purpose of carrying out such investigations as he may deem necessary under the circumstances.

The Veterinary Officer or any other Competent Officer would draw samples from any animal for the purposes of ascertaining whether the animal has been vaccinated against any disease, or whether the vaccination of the animal has been effective in conferring it immunity and have the samples examined, in such manner as he may deem necessary.

c) Resorting to euthanasia for infected animals

If the Veterinary Officer deems it necessary that in case of an animal, which is infected with a scheduled disease, euthanasia has to be resorted to, for preventing the spread of the disease to other animals in the area or to protect public health if the disease is of zoonotic importance, he/she may, notwithstanding anything contained in any other law for the time being in force, by an order in writing, direct euthanasia of the animal and the carcass disposed of immediately to his satisfaction.

d) Disposal of carcass

Every person in possession of carcass (or any part thereof) of any animal, which at the time of its death was infected with any scheduled disease or was suspected to have been infected, would dispose it of in such manner as prescribed.

e) Seizure and removal of certain animals

Where any animal which is infected or suspected to have been infected is found without any person claiming to be its owner, or where a valid order or direction given in relation to any such animal is not promptly complied with by the owner or other person in control of the animal, it would be open to the veterinary officer or any other competent officer to seize the animal and remove it to a place of isolation or segregation, as he/she may deem proper.

2.1.4 Enforcement and penalties

Orders under the Act should be promptly complied with. There is provision of penalties for contravening the provisions of the Act.

2.1.5 Precautionary measures on causative organism

a) *Prevention of escape of causative organism*: In every institution, laboratory or clinic, engaged in the manufacture, testing or research, related to vaccines, sera, diagnostics or chemotherapeutic drugs and aimed at the prevention or treatment of any scheduled disease, adequate precautionary measures have to be taken:

   - To ensure that the causative organism of any scheduled disease does not escape or otherwise get released;
   - To guard against any such escape or release; and
   - To warn and to protect everyone concerned in the event of any escape.

b) *Administartion of euthanasia to animals*: Every animal used for the manufacture, testing or research as referred above which is likely to carry or transmit any scheduled disease, would be promptly administered euthanasia and disposed of by the person in charge of or having control of the institution, laboratory or clinic, as the case may be, referred above if the other laws in place permit.

3. Animal Welfare Legislations

The Indian Constitution enshrines and casts upon every citizen of India, the duty to have compassion for all living creatures, as a fundamental duty. It reflects the importance, the country accords to the protection of animals and their rights. In keeping with this commitment, India is among the first countries to enact the Prevention of Cruelty to Animals Act, 1960 and many other legislative provisions.

3.1 The Prevention of Cruelty to Animals Act, 1960 (59 of 1960); amended in 1982

It is the Act to prevent infliction of unnecessary pain or suffering on animals and for that purpose to amend the law relating to the prevention of cruelty to animals. The Animal Welfare Board of India established under this Act advises the central government on making rules under this Act with a view to preventing unnecessary pain or suffering to animals generally, and more particularly when they are being transported from one place to another or when they are used as performing animals or when they are kept in captivity or confinement (GOI 1960). Some of the rules framed under this Act are briefly discussed below.

3.2 The Prevention of Cruelty to Animals (Slaughter House) Rules, 2001 (amended in 2010)

These rules are aimed at prevention of unnecessary pain and distress to animals meant for slaughter. Salient features of these rules (GOI 2001b, 2010b) are summarized below.

3.2.1 Animals not to be slaughtered except in recognized or licensed houses

No person should slaughter any animal within a municipal area except in a slaughter house recognized or licensed by the concerned authority. Any animal which is pregnant or has an offspring less than three months old, or is under the age of three months, or has not been certified by a veterinary doctor to be in fit conditions to be slaughtered should not be slaughtered.

3.2.2 Reception area or resting grounds

The slaughterhouse should have a reception area of adequate size sufficient for livestock subject to veterinary inspection. This area should have proper ramps for direct unloading of animals from vehicles or railway wagons. It should have adequate facility for feeding and watering of animals. Ante-mortem and pen area in slaughterhouse should be paved with impervious material such as concrete non-slippery herring-bone type suitable to stand wear and tear by hooves, or brick, and pitched to suitable drainage facilities.

3.2.3 Lairage

The lairage of the slaughterhouse should be adequate in size sufficient for the number of animals. The space provided in the pens of such lairage should not be less than 2.8 sq. m per large animal and 1.6 sq. m per small animal. The lairage should have adequate facilities for watering and post-mortem inspection.

3.2.4 Slaughter

- No animal should be administered any chemical, drug or hormone before slaughter except the drug for its treatment for any specific disease or ailment.
- Every slaughterhouse should provide a separate space for stunning of animals prior to slaughter, bleeding and dressing of the carcasses.
- A curbed-in bleeding area of adequate size as specified should be provided in a slaughterhouse and it should be so located that the blood does not splash on other animals being slaughtered or on the carcass being skinned.
- Dressing of carcasses in a slaughterhouse should not be done on floor and adequate means and tools for dehiding or pelting of the animals should be provided in a slaughterhouse with means for immediate disposal of hides or skins.

3.2.5 Slaughterhouse building

Slaughterhouse should be built and maintained by its owner in the manner as specified below:

a) *Plant building* : Materials used should be impervious, easily cleansable, and resistant to wear and corrosion.

b) *Floors* : The floors should be non-absorbent and nonslippery with rough finish and should have suitable gradient for drainage.

c) *Coves* : Coves with radii sufficient to promote sanitation should be installed at the juncture of floors and wall in all rooms which should not be less than 100 mm.

d) *Interior walls* : interior walls should be smooth and flat and constructed with impervious materials such a glazed brick, glazed tile, smooth surface Portland cement plaster, or other non-toxic, non-absorber material applied to a suitable base. Walls should be provided with suitable sanitary type bumpers to prevent damage by hand trucks, carcass shunks, and the like. The interior walls should have washable surface upto the height of 2 metres from the floor so that the splashes may be washed and disinfected.

e) *Ceilings* : Ceilings should be of the height of 5 metres or more in workrooms and so far as structure conditions permit, ceilings should be smooth and flat. Ceilings should be constructed with Portland cement plaster, large size cement asbestos boards with joint sealed with a flexible sealing compound, or other acceptable impervious material and finished so as to minimise condensation, mould development, flaking and accumulation of dirt. The walls above the glazed type portion and ceiling should be painted with water-resistant paint to maintain them clean.

f) *Doorways and doors* : Doorways through which product is transferred on rails or in hand trucks should be at least 1500 mm high and should be at least 1500 mm wide. Doors should either be of rust-resistant metal construction throughout, or made with rust-resistant metal having tight softwood.

g) *Screens and insect control* : All windows, doorways and other openings that may admit flies should be equipped with effective insect and rodent screens.

h) *Rodent proofing* : Except in the case of solid masonry; walls constructed of glazed tile, glazed brick, and the like, expanded metal or wire mesh not exceeding 12.5 mm mesh, should be embedded in walls and floor at their junction and such mesh shall extend vertically and horizontally to a sufficient distance to exclude the entrance of rats and other rodents.

i) *Drainage* : One drainage inlet should be provided for each 37 metre square of floor space and a slope of about 20 mm per metre to drainage inlets should be provided.

j) *Lighting and ventilation* : Unrefrigerated work rooms should be provided with adequate direct natural light and ventilation or ample artificial light and ventilation by mechanical means. Every abattoir should be provided with distributed artificial light of an overall intensity of not less than 200 lux at the distances as may be specified throughout the slaughter hall and workrooms and at places where meat inspection is carried out, the overall intensity of artificial light should not be less than 500 lux. Every abattoir should be provided with suitable and sufficient means of ventilation to the outside air and the construction of the slaughter hall should be so arranged that the dressed carcasses are not exposed to direct sunlight.

k) A sufficient, safe, potable and constant supply of fresh water should be available at adequate pressure through the premises. The pressure for the general purpose of floor washing may preferably be 200 to 330 kPa for thorough floor cleaning. For thorough and efficient washing of carcasses, a higher pressure between 1000 kPa to 1700 kPa should be maintained. A constant supply of clean hot water should be available in the slaughter hall and workrooms during working hours and the hot water required for frequent sterilising of equipment should not be less than 82°C.

l) The following materials should not be used in an abattoir

- Copper and its alloys in equipment used for edible products
- Cadmium in any form in equipment handling edible products
- Equipment with painted surface in product zone
- Enamel containers or equipment
- Lead

m) All permanently mounted equipment should either be installed sufficiently away from walls (minimum 300 mm) and above the floor (minimum 300 mm) to provide access for cleaning and inspection or be completely sealed (watertight) to the floor area.

3.3 Breeding of and Experiments on Animals (Control and Supervision) Rules, 1998 (Amended in 2001 and 2006)

These rules carry provisions for humane handling and treatment of experimental animals. The rules are meant for preventing unnecessary and unethical animal experimentation. Salient features of these rules (GOI 1998b, 2001a, 2006b) are given below.

3.3.1 Registration of establishment for breading of and experimentation on animals

No establishment is allowed to carry on the business of breeding of animals or trade of animals for the purpose of experiments and perform any experiment on animals unless it is registered.

3.3.2 Details of the experiments conducted

Every registered establishment has to maintain a register of particulars about the animals used from day to day for conducting experiments, with the number of animals, species, age, gender and other relevant particulars.

3.3.3 Stocking of animals

The animals have to be stocked by the breeder and the establishment in the following manner:

a) Animal houses must be located in a quiet atmosphere undisturbed by traffic, and the premises kept tidy, hygienic and the animals protected from drought and extremes of weather.

b) Animal cages for small animals and stables for large animals should be such that animals can live in comfort and overcrowding is avoided.

c) Where standards have been laid down by the Indian Standards Institution (now Bureau of Indian Standards), the cages or the stable, as the case may be, should conform to those standards.

d) Animals should be looked after before and after the experiments by a trained and experienced attendant.

3.3.4. Permission of the Committee required for conducting experiments

Every registered establishment before acquiring an animal or conducting any experiment on an animal/animals should apply for permission of the Committee or Institutional Animals Ethics Committee recognized for the purpose.

3.3.5 Performance of experiments

In conducting experiments on animals, regard must be had to the following conditions:

- Experiments have to be performed in every case by or under the supervision of a person duly qualified in that behalf.
- Experiments should be performed with due care and humanity.
- Animals intended for the performance of experiments must be properly looked both before and after experiments.
- Experiments involving operative procedure more severe than simple inoculation or superficial venesection should be performed under the influence of anaesthetic to prevent the animal feeling pain and it should remain so throughout the experiment.
- The experiment must not be performed for the sole purpose of attaining or retaining manual skill except in schools, colleges and programmes duly scrutinized and permitted in registered establishments by the Committee.

- No experiment, the result of which is already conclusively known, should be repeated without previous justification.
- Any chemical substance should not be applied to the eye of an animal by way of experiment for the purpose of absorption through the conjunctival membrane or through the cornea calculated to only give pain.
- Animals lowest on the phylogenetic scale which may give scientifically valid results should be first considered for any experimental procedure and the experiment should be designed using minimum number of animals.

3.4 The Transport of Animals Rules, 1978 (Amended in 2001 and 2009)

These rules are specified for transport and associated necessities for transport of dogs, cats, monkeys, cattle, equines, sheep, goats, poultry and pigs (GOI 1978, 2001d, 2009b). Salient features of these rules are presented below.

3.4.1 Issue of certificate before transportation

A valid certificate issued by an officer or any person or Animal Welfare Organisation duly recognised and authorised for this purpose by the Animal Welfare Board of India or the Central Government is to be procured by any person making transport of any animal before transportation of such animal verifying that all the relevant Central and State Acts, rules and orders pertaining to the said animals including the rules relating to transport of such animals have been duly complied with and that the animal is not being transported for any purpose contrary to the provision of any law. In the absence of such certificate, the carrier shall refuse to accept the consignment for transport.

3.4.2 General conditions of transport

- Animals to be transported should be healthy and in good condition and such animals should be examined by a veterinary doctor for freedom from infectious diseases and their fitness to undertake the journey; provided that the nature and duration of the proposed journey should be taken into account while deciding upon the degree of fitness.
- An animal which is unfit for transport should not be transported and the animals which are new born, diseased, blind, emaciated, lame, fatigued or having given birth during the preceding seventy two hours or likely to give birth during transport should not be transported.

- Pregnant and very young animals should not be mixed with other animals during transport.
- Different classes of animals should be kept separately during transport.
- Diseased animals, whenever transported for treatment, should not be mixed with other animals. Troublesome animals may be given tranquilisers before loading during transport.
- Animals should be transported in their on-farm social groups (established at least one week prior to journey).

3.4.3 Transport of dogs and cats

a) No dog or cat in an advanced stage of pregnancy should be transported.

b) Dogs or cats to be transported in the same container should be of the same species and breed.

c) Unweaned puppies or kittens should not be transported with adult dogs or cats other than their dams.

d) No female dog or cat in season (oestrus) should be transported with any male.

e) Any dog or cat reported to be vicious or exhibiting a vicious disposition should be transported individually in a cage, muzzled and labelled to give warning to the handlers. In extreme cases, the dogs and cats should be administered with sedative drugs by a qualified veterinary surgeon.

f) When dogs or cats are to be transported for long distances, they should be fed and given water at least two hours prior to their transport and should not be packed for transport if they are hungry or thirsty. They should be exercised as late as possible before dispatch. They should be given adequate water for drinking every four hours in summer or every six hours during winter. They should be fed once in twelve hours in the case of adult dogs or cats and once in four hours in the case of puppies and kittens in accordance with the instructions of the consignors, if any. Adequate arrangements should be made for their care and management during the journey. When the dogs or cats are to be transported by rail involving a journey of more than six hours, an attendant should accompany the dogs or cats to supply them with food and water on the way and the attendant should have access to the dogs or cats for this purpose at all stations and no dog or cat should be exposed to the direct blast of air during such journey.

g) Where dogs or cats are to be transported for short distance by road in a public vehicle, some precautions are to be taken. They should be put in a cage and the cage containing the dogs or cats should not be put on the roof of the vehicle but should be put inside the vehicle preferably near the end of the vehicle. The vehicle transporting the dogs or cats should as far as possible maintain constant speed, avoiding sudden stops and reducing effects of shocks and jolts to the minimum. At least one attendant should be present at all times during transit who would ensure that proper transit conditions are observed and would also replenish food and water whenever necessary.

h) Where dogs or cats are to be transported by air, the cages should be properly cleaned and disinfected before the dogs or cats are put in the cages. Sufficient paddy straw or saw dust or paper cuttings should be provided for cats in the cages as resting material. For international transport, the dogs or cats should be kept in pressurized compartment with regulated temperature. The size and type of crates for transport of dogs and cats should conform as clearly as may be to the size and type specified (Table 2).

Table 2 : The size of crates for transport of dogs and cats

Dimension	Dogs		Cats	
(in cm)	by rail/road/inland waterways, sea	by air	by rail/road/inland waterways, sea	by air
Length (L)	A x 1 ½	A + C + 10	A x 2	A x 2
Width (W)	A	D + 2 + 10	A	A
Height (H)	B + 15	B + 10	B + 15	B + 10

Where, Length - tip of nose to root of tail (A), Width - width across the shoulders (D), Height - tip of ears to toe while standing (B), Elbow size - toe to tip of elbow (C).

3.4.4 Transport of monkeys

a) Monkeys from one trapping area should not be allowed to mix with monkeys from any other trapping area for preventing the dangers of cross infection.

b) The time in transit from trapping area to the nearest rail-head should be as short as possible and factors causing stress to monkeys should be reduced to the minimum.

c) If the travel time is longer than six hours provision should be made to feed and to give water to the monkeys on the route.

d) During transit, precautions should be taken to protect the monkeys from extreme weather conditions and monkeys that die on route should be removed at the earliest available opportunity.

e) Monkeys that are not completely weaned, that is, less than 1.8 Kg in weight, should not be transported except when specifically permitted by the Central Government.

f) Pregnant and nursing monkeys should not be transported except when specifically permitted by the Central Government and such monkeys as well as monkeys weighing more than 5 Kg should be transported in compartmented cages.

g) All monkeys in the same cage should be of the same species and of approximately the same weight and size.

h) Monkeys captured within their natural habitat should be placed in new, sterilized or thoroughly cleaned cages and subsequent transfer, if any, should also be to new, disinfected or thoroughly cleaned cages.

i) Monkeys should be transported from trapping area to the nearest rail-head by the fastest means of transport available and the monkeys should not be left un-attended at any time during the journey. Monkeys should be transported in suitable wooden or bamboo cages as prescribed in these rules.

j) For transporting monkeys from a rail-head to another rail-head or from a rail-head to nearest airport, loading and unloading should be carried out quickly and efficiently. Cages should be stored in such a manner that ventilation is adequate and the monkeys are not exposed to drought and direct heat or cold. Monkeys found dead should be removed as quickly as possible for suitable disposal. Due provision should be made for sufficient supply of food and water during the journey. In case the journey is over six hours, an attendant should accompany to take care of the monkeys according to the provisions in these rules.

k) For transport of monkeys by air, monkeys should be brought to the airport sufficiently early. They should be provided with food and water immediately before loading on the aircraft. The time in transit should be as short as possible and factors causing stress to monkeys should be reduced to the minimum. The protection from infection and supply of feed and water should be provided according to the provisions made in these rules.

3.4.5 Transport of cattle

a) Veterinary first-aid equipment should accompany all batches of cattle.

b) The average space provided per cattle in Railway wagon or vehicle should be as shown in Table 3 and 4. Suitable rope and platforms should be used for loading.

c) Cattle should be loaded after they are properly fed and given water.

d) Cattle in advanced stage of pregnancy should not be mixed with young cattle in order to avoid stampede during transportation.

e) Watering arrangements on route should be made and sufficient quantities of water should be carried for emergency. Sufficient feed and fodder with adequate reserve should be carried to last during the journey.

f) Adequate ventilation should be ensured.

g) When cattle is to be transported by rail, an ordinary goods wagon should not carry more than ten adult cattle or fifteen calves on broad gauge, not more than six adult cattle or ten calves on metre gauge and not more than four adult cattle or six calves on narrow gauge. Every wagon carrying cattle should have at least one attendant. Material for padding, such as straw, should be placed on the floor to avoid injury if a cattle lies down and this should not be less than 6 cm thick. Two breast bars should be provided on each side of the wagon, one at height of 60 to 80 cm and the other at 100 to 110 cm. Cattle-in-milk should be milked at least twice a day and the calves should be given sufficient quantity of milk to drink.

Table 3 : Space allowance per cattle in railway wagon

Weight of the cattle	Space per cattle (Sq. m)
Cattle weighing upto 200 Kg	1.0
Cattle weighing 200-300 Kg	1.2
Cattle weighing 300-400 Kg	1.4
Cattle weighing above 400 Kg	2.0

Table 4 : Space requirement for transport of cattle in commonly sized road vehicles

Vehicle size Length x Width Sq. m	Floor area of vehicle in Sq. m	Number of cattle			
		Cattle weighing upto 200 Kg (1.0 Sq. m space per cattle)	Cattle weighing 200-300 Kg (1.2 Sq. m space per cattle)	Cattle weighing 300-400 Kg (1.4 Sq. m space per cattle)	Cattle weighing above 400 Kg (2.0 Sq. m space per cattle)
6.9 x 2.4	16.56	16	14	12	8
5.6 x 2.3	12.88	12	10	8	6
4.16 x 1.9	7.904	8	6	6	4
2.9 x 1.89	5.481	5	4	4	2

3.4.6 Transport of equines

a) The space requirement for horses when transported by road/ rail is given in Table 5.

b) Pregnant and young equines should not be mixed with other animals.

c) Different species of equines should be kept separately.

d) Equines should be loaded after being fed and given water adequately, watering arrangements should be made on route and sufficient food carried to last during the journey.

e) Veterinary first-aid equipment should accompany all batches of equines.

f) Adequate ventilation should be ensured.

g) For the transport of equines by rail, some precautions are to be taken. Equines should be transported by passenger or mixed trains only. Ordinary goods wagon when used for transportation should carry not more than eight to ten horses or ten mules or ten donkeys on broad gauge and not more than six horses or eight donkeys on metre-gauge. In extreme hot, water should be sprinkled over the wagons containing equines by the railway authorities to bring down temperature. Ice slabs in specially made containers may be placed inside the wagon, if recommended by a qualified veterinary surgeon. Material for padding, such as paddy straw, should be placed on the floor to avoid injury if an animal lies down and this should not be less than 6 cm thick. Two breast bars should be provided on each side of the wagon, one at a height of 50 to 80 cm and the other at 110 cm.

h) For the transport of equines by goods vehicles, the following precautions should be taken. Specially fitted vehicles with a special type of tail-board and padding around the sides should be used. Ordinary goods vehicles should be provided with anti-slipping material on the floor and the super structure, if low, should be raised. Bamboo poles of at least 8 cm diameter between each animal and two stout batons at the back should be provided to prevent the animal from falling. To prevent horses from being frightened or injured, their heads should face left, away from the passing traffic. Each vehicle should not carry more than four to six equines and these vehicles should be driven at a speed not more than 35 km per hour.

i) For the transport by sea, horses may normally be accommodated in single stalls and mules in pens, each pen holding four to five mules. Ample ventilation should be ensured by keeping portholes and providing permanent air trunks or electric blowers on all decks. Exhaust fans should be installed to blow out foul air. Colts and fillies should be kept on the exposed decks. A pharmacy and spare stalls for five per cent of equines should be available. Passage between two rows of pens should not be less than 1.5 metres.

Table 5 : Space requirement for transport of horses by road/ rail

Horses	Space in Sq. m
Stallion horses	2.25
Mares (including pregnant)	2.0
Ponies	1.5
6-12 months	1.4
12-18 months	1.6
Over 18 months and upto 2 years	2.0
Mares with foal at foot (upto 6 months)	2.25

3.4.7 Transport of sheep and goats

a) Sheep and goats should be transported separately, but if the lots are small, special partition should be provided to separate them.

b) Rams and male young stock should not be mixed with female stock in the same compartment.

c) Sufficient food and fodder should be carried to last during the journey and watering facility should be provided at regular intervals.

d) Material for padding, such as straw, should be placed on the floor to avoid injury if an animal lies down, and this should not be less than 5 cm thick.

e) The animals should not be fettered unless there is a risk of their jumping out and their legs should not be tied down.

f) Approximate space requirements for sheep and goat for transport by rail/ road is given in Table 6.

g) The maximum numbers of sheep or goats that can be accommodated in one railway wagon are given in Table 7.

h) Goods vehicles of capacity of 5 or 4 ½ tons, which are generally used for transporting animals, should carry not more than forty sheep or goats. In the case of large goods vehicles and wagons, partition should be provided at every two or three metres across the width to prevent crowding and trapping of sheep and goats. In the case of ewes, goats or lambs or kids under six weeks of age, separate panels should be provided.

Table 6 : Approximate space requirement for sheep and goat for transport by rail/ road

Approximate weight of animal in Kg	Space required in Sq. m.	
	Woolled	Shorn
Not more than 20	0.17	0.16
More than 20 but not more than 25	0.19	0.18
More than 25 but not more than 30	0.23	0.22
More than 30 but not more than 40	0.27	0.25
More than 40	0.32	0.29

Table 7 : Maximum Number of sheep and goat permitted in one railway wagon

Broad gauge		Metre gauge		Narrow gauge
Area of Wagon less than 21.1 sq.m	Area of wagon 21.1 sq.m and above	Area of wagon less than 12.5 sq. m	Area of wagon 12.5 sq. m and above	
70	100	50	60	25

3.4.8 Transport of poultry

a) The container should be properly cleaned and sterilised before the poultry is placed in them.

b) Poultry should not be exposed to sunlight, rain and direct blast of air during transport.

c) Poultry should not be transported when the temperature exceeds 25°C or when the temperature falls below 15°C.

d) For day-old chicks and turkey poults, chicks and poults should be packed and dispatched immediately after hatching and should not be stored in boxes for any length of time before dispatch. They should not be fed or watered before and during transportation. Every effort should be made to ensure they arrive as quickly as possible at the dispatching site. Personal attention should be given by the consignor or the forwarding agent to ensure that all consignments are kept out of direct sunlight, rain and heat; care should be taken to carry the boxes in a level position so that chicks are not in danger of falling over on to their backs. The putting up of other merchandise over and around chick boxes should be avoided.

e) The poultry to be transported should be healthy and in good condition and should be examined and certified by a veterinary doctor for freedom from infectious diseases and fitness to undertake the journey.

f) Poultry transported in the same container should be of the same species and of the same age group.

g) Poultry should be properly fed and watered before it is placed in containers for transportation and extra feed and water should be provided in suitable troughs fixed in the containers.

h) Arrangements should be made for watering and feeding during transportation and during hot weather, watering should be ensured every six hours.

i) Male stock should not be transported with female stock in the same container.

j) In transport of poultry by road, a container should not be placed on the top of the other and should be covered properly to protect from rain, heat and cold air, but to provide light and ventilation.

k) In transport of poultry by rail, in case the journey is for more than twelve hours, an attendant should accompany the consignment. Poultry should not be exposed to rain or direct blast of air and as far as possible poultry should be transported in wagons having adequate facilities for ventilation. No other merchandise which may result in mortality of birds should be loaded in the same wagon.

l) In transport of poultry by air or for international transport, the containers carrying poultry should be kept in pressurised compartments with regulated temperature and the container should preferably be kept near the door and should be unloaded immediately on arrival.

m) Containers used to transport poultry should be made of such material that does not collapse or crumble and they should be well ventilated and designed to protect the health of poultry by giving it adequate space and safety. The containers should be so designed as to render impossible for birds to crowd into the corners during transportation, and to avoid the danger of boxes being stocked so close together as to interfere with ventilation. All the containers should be clearly labelled showing the name, address and telephone number of the consignor and the consignee. The minimum floor space per bird and the dimension of the containers for transporting poultry is specified in the Table 8.

n) Special requirement of containers for chicks and poults for transport by road, rail or air include: wire mesh or a net of any material should not be used as a bottom for the containers; the container should be properly secured to avoid pilferage. A printed label marked "Care in Transit" should be fixed to the lid or printed directly on sides. Poultry should not be transported continuously for more than 6 hours and whole batch should be inspected at every 6 hours interval. The transportation should not remain stationary for more than 30 min and during this period, it should be parked in shade and arrangements should be made for feeding and watering. All precautions against fire should be taken and provision of fire extinguishers in transport should be provided.

Table 8 : Minimum floor space per bird and the dimension of the containers for transporting poultry

Kind of poultry	Minimum dimensions				Number in a container
	Floor space (per bird) (cm^2)	Length (cm)	Width (cm)	Height (cm)	
Month old chickens	75	60	30	18	24
Three month old chickens	230	55	50	35	12
Adult sock (excluding geese and turkeys)	480	115	50	45	12
Geese and turkeys	900	120	75	75	10 youngs
	1300	75	35	75	2 growing
	1900	55	35	75	1 grown up
Chicks	-	60	45	12	80
Poults	-	60	45	12	60

3.4.9 Transport of pigs

a) In transport of pigs by rail or road, first-aid equipment should accompany the pigs.

b) Male young stock should not be mixed with female stock in the same compartment.

c) Sufficient food and fodder should be carried to last during the journey and watering facility should be provided at regular intervals.

d) Material for padding, such as straw, should be placed on the floor to avoid injury if an animal lies down, and this should be not less than 5 cm thick.

e) The animals should not be fettered unless there is a risk of their jumping out and their legs should not be tied down.

f) No railway wagon should accommodate more than the number of pigs as specified in the Table 9.

g) Adequate ventilation should be provided in every wagon.

h) The maximum number of pigs permitted in commonly sized road vehicles is given in Table 10.

i) In the case of pigs under six weeks of age, separate panels should be provided.

Table 9 : Maximum number of pigs permissible in one railway wagon

Broad gauge	Metre gauge		Narrow gauge
VPU having floor area 63.55 sq. m	Area of wagon less than 12.5 sq. m	Area of wagon 12.5 sq. m and above	
104 pigs (0.61 sq. m per pig)	25 pigs	30 pigs	Not allowed

Table 10 : Maximum number of pigs permissible in commonly sized road vehicles

Type of animal	Maximum number of pigs permitted for road vehicles			
	Vehicles size			
	5.6 m x 2.35 m	5.15 m x 2.18 m	3.03 m x 2.18 m	2.9 m x 2.0 m
Weaner	43	37	22	19
Young	31	26	15	13
Adult	21	18	10	9

Where; Weaner is the piglet which has just been separated from the mother for the purpose of independent rearing and commonly in the weight range of 12-15 kg.
Young is a male or female pig between 3 to 6 months of age and commonly in the weight range of 15-50 kg.
Adult is a male or female pig above 6 months of age and having weight more than 50 kg.

3.5 Transport of Animals on Foot Rules, 2001

These rules apply to transport of animals on foot when the distance from the boundary of village or town or city of the origin of such transport to the last destination is 5 km or more than 5 km (GOI 2001c). Some major instructions are mentioned below.

3.5.1 Condition of health of animals transported on foot

- Every animal to be transported on foot should be healthy and in good condition for such transport.
- A certificate of a veterinary doctor in respect of each animal to the effect that such animal is in a fit condition for such transportation and is not suffering from any infectious, contagious or parasitic diseases and that it has been vaccinated against any infectious, contagious or parasitic diseases should accompany such animal.

3.5.2 Certain animals not to be transported on foot

New born animals of which the navel has not completely healed, diseased, blind, emaciated, lame, fatigued, or having given birth during the preceding seventy two hours or likely to give birth during transport are not to be transported on foot. Animal should be transported in their on farm social groups (established at least one week prior to journey).

3.5.3 First aid equipment to accompany animals transported on foot

The owner of the animals has to provide veterinary first aid equipment to be accompanied with animals.

3.5.4 Watering arrangement during transportation of animals

The owner of the animals has to make watering arrangement *en route.*

3.5.5 Feed and fodder arrangements during transportation of animals

Sufficient feed and fodder with adequate reserve is to be made available by their owner during transport.

3.5.6 Prohibition of the use of whip etc.

No person is allowed to use a whip or a stick or to apply chillies or any soft substance to any part of the body of the animal to hasten the pace of the animal.

3.5.7 Certain prohibitions on transport of animals on foot

- No person should transport an animal on foot before sunrise or after sunset.
- No animal should be made to walk under conditions of heavy rain, thunderstorms or extremely dry or sultry conditions.
- No animal should be transported on foot beyond the distance, time, rest interval and temperature specified for such animal in the rules.

3.5.8 Transportation of animals in certain cases not permitted without shoes

Animals whose hooves are not provided with shoes (as in the case of pack or draught animals) should not be transported on foot on hard cement, bitumen-coated or metalled roads, steep gradients or hilly and rocky terrain, irrespective of weather conditions (summer or winter).

3.6 Other rules

Apart from the rules discussed above, there exist several other rules framed under the Prevention of Cruelty to Animals Act, 1960. These are listed below and can be accessed at the website of the Ministry of Environment and Forests (GOI 2011b)..

- The Animal Birth Control (Dogs) Rules, 2001 (amended in 2009)
- The Performing Animals Rules, 1973
- The Performing Animals (Registration) Rules, 2001
- The Prevention of Cruelty to Animals (Establishment and Regulation of Societies for Prevention of Cruelty to Animals) Rules, 2001
- The Prevention of Cruelty (Capture of Animals) Rules, 1972
- The Prevention of Cruelty to Animals (Registration of Cattle Premises) Rules, 1978
- The Prevention of Cruelty to Animals (Application of Fines) Rules, 1978
- The Prevention of Cruelty to Animals (Licensing of Ferries) Rules, 1965
- The Prevention of Cruelty to Draught and Pack Animals Rules, 1965, amended 1968

All these rules are aimed at providing legal framework for preventing unnecessary pain or suffering to animals generally. However, over the last few decades there has been increasing concern that the legislation has not been as successful as it was intended, probably due to the provision of relatively weak penalties for violation and the absence of proactive and pre-emptive measures for the prevention of animal cruelty. The government of India now intends to enact **the Animal Welfare Act** that would provide, among other things, for steeper penalties for animal cruelty. This law intends to modify the approach of our authorities in dealing with animal protection by moving from a defensive position to a positive, welfare and wellbeing oriented approach through it. The Draft Animal Welfare Act, 2011 (GOI 2011a) has been prepared. Some of the salient features of this draft enactment are listed below.

- Augmenting animal welfare and wellbeing;
- Strengthening animal welfare organizations and conscientious citizens who wish to espouse the cause of animal welfare and wellbeing;
- Enhancing penalties for animal abuse;
- Altering and enlarging the definition of animal abuse, in keeping with the times, and in keeping with judicial pronouncements.

The Prevention of Cruelty to Animals Act, 1960, would stand repealed when this Act comes into force, but all actions already taken under the same, and rules and regulations already framed, would be saved to the extent and in the manner indicated in the (Draft) Animal Welfare Act, 2011.

4. Food Safety Legislations

Food safety regulations are essential to regulate the manufacture, storage, distribution, sale and import of safe and wholesome food for human consumption. The government of India has constituted the **Food Safety and Standards Authority of India (FSSAI)** which has been given this responsibility.

4.1 The Food Safety and Standards Act, 2006

The Food Safety and Standards Act, 2006 (GOI 2006a) has been made to consolidate various laws relating to food. The Act aims to establish a single reference point for all matters relating to food safety and standards, by moving from multi-level, multi-departmental control to a single line of command. It incorporates the salient features of the Prevention of Food Adulteration Act (PFA), 1954, Milk and Milk Products Order (MMPO) which is now renamed as Milk and Milk Products Regulations (MMPR) under Section 99 of the Food Safety and Standards Act, 2006, Meat Food Products Order (MFPO) etc. Some general provisions in the Act are given below in brief.

4.1.1 Use of food additive or processing aid

It prohibits the use of any food additives or processing aid unless it is in accordance with the provisions of the Act, and Regulations made there under.

4.1.2 Contaminants, naturally occurring toxic substances, heavy metals etc.

No article of food would contain any contaminant, naturally occurring toxic substances or toxins or hormone or heavy metals in excess of such quantities as may be specified by regulations.

4.1.3 Pesticides, veterinary drugs residues, antibiotic residues and microbiological counts

No article of food would contain insecticides or pesticides residues, veterinary drugs residues, antibiotic residues, solvent residues, pharmacologically active substances and microbiological counts in excess of such tolerance limit as may be specified by regulations. No insecticide would be used directly on article of food except fumigants registered and approved under the Insecticides Act, 1968.

4.1.4 Genetically modified foods, organic foods, functional foods, proprietary foods etc.

Save as otherwise provided under this Act and regulations made there under, it is prohibited to manufacture, distribute, sell or import any novel food, genetically modified articles of food, irradiated food, organic foods, foods for special dietary uses, functional foods, neutraceuticals, health supplements, proprietary foods and such other articles of food which the central government may notify.

4.1.5 Packaging and labelling of foods

Marking and labelling in the manner as specified by regulations is essential. It provides for restriction on advertisement of any food which misleads or contravenes the provisions of the Act or the rules and regulations made there under.

4.1.6 Imports of articles of food

All imports of food articles are subject to the provisions of the Act.

4.2 Food Safety and Standards Regulations, 2011

These regulations have been notified by the Food Safety and Standards Authority of India. Some major provisions included in these regulations are given below (GOI 2011c).

a) Licensing and registration of food businesses.

b) General hygienic and sanitary practices to be followed by food business operators.

c) Specific hygienic and sanitary practices to be followed by food business operators engaged in manufacture, processing, storing and selling of milk and milk Products - Sanitary requirements, personal hygiene requirements, sanitary requirements for storage, and wrapping and packaging requirements.

d) Specific hygienic and sanitary practices to be followed by food business operators engaged in manufacture, processing, storing and selling of meat and meat products - Slaughterhouse requirements, animal welfare requirements, ante-mortem inspection, post-mortem inspection, sanitary and hygienic requirements for meat processing units, and sanitary and hygienic requirements for the retail meat shops
e) Packaging and labeling regulations
f) Food product standards for individual food products
g) Regulations regarding food additives
h) Prohibition and regulation of sales
i) Contaminants, toxins and residues in foods
j) Laboratory and sample analysis
k) Limits of various food additives
l) Microbiological requirements of foods

4.3 Milk and Milk Products Order, 1992 (renamed as Milk and Milk Products Regulations under Section 99 of the Food Safety and Standards Act 2006)

These regulations (GOI 1992) were made under Section 3 of Essential Commodities Act, 1955, and have been amended six times in 1993, 1995, 2001 and 2002. It was done because it was felt that for maintaining and increasing the supply of liquid milk of the desired quality in interest of the general public, it was necessary to provide for regulating the production, supply and distribution of milk and milk product. Milk and Milk Products Advisory Board has been constituted under these orders to advise the Central Government on related matters. Some of the regulations are briefly described below.

4.3.1 Sanitary requirements for milk and milk products

The dairy establishment in which milk or any milk product is being handled, processed, manufactured, stored, distributed, the holder of registration certificate, and the persons handling them have to conform to the sanitary, hygienic requirement, food safety measures and other standards that are specified in the Fifth Schedule of these orders. These include the specifications for the following:

- Sanitary requirements for dairy establishments
- General conditions of hygiene applicable to staff
- Sanitary and hygienic requirements for storage
- Sanitary and hygienic requirements for wrapping and packaging

4.3.2 Certification, packing, marking and labelling

Every person engaged in the business of handling, processing or manufacturing milk or any milk product, in regard to the items of milk or milk product manufactured and the packing, marking and labelling of containers thereof, is liable to comply with the specified requirements.

5. Animal Biodiversity Legislations

5.1 Biological Diversity Act, 2002

India is party to the Convention on Biological Diversity (CBD), 1992 which recognizes the sovereign rights of states to use their own biological resources. In order to help in realizing the objectives of CBD, India has enacted an umbrella legislation called the **Biological Diversity Act, 2002** aimed at conservation of biological resources and associated knowledge as well as facilitating access to them in a sustainable manner and through a just process (GOI 2003b). The Central Government established a body called the National Biodiversity Authority (NBA) in Chennai to lay down procedures and guidelines and to advice the Government of India on related issues (GOI 2003d).

5.2 Biological Diversity Rules, 2004

The biological diversity rules, 2004 (GOI 2004) provide for the procedure for access to biological resources and associated traditional knowledge. The NBA may restrict or prohibit the request for access to biological resources for the following reasons:

- The request for access is for any endangered taxa;
- The request for access is for any endemic and rare species;
- The request for access is likely to result in adverse effect on the livelihoods of the local people;
- The request to access may result in adverse environmental impact which may be difficult to control and mitigate;
- The request for access may cause genetic erosion or affecting the ecosystem function;
- Use of resources for purposes contrary to national interest and other related international agreements entered into by India.

5.3 Constitution of Biodiversity Management Committees

Every local body constitutes a Biodiversity Management Committee (BMCs) within its area of jurisdiction. The main function of the BMC is to prepare People's Biodiversity Register in consultation with local people. The

Register contains comprehensive information on availability and knowledge of local biological resources, their medicinal or any other use or any other traditional knowledge associated with them (GOI 2004).

5.4 Repositories for biological resources under the Biological Diversity Act, 2002

The Ministry for Environment and Forests has designated various institutions to act as repositories under the Act for different categories of biological resources(GOI 2008b). The repositories for animal biological resources are listed in Table 11.

Table 11 : Repositories for biological resources

Name of the institution	Category of biological resource
Zoological Survey of India, Kolkata	Fauna
National Bureau of Animal Genetic Resources, Karnal, Haryana	Genetic Resources of domestic animals
National Bureau of Fish Genetic Resources, Lucknow, Uttar Pradesh	Fish Genetic Resources
National Institute of Oceanography, Goa	Marine flora and fauna
Indian Council for Forestry Research and Education, Dehradun (Forest Research Institute, Dehradun; Institute of Forest Genetics and Tree Breeding, Coimbatore and Tropical Forest Research Institute, Jabalpur)	Flora (angiosperms, gymnosperms, pteriodophytes, bryophytes, lichens, macrofungi, macroalgae). For TFRI only: Fauna (termites, butterflies, moths)
Wildlife Institute of India, Dehradun	Faunal resources in protected areas
Institute of Microbial Technology, Chandigarh	Microorganisms
National Institute of Virology, Pune	Viruses

6. Environment Protection Legislations

Decision was taken at the United Nations Conference on the Human Environment held at Stockholm in June, 1972, in which India participated, to take appropriate steps for the protection and improvement of human environment. It was, therefore, considered necessary to implement the decisions relating to the protection and improvement of environment and the prevention of hazards to human beings, other living creatures, plants and property. The Environment (Protection) Act was enacted in 1986. It empowers the Central Government to establish authorities charged with the mandate of preventing environmental pollution in all its forms and to tackle specific environmental problems that are peculiar to different parts of the country.

6.1 Environment (Protection) Act, 1986, amended subsequently

The Act provides for the protection and improvement of environment and for matters connected therewith (GOI 1986a). It empowers the Central government to take all such measures as it deems necessary or expedient for the purpose of protecting and improving the quality of the environment and preventing controlling and abating environmental pollution. Such measures may include the following matters:

- Coordination of actions by the State Governments, officers and other authorities;
- Planning and execution of a nation-wide programme for the prevention, control and abatement of environmental pollution;
- Laying down standards for the quality of environment in its various aspects;
- Laying down standards for emission or discharge of environmental pollutants from various sources;
- Restriction of areas in which any industries, operations or processes or class of industries, operations or processes shall not be carried out or shall be carried out subject to certain safeguards;
- Laying down procedures and safeguards for the prevention of accidents which may cause environmental pollution and remedial measures for such accidents;
- Laying down procedures and safeguards for the handling of hazardous substances;
- Examination of such manufacturing processes, materials and substances as are likely to cause environmental pollution;
- Carrying out and sponsoring investigations and research relating to problems of environmental pollution;
- Inspection of any premises, plant, equipment, machinery, manufacturing or other processes, materials or substances and giving directions to take steps for the prevention, control and abatement of environmental pollution;
- Establishment or recognition of environmental laboratories and institutes;
- Collection and dissemination of information relating to environmental pollution;

- Preparation of manuals, codes or guides relating to the prevention, control and abatement of environmental pollution;
- Securing the effective implementation of the provisions of the Act.

The Act empowers the government to make rules to regulate environmental pollution issue. Such rules may provide for the following matters:

- The standards of quality of air, water or soil for various areas and purposes;
- The maximum allowable limits of concentration of various environmental pollutants (including noise) for different areas;
- The procedures and safeguards for the handling of hazardous substances;
- The prohibition and restrictions on the handling of hazardous substances in different areas;
- The prohibition and restriction on the location of industries and the carrying on processes and operations in different areas;
- The procedures and safeguards for the prevention of accidents which may cause environmental pollution and for providing for remedial measures for such accidents.

6.2 Environment (Protection) Rules, 1986, amended subsequently

These rules (GOI 1986b) mainly deal with the following aspects.

- Standards for emissions or discharge of environmental pollutants
- Prohibitions and restrictions on the location of industries and the carrying on processes and operations in different areas
- Procedure of taking samples
- Procedure for submission of samples for analysis, and the form of laboratory report thereon
- Functions of environmental laboratories
- Manner of giving notice
- Furnishing of information to authorities and agencies in certain cases
- Prohibition and restriction on the handling of hazardous substances in different areas

7. Wildlife Protection Legislations

The Wild Life (Protection) Act, 1972. The Wild Life (Protection) Amendment Act, 2002 and The Wild Life (Protection) Amendment Act, 2010 (draft) provide for the protection of wild animals, birds and plants and for matters connected therewith or ancillary or incidental thereto with a view to ensuring the ecological and environmental security of the country. National Board for Wild Life and State Board for Wild Life have been constituted under this Act which are responsible for promotion of the conservation and development of wildlife and forests by appropriate measures (GOI 2003a). **Recognition of Zoo Rules, 2009** (GOI 2009c) provide for regulations regarding zoos and related places. The parent act provides for prohibition of hunting; protection of specified plants; declaration of sanctuaries, national parks and closed areas and game reserves; constitution of Central Zoo Authority and recognition of zoos and prohibition of trade or commerce in trophies, animal articles etc. derived from certain animals (GOI 2010a).

8. Biomedical Waste Legislations

The Bio-Medical Waste (Management and Handling) Rules, 1998 (Amended in 2003) are in place under the Environment Protection Act, 1986. These rules are meant for proper management and handling of bio-medical waste.

Biomedical waste means any waste, which is generated during the diagnosis, treatment or immunisation of human beings or animals or in research activities pertaining thereto or in the production or testing of biologicals, and including categories mentioned in Schedule I of the Bio-Medical Waste (Management and Handling) Rules, 1998. The methods of treatment and disposal of different categories of biomedical waste are shown in Table 12.

Schedule II of the Bio-Medical Waste (Management and Handling) Rules, 1998 lists the colour coding and type of container for disposal of bio-medical wastes (Table 13) and Schedule III of the Bio-Medical Waste (Management and Handling) Rules, 1998 describes label for bio-medical waste containers/ bags which is non-washable and prominently visible (Fig. 1).

Table 12 : Categories of biomedical waste and methods of their treatment and disposal

Option	Waste category	Treatment and disposal
Category No. 1	**Human anatomical waste** (human tissues, organs, body parts)	Incineration/deep burial
Category No. 2	**Animal waste** (animal tissues, organs, body parts carcasses, bleeding parts, fluid, blood and experimental animals used in research, waste generated by veterinary hospitals colleges, discharge from hospitals, animal houses)	Incineration/deep burial

Category No. 3	**Microbiology and biotechnology waste** (wastes from laboratory cultures, stocks or specimens of microorganisms live or attenuated vaccines, human and animal cell culture used in research and infectious agents from research and industrial laboratories, wastes from production of biologicals, toxins, dishes and devices used for transfer of cultures)	Local autoclaving/ microwaving/ incineration
Category No. 4	**Waste sharps** (needles, syringes, scalpels, blades, glass, etc. that may cause puncture and cuts. This includes both used and unused sharps)	Disinfection (chemical treatment/ autoclaving/ microwaving and mutilation/ shredding
Category No. 5	**Discarded medicines and cytotoxic drugs** (wastes comprising of outdated, contaminated and discarded medicines)	Incineration/destruction and drugs disposal in secured landfills
Category No. 6	**Solid waste** (Items contaminated with blood, and body fluids including cotton dressings, soiled plaster casts, lines, beddings, other material contaminated with blood)	Incineration autoclaving/ microwaving
Category No. 7	**Solid waste** (wastes generated from disposable items other than the waste shaprs such as tubings, catheters, intravenous sets etc).	Disinfection by chemical treatment autoclaving/ microwaving and mutilation/ shredding
Category No. 8	**Liquid waste** (waste generated from laboratory and washing, cleaning, house keeping and disinfecting activities)	Disinfection by chemical treatment and discharge into drains
Category No. 9	**Incineration ash** (ash from inc ineration of any biomedical waste)	Disposal in municipal landfill
Category No. 10	**Chemical waste** (chemicals used in production of biologicals, chemicals used in disinfection, as insecticides etc.)	Chemical treatment and discharge into drains for liquids and secured landfill for solids

Table 13 : Colour coding and type of containers for biological waste

Colour coding	Type of container -I	Waste category	Treatment options as per Schedule I
Yellow	Plastic bag	Cat. 1, Cat. 2, Cat. 3, Cat. 6	Incineration/deep burial
Red	Disinfected container/ plastic bag	Cat. 3, Cat. 6, Cat. 7	Autoclaving/microwaving/ chemical treatment
Blue/white translucent	Plastic bag/puncture proof container	Cat. 4, Cat. 7	Autoclaving/microwaving/ chemical treatment and destruction/ shredding
Black	Plastic bag	Cat. 5, Cat. 9 and Cat. 10 (solid)	Disposal in secured landfill

Biohazard Cytotoxic

Handle with Care

Fig. 1 : Label for biomedical waste containers/bags

9. Trade Legislation

Livestock Importation Act, 1898 (amended in 2001) is an Act to make better provision for the regulation of the importation of livestock. Under this Act the central government has the powers to regulate, restrict or prohibit the import of livestock into India which may likely be affected by infectious or contagious disorders, and of any fodder, dung, stable litter, clothing harness or fittings pertaining to livestock or that may have been in contact therewith (GOI 1898, 2001e). The Sea Customs Act, 1878 empowers the officers of customs in relation to the importation of livestock and associated articles. Under the Customs Act, 1962, the custom officers at every port, airport, inland container depot and land customs station have the same powers in relation to livestock and associated articles. The Act also provides for procedure for import of livestock products into India, sanitary conditions/ health protocols for various products. The Pet Food Products of Animal Origin (Import into India) order, 2008 under the principle Act regulates import of pet food products into India (GOI 2008a).

10. Fisheries Legislation

The Indian Fisheries Act, 1897 (GOI 1897) provides legislations for protection of fish. It contains penal provisions for destruction of fish by explosives or by poisoning of waters.

11. Drugs and Cosmetics Legislation

The Drugs and Cosmetics Act, 1940 amended many times is an Act to regulate the import, manufacture, distribution and sale of drugs and cosmetics (GOI 2003c). The Drugs and Cosmetics Rules, 1945 have also been made under the Act which also have been amended several times. The Act deals with the following:

- Constitution of the Drugs Technical Advisory Board, Central Drugs Laboratory and the Drugs Consultative Committee
- Import of drugs and cosmetics in terms of standards of quality, misbranded drugs, adulterated drugs, spurious drugs, misbranded cosmetics, spurious cosmetics and prohibition of import of certain drugs or cosmetics
- Manufacture, sale and distribution of drugs and cosmetics in terms of standards of quality, misbranded drugs, adulterated drugs, spurious drugs, misbranded cosmetics, spurious cosmetics and prohibition of manufacture of certain drugs or cosmetics including ayurvedic, siddha and unani drugs
- Standards to be complied with by the imported drugs and by the drugs manufactured for sale, sold, stocked or exhibited for sale or distributed
- Issues related to animal experimentation

12. Veterinary Education and Practice Legislations

The Indian Veterinary Council Act, 1984 is an Act to regulate veterinary practice and to provide, for that purpose, for the establishment of Veterinary Council of India and State Veterinary Councils and the maintenance of registers of the veterinary practitioners and for matters connected therewith (GOI 1984). Veterinary Council of India has been established under this Act to look after the issues related to veterinary education and practice.

12.1 Recognition of Veterinary Qualifications Granted by Veterinary Institutions in India

The recognized veterinary qualifications granted by any veterinary institution in India are included in the First Schedule of the Act. Any veterinary institution in India which grants a veterinary qualification not included in this schedule needs to apply to have such qualification recognized. The recognized veterinary qualifications granted by veterinary institutions outside India are included in the Second Schedule of the Act.

12.2 Minimum Standards of Veterinary Education

The Council may, by regulations, specify the minimum standards of veterinary education required for granting recognized veterinary qualifications by veterinary institutions in those states to which this Act extends.

12.3 Indian Veterinary Practitioners Register

The Council maintains a register of veterinary practitioners to be known as the Indian Veterinary Practitioners Register which contains the names of all persons who possess the recognized veterinary qualifications and who are for the time being enrolled on a State Veterinary Register of the state to which this Act extends.

12.4 Establishment of State Veterinary Councils

The State Veterinary Councils are constituted under the provisions of the Act. The State Governments have a register of veterinary practitioners known as the State Veterinary Register for the State.

13. Conclusion

Good governance is of critical importance in enabling veterinary services to improve animal health and welfare worldwide. In the first OIE Global Conference on Veterinary Legislation, with the theme 'Modernizing Veterinary Legislation for Good Governance' held in Djerba, Tunisia in December 2010, it has been noted that many countries, especially developing countries and those with 'in transition' economies, do not have up to date veterinary legislation and are not, therefore, well placed to meet the needs of current and future health challenges and societal expectations. Further, the important role of Veterinary Statutory Bodies to good governance of the veterinary profession is often overlooked.

The OIE Evaluation of Performance of Veterinary Services (PVS) Pathway is a global programme for sustainable improvement of a country's Veterinary Services for compliance with OIE standards. It has been recommended in the

Global Conference that the OIE Members should take steps to improve the quality of national Veterinary Services by following, when needed, the OIE PVS Pathway. The national veterinary authorities of countries that have done a PVS evaluation should apply the relevant next steps to address the shortcomings and modernize the national veterinary legislation (OIE 2011a). The recommendations include that the OIE Members should commence the process of creating an autonomous Veterinary Statutory Body (VSB) complying with the OIE *Terrestrial Code* and that the OIE Members should provide an enabling national legislation for the establishment of private veterinary sector organizations and their participation in all relevant animal health activities of the country.

The OIE has also developed Guidelines on Veterinary Legislation (OIE 2011b), setting out the essential elements that should be covered by legislation to meet the OIE quality standards. The OIE has a Veterinary Legislation Support Programme too to help governments that wish to modernize the national veterinary legislation and thereby help the veterinary services to meet the OIE standards.

References

1. GOI (1897). The Indian Fisheries Act, 1897. Government of India.
2. GOI (1898). The Live-stock Importation Act, 1898. Government of India.
3. GOI (1960). The Prevention of Cruelty to Animals Act, 1960. Ministry of Environment and Forests, Government of India, New Delhi.
4. GOI (1978). Transport of Animals, Rules, 1978. Ministry of Social Justice and Empowerment. Government of India, New Delhi.
5. GOI (1984). The Indian Veterinary Council Act, 1984. Ministry of Law, Justice and Company Affairs (Legislative Department), Government of India, New Delhi.
6. GOI (1986a). The Environment (Protection) Act, 1986. Ministry of Environment and Forests, Government of India, New Delhi.
7. GOI (1986b). Environment (Protection) Rules, 1986. Ministry of Environment and Forests (Department of Environment, Forest and Wildlife), Government of India, New Delhi.
8. GOI (1992). Milk and Milk Products Order, 1992. Ministry of Agriculture (Department of Animal Husbandry, Dairying and Fisheries), Government of India, New Delhi.
9. GOI (1998a). Bio-Medical Waste (Management & Handling) Rules, 1998. Ministry of Environment and Forests, Government of India, New Delhi.
10. GOI (1998b). Breeding of and Experiments on Animals (Control and Supervision) Rules, 1998. Ministry of Social Justice and Empowerment, Government of India, New Delhi.

11. GOI (2001a). Breeding of and Experiments on Animals (Control and Supervision) Amendment Rules, 2001. Ministry of Social Justice and Empowerment. Government of India, New Delhi.

12. GOI (2001b). Prevention of Cruelty to Animals (Slaughter House) Rules, 2001. Ministry of Social Justice and Empowerment. Government of India, New Delhi.

13. GOI (2001c). Prevention of Cruelty to Animals (Transport of Animals on Foot) Rules, 2001. Ministry of Social Justice and Empowerment. Government of India, New Delhi.

14. GOI (2001d). Transport of Animals (Amendment) Rules, 2001. Ministry of Social Justice and Empowerment. Government of India, New Delhi.

15. GOI (2001e). The Live-stock Importation (Amendment) Act, 2001. Ministry of Law, Justice and Company Affairs (Legislative Department), Government of India, New Delhi.

16. GOI (2003a). The Wild Life (Protection) Amendment Act, 2002. Ministry of Law and Justice (Legislative Department), Government of India, New Delhi.

17. GOI (2003b). The Biological Diversity Act, 2002. Ministry of Law and Justice (Legislative Department), Government of India, New Delhi.

18. GOI (2003c). The Drugs and Cosmetics Act and Rules; The Drugs and Cosmetics Act, 1940 and The Drugs And Cosmetics Rules, 1945. Ministry of Health and Family Welfare (Department of Health), Government of India, New Delhi.

19. GOI (2003d). Establishment of National Biodiversity Authority. Ministry of Environment and Forests, Government of India, New Delhi.

20. GOI (2004). Biological Diversity Rules, 2004. Ministry of Environment and Forests, Government of India, New Delhi.

21. GOI (2006a). Food Safety and Standards Act, 2006. Ministry of Law and Justice (Legislative Department), Government of India, New Delhi.

22. GOI (2006b). Breeding of and Experiments on Animals (Control and Supervision) Amendment Rules, 2006. Ministry of Environment and Forests, Government of India, New Delhi.

23. GOI (2008a). Pet Food Products of Animal Origin (Import into India) Order, 2008. Ministry of Agriculture (Department of Animal Husbandry, Dairying and Fisheries), Government of India, New Delhi.

24. GOI (2008b). Designation of Repositories under the Biological Diversity Act, 2002. Ministry of Environment and Forests, Government of India, New Delhi.

25. GOI (2009a). The Prevention and Control of Infectious and Contagious Diseases in Animals Act, 2009. Ministry of Law and Justice (Legislative Department), Government of India, New Delhi.

26. GOI (2009b). Transport of Animals (Amendment) Rules, 2009. Ministry of Environment and Forests, Government of India, New Delhi.

27. GOI (2009c). Recognition of Zoo Rules, 2009. Ministry of Environment and Forests, Government of India, New Delhi.

28. GOI (2010a). The Wild Life (Protection) Amendment Bill, 2010. Ministry of Environment and Forests, Government of India, New Delhi.

29. GOI (2010b). Prevention of Cruelty to Animals (Slaughter House) Amendment Rules, 2010. Ministry of Environment and Forests, Government of India, New Delhi.

30. GOI (2011a). Preamble of the Animal Welfare Act, 2011. Ministry of Environment and Forests, Government of India, New Delhi.

31. GOI (2011b). Ministry of Environment and Forests, Government of India, New Delhi. http://moef.nic.in/modules/rules-and-regulations/animal-welfare/. Accessed 16 June 2011.

32. GOI (2011c). Food Safety and Standards Regulations, 2011. Ministry of Law and Justice (Legislative Department), Government of India, New Delhi.

33. OIE (2011a). OIE Global Conference on Veterinary Legislation – Recommendations. Djerba, Tunisia, 7-9 December 2010. The World Organisation for Animal Health (OIE), Paris. http://www.oie.int/fileadmin/Home/eng/Conferences_Events/docs/pdf/recommendations/ANG_Recommendations.pdf. Accessed 14 June 2011.

34. OIE (2011b). Guidelines on veterinary legislation. The World Organisation for Animal Health (OIE), Paris. http://www.oie.int/support-to-oie-members/veterinary-legislation/veterinary-legislation-resources/. Accessed 14 June 2011.

□□□

Chapter 32

Future Needs of Veterinary Education

R. PRABAKARAN AND J. JOHN KIRUBAHARAN
Tamil Nadu Veterinary and Animal Sciences University, Chennai-600007

Contents

1. Introduction

Veterinary medicine is one of the two main aspects of veterinary education while animal husbandry/production constitutes the other. The role of a veterinarian does not stop with being a mere animal health provider but also includes that of a farm manager who has to ensure higher productivity, adopting good management practices and a technologist who takes care of the quality of animal products like meat, milk and egg and provides guarantee for food safety. Veterinary medicine is the only profession in the health and medical field that is trained in comparative medicine. Concern for animals, their health and well-being, and their interface with people keeps veterinarians as critical components of public health and as essential healthcare providers to society globally. As large and small ruminants and backyard poultry support rural people economically, the veterinarians play a major role in sustaining rural economy in the country. Veterinary medicine is not the same as it was. In fact, the profession is now more dynamic and changing more rapidly than ever before. There are major demographic, political, environmental, technological, economic and disease influences, all driving changes in the society. These changes will also have significant impacts on veterinary medicine and veterinary medical education in future. The role of veterinarians is expanding from ensuring animal health and production, to other areas of concern like public health, food safety etc. (Willis *et al.* 2007). Hence, the veterinary education has to be remodelled to fulfil more than one role. The veterinarian of 21st century should have craftsmanship coupled with an academic attitude. The graduates are expected to possess enthusiasm for the subject, an inquiring mind and a propensity for problem solving.

2. Minimum Standards of Veterinary Education

The notion of establishing minimum requirements for veterinary education throughout the world is not new. In 1987, the World Association of Veterinary Educators (WAVE) was created under the auspices of the World Veterinary Association (WVA). As one of its first actions, WAVE created a steering committee on veterinary education with the objectives of establishing a survey of veterinary education throughout the world and proposing recommendations to help teaching institutions achieve their goals, as well as establishing and maintaining expertise in the area of veterinary education. A draft of the minimum requirements was presented by this committee to the General Assembly of the World Veterinary Association and was adopted in May 1992 (Ruppanner 1994). The role of veterinarian varies, sometimes from country to country, but the veterinary profession, like most other professions, is always an amalgam of technical skills and conceptual abilities; both are important and necessary. Awareness of the dangers inherent to the loss of one or the other of these attributes is critical.

The minimum requirement for undergraduate veterinary education as suggested by WAVE in its education policy document is as follows (Ruppanner 1994).

- A veterinary education institution must be of university level and meet the standards specified by the World Veterinary Association (WVA) in its accreditation system. The veterinary curriculum must be under the immediate and sole direction of a veterinarian but non-veterinarians are not excluded from teaching. It must be adequately financed, housed, equipped and staffed.
- The duration of the veterinary curriculum must extend over a period of at least four years, not including pre-veterinary training, during which a minimum of eight months of instruction is given each year. The veterinary curriculum must cover in depth, and provide appropriate understanding of the subject matters in relation to the various animal species and animal production systems of importance in the area.
- Appropriate library and audiovisual facilities as well as sufficient clinical, laboratory and practical training must be provided. Students must be properly supervised and evaluated throughout the course of their studies.
- A veterinary education institution must be able to demonstrate that research activities are performed on its premises, contributing to the acquisition of new knowledge both at the applied and fundamental levels. A veterinary education institution must be able to assist veterinarians practising in whatever position, in whichever area or country, to cope with the quickly changing professional demands, by providing continuing education, for example.

2.1 Identification of skills for veterinarians

The role the veterinarians need to play in 21st century is diverse in nature. They are expected to be part of many systems like public service, research, private sector etc. The skills required for serving these sectors vary to a larger extent. Hence, the curriculum should concentrate on developing core skills, which are essential for serving in all these sectors and veterinarians of the 21st century and students may be allowed to decide on the area of their future employment and skills required for that may be provided as cocurricular activity. The topics identified for each as provided by the FAO (Ruppanner 1994) are provided below. Under every topic skills need to be identified as per the demands of the employer and the veterinary teaching institutions should assure that the passed out graduates possess all the skills.

2.2 Minimum basic veterinary curriculum

The following components have been suggested in the minimum basic veterinary curriculum (Ruppanner 1994, World Veterinary Association 1998).

- Macroscopic and microscopic anatomy
- Physiology (mammalian and avian)
- Biochemistry
- Pharmacology, parasitology
- Microbiology
- Pathology
- Theriogenology
- Diagnostics, treatment and prevention of diseases
- Surgery
- Veterinary economics
- Animal husbandry and production (genetics)
- Botany
- Cell biology
- Environment
- Professional ethics
- Animal welfare
- Population veterinary medicine
- Laboratory animal medicine
- Immunology, epidemiology, public health
- Meat inspection
- Food hygiene

2.3 Veterinary curriculum for private practice

Ruppanner (1994) suggested the following special constituents in the curriculum for preparing the veterinarians for private practice.

- Production economics
- Commerce
- Livestock and poultry farming systems

- Extension methodologies, including farmer organizational development
- Environmental management
- Management practices
- Book- and record-keeping
- Topics such as poultry, pig and cattle pathology; computer-based least ration formulation; meat handling and hygiene; virology etc. should be upgraded to provide the level of understanding of sophisticated technologies necessary for servicing modern livestock industries.

2.4 Veterinary curriculum for public service

The following area in the curriculum may be useful for the graduates opting for public service (Ruppanner 1994).

- Administration of animal welfare standards
- An understanding of the science of pain and stress assessment and of animal behaviour
- In-depth understanding of pharmacology and toxicology relative to the registration of veterinary chemicals and the control of chemical residues in food processing
- Keeping up to date with the emerging world and international regulatory homework for chemical residues, which has such an important impact on trade
- Risk assessment for quarantine and trade purposes
- Hazard analysis and critical control point (HACCP) methodology
- Total quality management (TQM) principles
- Contingency planning for exotic disease outbreaks and other disasters
- Management, organizational and communication skills

2.5 Veterinary curriculum for field research (Ruppanner 1994)

- *Surveys*: In advanced countries a mass of data has been accumulated on indigenous diseases of livestock and is being expanded to include aquatic species, wildlife and other animals for which most countries still do not have reliable data banks. As a result, there is a need to teach simple survey techniques and data analysis.
- *Epidemiological studies*: These should be designed to give detailed information on the prevalence, incidence, distribution and variability of specific diseases, in other words, disease dynamics.

- *Trials:* Assessment of vaccines or treatments and other intervention studies to show the value of a procedure in controlling disease, cost/ benefit analysis can be built into the experiment.
- *Productivity studies*: These must be concerned with the total farming system. Assessment of production indices is an important part of the work of veterinarians, whether animals are healthy or diseased, body-weight gain in young animals, milk or egg production and fertility are all important aspects of the production system. Underlying disease factors such as parasitism, bacterial or other diseases may be assessed as part of multidisciplinary studies.

3. Current Constraints

Veterinary medicine is a diverse and unique health profession contributing significantly to the welfare of the society through the enhancement of the health, value and productivity of livestock, poultry and other classes of animals. The noble profession also protects the society from the risks associated with animals and animal products, protects the quality of the environment besides assisting in the conservation of the germplasm. The major constraints hampering effective delivery of such services are apathy of many governments in funding, human resource issues like imbalance between the need and number available, poor quality human resources, poor infrastructure, rigid curriculum, lack of representation in the decision making bodies of the governments, non-functioning in relevance to social, economic and technological environment, service oriented problems in the field, unavailability of para-veterinary personnel, lack of continuing veterinary education programmes, lack of performance assessment system and technical auditing, change in the perception regarding animals in the society, rapid urbanization and loss of animal habitations – to name a few. Further, the focus of veterinary profession, which was merely providing animal health cover sometime back, today also includes augmentation of animal production, post harvest technology of animal products, animal business management, food safety, assuring safety from zoonotic diseases, marine medicine, honey bee diseases etc. Yet another major issue is the quality of students opting for veterinary education. Unlike western countries, in India it is not determined by the interest of the students but by the job avenues available in other professions and the social status one gets out of his profession. One more major issue is the relatively slow pace in which the veterinary profession progresses taking the developments in other fields like electronics, biomedical engineering, information technology and communication etc.

4. Guidelines for Future Veterinary Education

1. Reorient the veterinary curriculum to provide a basic holistic veterinary instruction to meet the challenges of the field and a specialized instruction on fields like pet animal medicine, companion animal medicine, animal and poultry production management, laboratory animal medicine, veterinary laboratory diagnostics, business management and rural economics etc.
2. Change the focus of veterinary curriculum from total concentration on clinical practice to include the needs of the society and industry in livestock and poultry production and entrepreneurship development equally.
3. Strengthen the knowledge base of veterinarians by including courses on basic science subjects.
4. Develop a strong education research and technology wing to suggest modifications and improvements to veterinary education and also to develop continuing veterinary education (CVE) programmes.
5. Utilize all the available developments in other fields for imparting veterinary education at colleges and also at off college CVE programmes.
6. Increase the scope for continuing veterinary education (CVE). Since veterinary medicine is dynamic, CVE programmes should be available in plenty for the practising veterinarians to choose from. For better efficiency, the extension wing should be strengthened to continuously evolve and develop new programmes and discard outdated ones.
7. Develop stringent quality accreditation norms for veterinary institutions.
8. Improve the image of veterinarians on compassion, expertise, humaneness, judgement, care and understanding.
9. Improve the relationship with sister disciplines like medicine, agriculture and engineering to improve the quality of veterinary education.
10. Influence upon the policymakers to provide a rational system of funding for veterinary education.

5. Pedagogy Tools for Future Veterinary Education

5.1 Problem solving teaching

Problem solving is a basic skill needed by today's learners. Guided by recent research in problem solving, changing professional standards, new workplace demands, and recent changes in learning theory, veterinary educators and trainers are revising curricula in most of the western countries to include integrated learning environments which encourage learners to use higher order thinking skills, and in particular, problem solving skills (Kirkley 2003).

Problem solving teaching becomes essential in the context of economic, organizational and technological forces that have changed the nature of most workplaces. Most of the veterinary employers feel that the new graduates lack necessary basic as well as higher order thinking skills. However, today's workplaces often demand high levels of both skill sets. According to the report of the U.S. Department of Labor's Secretary's Commission on Achieving Necessary Skills (SCANS), teaching should be offered in context, and students should learn content while solving realistic problems. With scientific knowledge doubling, it becomes increasingly important for students to develop higher order thinking skills. This involves basic skills, but also requires learners to use their knowledge in a variety of domains, perform critical analysis, and solve problems. As educators call for more integrated instruction, problem solving often serves as a core curriculum strand that joins together various disciplines, rules, concepts, strategies, and skills. For much of the 20th century, educators have devoted their attention to trying to define and teach problem solving skills. In the early 1900s, problem solving was viewed as a mechanical, systematic, and often abstract set of skills, such as those used to solve riddles or mathematical equations. These problems often have correct answers that are based on logical solutions with a single correct answer (convergent reasoning). Under the influence of cognitive learning theories, problem solving is shifted to represent a complex mental activity consisting of a variety of cognitive skills and actions. Problem solving includes higher order thinking skills such as visualization, association, abstraction, comprehension, manipulation, reasoning, analysis, synthesis, and generalization - each needing to be managed and coordinated. During the 1960s and 1970s, researchers developed general problem solving models to explain problem solving processes. By learning decontextualized problem solving skills, one could transfer these skills to any situation - context, later. However, the present day problem solving teaching differs from this method as a result of cognitive research done in the last two to three decades, which includes a complex set of cognitive, behavioural and attitudinal components. It is a multiple step process where the problem solver must find relationships between past experiences and the problem at hand and then act upon a solution. Instruction in problem solving teaching should be supplemented with supportive declarative knowledge in the form of facts, concepts and principles.

Instead of the conventional teaching methods, where the causes of a problem are explained under various subjects, a modified method where the problems and their solutions are explained in a holistic manner needs to be introduced. For example instead of explaining about respiratory problems under the subjects of clinical medicine and preventive medicine where the non-specific and specific causes respectively are explained separately, it should be approached on a single angle and solutions suggested. It can be achieved by the following methodologies.

a. *Interdepartmental teaching*: More emphasis needs to be laid on interdepartmental teaching where experts from different departments should be brought under a single roof and instruction rendered to the students.

b. *Expertise teaching*: Human resource development at the teachers level need to have experts on specific areas of a subject to render problem solving teaching. For example instead of developing more number of teachers in veterinary microbiology who can deliver instruction based on text book, efforts will be made to have teachers who are experts in a particular field by research to deliver instruction like respiratory viral infections of poultry, sheep viruses, bovine viruses etc. Such expertise teaching will no doubt inculcate a problem solving approach in the minds of students.

c. *Continuing education*: To abreast the knowledge of field veterinarians to emerging problems, CVE in the form of refresher courses needs to be introduced utilising the experts following multidisciplinary approach. It is suggested by the experts that a veterinarian has to refresh his knowledge once in every five years. Hence, a special impetus needs to be given to this area.

5.2 Modification of curriculum

a. A modified curriculum should be devised to ensure that every student studies an area of his choice (electives) besides the routine courses specified by the Veterinary Council of India (VCI). This elective subject study will provide the students to have sufficient depth of knowledge to derive deeper understanding than that available in the core courses. This will also be in the form of a mini project for three months in the chosen area/industry/commercial farm and preparation of a report.

b. To work in harmony with the demands of the society, knowledge on Hazard Analysis and Critical Control Points (HACCP) approach needs to be introduced in all the possible subjects.

c. The main frame curriculum of the VCI should be made into a base over which the universities should be allowed to build the curriculum emphasising on the needs of the region and developments that take place. This will help to revise the curriculum more often than now being done.

d. A modified examination system to assess the comprehension and problem solving ability of the student that promotes learning.

e. To support a curriculum that is more problem oriented than conventional, a radical appraisal of the time allotment and adoption of new teaching methods is essential. A suitable approach will be to reduce the formal teaching to less than 50 per cent of the timetable with much greater emphasis on student based teaching and problem solving. While proceeding with such an approach caution will have to be exercised not to reduce the amount of factual materials to be presented to the student.

f. According to the report of Riley Committee, the scientific base of the courses taught should be increased. The term scientific base here refers to basic and veterinary sciences and intercalation of basic science courses into veterinary science. Courses like molecular pathology, molecular epidemiology, genetic epidemiology, molecular genetics, nuclear medicine etc. need to be introduced where the basic science subject of molecular biology is introduced into applied subject like pathology. Such intercalated courses will also provide increased job opportunities for veterinary students.

g. In the present era, due to limited funding, animal experimentation regulations and such related issues, a big threat is looming large over the veterinary education. This scenario makes alternate teaching a mandatory. Hence, computer based learning (CBL) utilising artificial intelligence software, animal experiment simulation software, computer assisted clinical diagnosis software need to be introduced. Since, the modern computers provide the speed and interactivity, they reduce the burden of teachers besides making learning self-paced and self-motivated. The CBL also provides complex learning strategies and promote higher cognitive skills.

h. The most important function of the veterinary institutions besides producing expert veterinarians is to produce good citizens who are the building blocks of a law abiding and conscious society. Hence, ethical education should be imparted to inculcate good values among the students.

i. The stakeholders' (the teachers, students, potential employers, educationists, farmers, industrialised policy makers etc.) views on all these aspects need to be ascertained and applied while developing an appropriate curriculum for veterinary science education for the future.

j. The curriculum should also inculcate knowledge, skill and attitude to develop veterinarians into successful entrepreneurs. The veterinarians of 21st century should mould themselves to be "job providers rather than job seekers".

k. The educationists should also keep continuous watch on developing economic situation in the livestock and poultry industry and try to bring changes in the curriculum as fast as possible as any delay will make the entire curriculum obsolete.

l. There has to be provision for guest lectures and interaction with successful entrepreneurs, experts in specialised fields and the veterinarians employed in the industry with different assignments; transfer of credits among institutions; mutual exchange of students; associate faculty facilitation etc. to improve quality of veterinary education.

m. The existing system of evaluation at its best evaluates the students fully for their knowledge level, while skill is partially evaluated and attitude goes almost unevaluated. Effective systems need to be developed through appropriate expertise for evaluating the skill and attitude of the students also. Further, the teacher/teaching also has to be evaluated periodically. It is necessary to ascertain and measure the learning achievements, judge activities of teachers, and to assess the further needs for planning new courses.

5.3 Intercalation of basic sciences subjects

The prime requirement of veterinary education is to intercalate basic science subjects and clinical subjects in both teaching and research as per the Riley Report (1989 - Veterinary Education into 21st Century). Hence, the basic sciences need to be strengthened with adequate provision for students to even intercalate work for a science degree into veterinary course. In western countries students are permitted to opt to take a year out of their undergraduate veterinary studies in order to study a subject area in greater depth, before returning to complete the veterinary course. However, it is very difficult in Indian context. Hence, students may be permitted to opt for extra hours of study on a basic science subject of interest, for an undergraduate degree. While completing veterinary course, they will also have a degree in basic science subject. Such an intercalated degree provides an opportunity to acquire a better understanding of basic veterinary sciences, humanities, research methodologies and to pursue an additional qualification in a veterinary related subject that interests the student.

5.4 Vertical integration of subjects

A vertical relationship needs to be established between pre-, para- and clinical departments. In this way, a more logical approach to clinical features can be established earlier in the course and the students can be made more aware of a logical progression and accumulation of knowledge throughout the course rather than the teaching of subjects as discrete and distinct entities. A classic example of such integration is between anatomy, physiology, surgery and medicine leading to subjects like surgical anatomy, pathophysiology, pathobiology etc. which will provide practical and field oriented knowledge and skill to the students.

5.5 Establishment of centres of excellence

This concept originated from the Pew National Veterinary Education Program (1989) of USA to strengthen the health profession that issued the future directions for veterinary medicine. It is a logical development to manage limited resources and to rationalise expertise between veterinary colleges. This concept will have to be given more thrust in the era of limited funding.

6. Conclusion

Important challenges confront veterinary medicine. Most of these challenges also provide opportunities for the profession to improve the quality, effectiveness, and usefulness of its services to the society. Recognizing this fact, leaders in veterinary education need to develop strategies that address the changing needs of the profession and that will place it in a strong position.

References

1. Kirkley J (2003). Principles of problem solving teaching. Technical paper # 4, Indiana University, Plato Leaning Inc.
2. Pew National Veterinary Education Program (1989). Special report on future directions for veterinary medicine. Can Vet J 30:472-476.
3. Ruppanner R (1994). Veterinary education for public and private practice and research in developing countries - Creating, finding and exchanging information. World Animal Review (FAO) 80/81-1994/3-4, FAO, Rome, Italy, p. 25-33.
4. Willis NG, Monroe FA, Potworowski JA *et al.* (2007). Envisioning the Future of Veterinary Medical Education. Association of American Veterinary Medical Colleges Foresight Project, Final Report. J Vet Med Edu 34:1-41.
5. World Veterinary Association (1998). Education policies. http://www.worldvet.org/manuals/education.pdf. Accessed 20 January 2011.

□□□

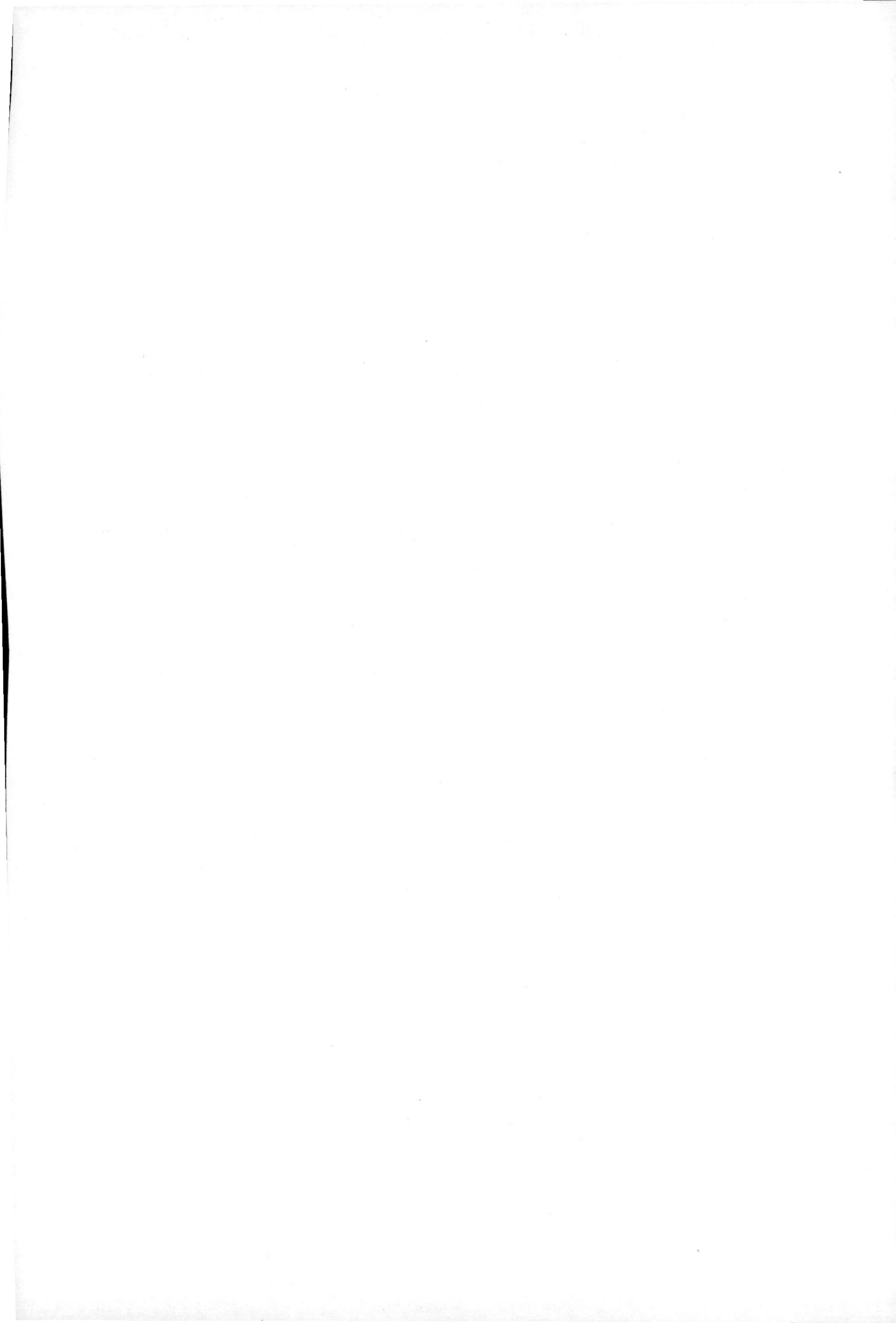